Macronutrients

Macronutrients

Investigating Their Role in Cancer

edited by
Marc S. Micozzi
National Museum of Health and Medicine
Armed Forces Institute of Pathology
Washington, D.C.

Thomas E. Moon
Arizona Disease Prevention Center
The University of Arizona Health Sciences Center
Tucson, Arizona

Marcel Dekker, Inc. New York • Basel • Hong Kong

ISBN: 0-8247-8593-2

This book is printed on acid-free paper.

MARCEL DEKKER, INC.
270 Madison Avenue, New York, New York 10016

Current printing (last digit):
10 9 8 7 6 5 4 3 2 1

PRINTED IN THE UNITED STATES OF AMERICA

Preface

The first phase of large-scale controlled scientific studies—including clinical trials and analytic epidemiology—on the role of diet and nutrition in cancer is near completion. Whether cancer incidence in the United States can be significantly effected by dietary modification remains an open question. This is due in large part to the limited scientific information and understanding of: (1) the person-to-person metabolic differences that influence nutritional status, (2) the interrelation between macro- and micronutrients and nutritional status, (3) whether macronutrients have a micronutrient effect in addition to their macronutrient effects, and (4) the time or times during carcinogenesis that macronutrients exert their effect. The role of dietary intake and of nutritional status in the etiology and prevention of cardiovascular disease provides an optimistic model for cancer researchers.

In the micronutrient area, a recent clinical trial of β-carotene supplementation—an abundant dietary constituent—did not demonstrate a protective effect against skin cancer at the levels administered (Greenberg et al., 1990). Perhaps higher levels of β-carotene may demonstrate an effect. However, studies on chronic β-carotene intake from foods and capsule supplements indicates significant variation in interindividual response to a given dose of β-carotene (Micozzi et al., in press). It is also interesting to note that foods associated with a lower risk for cancer, while initially thought to be consistently high in β-carotene (provitamin

A) content, are in fact much more consistently high in other carotenoids without vitamin A activity, low in fat and calories, high in fiber, and high in other micronutrients (Micozzi et al., 1990). The supporting rationale for β-carotene in the prevention of skin cancer, from either analytic epidemiology or animal studies, was virtually nonexistent when the intervention trial was initiated.

On the other hand, cancer prevention may be attempted by administration of micronutrient analogs such as isotretinoin, a biologically active vitamin A analog. A recently completed large-scale clinical trial on this agent indicated the appearance of detectable (if not clinically significant) toxicity at levels insufficient to prevent skin cancer in high-risk individuals (Tangrea, 1991). Another recently completed trial of this same agent, but at a dose previously shown to be clinically effective in controlling the skin lesions of acne, did demonstrate a lower incidence of second tumors in the head and neck and did not yield unacceptable toxicity (Hong et al., 1990).

In the macronutrient area, the question of the relationship among dietary modification, changes in nutritional status, and cancer prevention also remains open. The effect of dietary modification of macronutrients on cancer risk is proposed to be tested in large-scale clinical trials, particularly for breast and colon cancer (Chapters 15–17). A rationale is developing for clinical trials on prostate cancer as well (Chapter 18). Epidemiological and animal evidence is not clear or consistent as to the "nutritional causes" of breast, colon, or prostate cancer, and well-designed intervention trials may be an appropriate way to gain further information.

Relative to breast cancer, evolutionary biology (Chapter 3) would suggest that for the preponderance of human history most women spent much of their adult lives pregnant or lactating, a status associated with lower rates of breast cancer. Demographic transition theory posits that, through prehistory to modern times, human populations shifted from (1) high fertility/high mortality to (2) high fertility/low mortality to (3) low fertility/low mortality. The middle transition is held responsible for the tremendous world population growth of the last century, in which state much of the world remains, while Europe and northern North America have made the final transition to stage 3.

If the increasing rates of breast cancer, for example, in this country during this century are inevitable correlates of fundamental demographic shifts, what is the role of diet and nutrition? The interindividual variation in how people absorb and metabolize dietary constituents ("nutritional individuality" in evolutionary biology terms) has received little emphasis by cancer researchers. This is somewhat surprising when contrasted with cardiovascular disease (CVD) and its association with dietary cholesterol, and its greatly improved preventive measures provided by the understanding of nutritional individuality as quantified by serum lipids and lipoproteins. For CVD, the association with dietary intake of foods high in cholesterol (and other lipids) was an important first step. The identification of serum lipids, lipid metabolism, and cholesterol receptors provided a greatly improved understanding of the biological mechanisms and, more importantly, the focused hypotheses to be evaluated in intervention trials.

If we come to view diet as an adaptation to the environment, and the epidemiology of diet and cancer as evidence of human maladaptation (Chapter 3), may we begin to consider dietary experience for the preponderance of human history as a clue to the type of diet to which human metabolism may be adapted (and which may help prevent cancer if followed, or contribute to cancer if not)? Prehistoric archaeologists can reconstruct some human dietary patterns from ancient remains. Modern theories of human evolution and studies of primates and hunter-gatherer societies also provide some models. Certainly, until the development of agriculture and animal domestication approximately 10,000 years ago, omnivorous humans had available to eat only those plants and animals that appeared in the wild. While we tend to have a concept of "man the hunter" as somehow characteristic of early human experience, "woman the gatherer" may be a more accurate account. While big game hunting was a part of early human experience in some areas, its social significance may have been far greater than its nutritional significance, most of the time. In any event, wild game (with 4–6% body fat) is quite different nutritionally from modern domesticated animals (up to 40–60% body fat), the latter largely a phenomenon of the 20th century.

Is cancer the result of leaving behind the heritage of our primitive diet and lifestyle? The actual evidence for cancer in animals and humans in antiquity in the Old World before Byzantium, and the New World before Columbus, is vanishingly small or nonexistent, even under many circumstances where cancer could be readily detected paleopathologically where present (Micozzi, 1991). However, the national agenda for cancer research and prevention will not likely be set by greater understanding of human evolutionary biology or history. The controlled clinical trial remains as the means by which hypotheses on nutrition and cancer prevention will be tested. Having "assembled a powerful case for the intervention trial as an investigative tool free of the biases that hamper many etiological studies of nutrition and cancer" (Ershow, 1989) with our first volume on nutrition and cancer prevention (Moon and Micozzi, 1989), we will not disassemble it here.

The drug development and controlled clinical trial approach of pharmacology, as applicable to many areas of modern medical science, provides a useful model for scientific inquiry in cancer prevention, be it capsule supplementation or dietary change. Clinical trials emphasize the process of establishing results using the products of clinical pharmacology important to creating both a base for scientific knowledge and for regulatory affairs. This base has now become a familiar one from which public policy eventually proceeds in the interests of public health.

The large size, high cost, long duration, and widely publicized results of cancer prevention trials appear to require not only an exceptional rationale but also commensurate increases in knowledge of cancer etiology and prevention. The growing emphasis on intermediate or biologic markers is a result of not only the desire to lower costs and shorten trial duration but, equally important, the need to increase our understanding of carcinogenesis and cancer prevention in humans.

Cancer is generally recognized as a sequence of steps resulting in increased molecular changes and increased numbers of abnormal cells. If nutritional status or dietary intake, in the form of food constituents, macronutrients, or micronutrients, is to be recognized in the etiology of cancer, then a careful correspondence must be demonstrated between the sequence of steps that lead to clinical cancer and specific abnormalities or variations in nutritional status. Does excess fat in the diet yield only altered estrogen concentrations and metabolites? Also, does excess fat result in an increased oxidative stress? Must the altered estrogen metabolism precede the increased oxidative stress for the next carcinogenic step to occur? The interpretation of any one of these hypothetical steps may be incomplete (and misunderstood) if taken out of context or out of time sequence in carcinogenesis (Moon, 1992).

The chapters in this book summarize the role of macronutrients in cancer and begin to address the relationship between macro- and micronutrients and other risk factors, as well as illustrate the role of intervention trials in cancer prevention research on macronutrients.

Marc S. Micozzi
Thomas E. Moon

REFERENCES

Ershow, A. G. Book review: *Nutrition and Cancer Prevention: Investigating the Role of Micronutrients*. In *JNCI 81*:1186 (1989).

Greenberg, E.R., Baron, J.A., Stukel, T. A., et al. A clinical trial of beta-carotene to prevent basal cell and squamous-cell cancers of the skin. *N. Engl. J. Med. 323*;789–795 (1990).

Hong, W. K., Lippman, S. M., Itri, L. M. Prevention of second primary tumors with isotretinoin in squamous cell carcinoma of the head and neck. *N. Engl. J. Med. 323*:795–801 (1990).

Micozzi, M. S. Disease in antiquity: the case of cancer. *Arch. Path. Lab. Med. 115*: 1991.

Micozzi, M. S., Beecher, G. R., Taylor, P. R., Khachik, F. Carotenoid analyses of selected raw and cooked foods associated with a lower risk for cancer. *J. Natl. Cancer Inst. 82*:282–285 (1990).

Micozzi, M. S., Brown, E. D., Edwards, B. K., Bieri, J. G., Taylor, P. R., Khachik, F., Beecher, G. R., Smith, J. C. Plasma carotenoid response in men to chronic intake of selected foods and beta-carotene supplements. *Am. J. Clin. Nutr.* (in press).

Moon, T. E. Statistical considerations for chemoprevention trials. *Cancer Bulletin* (1992).

Moon, T. E., Micozzi, M. S. *Nutrition and Cancer Prevention: Investigating the Role of Macronutrients*. Marcel Dekker, New York, 1989.

Tangrea, J. *The Isotretinoin-Basal Cell Carcinoma Prevention Trial (The ISO-BCC Study): Results of the Three-Year Intervention Phase*. American Society for Preventive Oncology, Seattle, Washington, 1991.

Contents

Preface *iii*
Contributors *xi*

Part One
ROLE OF MACRONUTRIENTS IN CANCER

1. Mechanisms of Macronutrient Carcinogenesis 3
John H. Weisburger

2. Animal Experimental Evidence on Macronutrients and Cancer 33
Bandaru S. Reddy

3. Epidemiology of Diet and Cancer: Evidence of Human Maladaptation 55
John D. Potter

Part Two
METHODS FOR INVESTIGATING THE ROLE OF MACRONUTRIENTS

4. Dietary Assessment Methods for Macronutrients 87
Anne M. Hartman and Gladys Block

5. Assessment of Energy Intake and Expenditure 125
Johanna T. Dwyer

6. Anthropometry and Dietary Assessment in Nutrition and Cancer Studies 159
Marc S. Micozzi

7. Biomarkers of Macronutrient Intake 181
Anna R. Giuliano and Thomas E. Moon

Part Three
EVIDENCE FOR SPECIFIC MACRONUTRIENTS AND RELATED FACTORS

8. Energy Intake and Cancer 205
Demetrius Albanes

9. Dietary Fat 231
Anthony B. Miller

10. Alcohol 245
Robert A. Hiatt

11. Serum Albumin and the Risk of Cancer 283
Richard G. Stevens and Baruch S. Blumberg

12. Dietary Fiber 293
Elaine Lanza, Sharada Shankar, and Bruce Trock

13. Anthropometry, Body Composition, and Cancer 321
Loïc Le Marchand

14. Metabolic Effects and Micronutrient Interactions 343
David Kritchevsky

Part Four
CLINICAL TRIALS ON MACRONUTRIENTS AND CANCER

15. Rationale, Feasibility, and Design of a Low Fat Diet Intervention Trial Among Postmenopausal Women 355
Ross L. Prentice

16. Clinical Trials on Breast Cancer 377
Richard R. Love

17. Clinical Trials on Colorectal Cancer 407
Perla A. Vargas and David S. Alberts

18. Dietary Intervention Trials on Prostate Cancer 423
Laurence N. Kolonel and Abraham M. Y. Nomura

19. Participation in Macronutrient Trials 437
Barbara K. Rimer and Paul F. Engstrom

Index *469*

Contributors

Demetrius Albanes, M.D. Medical Epidemiologist, Cancer Prevention Studies Branch, National Cancer Institute, National Institutes of Health, Bethesda, Maryland

David S. Alberts, M.D. Professor of Medicine and Pharmacology, and Director of Cancer Prevention and Control, Arizona Cancer Center, The University of Arizona Health Sciences Center, Tucson, Arizona

Gladys Block, Ph.D.* Epidemiologist, Division of Cancer Prevention and Control, National Cancer Institute, National Institutes of Health, Bethesda, Maryland

Baruch S. Blumburg, M.D., Ph.D. Fox Chase Distinguished Scientist, Fox Chase Cancer Center, Philadelphia, Pennsylvania, and Master, Balliol College, Oxford, England

---

**Current affiliation*: Professor, School of Public Health, University of California, Berkeley, California

Johanna T. Dwyer, D.Sc., R.D. Professor of Medicine and Community Health, Tufts University Medical School, and Director, Francis Stern Nutrition Center, New England Medical Center Hospitals, Boston, Massachusetts

Paul F. Engstrom, M.D. Vice President for Population Science, Fox Chase Cancer Center, Cheltenham, Pennsylvania

Anna R. Giuliano, Ph.D. Post-Doctoral Fellow, Cancer Epidemiology and Prevention Training Program, and Department of Biochemistry, The University of Arizona Health Sciences Center, Tucson, Arizona

Anne M. Hartman, M.S. Health Statistician, Division of Cancer Prevention and Control, National Cancer Institute, National Institutes of Health, Bethesda, Maryland

Robert A. Hiatt, M.D., Ph.D. Assistant Director, Division of Research, Kaiser Permanente Medical Care Program, Oakland, California

Laurence N. Kolonel, M.D., Ph.D. Director of Epidemiology Program and Professor of Public Health, Cancer Research Center, University of Hawaii, Honolulu, Hawaii

David Kritchevsky, Ph.D. Associate Director, The Wistar Institute, Philadelphia, Pennsylvania

Elaine Lanza, Ph.D. Senior Investigator, National Cancer Institute, National Institutes of Health, Bethesda, Maryland

Loïc Le Marchand, M.D., Ph.D. Associate Researcher and Adjunct Associate Professor of Public Health, Epidemiology Program, Cancer Research Center of Hawaii, University of Hawaii, Honolulu, Hawaii

Richard R. Love, M.D. Associate Professor, Clinical Cancer Center, The University of Wisconsin, Madison, Wisconsin

Marc S. Micozzi, M.D., Ph.D. Director, National Museum of Health and Medicine, and Associate Director, Armed Forces Institute of Pathology, Washington, D.C.

Anthony B. Miller, M.B., FRCP Professor of Preventive Medicine, Department of Biostatistics, University of Toronto, Toronto, Canada

Thomas E. Moon, Ph.D. Director, Arizona Disease Prevention Center, and Professor of Epidemiology, College of Medicine, The University of Arizona Health Sciences Center, Tucson, Arizona

Abraham M. Y. Nomura, M.D., Dr.Ph. Director, Japan-Hawaii Cancer Study, Kuakini Medical Center, and Epidemiologist, Cancer Research Center, University of Hawaii, Honolulu, Hawaii

John D. Potter, M.D., Ph.D. Director, Cancer Prevention Research Unit, Division of Epidemiology, School of Public Health, University of Minnesota, Minneapolis, Minnesota

Ross L. Prentice, Ph.D. Director, Division of Public Health Sciences, Fred Hutchinson Cancer Research Center, Seattle, Washington

Bandaru S. Reddy, DVM, Ph.D. Chief, Division of Nutritional Carcinogenesis, Naylor Dana Institute, American Health Foundation, Valhalla, New York

Barbara K. Rimer, Dr. Ph.* Director, Behavioral Research, Fox Chase Cancer Center, Cheltenham, Pennsylvania

Sharada Shankar, Ph.D. Cancer Prevention Fellow, National Cancer Institute, National Institutes of Health, Bethesda, Maryland

Richard G. Stevens, Ph.D. Cancer Epidemiologist, Life Sciences Center, Pacific Northwest Laboratory, Richland, Washington

Bruce Trock, Ph.D. Cancer Epidemiologist, Fox Chase Cancer Center, Philadelphia, Pennsylvania

Perla A. Vargas, Ph.D. Research Specialist, Cancer Prevention and Control, Arizona Cancer Center, The University of Arizona Health Sciences Center, Tucson, Arizona

John H. Weisburger, Ph.D., M.D. (hon.) Senior Member, American Health Foundation, Valhalla, New York

**Current affiliation*: Director, Cancer Control, Duke Comprehensive Cancer Center, Durham, North Carolinia.

part one

ROLE OF MACRONUTRIENTS AND CANCER

1

Mechanisms of Macronutrient Carcinogenesis

John H. Weisburger
American Health Foundation
Valhalla, New York

INTRODUCTION

The history of intensive research associating nutritional elements with chronic diseases is almost 40 years old (Tannenbaum and Silverstone, 1953). In the meantime, much progress has also been made in the underlying sciences, especially as regards mechanisms of action of nutrients, and of greater relevance in carcinogenesis and cancer prevention, through the classification of carcinogens according to their individual mode of action. The early discoveries in the area of nutrition and health, and specifically nutrition and cancer, dealt with associations discovered in population and epidemiologic studies. The database is much broader now, involving deliberate studies in experimental models, including humans through the techniques of metabolic and biochemical epidemiology, and also in relevant animal models. Interpretation of the combined results, obtained through such multidisciplinary approaches, in light of the underlying mechanisms, provides an understanding of the role of specific dietary risk factors adequate to make recommendations on health promotion and disease prevention. This chapter will deal with select aspects of nutritional mechanisms as a basis for cancer prevention. It includes approaches to prevention of cancer recurrences applicable to patients with specific cancer types.

Causes of Cancer

Current concepts suggest that the optimal approach to uncovering etiologic factors is to consider each type of cancer as a specific disease entity with its own risk factors. In fact, in some instances, cancer in a given organ may have distinct risk factors affecting dissimilar targets within the organ. For example, it is not certain that breast cancer is a homogeneous disease, but rather that premenopausal breast cancer may involve causative elements distinct from those operating in postmenopausal breast cancer. Also, it is reasonably well established that large bowel or colorectal cancer represents actually three disease entities: (a) proximal, (b) distal colon cancer, and (c) rectal cancer, each with its own dietary risk factors. Studies on the association of nutrients and "large bowel cancer" are apt to have poor correlations, and even reach erroneous conclusions, since a given nutrient may not bear on all three types of large bowel cancer.

We will briefly review the overall carcinogenic process and then describe the underlying elements for each cancer type. Current knowledge requires that for each cancer, information be deliberately sought on the genotoxic causative elements This could be a single chemical, as is often true in occupational cancer, or a mixture of related chemicals, like the class of polycyclic aromatic hydrocarbons or the tobacco-specific nitrosamines associated with lung cancer. It could also be a mixture of closely related heterocyclic aromatic amines produced during cooking, which may bear on the nutritionally linked cancers to be discussed. Importantly, most types of cancer seen in humans require the presence of promoting or enhancing factors that are not genotoxic. In the nutritionally linked cancers, for example, this role is assumed by the total fat intake through specific metabolic mechanisms appropriate to each type of cancer. Effective prevention requires not only an appropriate lowering of the genotoxic carcinogens and promoting factors, but also discovery of suitable inhibiting elements for the operation of the genotoxic carcinogens as described in detail by Wattenberg (American Health Foundation, 1987) as well as elements that lower the effectiveness of promoting factors, like certain types of fiber, where the inhibitors most likely function in the later stages of the overall process.

MECHANISMS OF CARCINOGENESIS

Neoplastic Conversion

At least two distinct phases of carcinogenesis, namely an early stage and a late stage, or initiating agents and promoting agents, were recognized by early investigators (Berenblum, 1974). Now it is established that cancer is the result of a mutational event (Hayashi et al., 1986; Rosenkranz, 1988; Weinberg, 1989). Investigations at the molecular level permit definition of the precise nature of changes in the genome induced by carcinogens (Brown et al., 1988; Rosenkranz, 1988; Cavenee et al., 1989; Weinberg, 1989). The carcinogens leading to such mutational events are genotoxic (Williams, 1989). Such carcinogens have been associated with cancers of environmental or occupational origin, or important types of cancer related to lifestyle, because of use of tobacco products and exposure to tobacco smoke or their presence in foods as a result of cooking or salting or pickling. Genotoxic carcinogens undergo host-mediated biochemical activation and are thus converted to reactive electrophilic metabolites, which interact with nucleophilic centers in DNA and also RNA and protein (Fig. 1) (Witmer et al., 1990). There are techniques for assessing, with sensitive immunological procedures or through biochemical approaches like ^{32}P-postlabeling, to what extent such reactions have occurred (Randerath and Randerath, 1990). These procedures also permit assessment of prior exposure of individuals to genotoxic chemicals through marker studies (Rosenkranz, 1988; Shahin, 1989, Weinberg, 1989; Witmer et al., 1990).

The abnormal DNA can be repaired in a resting cell population. However, during cell duplications, the carcinogen-modified DNA template forms the basis for production of an altered DNA. The cells bearing such a changed DNA are considered typical of early neoplastic cells. Clearly, any endogeneous event or exogenous chemical that increases the rate of DNA synthesis and mitosis may potentiate the effect of a carcinogen, or vice versa, or attenuate it, if the rate is decreased (Brown et al., 1988; Clayson et al., 1989; Knight et al., 1989; Lipkin et al., 1989).

These cumulative series of events are neoplastic conversion (Williams, 1989; Weisburger, 1990). At the level of DNA and the gene, this set of reactions is carried out by genotoxic chemicals, by specific tumor viruses, or directly or indirectly by radiation. In addition to altering DNA through translocation and gene amplification, such actions can also affect tumor suppressor genes, and thus provide a template typical of neoplasia for DNA synthesis (Fig. 2).

Promotion, Growth, and Development

Later sequences, the growth and development of early neoplastic cells, are subject to a different set of endogenous and exogenous growth-controlling elements that operate through distinct mechanisms (Weisburger, 1990) (Table 1). This area of promotion and progression plays a key role in eventually leading to clinical, overt neoplasia. Additional alterations of the genome can take place during these stages, perhaps due to lack of fidelity of the DNA-polymerases in early cancer cells (Loeb and Cheng, 1990), but the main actions involve growth and development. Typical early neoplastic cells are under the influence of growth-controlling elements, transferred through intercellular gap junctions from surrounding normal cells. One role of promoters is to sever or constrict gap junctions, and thus neoplastic cells are subject to their intrinsic growth-enhancing elements. On the

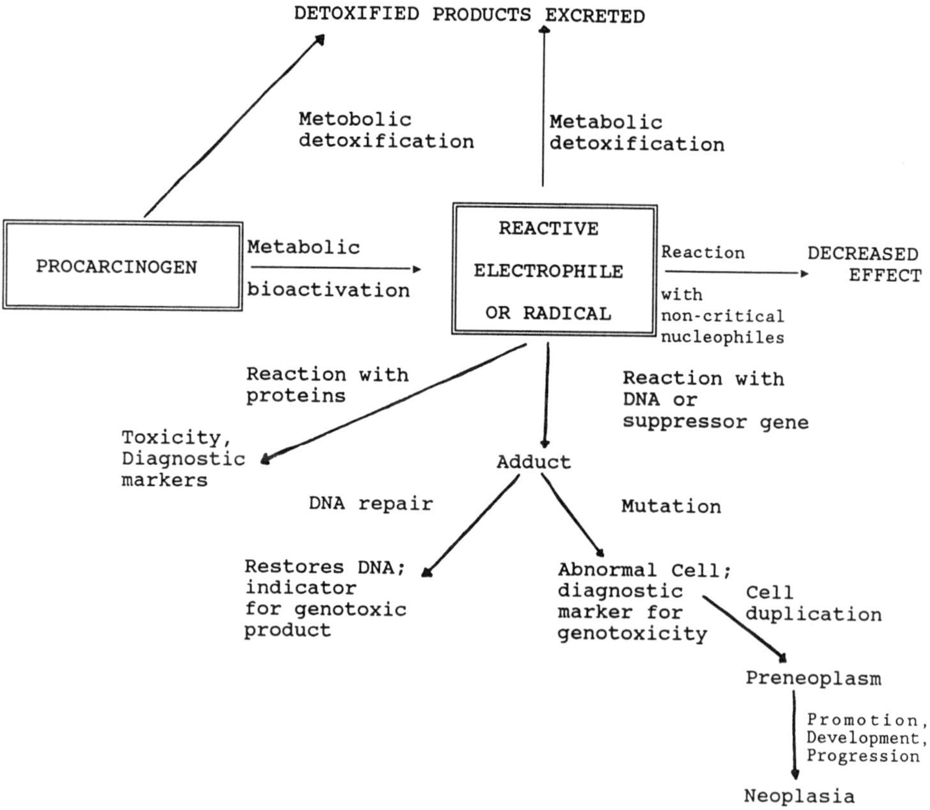

Figure 1 Most types of cancer stem from a complex sequence of steps, schematically outlined. Naturally occurring chemicals related to lifestyle undergo metabolic activation. The resulting ultimate carcinogen, a reactive molecule interacts with cellular macromolecules and, specifically, with the heritable element, DNA. This altered DNA undergoes further changes during replication, leading to codon (oncogene) rearrangements and amplification. Effects on tumor suppressor genes are also relevant. This sequence of reactions results from the presence of "genotoxic" elements. The cells with such abnormal DNA must grow and develop, subject to the control of diverse factors at the level of the cell, organ, tissue, whole animal or human being, and external environmental elements. This includes factors concerned with growth promotion or inhibition. This sequence of reactions is the result of nongenotoxic, epigenetic events that are highly dose-dependent, with a threshold no-effect dose. Duration of exposure is important as well. The effect of promoters is reversible, a key feature applicable to nutritional carcinogenesis.

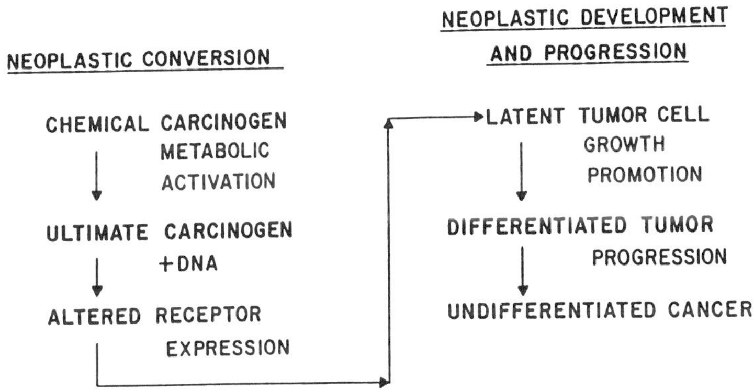

Figure 2 The overall process leading to cancer involves a complex sequence of steps. Carcinogens can undergo metabolic activation or are detoxified biochemically, usually the major set of reactions. The resulting ultimate carcinogen, a reactive electrophilic molecule (and also radiation or oncogenic viruses) interacts with nucleophilic sites in cellular macromolecules, and specifically in the competing reactions decreasing the effect with cellular nucleophiles and proteins, that can be used as markers. In a quiescent cell system, specific enzyme systems can repair the altered DNA. Another reaction serving to detect carcinogens. In growing cells the altered DNA serves as template for newly synthesized DNA, and leads to further changes in DNA structure, and thus in function, during replication. This altered DNA undergoes further changes during duplication, leading to codon, including oncogene rearrangements and amplification. Also, there can be effects of reactive carcinogen metabolites on suppressor genes. This sequence of reactions is the result of "genotoxic" elements, and represents an essential early event, neoplastic conversion. The latent precancerous cells with such abnormal DNA must grow and develop, subject to the control of diverse factors at the level of the cell, organ, or tissue and exogeneous nongenotoxic elements, neoplastic development. It includes factors with growth-promotion potential. This sequence of reactions is the result of epigenetic events, which are highly dose-dependent, with a threshold, no-effect dose level. Also, duration of exposure is important. Cessation of exposure with this class of agents often arrests progression to more advanced neoplasia and can even lead to regression.

other hand, vitamin A can enhance the patency of gap junction and facilitate intercellular transfer of growth-controlling elements, and thus serve to decrease promoting actions (Hossain et al., 1989). A major role of dietary components like fat, fiber, or certain micronutrients like vitamin A or calcium ions is to influence the growth and developmental aspects of neoplastic cell systems through specific effector mechanisms. This is important, since these actions are highly dose-dependent and are also reversible (Weisburger, 1990). Lowering the concentration of a growth-promoting substance by only 50% may exert a major delaying effect on the growth of neoplastic cells. Complete elimination of promoting

Table 1 Key Properties of Promoters

Do not react with DNA
Can bind to specific cellular receptors
Can be cytotoxic, lead to compensatory regeneration
Can affect hormonal balance
Can operate through immunosuppression
Usually display specific organotropism
Can affect intercellular communication
Can break gaps junctions
Can increase cell turnover rates and transformation
Can increase ornithine decarboxyase and protein kinase C

substances can almost immediately and sharply decrease the development of neoplastic cells. Smoking cessation, for example, progressively lowers the risk of the appearance of clinical cancer (Weisburger, 1990). It is possible to delay or abolish the growth of abnormal cells based on these well-documented properties inherent in the phenomenon of promotion. This is the foundation for dietary recommendations for the primary prevention of diet-related neoplasms. In patients with appropriate treated diet-sensitive neoplasms, a deliberate decrease of promoting phenomena is designed to prevent or delay recurrences, a sound means of adjuvant therapy (Hayashi et al., 1986; Boyar et al., 1988; Prentice, 1988; Greenwald, 1989; Palmer, 1989; Schatzkin et al., 1989; Cohen and Wynder, 1990).

DISCOVERY OF ETIOLOGIC FACTORS

Impressive progress in documenting specific etiologic factors resulted from multidisciplinary approaches (Table 2). The first set of data rests on population studies, using the classic techniques of epidemiology (Schottenfeld and Fraumeni, 1991). In the field of occupational health, or in the study of smoking and health, much has been learned from comparing groups of people exposed to carcinogens, such as smokers, with people not exposed, or nonsmokers. In the area of nutrition and health, and specifically nutrition and cancer, the approach needs to be more refined, since everyone eats. Thus, studies in a country with a given traditional diet often show few clear-cut differences in dietary habits between cases and controls. There may be certain quantitative differences, but within a given country, the group with the lowest compared with the highest intake of a nutrient may cover a fairly narrow range. Therefore, many studies in the area of nutrition and cancer examining the role of macronutrients like fat or fiber or micronutrients like vitamin A or calcium have not always yielded unambiguous

Table 2 Multidisciplinary Approaches to Ascertain Etiologic Factors

Epidemiology
Geographic pathology
Special populations
Time trends
Laboratory studies
Comparative metabolic and biochemical epidemiology in high and low risk populations
Comparative studies in animal models
Use of cell and organ cultures
Development of hypotheses and definition of mechansims
Established or suspected risk factors and their mode of action
Development of health-promotion programs
Control of genotoxic carcinogens
Control of promoting or enhancing agents
Use of protective or inhibiting factors

results (American Health Foundation, 1987; Simopoulos, 1987; Pariza, 1988; Berrino and Gatta, 1989; Committee on Diet and Health, 1989; Greenwald et al., 1989; Hulka, 1989; Moon and Micozzi, 1989; Schatzkin et al., 1989).

The most rewarding and relevant approach involved the study of populations with traditionally distinct nutritional habits (Table 3). Foods customarily consumed in Japan used to be quite different from those in the West, specifically North America or the United Kingdom (Bulbrook, 1986; Hayashi et al., 1986; Rose et al., 1986; Henderson et al., 1988; LaVecchia et al., Mills et a., 1989; Rogers and Longnecker, 1989; Toniolo et al., 1989; Howe, et al., 1990; Schottenfeld and Fraumeni, 1991). In Japan, the major nutrient was carbohydrate (rice) with some protein from fish, and a limited amount of total fat, approximately 15% of calories. In contrast, the typical Western diet consisted of 40–45% carbohydrates and 40–45% total fat (Table 4). These Japanese traditions were paralleled by a dramatically distinct lower incidence in mortality from cancer of the postmenopausal breast, distal colon, ovary, endometrium, pancreas, and prostate, and also myocardial infarction (Watanabe and Arimoto, 1989). Yet this striking association between dietary tradition and mortality from major types of cancer and heart disease has not been unanimously found satisfactory as a basis for drawing conclusions on etiology. It has been stated that there are many other elements in the lifestyle of the Japanese, compared to the Americans, that might account for the distinct lower incidence of these cancers and, indeed, also of coronary heart disease. Yet, key studies in migrants from China or Japan to Hawaii and the North American continent have revealed a sharp increase in risk for colon

Table 3 Low and High Risk Groups as a Function of Nutritional Traditions

Organ	Lower-risk population	Lower-risk factors	Higher-risk population	Higher-risk factors
Colon	Japan	Low fat diet	North America; Western Europe; New Zealand; Australia; southern Scandinavia	High-fat, high-cholesterol, low-fiber diets; fried foods
	Mormons	Higher fiber diet		
	7th Day Adventists	Low or no fried food, higher fiber diet		
	Finland	Higher fiber diet, lower intake of fried food (calcium??)		
Breast	Japan	Low fat diet	North America; Western Europe; New Zealand; Australia	High fat diet, low fiber
Endometrium	Japan	Low fat diet	California; Europe	High fat diet, obesity, estrogen use
Prostate	Japan	Low fat diet	United States; Scandinavia; Western Europe	High fat diet

Pancreas	Bombay, India		California; blacks	Early smoking habit, Western-style high fat, high cholesterol diet
Stomach	United States	Low pickled, salted foods, high fruits, salads, vitamins C, E	Japan; China; Chile; Colombia; Eastern Europe	Salted, pickled foods, geochemical nitrate and low intake of vitamins A, C, and E
Esophagus	Utah, rural Norway	Low alcohol and smoking habits	France (Calvados, Normandy); United States (lower socio-economic groups)	Alcohol and smoking
			India	Tobacco chewing
			Eastern Iran, Southern Soviet Union, Central China	Low vitamins A, C, and E; salted, pickled food?

Table 4 Macronutrient Intake as Percent of Calories in United States and Japan

Year	United States	Japan
1950	40.0	7.9
1955	41.5	8.7
1960	41.5	10.6
1965	41.6	14.8
1970	42.3	18.7
1975	41.9	22.3
1980	41.8	23.6
1985	43.5	24.5

Source: Wynder et al., 1990; personal communication.

cancer in migrants themselves and of breast or prostate cancer in the second generation (Hayashi, 1986; Rose et al., 1986; Mettlin, 1988; Rogers and Longnecker, 1989; Howe et al., 1990). Migrants adopted progressively the dietary traditions of their new host country. A reason for the delayed increase for the endocrine-related cancers like breast and prostate may stem from the fact that residency in a lower risk environment during the important developmental aspects at puberty biases these tissues toward maintenance of a certain resistance (Micozzi, 1985). On the other hand, cell turnover in the distal colon occurs at a relatively constant rate and may account for the sensitivity in the migrants themselves.

Currently, the best evidence of a major role for nutritional customs, especially fat intake, is the appreciable increase in cancer of the breast and the distal colon, but not the proximal colon in Japan (Fig. 3) (Tajima et al., 1985; Rose, 1986; Rose et al., 1986; Watanabe and Arimoto, 1989). The rise is particularly noteworthy in urban Japan, associated with the progressive introduction of Western dietary habits, essentially an increasing fat and decreasing carbohydrate intake (Table 4).

Other parts of the world provide supporting information. People in southern Italy have maintained the traditional Italian dietary pattern, whereas the diet of the industrial northern Italian population is virtually indistinguishable from that of the rest of Western Europe or the United States (LaVecchia et al., 1988). The southern Italian diet uses olive oil as the main lipid, and the total lipid intake is about 32% of calories. In northern Italy the fat intake also involves olive oil, but there is a more varied fat consumption, and the total linoleic acid intake is higher. Associated with this distinct dietary pattern is an appreciably lower rate of breast cancer in southern Italy compared to northern Italy or the United States. In animal models, olive oil is not a good promoter of mammary cancer formation (Cohen et al., 1986; Ip et al., 1986; Cohen and Wynder, 1990).

Another population that was exceptional was Finland, especially the rural area. As a rule the Finnish people consume appreciable amounts of total fat, mostly

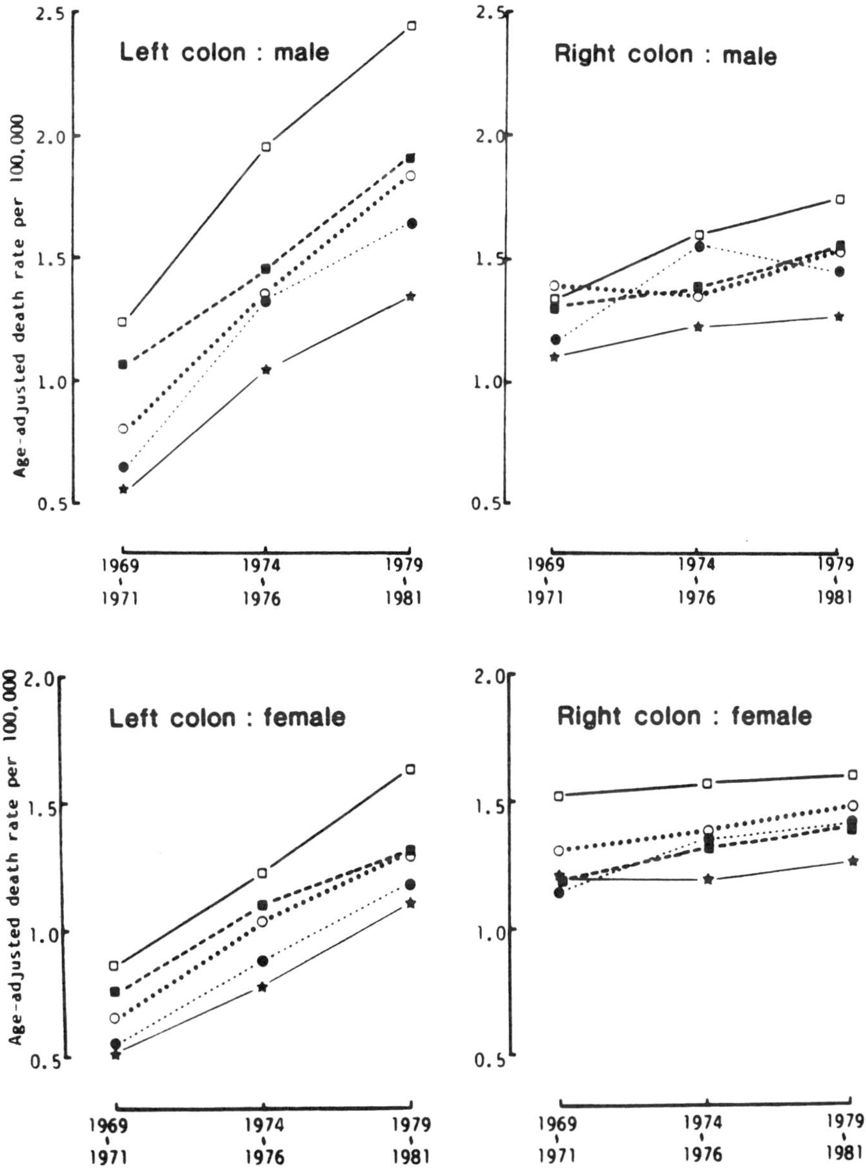

Figure 3 Time trends in the age-adjusted death rate for left-sided and right-sided colon cancer in five areas: metropolitan cities (□); large cities (■); medium-sized cities (○); small cities (●); countries (*). As the Japanese diet became more westernized, with an increasing fat intake, left-sided colon cancer, but not right-sided, increased. Thus, etiologic factors and mechanisms may be different. (From Tajima et al., 1985; with permission.)

saturated fats from extensive use of dairy products, a habit typical of a region at high risk for coronary heart disease (Reddy, 1988). Even so, Finnish people display a low incidence of distal colon cancer. Also, postmenopausal breast cancer mortality is lower than that in neighboring Denmark or the United States (Rose, 1986). An explanation rests on the fact that the Finnish people consume much higher amounts of foods rich in cereal fibers. The increased fiber intake yields a larger stool bulk, diluting the promoters for colon cancer—bile and fatty acids (Reddy, 1988). The lower breast cancer rate has not been fully clarified but may rest on a distinct enterohepatic cycling of estogrens. Similar trends are apparent in a study of vegetarian populations (Mills et al., 1989).

As noted, Japanese with a low risk for the Western nutritional cancers not only consume a low fat diet, but a fair proportion of their fat stems from fish oils, ω-3 polyunsaturated lipids (Hayashi et al., 1986; Karmali, 1989). Recent studies in several models of breast and colon cancer have observed that fish oil at any dose level is protective; parallel to these findings are those associated with atherosclerosis and heart disease, where regular intake of fish is also protective (Table 5) (Weisburger, 1988).

MODEL STUDIES

During the last 50 years, specific chemical carcinogens were found to induce cancer in target organs of relevance to the field of nutritional carcinogenesis. There are reliable means of inducing cancer of the mammary gland, colon, or pancreas in which dietary modulation can be studied and the underlying mechanisms explored (Russo and Russo, 1978; American Health Foundation, 1987; Nigro and Bull, 1987; Reddy, 1988; Birt, 1989; Rodgers and Longnecker, 1989; Wilpart, 1989; Shao et al., 1990). At this point, there is no reliable model for prostatic cancer (Kroes et al., 1986). Well-designed and executed studies in animal models have been powerful tools to outline the main role and mechanisms of action for components such as fat, fiber, and certain micronutrients, and have strengthened the database obtained through epidemiology and metabolic epidemiology.

GENOTOXIC CARCINOGENS IN NUTRITIONAL CARCINOGENESIS

In the context of a book on macronutrients concentrating on the role of fat, it is important to comment briefly on the specific genotoxic carcinogens in nutritional carcinogenesis, the effect of which is modified by macronutrients and which are essential in the overall process leading to important types of cancer in humans. Just as promoting agents have specific target organs, genotoxic carcinogens have similar distinctive propeties. Therefore, the following discussion will be orgnaized by key organs affected, the nutritional elements involved, and any modifiers of the action (Table 6).

Table 5 Mechanism of Major Risk Factors and Protective Elements for Western Nutritionally Linked Cancers

Disease	Risk factors	Mechanism	Protective elements	Mechanism
Endocrine-related cancers; prostate, breast	Total dietary fat (saturated + ω-6 polyunsatured lipids)	Complex multieffector elements: hormonal balances, membrane and intracellular effectors; genotoxic carcinogens: heterocyclic arylamines (HAA) in cooked foods (also for colon, pancreas)	Monounsaturated oil (olive); ω-3 polyunsaturated oils; medium chain triclycerides; cereal fiber and pectin	Neutral action on hormone metabolism; protective effect in hormone metabolism; caloric equivalent to carbohydrate; affects enterohepatic cycling of hormones
Endometrial and ovarian cancer	Same as above, and excessive body weight	Fat cells generate estrogen; high levels estrogen may yield reactive metabolite		
Colon cancer;				
proximal	?	?	?	?
distal	Same as endocrine-related cancers	Biosynthesis of cholesterol, thence bile acids, and colon cancer promotion, including higher cell cycling; HAA as genotoxic carcinogens	Cereal fiber, vegetables, pectins, calcium salts, medium-chain tryglycerides	Increases stool bulk, dilutes promoters, bind bile and fatty acids lower intestinal cell cycling equivalent to carbohydrates
Rectal cancer	Alcoholic beverages, especially beer	Increases cell cycling in rectum?	?	?
Pancreatic cancer	Same as endocrine, etc; cigarette smoking	Genotoxic carcinogens: tobacco-specific nitrosamines, or HAA; fat as enhancer through unknown mechanisms	?	?

Table 6 Questions to Be Resolved Relative to Types of Agents Associated with the Etiology of Human Cancer

Nature of genotoxic carcinogens or mixtures—can be chemical, viral, or radiation
Nature of any nongenotoxic promoting or enhancing stimulus—can be chemical or viral
Amount, duration of exposure, and potency for each kind or agent
Possibility of inhibition of the action of agents under A or B

Cancer of the Oral Cavity and Esophagus

In the Western world, these types of cancer are seen mainly in individuals who chew tobacco or who smoke and drink alcoholic beverages and are usually on a poor nutritional intake, especially as regards essential micronutrients. In a broad area, beginning in eastern Iran through the southern Soviet Union to parts of China, there is a high incidence of cancer of the esophagus, traced to general poor nutritional status and the probable formation in vivo or in foods of certain nitrosamines. Improvement in nutritional status would most likely lower the risk of this type of cancer.

Cancer of the Stomach

This type of cancer has declined sharply in the United States in the last 50 years and is beginning to decrease in importance in northern Europe and Japan. It is still a major type of cancer in Eastern Europe, Latin America, Japan, and parts of China. The associated etiologic factor stem from a relatively low intake of essential micronutrients, especially the traditional use of salted, pickled foods, or a geochemical environment with high soil, and therefore food, nitrate levels (Correa et al., 1990). Specific nitrosoindoles or diazophenols may be the associated risk factors. Salt, being cytotoxic to the stomach and increasing the mitotic rate, is an enhancing factor, and also a contributory cause of hypertension. Recommendations for prevention include lower intake of salted, pickled foods and better nutritional balance, including availability of foods containing micronutrients such as vitamins A, C, and E (Weisburger, 1991).

Cancer of the Breast, Colon, and Pancreas

The actual genotoxic carcinogens in foods for these Western-type neoplasms require further documentation. Cancer of the pancreas, in part associated with smoking, may stem from exposure to the tobacco-specific nitrosamines (Rivenson et al., 1988). Nonetheless, for all these types of cancer and perhaps cancer of the prostate, we have proposed that the newly discovered heterocyclic arylamines, formed during cooking, may be the relevant causative carcinogens. In animal models at high dose levels, these types of chemicals have specific target organs, including the mammary gland, colon, and pancreas (organs where the effect is powerfully enhanced by fat) and other organs like liver or urinary bladder not subject to promotion by dietary fat. Under the conditions of human consumption, usually meaning a low but daily intake of such compounds beginning in childhood, target organs like liver would not likely be affected. However, in those tissues where dietary fat exerts a decisive enhancing effect, there would be an increased risk of disease development.

Endometrium and Ovary

For these organs, the genotoxic carginogens have likewise not been fully documented. However, it has been suggested that specific metabolic steps affecting estrogen in these endocrine sensitive organs may yield a genotoxic intermediate (Degen and Metzler, 1987; Liehr, 1990). These types of cancer are more often seen in women who are obese, and therefore with higher levels of available estrogen, which could be thus modified in a specific way, yielding the reactive genotoxic compound. The effect would be powerfully enhanced by dietary fat and by estrogen biosynthesized by fat cells.

TYPE AND AMOUNT OF DIETARY FAT

Mammary Gland Cancer

An extensive series of studies by Carroll, by Cohen, by Ip, and others have usually compared the effect of different fats at 5 and 20% in the diet, or 10 and 40% of calories, approximating a low risk Japanese population and a high risk Western population (Ip et al., 1986; American Health Foundation, 1987). The models used were those discovered by Huggins, namely the administration of the polycyclic aromatic hydrocarbon 7,12-dimethylbenz(a)anthracene (DMBA) to female Sprague-Dawley rats at age 50 days, the time of sexual development, and maximum cell duplication rate (Russo and Russo, 1978; American Health Foundation, 1987; Russo et al., 1990). Another model, discovered by Gullino, involved administration of N-nitrosomethylurea (NMU) to female Sprague-Dawley rats, and also to F344 rats, which are somewhat less sensitive. The mammary gland has a low level of the DNA-repair enzyme methyltransferase and therefore is highly susceptible to NMU (Fong et al., 1990). In both models, the high level of fat yields more and a greater multiplicity of neoplasms in the mammary glands than the low fat diet. Fat affects the proliferative activity of the gland, and calcium lowers it, as is true in the colon (Zhang et al., 1987; Lipkin et al., 1989).

It was discovered, however, that not every type of fat has an identical promoting effect at the high dosage (Ip et al., 1986; American Health Foundation,

1987; Clayson, 1989). Fully saturated fats like coconut oil failed to enhance, perhaps because of a partial deficiency in essential fatty acids (EFA) of the polyunsaturated type. Ip et al. (1986) observed that in these systems, the minimal requirement for essential fatty acids (EFA) measured by linoleic acid was 3.4%. Also, these oils contain esters of short-chain fatty acids, without promoting action. Carroll (Ip et al., 1986, American Health Foundation, 1987) found that with the minimal amount of EFA, even a saturated fat displayed a full promoting potential when the total fat intake was 20% of the diet. On the other hand, the omega-6 polyunsaturated oils like safflower, cotton seed, or corn oil had the highest promoting potential, meaning a higher yield of multiple mammary gland cancers than fats such as lard or beef fat. Importantly, an oil rich in monounsaturated lipid, olive oil, also was a poor promoter (Cohen et al., 1986). In part, this property may also be due to lower levels of EFA. Importantly, however, this limitation is not severe, and growth and survival is quite normal. In the Mediterranean countries, particularly southern Italy and Greece, where olive oil is the main dietary lipid, the postmenopausal breast cancer incidence is appreciably lower than in northern Italy (LaVecchia et al., 1988; LaVecchia, 1989). Thus, the animal data have a parallel in the human situation.

With corn oil, a standard oil frequently used in the West, an important dose-response relationship was established by Cohen et al. (1986). After an initiating dose of carcinogen, female Sprague-Dawley rats were fed diets containing 10, 20, 32, of 46% of calories in fat under highly controlled conditions (Fig. 4). The "low" level of 32% of fat, often recommended because it requires only slight adjustments in dietary habits, gave as high a yield as 46% of mammary gland tumors. The human equivalent was a key study by Willett et al. (1987), who observed a similar incidence of breast cancer in a prospective study involving the intake of 32–46% of calories as fat. Thus, the human data of Willett et al. (1987) agree with the experimental findings of Cohen et al. (1986). Especially noteworthy, therefore, is the finding that 20% of fat calories gave the same low incidence of mamary gland tumors as the lowest amount used, 10%. These data imply that a meaningful, significant decreased risk of the nutritionally linked cancers would involve a regimen with about 20%, at the most 25%, fat calories (Fig. 4).

The role of fat in promoting breast cancer is complex (Bulbrook, 1986; Willett, 1987; Henderson et al., 1988; deWaard, 1989; Holm et al. 1989; Cohen et al., 1990; Russo et al., 1990). Clearly, the growth and development of the mammary gland and other endocrine neoplasms are controlled by endocrine balancies, including free estrogen, estrogen-binding globulin, and pituitary, adrenal, and thyroid hormones. Their amounts and their relative ratios are a function of diet and dietary fat.

Women on a high fat diet had more free serum estrogen than women on a low fat diet (Woods et al., 1989). Also the level of the estrogenic 16-hydroxy metabolite

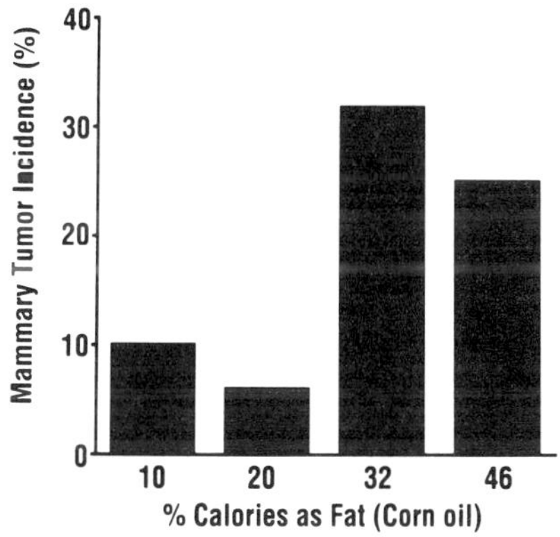

Figure 4 Female F344 rats, 50 days old, were given a single i.v. dose of N-nitrosomethylurea. They were placed on semipurified diets providing 10, 20, 32, and 46% fat-calories, given as corn oil. Mammary gland carcinomas were evaluated after 22 weeks. There was no difference between 10 and 20% fat-calories, or 30 and 40%. There is a major difference between 20 and 32% fat-calories. (From Cohen et al., 1986.)

was a function of fat calories (Michnovicz and Bradlow, 1990). These findings reflect not only the production of hormones but also their further metabolism by nonendocrine organs like liver, which are in turn under the influence of lipid as regards to the operation of specific enzymes of the complex cytochrome P-450 enzyme system. Another area requiring further investigation is the role of fat in modifying DNA synthesis and cell duplication rates in the mammary gland, an aspect clearly relevant in the overall development of neoplasia. Also, Liehr (1990) has described genotoxic metabolites of estrogen, although these may apply more to endometrial and perhaps ovarian cancer than to breast cancer. This topic will be discussed when reviewing the role of dietary restriction.

Colon Cancer

Colon cancer can be induced specifically by a number of carcinogens, such as 1,2-dimethylhydrazine and the related azoxymethane or methylazoxymethanol, and also 2′,3-dimethyl-4-aminobiphenyl, which also causes cancer in the mammary gland, pancreas, and prostate (in situ cancer only) (Reddy, 1988; Rogers and Longnecker, 1989; Wilpart, 1989). Newly discovered are carcinogens with a similar structure, belonging the class of heterocyclic aromatic amines, formed during cooking and especially browning of meat or fish (American Health Foundation, 1987; Weisburger, 1990). These chemicals induce cancer in several tissues, including the colon, mammary gland, and pancreas. A general means of inducing colon cancer, the intrarectal infusion of N-nitrosoalkylureas, was discovered by Narisawa (American Health Foundation, 1987; Reddy,1988). These carcinogens are direct-acting, highly potent, and require only one or a few doses, and are therefore useful in any species, from mouse to dog. Thus, they are ideal to study dietary modification by components such as fat, fiber, or micronutrients, since the experiment can be designed to investigate the modifying effects of the nutritional component (see Chap. 2).

Irrespective of the genotoxic carcinogen used, it has been found that dietary levels of 40% of calories of most types of fat have a promoting effect, compared to 10% of calories, paralleling without exception the findings made in models for mammary gland cancer. For example, safflower or corn oil were more efficient promoters than olive oil or a saturated fat (American Health Foundation, 1987; Reddy, 1988). Modulators such as vitamin A or carotene may affect the end point, cancer, to some extent, but clearly the fat level is the controlling element (Weisburger and Jones, 1989; Newberne et al., 1990).

The underlying mechanisms are reasonably secure, especially as a result of the extensive documentation produced by Reddy and collaborators (Reddy,1988). The fat type and amount controls the biosynthesis of cholesterol, and that in turn is converted further to primary bile acids. The ω-6-polyunsaturated fats yield higher levels of bile acids than the monounsaturated fats or saturated fats. The ω-6 fats stimulate the enzymes producing bile acids from cholesterol, a fact that is well established from studies in man and animals where these kinds of fats have a demonstrated cholesterol-lowering action. In this connection, there is a small proportion of individuals on a Western high fat intake that have a low serum cholesterol level. Their hepatic enzyme pattern may favor the production of bile acids and hence they may be at a higher risk of colon cancer (Cowen et al., 1990). Also, they may be on a higher intake of ω-6-polyunsaturated lipids, yielding a lowered serum cholesterol, but an increased risk of colon cancer. For such individuals at a low risk of atherosclerosis, an obvious protective element in colon cancer would be to consume regularly adequate bran cereal fiber to produce stool bulk and dilute bile acids, as discussed by Reddy (see Chapter 2) and through the mechanism outlined in this chapter.

Bile acids are not genotoxic. Rather, at higher levels they, and also fatty acids, are cytotoxic and thus exert a promoting effect through these mechanisms (American Health Foundation, 1987; Reddy, 1988; Wilpart, 1989). An old proposal states that bile acids are converted to a carcinogen like 3-methylcholanthrene. However, there is no known biochemical mechanism to account for such a reaction.

The amount of total bile acids in the intestinal tract and in the stool is a function of the type and amount of fat consumed in animal models and in humans. Importantly, studies in metabolic epidemilogy showed that switching people from a high fat intake to a low fat intake lowers the amount of bile acids within days

(Hill, 1971). Upon return to a high fat diet, the amount of stool bile acids returned to its former level. Since bile acids are the key promoters, it is obvious that the risk for colon cancer development can be sharply reduced within days by switching from a high fat to a low fat diet. The old dogma that carcinogenesis is determined through early events, and therefore would take decades for an alteration of risk does not apply to situations where the essential controlling factor depends on a promoting effect.

Cancer of the Pancreas

Three animal models have been found useful. One is the induction of pancreatic cancer in rats by the antimetabolite azaserine, another is the induction of pancreatic cancer in hamsters by nitrosamines such as N-nitroso-bis(isopropyl)amine and 2,6-dimethylnitrosomorpholine. In either of these models administration of a diet containing 20% by weight of ω-6-polyunsaturated fats yields more pancreatic cancers than 5% (Birt et al., 1989; Rogers and Longnecker, 1989). The precise mechanism whereby the fat increased pancreatic cancer development remains to be outlined (Howe et al., 1990). The pancreas is one target organ in smokers of cigarettes. A new model mimicking this fact is based on the finding that low level adminsitration to rats of NNK, a specific nitrosamine in tobacco and its smoke, induced cancer of the pancreas (Rivenson et al., 1988). Higher levels of NNK killed the animals earlier with competing cancers, and thus pancreatic cancer, with a longer latent period, was not seen.

MECHANISMS OF ACTION OF MODIFYING FACTORS

Fiber and Calcium

The people in rural Finland consume a high saturated fat diet and thus have an elevated incidence of heart disease. In sharp contrast, they display a low distal colon cancer risk (Reddy, 1988). The underlying mechanism is a regular high wheat bran intake, leading to a large stool bulk, 200–280 grams, in one or more passes. For that reason, fatty and bile acids, that are promoters in colon carcinogenesis, occur at a threefold lower concentration than what is found in high risk populations (Reddy et al., 1989). This situation has been reproduced in animal models for colon cancer, where fiber has reduced the multiplicity of colon cancer (Kroes, 1986; Nigro and Bull, 1987; Reddy, 1988). Fat and fiber actually interact, the effect depending on the ratio (Sinkeldam et al., 1990). The rate of breast cancer in Finnish women is also lower than in Western women (Rose, 1986). Fibers and especially specific lignin type of compounds appear to be protective. Also, food fibers contain complex chemicals, which after intestinal hydrolysis of glycosides yield components with antiestrogenic activity. Fibers also affect the microflora, intestinal pH, and activity of bacterial enzymes, in turn altering the enterohepatic cycling of estrogen conjugates and yield hormonal patterns with a protective mode (Bulbrook, 1986; Woods et al., 1989; McBurney and Thompson, 1990; Trock et al., 1990; Van't Veer et al., 1990).

Supplemental calcium salts and wheat bran lowered the rate of cell cycling in the intestinal tract of high risk patients (Lipkin et al., 1989; Alberts et al., 1990). The rate of cellular DNA-biosynthesis and mitosis controls the overall sequence of events leading to clinical cancer. Currently, the potential benefits of calcium and vitamin D in the fat-associated cancers is under active investigation in humans and in model systems (Garland et al., 1989; Wargovich and Baer, 1989; Negri et al., 1990; Reschef et al., 1990). Wheat bran also lowered cell duplication rates in the rectum in high risk patients, an indicator of beneficial effects that deserves not only detailed study, but prompt application to disease prevention (Alberts et al., 1990).

Dietary Restriction

Investigators in the field of nutrition and cancer recorded that moderate to severe dietary restriction in a number of animal models, particularly in mammary gland carcinogens, uniformly yielded fewer neoplasms (Reddy, 1988; Weindruch and Walford, 1988; Rogers and Longnecker, 1989; Albanes et al., 1990). This situation may have prevailed in humans when there was hunger, such as in The Netherlands or Norway during World War II, where fat intake was especially depressed. This has resulted in an apparent lowering of the nutritionally linked cancers (delayed puberty?) and of fatal heart attacks. The last condition may have also been decreased because of an absence of cigarettes, a major risk factor for heart disease.

In breast cancer induction a dietary restriction may have an indirect explanation, based on altered endocrine balances (Weindruch and Walford, 1988). Also to be considered is a more general mechanism. Several investigators, but especially Clayson et al. (1989), reported that dietary restriction results in a dramatic decrease in DNA synthesis, mitosis, and cell cycling. Thus, the view that dietary restriction inhibits carcinogenesis, through various mechanisms, is no doubt true. A high fat diet fed at moderate restrictive levels would not lead to promotion, mediated by an increased rate of cell cycling, because the dietary restriction would have the opposite effect. This finding could obviously be transferred to humans.

However, the important point is that most human populations do not voluntarily undergo lifelong dietary restriction but rather eat ad libitum, and indeed overeat, considering that modern humans are often sedentary and their caloric requirements are lower. Exceptional situations like war temporarily would have restrictive effects, with a consequent lower risk. Thus, the experimental findings, while giving valuable mechanistic insights, cannot be applied to a free living population with reasonable access to a variety of foods, as is true in the developed world. For such populations, other means of lowering disease risk are needed. This includes the adoption of a new nutritional tradition, with an energy-need balanced intake of foods including a high complex carbohydrate component (65–70%), protein (10–15%), and especially a moderate total fat intake (20–25%).

Exercise

People who had regular occupational or avocational exercises had lower risk of colon cancer than sedentary individuals (Ballard-Barbash et al., 1990; Boffetta et al., 1990; Kune et al., 1990). Also interesting: women who were athletic in the first 25 years appeared later to have a lower breast cancer rate than women who were not. Thus, an early lifestyle was carried over as a benefit to a subsequent period of life. These situations were mimicked in rats who had free access to a wheel cage while controls did not (Cohen and Wynder, 1990). Some rats were active runners and others were less frequent users. Younger animals ran longer than the same animals as they aged. The key finding was that even on a high fat diet, the percentage of rats with NMU-induced mammary gland cancer and the tumor multiplicity was lower in rats that were moderate runners than in rats that were low and high runners. Similar results were obtained for colon cancer. The protective effect of exercise was not due to a lower food intake or a lower weight gain. The animals on the exercise wheel weighed as much or more than the sedentary controls, but their body contained less fat and more protein and especially more water.

Comments, with Application to Health Promotion

Cancer affecting certain target organs is clearly a multistep disease providing the opportunity to block or at least decrease the action at a number of points and therefore lead to a lower overall risk, and thus incidence, of a specific type of cancer. The data on mortality show that nutritional factors account for 35% of all cases and lifestyle for the majority (Table 7). Directly linked with macronutrients, dietary fat, and fiber are cancers in the postmenopausal breast, ovary and endometrium, and prostate, pancreas, and distal colon. Our view is that the cancers of the breast, colon, and pancreas, and perhaps others for which evidence remains to be acquired, may involve genotoxic carcinogens in the form of the heterocyclic amines formed during cooking. It is possible that cancer of the prostate likewise is caused by such chemicals. The genotoxic events as regards cancer of the ovary and endometrium are ill-defined, but it may be that estrogen can be converted through metabolism to DNA-reactive metabolites (Degen and Metzler, 1987; Liehr, 1990). With all these cancers, the amounts of genotoxic carcinogens are small, but clearly exposure to such agents occurs beginning early in life, when rapid growth of tissues involving high levels of DNA synthesis and mitosis facilitates transformation of normal cells to early neoplastic cells.

Table 7 Analysis of Causes of Cancer Mortality in North America

Type	% of total
Lifestyle cancers	
Tobacco-related—lung, pancreas, bladder, kidney	32
Nitrate-nitrite (salted, pickled foods), low vitamin C—stomach	2.7
High fat, lower fiber, broiled or fried foods—colon, pancreas, breast, prostate, ovary, endometrium	31
Alcohol—rectum; mycotoxin, hepatitis B—liver	3.8
Sunlight—skin (melanoma)	1.7
Transplacental chemicals—brain	2.2
Occupational cancers—various organs	1
Cryptogenic cancers (virus?)	
Lymphomas, leukemias, sarcomas, cervix	11
Tobacco and alcohol—oral cavity, esophagus	3.5
Tobacco and asbestos, tobacco and mining, tobacco and uranium and radium—lung, respiratory tract	3.0
Iatrogenic cancers	
Radiation, drugs—diverse organs	1
Unspecified—diverse organs	7

Source: Calculated from American Cancer Society Statistics, 1990.

Yet without promotion or enhancing effects, it is likely that these effects would not translate to clinically overt cancer. The in situ cancer of the prostate seen in older Japanese men represents such an early effect leading to dormant tumor cells (Akazaki and Stemmerman, 1973). On the other hand, promotion due to higher intake of dietary fat as occurs in the Western world, and other as yet undefined factors such as sedentary lifestyle, causes the clinically overt invasive disease. Therefore, one key element in the control and prevention of the nutritionally linked types of cancer rests on a definition of the maximal amount of dietary fat that would not increase appreciably the risk of these cancers. About 10 years ago, a special committee under the auspices of the National Academy of Sciences recommended in a preliminary way that the intake of total fat, traditionally about 38–44% of calories in the United States and in Western Europe, be lowered to about 30% of calories (Committee on Diet, Nutrition and Cancer, 1982). This decision was based on the parallel recommendation of the consultants to the American Heart Association and federal agencies concerned with heart disease risk, which had adopted 30% of fat calories and also an increase of the P/S ratio from 0.3 to 1.0 as a desirable goal.

Data generated in the last 10 years, however, in models for colon and breast cancer and observations in humans indicated that 30% is not likely to have a preventive effect. For example, a prospective study on breast cancer incidence in nurses as a function of dietary fat indicated no effect (Willett et al., 1987). The explanation rested on the fact that in the five subgroups, the one with the lowest fat intake consumed diets with about 32% fat calories, and the highest 46%. Therefore, based on current knowledge, there is a sharp nonlinearity in the effect of fat in at least two target organs, breast and colon, between 20–30% of fat. Hence, based on these facts and the underlying mechanisms, the promoting aspects of dietary fat in humans would be minimized by a recommendation that the total fat by humans optimally approach 20% of calories. Public education, especially as regards information on sources of fat, on foods, high or low in fat, and likewise desirable substitutes such as bran cereal fibers, other carbohydrates, vegetables, and fruits is important (Hirayama, 1988; Engle et al., 1990). Production and marketing of low fat–high fiber foods is an essential component of

Table 8 Approaches to Chronic Disease Prevention Based on Mechanisms

Action	Lower Risk
Control smoking	Coronary heart disease; cancers of the lung, kidney, bladder, pancreas, and head and neck (chewing tobacco)
Lower total fat intake (aim for 20% of calories)	Coronary heart disease; cancers of the colon, pancreas, breast, prostate, ovary, endometrium
Increase fiber, vegetables, fruits, and Ca^{2+}	Cancer of the colon, breast; constipation, diverticulosis, appendicitis
Have regular moderate exercise	Coronary heart disease; cancer of the colon, breast
Avoid obesity	Coronary heart disease; cancer of the endometrium, kidneys
Moderate or no use of alcoholic beverages	Liver cirrhosis, cardiomyopathy; male impotence, head and neck cancers (in smokers)
Lower intake of fried foods	Cancers of colon, breast, pancreas (?)
Lower salt Na^+ intake; Balance $K^+ + Ca^{2+}/Na^+$ ratio	Hypertension, stroke, cardiovascular disease
Avoid pickled, smoked, salted foods	Cancer of the stomach, esophagus, nasopharynx, liver (?); hypertension stroke
Practice sexual hygiene	Cancer of the cervix, penis

a more wholesome lifestyle, which would also reduce the risk of cardiovascular diseases (Table 8). Perhaps imaginative research and development by the food and agricultural industries can find a profitable nonfood application of unavoidably produced fats.

As discussed, micronutrients can modulate, sometimes quite appreciably, the effect of macronutrients. For example, vitamin A appears to reduce the risk of breast cancer associated with dietary fat or of lung cancer in smokers. Therefore, it is necessary to define the optimal composition of the total diet as regards protein, fat, fiber, carbohydrate, and micronutrients to minimize cancer risks and indeed chronic disease risks generally.

REFERENCES

Akazaki, K., and Stemmerman, G. N. Comparative study of latent carcinoma of the prostate among Japanese in Japan and Hawaii. *JNCI 50*: 1137–1144 (1973).

Albanes, D., Salbe, A. R., Levander, O. A., Taylor, P. R., Nixon, D. W., Winick, M. The effect of early caloric restriction on colonic cellular growth in rats. *Nutr. Cancer 13*: 73–80 (1990).

Alberts, D. S., Einspahr, J., Rees-McGee, S., Ramanujam, P., Buller, M. K., Clark, L., Ritenbaugh, C., Atwood, J., Pethigal, P., Earnest, D., Villar, H., Phelps, J., Lipkin, M., Wargovich, M., Meyskens, Jr., F. L. Effects of dietary wheat bran fiber on rectal epithelial cell proliferation in patients with resection for colorectal cancers. *JNCI 82*: 1280–1285 (1990).

American Health Foundation. Workshop on new developments on dietary fat and fiber in carcinogenesis (optimal types and amounts of fat or fiber). *Prev. Med. 16*: 449–595 (1987).

Ballard-Barbash, R., Schatzkin, A., Carter, C. L., Kannel, W. B. Kreger, B. E., D'Agostino, R. B., Splansky, G. L., Anderson, K. M., and Helsel, W. E. Body fat distribution and breast cancer in the Framingham study. *JNCI 82*: 286–290 (1990).

Ballard-Barbash, R., Schatzkin, A., Albanes, D., Schiffman, M. H., Kreger, B. E., Kannel, G. L., Anderson, K. M., and Helsel, W. E. Physical activity and risk of large bowel cancer in the Framingham study. *Cancer Res. 50*: 3610–3613 (1990).

Berenblum, I. Carcinogenesis as a biological problem. North-Holland Publ. Co., Amsterdam, 1974.

Berrino, F., and Gatta, G. Energy-rich diet and breast cancer risk. *Int. J. Cancer 44*: 186–187 (1989).

Birt, D. F., Julius, A. D., White, L. T., Pour, P. M. Enhancement of pancreatic carcinogenesis in hamsters fed a high-fat diet ad libitum and at a controlled calorie intake. *Cancer Res. 49*: 5858–5851 (1989).

Birt, D. F. The influence of dietary fat on carcinogenesis: Lessons from experimental models. *Nutr. Reviews 48*(1):1–5 (1990).

Boffetta, P., Barone, J., Wynder, E. L. Leisure time physical activity in a hospital-based population. *J. Clin. Epidemiol. 43*(6): 569–577 (1990).

Boyar, A. P., Rose, D. P., Wynder, E. L. Recommendations for the prevention of chronic disease: the application for breast disease. *Am. J. Clin. Nutr. 48*: 896–900 (1988).

Boyar, A. P., Rose, D. P., Loughridge, J. R., Engle, A., Palgi, A., Laakso, K., Kinne, D., Wynder, E. L. Response to a diet low in total fat in women with postmenopausal breast cancer: A pilot study. *Nutr. Cancer 11*: 93–99 (1988).

Brown, K., Buchmann, A., Balmain, A. Carcinogen-induced mutations in the mouse c-Ha-*ras* gene provide evidence of multiple pathways for tumor progression. *Proc. Natl. Acad. Sci USA 87*: 43–51 (1988).

Bulbrook, R. D. (ed.) Hormones and cancer; 90 years after Beatson. *Cancer Surv. 5*: 435–687 (1986).

Cavenee, W. K., Hastie, N. D., Stanbridge, E. J. (eds.). Recessive oncogenes and tumor suppression. Cold Spring Harbor Univ Press, Cold Spring Harbor, NY, 1989.

Clayson, D. B., Nera, E. A., Lok, E. The potential for the use of cell proliferation studies in carcinogen risk assessment. *Regul. Toxicol. Pharmacol. 9*: 284–295 (1989).

Cohen, L. A., Choi, K., Weisburger, J. H., Rose, D. P. Effect of varying proportions of dietary fat on the development of N-nitrosomethylurea-induced rat mammary tumors. *Anticancer Res. 6*: 215–218 (1986).

Cohen, L. A., Wynder, E. L. Do dietary monounsaturated fatty acids play a protective role in carcinogenesis and cardiovascular disease. *Med. Hypotheses 31*: 83–89 (1990).

Committee on Diet and Health, Food and Nutrition Board. *Diet and Health: Implications for Reducing Chronic Disease Risk*. National Academy Press, Washington, DC, 1989.

Committee on Diet, Nutrition and Cancer, National Research Council. *Diet, Nutrition and Cancer*. National Academy Press, Washington, DC, 1982.

Correa, P., Haenszel, W., Cuello, C., Zavala, D., Fontham, E., Zarama, G., Tannenbaum, S., Collazos, T., Ruiz, B. Gastric Precancerous process in a high risk population: Cross-sectional studies. *Cancer Res. 50*: 4731–4736 (1990).

Cowen, L. D., O'Connell, D. L., Criqui, M. H., Barrett-Connor, E., Bush, T. L., Wallace, R. B. Cancer mortality and lipid and lipoprotein levels. *Am. J. Epidemiol. 131*: 468–482 (1990).

Degen, G. H., Metzler, M. Sex hormones and neoplasia: Genotoxic effects in short term assays. *Arch. Toxicol.* (Suppl.) *10*: 264–278 (1987).

deWaard, F., Trichopoulos, D. Unifying concept of the aetiology of breast cancer. *Int. J. Cancer 41*: 666–669 (1988).

Engle, A., Hebert, J. R., Reddy, B. S. Relationships between food consumption and dietary intake among healthy volunteers and implications for meeting dietary goals. *J. Amer. Dietetic Assoc. 90*: 526–533 (1990).

Fong, L. Y. Y., Jensen, D. E., Magee, P. N. DNA methyl-adduct dosimetry and O^6-alkylguanine-DNA alkyl transferase activity determinations in rat mammary carcinogenesis by procarbazine and N-methylnitrosourea. *Carcinogenesis 1*: 411–417 (1990).

Franceschi, S. Productive factors and cancers of the breast, ovary and endometrium. *Eur J. Cancer Clin. Oncol. 25*: 1933–1943 (1989).

Garland, C. F., Garland, F. C., Shaw, E. K., Comstock, G. W., Helsing, K. J. Gorham, E. D. Serum 25-hydroxyvitamin D and colon cancer: Eight-year prospective study *Lancet ii*: 1176–1178 (1989).

Greenwald, P. Strengths and limitations of methodologic approaches to the study of diet and cancer: Summary and future perspectives with emphasis on dietary fat and breast cancer. *Prev. Med. 18*: 163–166 (1989).

Greenwald, P., Nixon, D. W., Malone, W. F., Kelloff, G. J., Stern, H. R., Witkin, K. M. Concepts in cancer chemoprevention research. *Cancer 65*: 1483–1490 (1990).

Hayashi, Y., Nagao, M. Sugimura, T., Takayama, S., Tomatis, L., Wattenberg, L. W., Wogan, G. N. (eds.). *Diet and Nutrition and Cancer*. Japan Scientific Societies Press and VNU Science Press BV, Tokyo and Utrecht, 1986, pp. 3–345.

Henderson, B. E., Ross, R., Bernstein, L. Estrogens as a cause of human cancer. *Cancer Res. 48*: 246–253 (1988).

Hill, M. J. The effects of some factors on the faecal concentration of acid steroids, neutral steroids and urobilins., *J. Pathol. 104*: 239–245 (1971).

Hirayama, T. Eylenbosch, W. J., Van Larebeke, N., Depoorter, A. M. (eds.). *Primary Prevention of Diet Related Cancers*. Pri. Prev. Cancer/Raven Press, New York, 1988, pp. 159–175.

Holm, L. E., Callmer, E., Hjalmar, M. L., Lidbrink, E., Nilsson, B., Skoog, L. Dietary habits and prognostic factors in breast cancer. *JNCI 81*: 1218–1223 (1989).

Hossain, M. Z., Wilkens, L. R. Mehta, P. P., Loewenstein, W., Bertram, J. S. Enhancement of gap junctional communication by retinoids correlates with their ability to inhibit neoplastic transformation. *Carcinogenesis 10*: 1743–1748 (1989).

Howe, G. R., Hirohata, T., Hislop, T. G., Iscovich, J. M., Yuan, J. M., Katsouyanni K., Lubin, F., Marubini, E., Modan, B., Rohan, T., Toniolo, P., Shunzhang, Y. Dietary factors and risk of breast cancer: Combined analysis of 12 case-control studies *JNCI 82*: 561–569 (1990a).

Howe, G. R., Jain, M., Miller, A. B. Dietary factors and risk of pancreatic cancer: Results of a Canadian population-based case-control study. *Int. J. Cancer 45*: 604–608 (1990b).

Hulka, B. S. Dietary fat and breast cancer: Case-control and cohort studies. *Prev. Med. 18*: 180–193 (1989).

Ip, C., Birt, D. F., Rogers, A. E., Mettlin, C. (eds.) *Dietary Fat and Cancer. Progress in Clinical and Biological Research*, Vol. 222, Liss, New York, 1986.

Karmali, R. A. n-3 fatty acids and cancer. *J. Intern Med. Suppl. 225*(731): 197–200 (1989).

Knight, G. B., Gudas, J. M., Pardee, A. B. Coordinate control of S phase onset and thymidine kinase expression. *Jpn. J. Cancer Res. 80*: 493–498 (1989).

Kroes, R., Beems, R. B., Bosland, M. C., Bunnik, G. S. J., Sinkeldam, E. J. Nutritional factors in lung, colon, and prostate carcinogenesis in animal models. *Federation Proc. 45*: 136–141 (1986).

Kune, G. A., Kune, S., Watson, L. F. Body weight and physical activity as predictors of colorectal cancer risk. *Nutrition and Cancer 13*: 9–18 (1990).

LaVecchia, C. Nutritional factors and cancers of the breast, endometrium and ovary. *Eur. J. Cancer Clin. Oncol. 25*: 1945–1951 (1989).

LaVecchia C., Harris, R. E., and Wynder, E. L. Comparative epidemiology of cancer between the United States and Italy. *Cancer Res. 48*: 7285–7293 (1988).

Lerman, C., Rimer, B., and Engstrom, P. F. Reducing avoidable cancer mortality through prevention and early detection regimens. *Cancer Res. 49*: 4955–4962 (1989).

Liehr, J. G. Genotoxic effects of estrogens. *Mutation Res. 238*: 269–276 (1990).

Lipkin, M., Friedman, E., Winawer, S. J., Newmark H. Colonic epithelial cell proliferation in responders and nonresponders to supplemental dietary calcium. *Cancer Res. 49*: 248–254 (1989).

Loeb, L. A., Cheng, K. C. Errors in DNA synthesis: A source of spontaneous mutations. *Mutation Res. 238*: 297–304 (1990).

McBurney, M. I., Thompson, L. U. Fermentative characteristics of cereal brans and vegetable fibers. *Nutr. Cancer. 13*: 271–280 (1990).

McGinnis, J. M. National priorities in disease prevention. *Issues Science Technol. 5*: 46–92 (1988–89).

Mettlin, C. Level of epidemiologic proof in studies of diet and cancer with specific reference to dietary fat and vitamin A. *Prog. Clin. Biol. Res. 259*: 149–159 (1988).

Michnovicz, J. J., Bradlow, H. L. Induction of estradiol metabolism by dietary indole-3-carbinol in humans. *JNCI 82*: 947–949 (1990).

Micozzi, M. S. Nutrition, body size, and breast cancer. *Yearbook of Physical Anthropology 28*: 175–206 (1985).

Mills, P. K., Deeson, W. L., Phillips, R. L., Fraser, G. E. Dietary habits and breast cancer incidence among Seventh-Day Adventists. *Cancer 64*: 582–590 (1989).

Moon T., Micozzi, M. S. (eds). *Nutrition and Cancer Prevention: Investigating the Role of Micronutrients*. Marcel Dekker, New York, 1989.

Negri, E., La Vecchia, C. D'Avanzo, B., Franceschi, S. Calcium, dairy products, and colorectal cancer *Nutr. Cancer 13*: 255–262 (1990).

Newberne, P. M. Beuche, D., Riengropitak, S., Schrager, T. F. The influence of dietary levels of vitamin A and fat on colon cancer. *Nutr. Cancer 13*: 235–242 (1990).

Newmark, H. L. Lipkin, M., Maheshwari, N. Colonic hyperplasia and hyperproliferation induced by a nutritional stress diet with four components of Western-style diet. *JNCI 82*: 491–496 (1990).

Nigro, N. D., Bull, A. W. The impact of dietary fat and fiber on intestinal carcinogenesis. *Prev. Med. 16*: 451–459 (1987).

Palmer, S. The implications of dietary recommendations for dietary patterns and health. *In Vivo 3*: 135–142 (1989).

Pariza, M. W. Dietary fat and cancer risk: Evidence and research needs. *Annu. Rev. Nutr. 8*: 167–183 (1988).

Parkin, D. M. Cancers of the breast, endometrium and ovary: Geographic correlations. *Eur. J. Cancer Clin. Oncol. 25*: 1917–1925 (1989).

Prentice, R. L., Kakar, F., Hursting, S., Sheppard, L., Klein, R., Kushi, L. H. Aspects of the rationale for the Women's Health Trial. *JNCI 80*: 802–814 (1988).

Prentice, R. L., Pepe, M., Self, S. G. Dietary fat and breast cancer: A quantitative assessment of the epidemiological literature and a discussion of methodological issues. *Cancer Res. 49*: 3147–3156 (1989).

Randerath, K., Li, D., Randerath, E. Age-related DNA modifications (I-compounds): Modulation by physiological and pathological processes. *Mutation Res. 238*: 245–253 (1990).

Reddy, B. S. Overview of diet and colon cancer. *Prog. Clin. Biol. Res. 279*: 111–121 (1988).

Reddy, B., Engle, A., Katsifis, S., Simi, B., Bartram, H. P., Perrino, P., Mahan, C. Biochemical epidemiology of colon cancer: Effect of types of dietary fiber on fecal mutagens acid, and neutral sterols in healthy subjects. *Cancer Res. 49*: 4629–4635 (1989).

Reshef, R., Rozen, P., Fireman, Z., Fine, N., Barzilai, M., Shasha, S. M., Shkolnik, T. Effect of a calcium-enriched diet on the colonic epithetial hyperproliferation induced by N-methyl-N′-nitro-N-nitrosoguanidine in rats on a low calcium and fat diet. *Cancer Res. 50*: 1764–1767 (1990).

Rivenson, A., Hoffman, D., Prokopczyk, B., Amin, S., Hecht, S. S. Induction of lung and exocrine pancreas tumors in F344 rats by tobacco-specific an areca-derived N-nitrosamines, *Cancer Res. 48*: 6912–6917 (1988).

Rogers, A. E., Longnecker, M. P. Dietary and nutritional influences on cancer: A review of epidemiologic and experimental data. *Path. Rev.* 215–245 (1989).

Rose, D. P. Dietary factors and breast cancer. *Cancer Surv. 5*: 671–687 (1986).

Rose, D. P., Boyar, A. P., Wynder, E. L. International comparisons of mortality rates for cancer of the breast, ovary, prostate, and colon, and per capita food consumption. *Cancer 58*: 2363–2371 (1986).

Rosenkranz, H. S. (ed.). Strategies for the deployment of batteries of short-term tests. *Mutat. Res. 205*: 1–424 (1988).

Russo, I. H., Russo, J. Developmental stage of the rat mammary gland as determinant of its susceptibility of 7,12-dimethylbenz(a)anthracene. *JNCI 61*: 1439–1449 (1978).

Russo, I. H., Koszalka, M., Russo, J. Human chronic gonadotropin and rat mammary cancer prevention. *JNCI 82*: 1286–1289 (1990).

Schapira, D. V., Kumar, N. B., Lyman, G. H., McMillan, S. C. The value of current nutrition information. *Prev. Med. 19*: 45–53 (1990).

Schatzkin, A., Greenwald, P., Byar, D. P., Clifford, C. K. The dietary fat-breast cancer hypothesis is alive. *JAMA 261*: 3284–3287 (1989).

Schottenfeld, D., Fraumeni, J. F., Jr. *Cancer Epidemiology and Prevention*. Oxford University Press, Oxford, New York, Tokyo, 1991.

Shahin, M. M. (ed.) Structure-activity relationships in chemical mutagenesis. *Mutat. Res. 221*: 163–286 (1989).

Shao, R., Dao, M. L., Day, N. K., Good, R. A. Dietary manipulation of mammary tumor development in adult C3H/Bi mice. *Proc. Soc. Exp. Biol. Med. 193*: 313–317 (1990).

Simopoulos, A. P. Diet and Health: Scientific concepts and principles. *Am. J. Clin. Nutr. 45*: 1027–1414 (1987).

Sinkeldam, E. J., Kuper, C. F., Bosland, M. C. Hollanders, V. M. H., Vedder, D. M. Interactive effects of dietary wheat bran and lard on N-Methyl-N′-nitro-N-nitrosoguanidine-induced colon carcinogenesis in rats. *Cancer Res. 50*: 1092–1096 (1990).

Tajima, K., Hirose, K., Nakagawa, N., Juroshishi, T., Tominaga, S. Urban-rural difference in the trend of colo-rectal cancer mortality with special reference to the subsites of colon cancer in Japan. *Gann 76*: 717–728 (1985).

Tannenbaum, A., Silverstone, H. Nutrition in relation to cancer, *Adv. Cancer Res. 1*: 451 (1953).

Thijssen, J. H. H., Blankenstein, M. A. Endogenous oestrogens and androgens in normal and malignant endometrial and mammary tissues. *Eur. J. Cancer Clin. Oncol. 25*: 1953–1959 (1989).

Toniolo, P., Riboli, E., Protta, F., Charrel, M., Cappa, A. P. M. Calorie-providing nutrients and risk of breast cancer. *JNCI 81*: 278–286 (1989).

Toporoff, E., Hebert, J. R. A proxy approach to the determination of total caloric intake for use in cancer epidemiology. *Nutr. Cancer 13*: 35–50 (1990).

Trock, B., Lanza, E., Greenwald, P. Dietary fiber, vegetables, and colon cancer: Critical review and meta-analyses of the epidemiologic evidence. *JNCI 82*: 650–661 (1990).

United States Deparatment of Health and Human Services. *The Surgeon General's Report on Nutrition and Health*. Public Health Service, DHHS, Publication No (PHS) 88-50210, Washington, DC, 1988.

Van't Veer, P., Kolb, C. M., Verhoef, P., Kok, F. J. Schouten, E. G., Hermus, R. J. J., Sturmans, F. Dietary fiber beta-carotene and breast cancer: Results from a case-control study. *Int. J. Cancer 45*: 825–828 (1990).

Wargovich, M. J., Baer, A. R. Basic and clinical investigations of dietary calcium in the prevention of colorectal cancer. *Prev. Med. 18*: 672–679 (1989).

Watanabe, S., Arimoto, H. Long term trends in cancer mortality rates from 1955 to 1987 in Japan. *Jpn. J. Clin. Oncol. 19*: 305–317 (1989).

Weinberg, R. A. Oncogenes, antioncogenes, and the molecular bases of multistep carcinogenesis. *Cancer Res.49*: 3713–3721 (1989).

Weindruch, R., Walford, R. L. (eds.) *The Retardation of Aging and Disease by Dietary Restriction*. Charles C. Thomas, Springfield, IL, 1988.

Weisburger, J.H. Comparison of nutrition as customary in the Western world, the Orient, and northern populations (Eskimos) in relation to specific disease risks. *Arctic Medical Research 47*(Suppl. 1):110–120 (1988).

Weisburger, J. H. The mechanisms of lung carcinogenesis and smoking cessation. *Epidemiology 4*: 314–317 (1990).

Weisburger, J. H. Nutritional approach to cancer prevention with empahsis on vitamins, antioxidants, and carotenoids. *Am. J. Clin. Nutr. 53*:226S–237S (1991).

Willett, W. C., Stampfer, M. J., and Colditz, G. A., et al. Dietary fat and the risk of breast cancer. *N. Engl. J. Med. 316*: 22–28 (1987).

Willett, W. The search for the causes of breast and colon cancer. *Nature 338*: 389–394 (1989).

Williams, G. M. Methods of evaluating chemical genotoxicity. *Annu. Rev. Pharmacol. Toxicol 29*: 189–211 (1989).

Wilpart, M. Dietary lipids and experimental colonic carcinogenesis. Critical review of the literature. *Acta Gastroenterol Belg. 51*: 357–364 (1989).

Witmer, M. C., Snyder, R., Jollow, D. J., Kalf, G. F., Kocsis, J., Sipes, I. G. (eds.) *4th International Symposium, Biological Reactive Intermediates*. Adv. Exptl. Med. Biol. Vol. 283. Plenum Press, New York and London, 1990.

Woods, M. N., Gorbach, S. L., Longcope, C., Goldin, B. R., Dwyer, J. T., Morrill-LaBrode, A. Low-fat, high-fiber and serum estrone sulfate in premenopausal women. *Am. J. Clin. Nutr. 49*: 1179–1183 (1989).

Wynder, E. L., Rose, D. P., Cohen, L. A. Diet and breast cancer in causation and therapy. *Cancer 58*: 1804–1813 (1986).

Wynder, E. L., Cohen, L. A. A rationale for dietary intervention in the treatment of postmenopausal breast cancer patients. *Nutr. Cancer 3*(4): 195–199 (1982).

Zhang, L., Bird, R. P., Bruce, W. R. Proliferative activity of murine mammary epithelium as affected by dietary fat and calcium. *Cancer Res. 47*: 4905–4908 (1987).

2

Animal Experimental Evidence on Macronutrients and Cancer

Bandaru S. Reddy
Naylor Dana Institute
American Health Foundation
Valhalla, New York

INTRODUCTION

During the past three decades, epidemiologic studies have demonstrated the influence of the environment and lifestyles on the development of certain forms of cancer, and these findings have led to the conclusion that cancer may not be an inevitable consequence of aging (1). These encouraging observations have led several investigators to identify the ways in which environmental factors increase the risk of cancer and to manipulate the environment and reduce the risk to a minimum. The effect of environmental factors on cancer incidence and mortality has been investigated by several investigators using both ecologic and case-control studies. The consistency of these findings suggests that environmental rather than genetic factors play a predominant role in the etiology of several types of cancer in men and women worldwide.

The observation that the causes of several types of cancer may be mainly environmental in origin has led to a great deal of interest on the role of diet in cancer etiology. Interest in the role of nutrition in human cancer was renewed in the 1960s when a report from the World Health Organization (WHO) examined lifestyle and environmental factors associated with cancer (2). Although the exact proportion of diet involvement in cancer causation is unknown, Wynder and Gori (1) estimated that as many as 60% of cancer in women and more than 40% of cancers in men are related to nutritional factors. Doll and Peto (3) also estimated that about 35% (range 10–70%) of all cancer mortality in the United States may be attributable to dietary factors. Because few relationships between specific dietary components and cancer risk are well established, it is not possible to quantify precisely the contribution of diet to individual cancers and thus to total cancer rates (4). Nevertheless, these estimates help to emphasize the importance of nutritional factors in the etiology and prevention of several types of cancer in the United States and other countries (4).

Following up on leads advanced by the epidemiologists, experimentalists using laboratory animal models have found that nutritional factors have a major etiologic role. Nutritional factors may relate to the development of cancer in several ways and include the following: (a) food additives, contaminants, or a particular dietary component may act as a carcinogen, cocarcinogen, and/or promoter, (b) a dietary constituent acts as an anticarcinogen, (c) nutrient deficiencies and excesses may lead to biochemical alterations that promote neoplastic processes, and (d) changes in the intake of selected macronutrients may induce metabolic and biochemical abnormalities, which increase the risk of cancer. Although the relationship of nutrition and cancer is complex and sometimes perplexing to those who visualize carcinogenesis in terms of a specific carcinogen, it is important to understand that specific carcinogens play only a minor role in the relationship between nutrition and the development of cancer.

The literature relating macronutrients to cancer has been reviewed several times in recent years (5,6). The purpose of this chapter is (a) to provide an overview of the results thus far generated in laboratory animal model studies on the relationship between macronutrients (fat, protein, calories, and fiber) and the development of cancer and (b) to define more precisely some inadequacies of information, with the hope that this will lead to further research in this area. The discussion is presented by specific cancer sites because the dietary associations are not the same for all cancer types. Although the primary emphasis of this review article will be on laboratory animal model studies, reference will be made to human studies where appropriate. Future research will undoubtedly produce abundant evidence for the etiologic role of nutrition and diet in all types of cancer included in this chapter.

MACRONUTRIENTS AND COLON CANCER

A variety of compounds, namely, 1,2-dimethylhydrazine (DMH), azoxymethane (AOM), methylazoxymethanol acetate (MAM acetate), 3,2′-dimethyl-4-aminobiphenyl (DMAB), methylnitrosourea (MNU), and N-methyl-N′-nitro-N-nitrosoguanidine (MNNG), that are carcinogenic for the colon have been used in a number of animal models to study the effect of dietary macronutrients on tumorigenesis at the site (7,8). Additionally, these animal models have been used as unique tools for systematic studies of risk factors observed in the human setting and for determining whether or not suspected etiologic factors can be reproduced under controlled laboratory conditions. Thus, as is described here, a number of major elements observed in humans could not have been established without careful, deliberate investigations carried out in laboratory animals.

Dietary Fat

Dietary fat has received considerable attention as a possible risk factor in the etiology of colon cancer. Based on Japanese data and case-control studies, Wynder et al. (9) proposed in the late 1960s that colon cancer incidence is mainly associated with dietary fat and further suggested that dietary fat influences the composition of the gut flora and thus may be involved in the pathogenesis of cancer of the colon. These pioneering studies led to several correlation and case-control studies on the relationship of dietary fat and colon cancer. Since then, a substantial amount of progress has been made in understanding the relation between dietary factors and the development of colon cancer in man, but the conduct and interpretation of some studies is complicated by inherent problems in testing the dietary hypothesis for their reliability, validity, and sensitivity to reveal narrow but biologically significant differences, and to achieve some degree of dose stratification. For example, the major difficulty with several studies has been the lack of accurate methods of measurement of types of dietary fat and fiber content of foods in the populations being studied. The importance of types of fat with different fatty acid compositions rather than total fat can also not be discounted since animal model studies provided evidence that the colon tumor–promoting effect of dietary fat depends not only on the total fat but on the types of fat (8). Several epidemiologic studies have combined cases of colon and rectal cancer, as well as proximal and distal colon cancer, despite the evidence that these conditions do not have identical etiology.

Every scientific discipline including epidemiology has unique methodologic constraints. Therefore, the lack of consistent findings does not necessarily mitigate a dietary etiology of colon cancer since the discrepancies may have arisen, at least in part, from methodologic limitations of the studies. However, recent case-control studies have demonstrated that colon cancer risk increases with increased intake of dietary fat (10–12). Laboratory animal model studies provided evidence that not only the amount but also the types of fat (differing in fatty acid composition) are important factors in determining the enhancing effect of this nutrient in colon tumor development (8). In addition, the stage of carcinogenesis at which the effect of dietary fat is exerted appears to depend on the fatty acid composition (6). In several earlier animal model studies on dietary fat and colon cancer, interpretation of results between high fat and low fat diets was complicated by the use of diets of varying caloric density and confounded by different intakes of other nutrients. For example, in experiments comparing a relatively low fat diet with a high fat diet, there will be major changes in the consumption of other dietary components unless the content has been changed isocalorically. Generally, laboratory animals adjust their food intake so that similar energy intake is maintained even with diets containing substantially different energy density (13). Therefore, a diet with a low energy value per unit weight (low fat) will be consumed at a greater rate than a diet with more highly concentrated energy (high fat). Accordingly, in addition to the changes in fat and carbohydrate intake, the intakes of protein, minerals, vitamins, and fiber will be lower in animals fed the high fat diet. Therefore, it is necessary to formulate high fat diets that ensure an intake of protein, vitamins, minerals, and fiber comparable to a low fat diet so that the effect of high fat on tumorigenesis can be measured.

With the above limitations, numerous experiments in animal models have shown that certain dietary lipids influence tumorigenesis in the colon. This promoting effect can be modified, however, by the type of dietary fat. In general, the overall evidence from the animal model studies is consistent with the epidemiologic data.

Effect of Type and Amount of Fat During Initiation and Postinitiation Phases of Carcinogenesis

Multifactorial and multistage model systems of cancer induction in experimental animals were first discovered more than 40 years ago (14). It was shown that tumor induction can be divided into two distinct treatment stages, i.e., initiation and promotion, and that the promotion stage is reversible. Initation of carcinogenesis alters the genetic information of the cell, whereas the promotion then leads to expression of genetic changes and malignancy which involves loss of control over cellular proliferation. Evidence for two-stage carcinogenesis has also been obtained for colon tumors (15). The concept of tumor progression has been distinguished from tumor promotion, although experimentally absolute distinction between the two is difficult. Many factors, including dietary factors, may enhance these processes at certain stages. Although our early experiments and those of others did not distinguish the effect of dietary fat between the initiation and postinitiation (promotion) phases of carcinogenesis, these studies, however, indicated a strong relationship between the amount of dietary fat and colon cancer in animal models (16–19).

Investigations were also carried out to test the effect of diets comprising 20% and 5% beef fat on colon carcinogenesis by a variety of carcinogens—DMH, MAM acetate, DMAB, or MNU—which differ in metabolic activation (20,21). In these studies, semipurified diets containing high and low levels of fat were fed to animals before, during, and after carcinogen treatment to study the specific effects on the initiation and promotion stages of colon carcinogens. Combined results of these two studies indicate that, irrespective of colon carcinogens used, animals fed the diet containing a high amount of beef fat had a greater incidence of colon tumors than did rats fed a low beef-fat diet (Table 1).

Table 1 Effect of Type and Amount of Dietary Fat During Initiation and Postinitiation Phase of Colon Carcinogenesis in F344 Rats

Experiment no.	Type and amount of dietary fat	Carcinogen dosage (%)	Male (M) or female (F)	% Animals with colon tumors
1[a]	5% Corn oil	DMH, 10 mg/kg body wt, once weekly for 10 weeks, s.c.	F	36[d]
	20% Corn oil	DMH, 10 mg/kg body wt, once weekly for 10 weeks, s.c.	F	64
	5% Lard	DMH, 10 mg/kg body wt, once weekly for 10 weeks, s.c.	F	17[d]
	20% Lard	DMH, 10 mg/kg body wt, once weekly for 10 weeks, s.c.	F	67
2[b]	5% Beef fat	DMH, 150 mg/kg body wt, once, s.c.	M	27[d]
	20% Beef fat	DMH, 150 mg/kg body wt, once, s.c.	M	60
	5% Beef fat	MNU, 2.5 mg/rat, twice a wk for 2 weeks, i.r.	M	33[d]
	20% Beef fat	MNU, 2.5 mg/rat, twice a wk for 2 weeks, i.r.	M	73
	5% Beef fat	MAM acetate, 35 mg/kg body wt, once, i.p.	M	45[d]
	20% Beef fat	MAM acetate, 35 mg/kg body wt, once, i.p.	M	80
3[c]	5% Beef fat	DMAB, 50 mg/kg body wt, once weekly for 20 weeks s.c.	M	26[d]
	20% Beef fat	DMAB, 50 mg/kg body wt, once weekly for 20 weeks s.c.	M	74

[a] From Ref. 22.
[b] From Ref. 20.
[c] From Ref. 21.
[d] Significantly different from their respective high fat (20%) diets.

Nigro et al. (16) studied the effect of diets containing 5 and 35% beef fat on azoxymethane (AOM)-induced intestinal tumors in Sprague-Dawley rats. Animals fed the high beef-fat developed more intestinal tumors and more metastases in the abdominal cavity, lungs, and liver than did rats fed the low fat diet. Howarth and Pihl (18) demonstrated that DMH-induced colon tumors were increased in male D/A rats fed a high fat diet compared with those in such rats fed a low fat diet. Studies conducted in our laboratory indicate that animals fed 20% lard or 20% corn-oil diets were more susceptible to DMH-induced colon tumors than those fed 5% lard or 5% corn oil diets (22). The type of fat appears to be immaterial at the 20% level; however, at the 5% fat level, unsaturated fat (corn oil) induced more colon tumors than did saturated fat (lard) (22). Recent studies by Nutter et al. (23) demonstrated that Sprague-Dawley rats fed the beef-fat diet had a higher colon tumor incidence than those fed the corn-oil diet. Sakaguchi et al. (24) demonstrated a significantly higher incidence of colon tumors in rats fed 5% linoleic acid than in those fed 4.7% stearic acid + 0.3 linoleic acid. A recent study by Pence and Buddingh (25) indicated that DMH-induced colon carcinogenesis was increased in F344 rats fed a high-fat (corn oil) diet. However Nauss et al. (26) showed that a high fat diet containing 24% corn oil, 24% beef fat, or 24% Crisco had no promoting effect on colon tumors induced by DMH in rats.

Effect of Type and Amount of Fat During Initiation Phase of Carcinogenesis

The pioneering study of Bull et al. (27) indicated that ingestion of a high amount of beef fat increased the intestinal tumor incidence in rats when fed after AOM treatment, but not during or before the carcinogen administration, suggesting that excess dietary beef fat acts at the postinitiation phase of colon carcinogenesis. We investigated the effect of various levels of polyunsaturated (corn oil) and saturated (lard) fats fed during the initiation phase of colon carcinogenesis (28). The results of this study are of interest in several respects. When the animals were fed the diets containing 23.5% corn oil during the stage of initiation (before and during carcinogen treatment), there was no increase in the incidence of colon tumors compared with that of animals on a 5% corn oil diet. When the 23.5% corn-oil diet was fed during the promotion (postinitiation) stage of carcinogenesis (after carcinogen treatment), there was a significant increase in colon tumor incidence compared with that of animals fed either the 5% corn-oil diet or the 23.5% corn-oil diet during the initiation stage. These results thus suggest that the effect of a high corn-oil diet in colon carcinogenesis is observed mainly during the promotion stage, rather than during the initiation stage of carcinogenesis. In contrast, animals fed the 23.5% lard diet during the initiation period showed an increase in colon tumor incidence. Animals fed the 23.5% lard diet during the promotion period also had a higher colon tumor incidence than did those fed the

23.5% lard diet during initiation as well as those fed the 5% lard diet during the promotion stage.

In contrast to dietary corn oil and lard, high dietary fish oil rich in omega-3 fatty acids (docosahexaenoic acid and eicosapentacnoic acid) had no colon tumor-promoting effect (29,30). The effect of high dietary fish oil during the initiation phase of colon carcinogenesis was also investigated in our laboratory. These results indicate a significant reduction in colon tumor incidence in animals fed the high fish-oil diet as compared to those fed the high corn-oil diet during the initiation phase of carcinogenesis. These results thus indicate that the enhancing effect of colon carcinogenesis by the dietary fat during the initiation phase depends on the types of fat and their fatty acid composition.

Effect of Type and Amount of Fat During Postinitiation Phase of Carcinogenesis

The role of type and amount of dietary fat during the promotional phase of colon carcinogenesis has been studied in our laboratory (28–30). In these studies, the effect of corn oil, coconut oil, olive oil, safflower oil, and fish oil was investigated. Body weights and consumption of total calories, protein, micronutrients, and fiber, except the amount of calories from fat were comparable between high and low fat fed animals irrespective of type of fat. The animals fed the high corn oil or high safflower oil (23.5%) diets had a higher incidence of AOM-induced colon tumors than did those fed the diets low in fat (5%) (Table 2). By contrast, diets high in coconut oil, olive oil, or menhaden fish oil had no colon tumor–promoting effect compared with diets high in corn oil or safflower oil. The varied effects of different types of fat on colon carcinogenesis suggest that fatty acid composition is one of the determining factors in colon tumor promotion. Corn oil and safflower oil are very high in omega-6 fatty acids (linoleic acid), olive oil is rich in monounsaturated fatty acid (oleic acid), coconut oil is high in medium-chain fatty acids (lauric acid), and fish oil is rich in omega-6 fatty acids (docosahexaenoic acid and eicosapentaenoic acid).

Although high dietary fat oil (22.5%) inhibited colon carcinogenesis in the above study (29), large amounts of fish oil may induce a variety of physiopathologic conditions and harmful side effects. Therefore, we have conducted another study to investigate the efficacy of varying levels of fish oil and corn oil on colon carcinogens to determine the optimum dietary levels at which the combination of two sources of fat elicits maximum inhibition (30). In this study, feeding of high fat diets containing 17.6% corn oil + 5.9% fish oil, 11.8% corn oil + 11.8% fish oil, or 5.9% corn oil +17.6% fish oil significantly inhibited colon carcinogenesis as compared to 23.5% corn oil diet (Table 2). High fat diets containing high levels of fish oil and low levels of corn oil induced fewer colon adenocarcinomas than did the diet containing high oil alone (not shown in the table). Further studies in our laboratory demonstrated that feeding of increasing levels of

Table 2 Effect of Type and Amount of Dietary Fat During Initiation and Postinitiation Phase of Colon Carcinogenesis in F344 Rats

Experiment no.	Type and amount of dietary fat	Carcinogen dosage (%)	Male (M) or female (F)	% Animals with colon tumors
1[a]	5% CO	AOM, 20 mg/kg body wt, once, s.c.	F	17[e]
	23.5% CO	AOM, 20 mg/kg body wt, once, s.c.	F	46
	5% SO	AOM, 20 mg/kg body wt, once, s.c.	F	13[e]
	23.5% SO	AOM, 20 mg/kg body wt, once, s.c.	F	36
	5% OO	AOM, 20 mg/kg body wt, once, s.c.	F	10[e]
	23.5% OO	AOM, 20 mg/kg body wt, once, s.c.	F	13
	23.5% CN	AOM, 20 mg/kg body wt, once, s.c.	F	13
2[b]	4% MFO + 1% CO	AOM, 15 mg/kg body wt, once weekly for 2 weeks, s.c.	M	50
	22.5% MFO + 1% CO	AOM, 15 mg/kg body wt, once weekly for 2 weeks, s.c.	M	33
	5% CO	AOM, 15 mg/kg body wt, once weekly for 2 weeks, s.c.	M	54[e]
	23.5% CO	AOM, 15 mg/kg body wt, once weekly for 2 weeks, s.c.	M	92
3[c]	5% CO	AOM, 15 mg/kg body wt, once weekly for 2 weeks, s.c.	M	70[f]
	23.5% CO	AOM, 15 mg/kg body wt, once weekly for 2 weeks, s.c.	M	93
	4% MFO + 1% CO	AOM, 15 mg/kg body wt, once weekly for 2 weeks, s.c.	M	59[f]
	5.9% MFO + 17.6% CO	AOM, 15 mg/kg body wt, once weekly for 2 weeks, s.c.	M	70[f]
	11.8% MFO + 11.8% CO	AOM, 15 mg/kg body wt, once weekly for 2 weeks, s.c.	M	63[f]
	17.6% MFO + 5.9% CO	AOM, 15 mg/kg body wt, once weekly for 2 weeks, s.c.	M	63[f]

[a]From Ref.30.
[b]From Ref. 29.
[c]From Ref. 28.
[d]Abbreviations: CO, corn oil; SO, safflower; OO, olive oil; CN, coconut oil, MFO, menhaden fish oil.
[e]Significantly different from their respective high fat diets.
[f]Significantly different from 23.5% corn-oil diet.

fish oil altered the incorporation of fatty acids into the microsomes of colonic mucosal cells and tumors (30). Compared to microsomes prepared from rats fed the 23.5% corn oil diet, microsomes from the animals fed the increasing levels of fish oil diets were enriched with omega-3 fatty acids at the expense of omega-6 fatty acids such as linoleic acid and arachidonic acid in mucosa and tumors (Table 3).

There has been an increase in per capita consumption of fat for the last 50 years in the United States, and this increase can be partly accounted for by a trend toward greater use of vegetable oils, which include partially hydrogenated fats and processed vegetable oils that contain *trans* fatty acids. The most common isomers that occur in processed fats are 9-*trans*-18:1 (elaidic acid) and *cis-trans*-octadecadienoic acid. Experiments conducted in colon cancer model failed to support the hypothesis that *trans* fatty acids increase tumorigenesis (13). High fat diets (23.5%) containing low *trans* fat (5.8% corn oil + 5.9% *trans* fat + 11.8% oleate), intermediate level of *trans* fat (5.8% corn oil + 11.8% *trans* fat + 5.9% oleate), high level of *trans* fat (5.8% corn oil + 17.6% *trans* fat), and no *trans* fat (23.5% corn oil) were tested for colon tumor-promoting effect (13). Animals fed the high fat diets containing different levels of *trans* fat developed significantly fewer colon tumors than did the rats fed the high corn-oil diet. Thus, high *trans* fat had little or no promoting effect in colon carcinogenesis when used in a diet that contained about 5.9% corn oil.

In summary, laboratory animal studies have provided useful data for evaluating the role of dietary fat in the development of colon carcinogenesis. A majority of studies in colon cancer models in which the intakes of all nutrients and total calories were controlled in both high and low fat diet groups clearly suggest that not only the amount but also the type of fat (differing in fat acid composition) are important factors in determining the modulating effect of dietary fats in colon tumor development. The stage of carcinogenesis at which the effect of dietary fat is exerted appears to be mainly the promotional phase of carcinogenesis; however, certain dietary fats such as lard or fish oil also act during the initiation phase of colon carcinogenesis. The strength of the association between dietary fat and colon cancer risk is supported by experimental evidence as well as biological plausibility.

Dietary Fiber

The hypothesis that a diet high in fiber may protect against colon cancer was first proposed by Burkitt (31), who observed that African Blacks consuming high fiber and low fat foods had lower death rates due to colon cancer than their white counterparts eating low fiber and high fat diets. Subsequent studies demonstrated that, in certain populations consuming diets high in total fat, the intake of diets high in total fiber, fibrous foods, and certain whole grain foods has been

Table 3 Percentage Composition of Fatty Acids in the Microsomal Fraction of Colonic Mucosa and Tumors of Male F344 Rats Fed Corn Oil and Fish Oil

	CO diets[a]				MFO diets	
	Colon mucosa		Colon tumor		Colon mucosa	Colon tumor
Fatty acids	5% CO	23.5% CO	5% CO	23.5% CO	5.9% CO + 17.6% MFO	5.9% CO + 17.6% MFO
Palmitic acid (16:0)	14.1	13.9	15.4	14.6	15.4	18.1
Palmitoleic acid (16:1)	1.5	1.8	2.1	1.9	4.0	6.4
Stearic acid (18:0)	20.6	21.9	13.8	12.9	19.6	12.9
Oleic acid (18:1)	12.6	11.4	14.1	14.2	15.1	19.7
Linoleic acid (18:2)	26.4	26.6	10.0	13.6	15.2	3.0
Linolenic acid (18:3)	1.9	2.2	0.61	0.69	0.6	0.60
Arachidoic acid (20:4)	16.5	19.6	11.0	12.4	5.7	4.2
Ecosapentaenoic acid (20:5, n-3)	0.2	0.3	0.2	0.2	11.9	5.1
Docasapentaenoic acid (22:5, n-3)	0.2	0.2	1.0	0.8	1.8	3.2
Docosahexaenoic acid (22:6, n-3)	0.3	0.4	1.9	2.2	7.1	7.2
Others	5.5	1.7	29.1	26.5	3.6	19.6

[a] Abbreviations: CO, corn oil; MFO, menhaden fish oil.
Source: Ref. 30.

associated with a reduced risk for colon cancer (32,33). Intracountry comparisons of dietary fiber and colon cancer mortality rates strongly supported the hypothesis that dietary fiber protects against colon cancer (34). Case-control studies on the relationship between the dietary fiber and colon cancer provided conflicting results (35). Out of 19 case-control studies to assess the role of fiber and fiber-containing foods, 3 studies reported no protective effect, 2 found an increased risk, and 13 studies reported a protective effect of fiber-containing foods and vegetables (35).

Dietary fiber includes nonstarch polysaccharides (both soluble and insoluble) and lignin, which are resistant to the endogenous secretions of the human digestive tract. Although the concept of dietary fiber involvement in colon carcinogenesis is of great importance, studies examining the possible role of various types of dietary fiber in animal models appear to have provided some conflicting results (8). This discrepancy might be due, in part, to the nature and amount of the carcinogen used, to differences in the susceptibility of rat strain to carcinogen treatment, to variation in the composition of the diets, to qualitative and quantitative differences in the intact fibers and their components administered, to relative differences in food intake by the animals, and/or to differences in experimental design and duration. In addition, part of the discrepancy in several studies may be attributed to failure to define the source of dietary fiber and/or the intake of other nutrients, such as fat and trace minerals.

The protective effect of dietary fiber, which comprises a heterogeneous group of nonstarch polysaccharides such as cellulose, hemicellulose, pectin, and gums and a noncarbohydrate substance (lignin), depends on the nature and source of fiber in the diet. Possible mechanisms by which certain dietary fibers may reduce the risk of the development of colon cancer include dilution and adsorption of carcinogens, cocarcinogens, and/or promoters present in the gut by the dietary fiber (8). In addition, dietary fiber affects the gut microflora by modifying both its metabolic activities and its composition (36,37), which, in turn, alters the breakdown products of nonstarch polysaccharides, fat, and protein in the gut. The amount and type of breakdown products produced by the gut microflora may depend partly on the intake of certain dietary fibers. These breakdown products act as promoters and/or inhibitors in the colon. Thus, the intake of certain dietary fibers may be important in the activation and detoxification of carcinogens and promoters. Also, certain dietary fibers induce structural and functional alterations in the gut epithelium and modify rates of colonic cell proliferation and migration.

The effect of a semipurified diet containing 15% alfalfa, pectin, or wheat bran and 20% fat on colon carcinogenesis induced by N-methylnitrosourea (MNU) or azoxymethane (AOM) was studied in F344 rats by Watanabe et al. (38). The control and experimental diets were fed to rats before, during, and after carcinogen treatment and then until termination of the experiment. The addition of pectin or wheat bran to the diet greatly inhibited colon tumor incidence induced by AOM, a carcinogen requiring host-mediated metabolic activation. However, the incidence of AOM-induced colon tumors was not influenced by the addition of alfalfa to diet. The diets containing wheat bran and pectin did not protect against MNU-induced colon carcinogenesis. Watanabe et al. (39) showed that carrageenan, a product of seaweed, fed at a 15% level in the diet of rats increased both AOM- and MNU-induced colon tumors in rats.

The effect of dietary wheat bran and dehydrated citrus fiber at levels of 15% on intestinal carcinogenesis induced by AOM and DMAB was studied in male F344 rats (40,41). The composition of diets was adjusted so that all animals in different experimental groups consumed approximately the same amount of protein, fat, minerals, and vitamins. Experimental diets were begun before carcinogen administration and continuation until the termination of the experiment. The animals fed the wheat bran or citrus fiber and treated with AOM had a lower incidence (number of animals with tumors) and multiplicity (number of tumors/tumor-bearing rat) of colon tumors and tumors of the small intestine than did those fed the control diet and treated with AOM. Since citrus fiber contains only about 22% pectin, its colon tumor inhibitory effect may have been due to factors other than the pectin content. The animals fed the wheat bran and treated with DMAB had a lower incidence and multiplicity of colon tumors than those fed the control diet and treated with DMAB. Dietary citrus fiber had no effect on DMAB-induced colon tumors.

In another study, we tested the effect of dietary corn bran (high in hemicellulose) or lignin on DMAB-induced colon carcinogenesis in rats. Animals fed a semisynthetic diet containing 10% corn bran showed an increase in the multiplicity of colon adenocarcinomas, whereas the diet containing 7.5% lignin inhibited the multiplicity of colon adenocarcinomas compared with control diets containing 5% alphacel (42).

Nigro and Bull (43) reported that diets containing 35% beef fat plus 10% alfalfa, wheat bran, or cellulose showed no inhibitory effect on AOM-induced colon carcinogenesis, whereas the diets containing 5% fat plus either 20 or 30% wheat bran or cellulose inhibited colon carcinogenesis in rats. While the fat and fiber levels were extreme in this study, the data indicate that in assessing the effect of fiber on colon cancer, the amount of fat in the diet is important, because dietary fat in large amounts appears to be a stronger promoter of colon cancer than dietary fiber is an inhibitor.

Bauer et al. (44) studied the effect of 20% wheat bran or 6.5% pectin in a fiber-free semisynthetic diet containing 20% peanut oil as source of fat on DMH-induced colon carcinogenesis. Unfortunately, the diets were deficient in selenium, since the mineral mixture used excluded it. The experimental wheat bran and pectin diets were fed to animals only before, during, and until 2 weeks after carcinogen injection. Diets containing 20% wheat bran had no effect on colon tumor incidence, whereas those containing 6.5% pectin increased the colon tumor incidence compared with the fiber-free control diet. Jacobs (45) reported a study on the effect of feeding rats a 20% wheat-bran diet during and/or after DMH treatment and found an increase in colon tumor incidence in rats fed the wheat-bran diet during carcinogen treatment. However, in those animals fed the wheat bran after DMH administration, tumor incidence was inhibited compared with that in the fiber-free control group. It can be concluded from these studies that dietary wheat bran protects against colon cancer when fed during the stage of promotion (postinitiation).

Barnes et al.(46) studied the effects of 20% wheat bran, rice bran, corn bran, and soybean bran in a semipurified diet containing 20% corn oil on DMH-induced colon tumors in rats. Colon tumors were inhibited in rats fed wheat bran, rice bran, and soybean bran but increased in those fed corn bran. In this study, all experimental diets were fed before, during, and after carcinogen treatment.

The effect of fiber fractions such as cellulose and guar gum on DMH-induced colon carcinogenesis has also been examined (47,48). Experiments in which guar gum was present at a 5% level and fat at a 19% level demonstrated no effect on colon carcinogenesis (47), whereas another with 10% guar gum in a 7% fat diet showed an increase in colon tumors (48). Several studies have shown an inhibitory effect of dietary cellulose on DMH-induced colon carcinogenesis (47). In a separate study, dietary cellulose had no effect on colon carcinogenesis (48). Several of these studies are difficult to interpret, because several dietary components such as fat, minerals, and other nutrients were different in the experimental diets compared with those in the control diets. The results of several of these studies have been complicated by the use of very high doses of carcinogen.

In conclusion, the results of studies thus far generated on the effect of dietary fiber in colon carcinogenesis suggest that (a) the inhibitory effect depends on the type of fiber, and (b) wheat bran appears to inhibit colon tumor development more consistently in animal models. The varied conclusions on the other types of fiber appear to be due to differences in the experimental protocols, the amount and type of carcinogen used to induce colon tumors and, perhaps even more importantly, elements of the diet other than the fiber. Several of the diets used to study the effect of fiber were deficient in certain micronutrients that are involved in carcinogen metabolism or detoxification.

Dietary Protein

Dietary protein has often been associated with colon cancer risk. Since the major dietary sources of protein such as meat contain a variety of other nutrients such as fat, the association of protein with colon cancer risk may not be direct but could reflect the action of another constituent of protein-rich foods. Nevertheless, the evidence does not completely preclude an independent effect. Armstrong and Doll (49) reported that per capita intake of total protein and animal protein were strongly associated with the incidence and mortality of colon cancer. A case-control study conducted by Jain et al. (10) demonstrated a direct association between consumption of high levels of protein and risk of colon cancer.

There have been very few studies with laboratory animal models on the effect of dietary protein in colon carcinogenesis. The possible role of dietary protein in DMH-induced colon carcinogenesis in Sprague-Dawley rats was studied by Visek et al. (50). Protein source as a modifying factor in colon carcinogenesis was studied using semipurified diets containing 20% protein as freeze-dried raw beef, charcoal-broiled beef or soybean protein, and 20% beef fat. It was concluded that the source of protein was not a factor in the DMH-induced colon carcinogenesis in rats. In another sutdy, rats fed 15% and 22.5% protein had a greater number of DMH-induced intestinal tumors than those fed 7.5% protein (51). However, the percentage of animals with colon tumors was not significantly different between various dietary groups. Whether the reduced number of tumors in rats fed 7.5% protein diet was due to suboptimal protein intake during the period of rapid body growth could not be answered from this study, although the evidence seems compatible with the conclusion that the time of appearance of tumors and their size and number was influenced by protein intake (51)

Calories

Currently there is considerable interest in the relationship between calorie intake and carcinogenesis. The question of whether the effect of dietary fat on carcinogenesis is due to a specific action of fat or to an associated caloric effect has been raised several times and is a subject to recent discussion (52,53). Pioneering studies by Tannenbaum and others indicated the calorie restriction reduces the formation of spontaneous and chemically induced tumors in mice (54,55). Epidemiologic evidence indicating the role of calories on colon carcinogenesis came from case-control studies (11,12).

Klurfeld et al. (56) demonstrated that DMH-induced colon tumors could be inhibited by 40% calorie restriction in rats, although the calorie-restricted rats ingested twice as much fat as ad libitum fed animals. They concluded that calorie ingestion may be a greater determinant than dietary fat in enhancing tumorigenesis. Pollard and Luckert (57) demonstrated the calorie restriction by 25% exerted an inhibiting effect on colon carcinogenesis when the initiating agent was MAM acetate (requiring host activation) but not when it was MNU (direct-acting carcinogen) suggesting that the metabolic activation of MAM was interrupted in the rats on the restricted dietary regimen.

Studies conducted in our laboratory demonstrated an effect of calorie restriction on colon carcinogenesis in F344 rats. In the first study, we investigated the effect of a high-fat semipurified diet fed ad libitum and of 30% calorie-restricted diet on AOM-induced colon carcinogenesis during the postinitiation phase (58).

In this study, the animals on the calorie-restricted diet consumed about 30% fewer calories from carbohydrate, protein, and fat, but consumed the same amount of vitamins, minerals, and fiber. The animals in the calorie-restricted group developed significantly fewer colon tumors and had a lower colon tumor incidence than did the rats in the ad libitum group. In the second study, we investigated the dose-response effect of different levels of calorie-restriction (59). In this study, the animals were restricted to 90, 80, and 70% of calories consumed by the high-fat ad libitum group (i.e., 10, 20, and 30% calorie restriction, respectively). The incidence and multiplicity of colon tumors were significantly inhibited in animals fed 20 and 30% calorie-restricted diets. The regression coefficient representing the dose-response effect of different levels of calorie restriction is significant.

MACRONUTRIENTS AND MAMMARY CANCER

Despite some inconsistencies in the epidemiologic data relating dietary fat to breast cancer causation, animal studies show a cancer-promoting role for the dietary fat. The risk of breast cancer is correlated with total fat intake in international comparisons (60). Case-control and cohort studies relate the risk for breast cancer to total fat consumption in several studies (61,62), but not in other studies (63). A recent case-control study by Ross (64) in Shanghai, China, suggests a positive association with total fat and fat from animal sources. The methodologic problems might have obscured a true risk association in these negative studies (65).

Dietary Fat

Pioneering studies of Tannenbaum and colleagues (54) demonstrated that high fat diet (12% hydrogenated cottonseed oil) increased spontaneous mammary tumors in mice more than in animals fed a low-fat diet (3% hydrogenated cottonseed oil) and that the effect of a high fat diet was not based on caloric intake. The discovery by Huggins (66) in the early 1960s that a single dose of 7,12-dimethylbenz(a)anthracene (DMBA) could induce mammary carcinomas in rats within 6 months led to the studies of environmental factors that play a role in tumorigenesis. The tumors produced were hormone-responsive and resembled human breast cancers histologically; however, they failed to metastasize. The DMBA model provided an operational means to separate out those factors that act during the initiation phase and those that act during the postinitiation (promotion) phase of mammary carcinogenesis. Tannenbaum's early work brought to light that the time of initiaton of diet influenced the course of tumor development and that the reproductive history of the animals as an important experimental variable (54). In the ensuring four decades, Tannenbaum's observations have been confirmed by a variety of investigators in both rats and mice. Early studies of Carroll and colleagues (67,68) using a DMBA model demonstrated that the primary effect of dietary fat was to enhance DMBA-induced mammary carcinogenesis during the postinitiation phase and that the amount of dietary fat given prior to DMBA treatment (initiation phase) was of minimal significance. Carroll and Khor (68) showed that, in the DMBA model, the high-fat effect could be demonstrated only when the diet was administered after initiation with DMBA. When a high fat diet was fed before DMBA administration and then replaced by a low fat diet, no tumor enhancement was observed. Hence, it appears that the enhancing effect of dietary fat is exerted at the postinitiation but not at the initiation phase of mammary carcinogenesis. However, recent studies suggest that high dietary fat may also influence the initiation stage as well (69,70). The type of fat that affects the initiating stage of mammary carcinogenesis appears to be of animal origin, i.e., lard and beef tallow.

Effect of Type and Amount of Dietary Fat

Dietary fats and oils containing higher levels of polyunsaturated fatty acids of n-6 series such as linoleic acid have been shown to be more tumorigenic than the higher levels of saturated fatty acids or of polyunsaturated fatty acids of n-3 series such as docosahexaenoic acid and ecosapentaenoic acid (71). The tumor-promoting effects of various dietary fatty acids have been investigated by several investigators, but only linoleic acid has been consistently shown to enhance rat mammary tumorigenesis (68,72–75). For example, Carroll and Khor (68) demonstrated lower DMBA-induced mammary tumor incidence and longer latent periods in rats fed the diets containing 20% by weight beef tallow as compared to those fed corn oil. Saturated fat was as effective as polyunsaturated fat when a small quantity of polyunsaturated fat (3% sunflower seed oil) was added to 17% cocount oil (72,73). McCay et al. (76) demonstrated that rats fed a diet containing 20% corn oil had an increase in DMBA-induced mammary tumor yield as compared to those fed a diet containing 18% coconut oil and 2% linoleic acid. These studies have also shown that polyunsaturated fat used must provide sufficient amounts of essential fatty acids such as linoleic acid and that diet must contain high levels of total fat to enhance the mammary tumor yield. Ip et al. (73) demonstrated that about 4% (wt/wt) dietary linoleic acid is needed for optimal tumor promotion in DMBA-induced rat mammary tumor model and that beyond 4% dietary linoleic acid, different dietary fats have similar effects on tumor promotion. Growth of transplantable tumors is also influenced by dietary fat (77). A recent study also demonstrated that 20% olive oil in the diet induced fewer DMBA-induced mammary tumors in rats than in those fed 20% safflower oil or olive oil supplemented with safflower oil (78). Cohen et al. (79) showed that dietary olive oil had no mammary tumor–promoting effect as compared to safflower oil. They suggested that oleic acid and linoleic acid content of diets might be responsible for the observed results on olive oil and safflower oil. Other studies used rapeseed oil, which contains about 50% c-22 monoenoic erucic acid. These studies also indicate that rapeseed oil had no DMBA-induced mammary tumor–promoting effect (80).

Recently, Cohen and Thompson (81) demonstrated that a medium-chain triglyceride–containing diet was less tumorigenic in a MNU tumor model than corn oil containing longer-chain unsaturated fatty acids. Medium-chain triglycerides are an unique class of lipids derived from cocount oil and consist mainly of c-8:0 (75–75%). and c-10:0 (25–35%) fatty acids. In addition, *cis*-isomerization of fatty acids appears to be an important aspect of mammary tumor enhancement. Diets rich in unsaturated fatty acids with a large proportion of *trans*-isomerization act like saturated fat diets in the promotion of mammary tumors (82).

There are several reports in the literature associating decreased mammary tumorigenesis with fish oils. Marine oils contain high levels of c-20 and c-22 polyunsaturated fatty acids of n-3 series such as ecosapentaenoic acid (20:5) and docosahexaenoic acid (22:6). In mammary carcinogenesis, Karmali (83) demonstrated that daily supplementation of the rat chow diet with 17, 33, and 67 mg eicosapentaenoic acid and 16, 32, and 64 mg docosahexaenoic acid significantly inhibited the size of the transplantable R3230 AC mammary tumors. Subsequent study using semipurified diets demonstrated a marginal reduction in size of mammary tumors only in the group receiving a diet with omega-3 to omega-6 ratio 2.0 (83). Interestingly, the animals fed the 23.5% fish oil had larger mammary tumors than those fed the 23.5% corn oil diet.

The effect of dietary fish oil on chemically induced mammary carcinogenesis has been studied by several investigators. Carroll and Braden (84) demonstrated that dietary menhaden fish oil at 10 and 20% inhibited DMBA-induced mammary carcinogens in female Sprague-Dawley rats. Ip et al. (85) reported that compared to a 20% corn oil diet, 20% fat diets containing either 12% menhaden fish oil + 8% corn oil or 19% menhaden fish oil + 1% corn oil significantly inhibited DMBA-induced mammary carcinogenesis. This decrease in tumorigenesis is not due to insufficient essential fatty acid (linoleic acid) levels since the lowest tumor incidence in this study was observed in rats receiving 12% menhaden fish oil plus 8% corn oil. There was also a much larger number of tumor regressions observed in the menhaden fish oil groups. Using the mammary tumor model induced by methylnitrosourea, Jurkowski and Cave (71) reported that mammary tumor development in female Buffalo rats were inversely related to the amount of menhaden fish oil in the diet.

Dietary Protein

There have been few studies with animals on the effect of dietary protein on mammary carcinogenesis. Early studies by Tannenbaum and Silverstone (86) and Ross and Bras (87) showed no effect of increasing dietary protein on mammary carcinogenesis, whereas others (88,89) demonstrated an enhancement. Hawrylewicz et al. (89) demonstrated that increasing amounts of dietary protein during the initiation and postinitiation phases enhanced DMBA-induced mammary carcinogenesis in female rats. Increasing dietary protein from 8 to 15% of calories during the initiation phase was associated with a reduction in DMBA-induced mammary tumorigenesis (90). There was, however, no effect of dietary protein on mammary carcinogenesis when increasing levels of protein were fed during the postinitiation phase (91).

MACRONUTRIENTS AND PANCREATIC CANCER

Animal models have been developed to study pancreatic carcinogenesis. Pancreatic duct neoplasms were induced in Syrian golden hamsters after subcutaneous injections of N-nitrosobis (2-oxopropyl) amine (BOP) (92). In contrast to the hamster model, the significant feature of azaserine-induced pancreatic cancer in the rat model is the appearance of atypical acinar cell foci and nodules with the subsequent development of adenocarcinomas (93). While most human pancreatic cancers are ductal adenocarcinomas, the total spectrum of histologic types is best matched by a combination of the tumor types induced in Syrian golden hamster and rat models (94).

Dietary Fat and Protein

In the hamster model, Birt et al. (95,96) investigated the effect of different levels of dietary fat (4.5, 9.0, and 18.0 g/385 kcal) and protein (9, 18, and 35 g/385 kcal) at the initiation stage of BOP-induced pancreatic carcinogenesis. Among all dietary groups, the lowest rate of pancreatic cancer was observed in animals fed the low fat/low protein diet, whereas the highest rate of pancreatic cancer was seen in hamsters fed the high protein/medium fat diet. There was, however, not a strong consistent effect of dietary fat during the initiation phase of BOP-induced pancreatic carcinogenesis in the hamster model.

The effect of type of dietary fat on azaserine-induced pancreatic cancer was studied in the rat model. Feeding of diets high in unsaturated fat (20% corn oil) and saturated fat (18% hydrogenated coconut oil plus 2% corn oil) during the initiation phase produced no differences in pancreatic carcinogenesis (97). In addition, there was no difference in pancreatic carcinogenesis among the groups fed the high corn oil, low corn oil, and high coconut oil diets.

The effect of dietary fat and protein during the postinitiation phase of pancreatic carcinogenesis was studied. A high fat diet with medium and high protein levels given during the postinitiation phase increased the incidence of multiplicity of BOP-induced pancreatic carcinogenesis (95,96). A high fat diet in combination with low protein, however, had no enhancing effect in hamster model. Using the rat model, Roebuck et al. (98) demonstrated an increase in azaserine-

pancreatic acinar cell foci in animals fed 20% corn oil or safflower oil diets as compared to those fed 20% coconut oil diet. When compared to 5% corn oil diet, 20% corn oil diet enhanced azaserine-induced pancreatic carcinogenesis.

The effect of fish oil on the development of pancreatic cancer in rats was examined by O'Connor et al. (99). A diet containing 20% menhaden fish oil produced a significant decrease in the development of azaserine-induced pancreatic preneoplastic lesions when compared to a 20% corn oil diet in rats.

CONCLUSIONS

The role of nutritional factors, especially macronutrients, in the etiology of cancer has become increasingly apparent. In recent years, scientific investigations have produced considerable information on the relationship between the macronutrients and cancers of colon, breast, and pancreas.

The information base is sufficiently convincing with respect to an enhancing effect as a function of total fat intake and certain types of fat in breast, colon, and pancreatic cancers, and a protective effect of certain dietary fibers in colon cancer. The available evidence suggests that high intake of dietary protein over long periods increases risk of certain types of cancer.

The first *Surgeon General's Report on Nutrition and Health* concluded that "overconsumption of certain dietary components is now a major concern for Americans. While many food factors are involved, chief among them is the disproportionate consumption of foods high in complex carbohydrate and fiber that may be more conductive to health" (100). The conclusions drawn by the National Research Council include that "in several types of epidemiologic studies, a high-fat intake is associated with increased risk of certain cancers, especially cancers of the colon, breast, and prostate. The epidemiologic evidence is not totally consistent, but it is supported by experiments in animals. The combined epidemiologic and laboratory evidence suggests that a reduction in total fat is likely to decrease the risk of these cancers" (101).

REFERENCES

1. E. L. Wynder and G. B. Gori, *JNCI 58*, 825 (1975).
2. World Health Organization, *Prevention of Cancer*, Technical Report Series *276*, Geneva, World Health Organization, 1964.
3. R. Doll and R. Peto, *JNCI, 66*, 1191 (1981).
4. Committee on Diet and Health, Food and Nutrition Board, *Diet Health*, National Research Council, National Academy of Sciences, Washington, DC, 1989, p. 593.
5. C. Welsch, in *Carcinogenesis and Dietary Fat* (S. Abraham, ed.), Kluwer Academic Publishers, Boston, 1989, p. 115.
6. B. S. Reddy and L. A. Cohen (eds.), *Diet, Nutrition, and Cancer; A Critical Evaluation*, Vol., 1, CRC Press, Boca Raton, FL, 1986.

7. A. K. Shamsuddin, in *Experimental Colon Carcinogenesis* (H. Autrup and G. M. Williams, eds.), CRC Press, Boca Raton, FL, 1983, p. 51.
8. B. S. Reddy, in *Diet, Nutrition, and Cancer: A Critical Evaluation*, Vol 1 (B. S. Reddy and L. A. Cohen, eds.), CRC Press, Boca Raton, FL 1986, p. 47.
9. E. L. Wynder, T. Kajitani, S. Ishikawa, H. Dodo, and A. Takano, *Cancer, 23*, 1219 (1969).
10. M. Jain, G. M. Cook, F. G. Davis, M. G. Grace, G. R. Howe, and A. B. Miller, *Int. J. Cancer, 26*, 757 (1980).
11. A. B. Miller, G. R. Howe, and M. Jain, *Int. J. Cancer, 32*, 155 (1983).
12. S. Graham, J. Marshall, B. Haughey, A. Mittleman, M. Swanson, M. Zielexny, T. Byers, G. Wilkinson, and D. West, *Am. J. Epidemiol, 128*, 490 (1988).
13. B. S. Reddy, T. Tanaka, and B. Simi *J. Natl. Cancer Inst., 75*, 791 (1985).
14. L. Diamond, T. G. O'Brien, and W. M. Baird, *Adv. Cancer Res., 32*, 1 (1980).
15. A. P. Maskens, *Cancer Res., 41*, 1240 (1981).
16. N. D. Nigro, D. V. Singh, R. L. Campbell, and M. S. Pak, *JNCI, 54*, 439 (1975).
17. S. A. Broitman, J. J. Vitale, E. Vavrousek-Jakuba, and L. S. Gottlieb, Cancer, 40, 2455 (1977).
18. A. E. Howarth and E. Pihl, *Nutr. Cancer, 6*, 229 (1985).
19. B. S. Reddy, S. Mangat, J. H. Weisburger, and E. L. Wynder, *Cancer Res., 37*, 3533 (1977).
20. B. S. Reddy, K. Watanabe, and J. H. Weisburger, *Cancer Res., 37*, 416 (1977).
21. B. S. Reddy and T. Ohmori, *Cancer Res., 41*, 1363 (1981).
22. B. S. Reddy, T. Narisawa, D. Vukusich, J. H. Weisburger, and E. L. Wynder, *Proc. Soc. Exp. Biol. Med., 151* 237 (1976).
23. R. L. Nutter, J. D. Kettering, R. M. Apprecio, D. A. Weeks, and D. S. Gridley, *Nutr. Cancer, 13*,141 (1990).
24. M. Sakaguchi, Y. Hiramatsu, H. Takada, M. Yamamura, K. Kioki, K. Sato, and M. Yamamoto, *Cancer Res., 44*, 1472 (1984).
25. B. C. Pence and F. Buddingh, *Carcinogenesis, 9*, 187 (1988).
26. K. M. Nauss, M. Locniscar, and P. M. Newberne, *Cancer Res., 43*, 4083 (1983).
27. A. W. Bull, B. K. Soullier, P. S. Wilson, M. T. Haydon, and N. D. Nigro, *Cancer Res., 39*, 4956 (1979).
28. B. S. Reddy and H. Maruyama, *JNCI, 77*, 815 (1986).
29. B. S. Reddy and H. Maruyama, *Cancer Res., 46*, 3367 (1986).
30. B. S. Reddy and Y. Maeura, *JNCI, 72*, 745 (1984).
31. D. P. Burkitt, *Cancer, 28*, 3 (1971).
32. O. M. Jensen, R. MacLennan, and J. Wahrendorf, *Nutr. Cancer, 4*, 5 (1982).
33. B. S. Reddy, C. Sharma, B. Simi, A. Engle, K. Laakso, P. Puska, and R. Korpela, *Cancer Res., 47*, 644 (1987).
34. G. E. McKeown-Eyssen and E. Bright-See, *Nutr. Cancer, 6*, 160 (1984).
35. S. M.Pilch (ed)., *Physiological Effects and Health Consequences of Dietary Fiber*, Life Sciences Research Office, FASB, Bethesda, MD, 1987.
36. B. R. Goldin and S. L. Gorbach, *JNCI, 47*, 371 (1976).
37. A. A. Salyers, in *Dietary Fiber: Basic and Clinical Aspects* (G. V. Vahouny and D. Kritchevsky, eds.), Plenum Press, New York, 1986, p. 119.

38. K. Watanabe, B. S. Reddy, J. H. Weisburger, and D. Kritchevsky, *JNCI 63*, 151 (1979).
39. K. Watanabe, B. S. Reddy, C. Q. Wong, and J. H. Weisburger, *Cancer Res., 38*, 4427 (1978).
40. B. S. Reddy and H. Mori, *Carcinogenesis, 2*, 21 (1981).
41. B. S. Reddy, H. Mori, and M. Nicolais, JNCI, 66, 553 (1981).
42. B. S. Reddy, Y. Maeura, and M. Wayman, *JNCI, 71*, 419 (1983).
43. N. D. Nigro and A. W. Bull, Jr., in *Dietary Fiber: Basic and Clinical Aspects* (G. V. Vahouny and D. Kritchevsky, eds.), Plenum Press, New York, 1986, p. 467.
44. H. G. Bauer, R. Asp, A. Oste, A. Dahlquist, and P. E. Fredlund, *Cancer Res., 39*, 3752 (1979).
45. L. R. Jacobs, *Cancer Res., 43*, 4057 (1983).
46. D. S. Barnes, N. K. Clapp, D. A. Scott, D. L. Oberst, and S. S. Berry, *Nutr. Cancer, 5*, 1 (1983).
47. H. J. Freeman, in *Dietary Fiber in Health and Disease* (G. V. Vahouny and D. Kritchevsky, eds)., Plenum Press, New York, 1982, p. 287.
48. L. R. Jacobs and J. R. Lupton, *Cancer Res., 46*, 1727 (1986).
49. D. Armstrong and R. Doll, *Int. J. Cancer, 15*, 617 (1975).
50. W. J. Visek, S. K. Clinton, and C. R. Truex, *Cornell Vet., 68*, 3 (1978).
51. D. C. Topping and W. J. Visek, *J. Nutr., 106*, 1583 (1976).
52. K. K. Carroll, *J. Nutr., 116*, 1130 (1986).
53. B. S. Reddy, *J. Nutr., 116*, 1132 (1986).
54. A. Tannenbaum and H. Silverstone, *Adv. Cancer Res., 1*, 451 (1953).
55. M. H. Ross and G. Bras, *J. Nutr., 47*, 1095 (1971).
56. D. M. Klurfeld, M. M. Weber, and D. Kritchevsky, *Cancer Res., 47*, 2759 (1987).
57. M. Pollard and P. H. Luckert, *JNCI, 74*, 1347 (1985).
58. B. S. Reddy, C. X. Wong, and H. Maruyama, *Cancer Res., 47*, 1226 (1987).
59. S. P. Kumar, S. J. Roy, K. Tokumo, and B. S. Reddy, *Cancer Res.*, 50 (1990).
60. D. P. Rose, A. P. Boyar,and E. L. Wynder, *Cancer, 58*, 2363 (1986).
61. A. B. Miller, A. Kelly, N. W. Choi, V. Matthews, L. W. Morgan, L. Munan, J. D. Burch, J. Feather, G. R. Howe, and M. Jain, *Am. J. Epidemiol., 107*, 499 (1978).
62. J. H. Lubin, Y. Wax, and B. Modan, *JNCI, 77*, 605 (1986).
63. W. C. Willet, M. J. Stampfer, G. A. Colditz, B. A. Rosner, C. H. Hennekens, and F. E. Speizer, *New Engl. J. Med., 316*, 22 (1987).
64. B. E. Henderson, *JNCI, 82*, 117 (1990).
65. J. R. Hebert and E. L. Wynder, *New Engl. J. Med., 317*, 165 (1987).
66. C. Huggins, L. C. Grand, and F. P. Brillantes, *Nature* (Lond.), *189*, 204 (1961).
67. K. K. Carroll and H. T. Khor, *Cancer Res., 30*, 2260 (1970).
68. K. K. Carroll and H. T. Khor, *Prog. Biochem. Pharmacol., 10*, 308 (1975).
69. P. W. Sylvester, M. Russell, M. M. Ip, and C. Ip, *Cancer Res., 46*, 757 (1986).
70. T. L. Dao and P. C. Chan, *JCNI, 71*, 201 (1983).
71. J. J. Jurkowski and W. T. Cave, *JNCI, 74*, 1145 (1985).
72. K. K. Carroll and G. J. Hopkins, *Lipids, 14*, 155 (1979).
73. C. Ip, C. A. Carter, and M. M. Ip, *Cancer Res., 45*, 1997 (1985).
74. L. A. Cohen, in *Diet, Nutrition, and Cancer: A Critical Evaluation* (B. S. Reddy, and L. A. Cohen, eds.), CRC Press, Roca Raton, FL, 1987, p. 77.

75. G. J. Hopkins and K. K. Carroll, *JNCI, 62*, 1009 (1979).
76. P. B. McCay, M. King, L. R. Rikins, and J. V. Pitha, *J. Environ. Pathol. Toxicol., 3*, 451 (1980).
77. S. Abraham and G. A. Rao, *JNCI, 56*, 431 (1976).
78. J. B. Lasekan, M. K. Clayton, A. Gendron-Fitzpatrick, and D. M. Ney, *Nutr. Cancer, 13*, 153 (1990).
79. L. A. Cohen, D. O. Thompson, Y. Maeura, K. Choi, M. E. Blank, and D. P. Rose, *JNCI, 77*, 33 (1986).
80. I. J. Tinsley, J. A. Schmitz, and D. A. Pierce, *Cancer Res., 41*, 1460 (1981).
81. L. A. Cohen and D. O. Thompson, *Lipids, 22*, 455 (1987).
82. S. L. Selenskas, M. M. Ip, and C. Ip, *Cancer Res., 44*, 1321 (1984).
83. R. A. Karmali, in *Proceedings of the AOAC Short Course on Polyunsaturated Fatty Acids and Ecosanoids* (W. E. M. Lands, ed.), American Oil Chemists' Society, Champaign, IL, 1987, p. 222.
84. K. K. Carroll and L. M. Braden, *Nutr. Cancer, 6*, 254 (1984).
85. C. Ip, M. M. Ip, and P. Sylvester, *Prog. Clin. Biol., Res., 222*, 283 (1986).
86. A. Tannenbaum and H. Silverstone, *Cancer Res., 9*, 162 (1949).
87. M. Ross and G. Bras, *J. Nutr., 130*, 944 1973).
88. H. Shay, M.Gruenstein, and M. Shimkin, *JNCI, 33*, 243 (1964).
89. E. Hawrylewicz, H. Huang, J. Kissane, and E. Darb, *Nutr. Rep. Int., 26*, 793 (1982).
90. S. K. Clinton and W. J. Visek, in *Dietary Fat and Cancer* (C. Ip, D. F. Birt, A. E. Rogers and C. Mettlin, eds.), A. R. Liss, New York, 1986, p. 377.
91. S. K. Clinton, J. M. Alster, P. B. Imrey, J. Simon, and W. Visek, *J. Nutr., 118*, 1577 (1988).
92. P. Pour, R. Runge, D. Birt, R. Gingell, T. Lawson, D. Nagel, L. Wallcave, and S. Z. Salmasi, *Cancer, 47*, 1573 (1981).
93. D. S. Longnecker, B. D. Roebuck, J. D. Yager, and H. S. Lilja, *Cancer, 47*, 1562 (1981).
94. D. S. Longnecker, in *Experimental Pancreatic Carcinogenesis* (D. G. Scarpelli, J. K. Reddy, and D. S. Longnecker, eds.), CRC Press, Boca Raton, FL, 1987, p. 117.
95. D. F. Birt, S. Salmasi, and P. M. Pour, *JNCI, 67*, 1327 (1981).
96. D. F. Birt, K. R. Stepan, and P. M. Pour, *JNCI, 71*, 355 (1983).
97. B. D. Roebuck, D. S. Longnecker, and D. F. Birt, in *Carcinogenesis and Dietary Fat* (S. Abraham, ed.), Kluwer Academic Press, Boston, 1989, p. 135.
98. B. D. Roebuck, J. D. Yagar, and D. S. Longnecker, *Cancer Res., 41*, 888 (1981).
99. T. P. O'Connor, B. D. Roebuck, and T. C. Campbell, *JNCI, 75*, 955 (1985).
100. *The Surgeon General's Report on Nutrition and Health*, U.S. Department of Health and Human Servies, Public Health Service, DHHS (PHS) Publication No. 88-50210, U.S. Government Printing Office, Washington, DC, 1988.
101. National Research Council, *Diet and Health, Implications for Reducing Chronic Disease Risk*, National Academy Press, Washington, DC, 1989.

3

Epidemiology of Diet and Cancer: Evidence of Human Maladaptation

John D. Potter
University of Minnesota
Minneapolis, Minnesota

INTRODUCTION

A simple objection to a connection between chronic disease and diet might be to argue that humans have always had to eat, and have always eaten the same nutrients—protein, fat, carbohydrates, vitamins, minerals. Therefore, the argument would go, the present pattern of disease and any changes in that pattern cannot be causally linked to food consumption. This argument, despite its naiveté, raises issues for nutrition and epidemiology. Current research investigating the relationship between specific dietary patterns and specific diseases is obviously based on the assumption that the above argument is false. This chapter examines the evidence for a significant and causal association between eating patterns and cancer. Far from being an implausible link, it is proposed that much of the explanation for the relation between diet and cancer comes from an intimate dependence of humans on their food supply. This dependence is not confined to the obvious provision of fuel for the organism but derives from long-standing adaptive patterns of dietary intake.

As a starting point, this chapter considers a seasonally variable diet to which humans are adapted, noting especially intakes of substances for which we are dependent on the environment and intakes of substances to which we have little or infrequent exposure.

There are four broad ways in which aberrations in the dietary pattern of humans could produce disease and perhaps cancer. There may be an imbalance in energy intake and output; there may be an alteration of the pattern of nutrients—both macro and micro—in the diet; specific deficiencies may occur; the food supply may contain substances to which the organism is almost never exposed and, therefore, for which they may not be the relevant metabolic responses. This chapter will focus *primarily* on the first two of these. The reader is referred to Moon and Micozzi (1989) and Potter and Graves (1991) for further data on the other two. Note, however, that there is a difficulty in considering only macronutrients, especially when a general argument related to *food* patterns is being developed. Accordingly, there will be some reference to the general issue of deficiencies of potentially protective substances—micronutrient but, more importantly, nonnutrient.

HUMAN DIETARY ADAPTATION?

Evoking a lost Golden Age to compare with present difficulties or explain current misfortunes is a human trait: from Eden (where fruit-eating habits were a part of the problem) through Rousseau's noble savage to the recent attention to paleolithic diets (Eaton and Konner, 1985). We cannot be certain as to what kind of diets humans are well adapted biologically (although the length and morphology of the GI tract, dentition, and enzyme patterns provide some clues). Further, most of us would probably find the associated living conditions unacceptable and perhaps nonsurvivable. Nonetheless, it is appropiate to ask if it is possible to essay some tentative description of our early diet. It should be taken into account that extensive variability in details must have existed in the same way that we can describe extensive geographic and temporal variability in contemporary diets. Some common features are proposed, including a high intake of a wide variety of foods—roots, leaves, nuts, seeds, fruit (grains could have only become a *staple* in the last 10,000–15,000 years but were probably gathered regularly in season); sporadic intake of lean meat low in saturated fat (a more secure and regular supply of fish and seafood for coastal dwellers); an intake of insects, grubs (high in protein) and bone marrow and organ meats; very low intake of alcohol; little refining or fractionation of food; low and irregular intake of eggs and very little nonhuman milk; variability, by season, both of total amount of food available and of kinds of foods resulting in variability in intake of particular nutrients. Other variations in this overall intake pattern would have been defined by climate as it varied over time and from place to place including the consumption of high fat (but not high saturated-fat) diets in extreme northern populations. In general, until very recently, saturated fat and alcohol intake would have been low, plant food (but not grain) intake high, and food sources highly varied.

If, as I argue here, there is a diet to which humans are more than trivially adapted, that adapation is not just a shopping list of taste preferences (to be discarded as easily as last year's fashions) but a specrum of human-environment dependencies, deviation from which will have significant consequences for health. There is a risk of circularity here, as with many adaptation arguments, of which both author and reader should be wary.

One important argument in favor of human adaptation to specific kinds of foods and eating habits is that there are many substances for which the organism is known to be dependent on the environment. This well-established concept in nutrition has, as we have also argued elsewhere (Potter and Graves, 1991), some important implications for cancer etiology. The consequences of a variety of nutrient deficiencies is a range of well-described disorders. Consider, though, that deficiency disorders can only arise if an organism is incapable of synthesis. This argues that there has been no selection pressure for such a capacity and, therefore, that the essential substances are widely available in the environment. Therefore, because certain nutrients are widely available in nature, deficiencies are possible. Essential amino acids, essential fatty acids, microelements, and vitamins are examples. The fact that what is essential varies among mammalian species underlines the importance of the adaptation process.

The adaptation argument, in short, is: The essential nutrients—both energy-bearing and micronutrients—are available to varying degrees in nature; they have important functions in growth, development, and reproduction; the organism is dependent on their ubiquity; deficiencies or excesses impair growth, development, and reproduction.

There is a plausible analogy for this argument in relation to the presence of substances necessary for the *maintenance* of the organism including dietary patterns that reduce the risk of carcinogensis: Normal long-term function of cells is dependent on the presence of a variety of widespread dietary constituents including, but not confined to, those necessary for growth and development. In their absence, cells malfunction. This malfunctioning state may make the cells more susceptible to exposure to carcinogens or may impair some specific protective mechanisms such as enzyme induction. It may also be characterized by higher cell replication rates as somatic cells seek to adapt to the new conditions. Consider that maintenance is a continuous function from birth but growth, development, and reproduction are time-limited.

A converse argument applies to those dietary constituents which are rare in nature: If substances are normally met with only occasionally (or not at all), intensive ingestion may have untoward consequences. This applies to very rare exposures that produce acute toxicity and to unaccustomed intake levels that overwhelm the metabolic processes which normally handle the exposure. Bacterial, plant, and fungal toxins are members of the first class. Several examples exist of the second: A high fat/calorie intake has consequences for cholesterol and insulin metabolism, adipose storage, and sex steroid hormone production; a high grain diet (such as that found in predominantly agricultural communities) is often associated with a reduced intake of other plant foods (and a lower intake of animal foods) and contains large amounts of abrasive material that may increase cell replication rates particularly in the upper digestive tract; a high intake of alcohol, which together with a generally reduced range of foods is associated with a wide variety of metabolic abnormalities. There may be differing degrees of adaptation in long-exposed vs. unexposed populations in each of these cases.

An objection to an adaptation argument, in relation to chronic disease, is that natural selection influences reproductive success and that, as chronic diseases are largely diseases of postreproductive years, a dietary adaptation is an unnecessary postulate. There are four responses to this: The first is to argue that humans have a long period of infant and juvenile dependence and that survival of parents and grandparents in a healthy state (i.e., longevity) is likely to be selected for.

The second response requires consideration of the unit of selection. If the issue is the survival of tribes or bands, then those bands would have survived better that had sufficient elders who knew how to respond to infrequently met hazards—food or water shortage, epidemic disease, and natural hazards such as fire or extreme weather. The tribal wisdom maintained by the old would have meant suvival of the tribe. Tribes without elders and without knowledge would be more likely to perish. Therefore the tribes in which longevity was selected would, in turn, have survived other threats to pass on their wisdom, their adaptive eating habits, their adapted metabolisms, and their genes.

Third, to argue that chronic diseases are a phenomenon of older age and therefore that resistance to them cannot have been selected for is to forget that these diseases are *not* a phenomenon of younger ages and that, therefore, some resistance (at least to the point of postponing them to older ages) has been selected for.

Finally, a diet that reduces risk of cancer may also improve reproductive success. There are a wide variety of substances that are both teratogenic and carcinogenic. So selection for improved reproductive success could directly select for reduced risk of cancer.

This chapter will explore the empirical evidence for the existence of unaccustomed exposures and protective dietary constituents and for risks associated with nutrient and energy imbalance. Some evidence for likely biologic mechanisms and the implications for further research are considered.

DIETARY EXPOSURE AND CANCER RISK

The available empirical epidemiologic and biologic data on diet and cancer are not readily summarized in a single chapter. The adaptation argument outlined above is used as a framework in order to show that some of the empirical relationships that have been established in the epidemiologic literature are explainable in relation to three kinds of aberration in dietary behavior—energy imbalance, nutrient imbalance, and specific deficiency. These relationships will be illustrated in relation to certain cancers, particularly breast, colon, and pancreas. Possible mechanism will be outlined.

Energy Imbalance

Evidence

Energy imbalance is a major topic. Therefore, we will consider only one or two aspects of it here; it is not intended to unravel its causes. Three measures relevant to energy balance (Pariza and Simopoulos, 1986) have been explored in epidemiologic studies of cancer—total intake (Potter and McMichael, 1986; Willett and Stampfer, 1986; Lyon et al., 1987), energy output (Garabrant et al., 1984) and a variety of measures of growth (Micozzi, 1985) and obesity (Paffenbarger et al., 1980; Helmrich et al., 1983). No simple established relationship exists between any of these measures and all cancers, and even for some specific cancers the empirical data are not clear. Further, there are some paradoxes.

The present evidence suggests that higher physical activity is related to a lower risk of colon cancer (Garabrant et al., 1984; Vena et al., 1985; Gerhardsson et al., 1986; Wu et al., 1987; Paffenbarger et al., 1987; Slattery et al., 1988a) but that obesity is probably not a risk factor (Potter and McMichael, 1986). For endometrial cancer (Elwood et al., 1977; LaVecchia et al., 1984; Folsom et al., 1989) and postmenopausal breast cancer, (Lew and Garfinkel, 1979; Helmrich et al., 1983), obesity is a risk factor. For premenopausal breast cancer, however, obesity is associated with a lower risk (Paffenbarger et al, 1980; Helmrich et al., 1983). Physical activity bears an uncertain but possibly negative relationship to risk of breast cancer (Frisch et al., 1985). Total energy intake is an inconsistent risk factor for all three cancers, but it is worth noting that dietary instruments vary widely in their capacity to measure total energy. There are no established relationships with other specific cancers; there is a general association between obesity and overall cancer risk (Lew and Garfinkel, 1979). Fat distribution (known to be related to diabetes and CHD (Vague et al., 1956; Feldman et al., 1969; Larsson et al., 1984; Donahue et al., 1987; Selby et al., 1989) is increasingly under investigation as a cancer risk factor (Le Marchand et al., 1988; Folsom et al., 1989,1990; Ballard-Barbash et al., 1990).

Mechanisms

Three plausible mechanisms can be advanced, characterized here as hormonal, mechanical, and total cellular workload arguments. Peripheral adipose tissue is the major source of postmenopausal estrogens (Grodin et al., 1973) via conversion of adrenal androstenedione; this provides a plausible explanation for the association with endometrial and postmenopausal breast cancer, both of which are thought to be causally associated with higher (perhaps cumulative) lifetime estrogen exposures. The association of obesity with a lower risk of premenopausal breast cancer is one of the paradoxes (but see below)—it does not seem to be merely a matter of a lower likelihood of detecting lesions in large breasts (Willett et al., 1985).

The role of physical activity in colon cancer is plausibly a mechanical effect—higher activity results in shorter mouth-to-anus transit time. However, shorter transit time is not an established negative risk factor for colon cancer (higher fecal weight is). Because obesity is not a risk factor for colon cancer (while high energy intake and low energy output are), it suggests that there may be metabolic differences in those who get colon cancer compared with those who do not. Other aspects of host differences relevant to colon cancer risk have also been proposed (McMichael and Potter, 1980,1983,1985). The total amount of food passing through the colon may represent a measure of total cellular work load (absorption, mucus and enzyme production, and detoxification) and therefore could determine cell replication rates (Potter, 1989b).

The complex relation among dietary intake, obesity, and physical activity on the one hand, and cancer risk on the other, will probably only be fully explicated when some of the relevant metabolic intermediate steps including the effects on gut function, on cell turnover, and on hormone production have been clarified. However, the empirical observation that aspects of energy imbalance are related to cancer risk is clearly established.

Adaptation

The human organism, it was argued above, is adapted to a high degree of variability in food intake and is able to make rapid use of a sudden increase in food supply in order to better survive through lean periods. This is the thrifty gene hypothesis, originally proposed as an explanation for the survival advantage of the predisposition to diabetes (Neel, 1969). More generally, a high intake of food as a regular, rather than sporadic, phenomenon is also likely to "jam open" other processes than insulin response. Thus, as low intakes of food, say at the end of winter, gave way to a more plentiful supply, reproductive success might plausibly be higher in those (females particularly) who gained sufficient body fat rapidly not only via insulin response but also by increasing intestinal tract surface area. Further, colonic surface area would be particularly valuable in extracting energy via bacterial fermentation from relatively energy-poor food. Such changes may also increase peripheral adipose production of estrogen, a factor perhaps originally associated with reproductive success—sufficient body fat, plus hormonal support to carry a child to term. Does this help explain why obesity is actually protective against premenopausal breast cancer and only a liability later?

Animal data show that on a low intake or in a fasting stage, the structure of the gut epithelium is much simpler and cell replication rates much lower (Stragand and Hagemann, 1977). With refeeding, the replication rates increase as do the complexity of the epithelial surface and the total surface area. This appears to be a highly adaptive response to marked variability in food availability—high cell turnover and large absorptive area in times of abundance; low activity during shortage to conserve energy. In the presence of a high intake diet as a regular phenomenon, however, high cell turnover and maximal epithelial surface area provide a favorable environment for carcinogenesis—via increased ingestion of initiator or promoter substances, via maximal absorptive surface area, and via increased probability of a "hit" in maximally replicating tissue.

The originally described association between increased frequency of food consumption and risk of colon (but not rectal) cancer (Potter and McMichael, 1986) has now been confirmed in two other studies (LaVecchia et al., 1988a; Young and Wolf, 1988). This provides additional evidence for the idea that there is a cost for frequent food intake (one concomitant of a high food intake).

Thus, although obesity itself was almost certainly uncommon in our ancestors, the capacity to assimilate food rapidly and store energy when it was available has probably been selected for. Inheritance of this metabolic profile in a society where food is widely available appears to have consequences for cancer risk at a number of sites.

Imbalance of Food/Nutritional Intake

Evidence

Current dietary epidemiology of cancer has largely been focused on elevated intakes of specific macronutrients, especially fat and alcohol. The evidence for a role of fat in the etiology of breast cancer is relatively poor and inconsistent but that for alcohol is suprisingly consistent.

Several ecologic studies of fat and breast cancer have been published. Stocks' (1970) regional study in Great Britain found that dairy products were positively associated with risk but that other sources of fat were inversely associated. Hirayama (1978) reported that pork consumption (but not fat) correlated with risk over 12 regions in Japan. A study of ethnic groups within Hawaii found a strong relation between fat and breast cancer: An approximately 35% difference in fact was associated with about a 200% difference in risk of breast cancer (Kolonel et al., 1981).

In subpopulations where the known intakes of animal fat and animal protein are lower than that of the general community—vegetarian nuns (Kinlen, 1982) and Seventh-day Adventists (Phillips et al., 1980) (the majority of whom are lacto-ovo-vegetarians)—the risk of breast cancer is not lower than in the general population. Although it may be argued that, in both these groups, the reproductive rate is lower than in comparison populations, neither study provides strong evidence for the importance of dietary fat in the genesis of breast cancer.

There have been at least 10 case-control studies on the relationship between meat or fat consumption and breast cancer (Table 1). The study of Lubin et al.

Table 1 Case-Control Studies of Consumption of Fat, Meat and Dairy Products in Relation to Breast Cancer

Specific exposure	Relative risk (95% confidence limits) high vs. low	Ref.
Fat		
hard frying fat	2.0 (0.0–4.6)[b]	Phillips, 1975
total fat	1.8 (N/A)	Miller et al., 1978
saturated fat	1.2 (N/A)	
animal fat	0.0 (0.7–1.2)	Graham et al., 1982
total fat	1.3 (N/A)	Howe, 1985[a]
saturated fat	1.5 (N/A)	
total fat	1.0 (0.6–17)	Hirohata et al. 1985
animal fat	1.3 (0.8–2.2)	
fat at age ≥ 50	1.6 (0.9–2.7)	Lubin et al., 1986
oils, fats	0.6 (0.2–1.4)[b]	Katsouyanni et al., 1986
total fat (per 75.8 g/day)	1.7 (1.0–2.1)	Shun-Zhang et al., 1990
saturated fat (per 20.8 g/day)	0.9 (0.5–1.4)	
monounsaturated fat (per 54.3 g/day)	1.9 (1.1–3.2)	
Meat		
beef	1.5 (1.1–2.1)	Lubin et al., 1981
pork	2.2 (1.6–2.9)	
meat	1.6 (1.2–2.6)	Talamini et al., 1984
meat, fish, eggs	1.2 (0.4–3.3)	Katsouyanni et al., 1986.
Dairy products		
dairy products	3.4 (2.0–5.8)	Talamini et al., 1984
milk	1.8 (1.3–2.4)	Le et al., 1986
cheese	1.5 (1.0–2.3)	
butter	0.9 (0.7–1.1)	
yogurt	0.7 (0.3–1.6)	
dairy products	0.7 (0.3–1.6)	Katsouyanni et al., 1986
Fried foods		
fried foods	1.8 (0.9–3.5)[b]	Phillips, 1975
fried potatoes	2.4 (1.1–5.2)[b]	

[a]Reanalysis of Miller et al., 1978.
[b]95% confidence limits from Rohan and Bain, 1987.
N/A = not available.

(1981)—one of only two case-control studies showing a significant increase in risk associated with consumption of fat—was based on frequency of consumption of just eight food items; the other positive finding was recently reported from Shanghai (Shun-Zhang et al., 1990). Two of three studies reporting on dairy products consumption found positive associations with risk.

Of the three cohort studies (Table 2), only that of Hirayama (1978) found an association between daily consumption of meat and risk of breast cancer (after age 54); this finding was based on just 14 cases in this category.

The findings for breast cancer are in sharp contrast to those for colorectal cancer (Table 3). In 16 case-control studies where saturated fat or total fat were studied, nine found a significantly increased risk. Meat has also been shown to be a significant risk factor in 9 of the 14 studies in which its consumption was reported. Protein was positively associated with risk in five of six studies. Similar results have recently been reported from the prospective Boston Nurses Health Study (Willett et al., 1990).

Pancreas cancer shows an even more consistent relationship with meat and fat. All of the six reported studies show an increased risk in association with higher consumption of meat, fat, or fried foods (Table 4). The recent study of Howe et al. (1990) found total energy intake (particularly from carbohydrate) sources to be a major predictor of risk.

Alcohol consumption has been shown in ecologic studies to be related to colon and rectal cancer (Potter et al., 1982) and to cancers to the larynx and esophagus (McMichael et al., 1979).

Among analytic studies, there is a consistent but not strong relationship with breast cancer (Table 5) and somewhat less consistent association with cancers of

Table 2 Cohort Studies of Fat and Meat Consumption in Relation to Breast Cancer

Specific exposure	Relative risk (95% confidence limits) high vs. low	Ref.
Fat		
fat	0.9 (0.7–1.1)	Willett et al., 1987a
saturated fat	0.9 (0.7–1.1)	
Meat		
age 40–54	1.3 (0.6–2.2)[a]	Hirayama, 1978
aged ≥ 55	2.3 (1.5–3.0)[a]	
meat, poultry	1.2 (N/A)	Phillips and Snowdon, 1983

[a]95% confidence limits from Rohan and Bain, 1987.
N/A = not available.

Table 3 Case-Control Studies of Dietary Factors in Relation to Cancer of Colon and Rectum

Factor	Relationship to risk	No. of studies showing relationship	No. of studies done
Meat, fat, protein, energy			
meat	+	9	14
saturated fat/total fat	+	9	16
protein	+	5	6
energy	+	5	6
Vegetables			
vegetables	−	12	15
string beans	+	1	2
Fiber			
fiber	−	5	11
fiber	+	2	11
Cereals			
rice	−	1	4
rice	+	2	4
pasta/past and rice	+	3	3
cereals	+	2	7
Fruit			
fruit	−	2	9
fruit	+	1	9
vitamin C	−	3	4
vitamin A	−	1	4

Sources: Stocks, 1957; Pernu, 1960; Higginson, 1966; Wynder and Shigematsu, 1969; Wynder et al., 1969; Haenszel et al., 1969; Bjelke, 1973; Philips, 1975; Modan et al., 1975; Graham et al., 1978; Dales et al., 1979; Martinez et al., 1979; Haenszel et al., 1980; Jain et al., 1980; Miller et al., 1983; Manousos et al., 1983; Berta et al., 1985; Bristol et al., 1985; Macquart-Moulin et al., 1986; Potter and McMichael, 1986; Lyon et al., 1987; Graham et al., 1988; LaVecchia et al., 1988a; Young and Wolf, 988; Tuyns et al., 1988; Benito et al., 1989; Heilburn et al., 1989 (among *low* fat intake males only); Benito et al., 1990.

Table 4 Studies of Meat and Fat in Relation to Pancreatic Cancer

Study type	Comparison	Relative Risk		Ref.
Case control	Fat per 10 gm/day	1.8		Durbec et al., 1983
		H	P	
Case-control	Butter ≥ 2 vs. < 2/wk	2.4	1.1	Gold et al., 1985
	Deep fried foods	< 1.0		
	Beef	< 1.0		
		D	A	
Case-control	Beef ≥ 5/wk vs. 5 < wk	2.1	1.2	Mack et al., 1986
	Eggs ≥ 5/wk vs. 5 </wk	0.7	0.8	
	Fried bacon/ham ≥ 5/wk vs. < 5/wk	1.4	0.9	
		H	P	
Case-control	Fried/grilled meat			
	< 1/week	1.0	1.0	Norell et al., 1986
	Every week	1.5	1.7	
	Almost daily	4.6	13.4	
		M	F	
Case-control	Beef 6/month	1.0	1.0	Falk et al., 1988
	6–15/month	1.2	0.8	
	≥ 16/month	1.1	0.7	
	Pork < 9/month	1.0	1.0	
	9–30 month	1.4	1.6	
	≥ 31/month	1.7	1.3	
	Dairy < 34/month	1.0	1.0	
	34–67/month	1.6	1.6	
	≥ 68/month	2.2	1.0	
	Seafood < 2/month	1.0	1.0	
	2–7/month	1.0	1.2	
	≥ 8/month	1.0	1.9	
Cohort	Current use of meat, poultry, fish			Mills, et al., 1988
	< 1/wk	1.0		
	1–2/wk	0.8		
	≥ 3/wk	2.2		
	Current use of eggs			
	< 1/wk	1.0		
	1–2/wk	1.5		
	≥ 3/wk	2.5		
	Butter	~ 1.0		
	Milk	~ 1.0		

H = Hospital controls; P = Population controls; D = Directly Interviewed; A = All; M = Male; F = female.

Table 5 Studies on Alcohol and Breast Cancer

Comparison	Relative Risk (95% confidence levels)	Ref.
Cohort studies		
≥ 3 drinks/day vs. never	1.4 (N/A)	Hiatt and Bawol, 1984
≥ 5 g/day vs. none	2.0 (1.1–3.7)	Schatzkin et al., 1987
≥ 15 g/day vs. none	1.6 (1.3–2.0)	Willett et al., 1987b
≥ 5 g/day vs. none	0.8 (0.5–1.2)	Schatzkin et al., 1989
Case-control studies		
> 50 ounce-years vs. never	1.6 (N/A)	Williams and Horm, 1977
ever vs. never	1.9 (1.5–2.4)	Rosenberg et al., 1982
≥ 26 drinks/month vs. never	1.1 (N/A)	Byers and Funch, 1982
≥ 1 drink/day vs. never	1.4 (0.9–2.0)	Begg et al., 1983
≥ 2 drinks/day vs. never	1.0 (N/A)	Paganini-Hill and Ross, 1983
ever vs. never	1.0 (0.8–1.2)	Webster et al., 1983
≥ 300 g/wk vs. never	1.1 (0.6–1.8)	
ever vs. never	2.5 (1.7–3.7)	Talamini et al., 1984
≥ 0.5 liters wine s. no wine	16.7 (3.1–89.7)	
alcohol with meals vs. not	1.5 (1.3–1.7)	Le et al., 1984
≥ 240 g/wk vs. never	1.2 (0.7–2.0)	
≥ 4 drinks/day vs. never	2.1 (1.1–4.0)	LaVecchia et al., 1985
≥ 1 drink/wk vs. < 1/wk	1.5 (0.99–2.1)	O'Connell et al., 1987
> 2 drinks/day vs. never	1.7 (1.2–2.4)	Harvey et al., 1987
> 9.3 g/day vs. never	1.6 (0.99–2.5)	Rohan and McMichael, 1988
ever vs. never	0.9 (N/A)	Harris and Wynder, 1988
10 vs. 0 drinks/wk		
early age drinking	2.1 (1.3–3.5)	Young, 1989
later age drinking	1.9 (1.3–3.0)	

N/A = not available.

colon and rectum (Table 6). The evidence in favor of a causal association with pancreas cancer is weak (Velema et al., 1986). Alcohol is, however, extensively implicated in cancers of the upper digestive and respiratory tracts; it is regarded by IARC as an established human carcinogen largely because of this association (IARC, 1988).

High grain-consuming areas are at high risk of esophageal or stomach cancer or both. Van Rensberg (1981) has shown that there is a consistently higher risk for esophageal cancer among populations with high corn and wheat consumption compared with those with high sorghum, millet, cassava, yam, or peanut consumption. A reduced risk of colon cancer in high risk areas (e.g., the United States, Western Europe, Australia) is much more consistently found with high vegetable rather than high cereal intake (see Table 3) although, in international comparisons cereal-eating communities are at lower risk of cancer at this site.

Some data suggest that an elevated intake of simple carbohydrate is associated with increased risk of colorectal cancer (Bristol et al., 1985, Tuyns et al., 1988). Note also the above-mentioned association of total carbohydrate and risk of pancreatic cancer (Howe et al., 1990).

Mechanism

A variety of mechanisms have been proposed to account for an association between dietary fat, etc., and cancer. The explanations have been most prolific for the cancer—breast—for which the empirical analytic study evidence is weakest. Direct and indirect mechanisms have been proposed. The suggested direct mechanisms are all via effects of (a) unsaturated fatty acids on cell membrane structure and function (Welsch and Aylsworth, 1983), epithelial proliferation (Kidwell et al., 1982), immune responsiveness (Vitale and Broitman, 1981), and cell-to-cell communication (Welsch and Aylsworth, 1983) or (b) fatty acid and cholesterol metabolites (epoxides and peroxides) on promotion of transformed cells (Petrakis et al., 1980, Gruenke et al., 1987). Given that neither class of

Table 6 Studies of Alcohol and Colorectal Cancer

Study Type	No. of studies done	No. showing increased risk
Case-control	8	5
Cohort	4	4
Cohort (brewery workers)	2	1[a]

[a]The other study (Jensen et al., 1979) shows a higher risk than would be expected for rectal cancer in this blue-collar workforce.

Sources: Stocks, 1957; Pernu, 1960, Higginson, 1966; Wynder and Shigematsu, 1967; Wynder et al., 1967; Bjelke, 1973; Graham et al., 1978; Potter and McMichael, 1986; Sundby, 1967; Bjelke, 1974; Wu et al., 1987; Klatsky et al., 1988; Dean et al., 1979; Jensen et al., 1979.

explanation involves total fat intake, this may partly explain the mismatch between the plausibility of mechanisms and the absence of data: The wrong exposure is being measured in epidemiologic studies.

The proposed indirect mechanisms are (a) via the effects of fat on hormone receptors (Welsch and Aylsworth, 1983), on prolactin production (Hill et al., 1980), or on bowel flora (Hill et al., 1970) which, it is suggested, may alter the bioavailability of estrogens through effects on steroid deconjugation (Gorbach, 1984) or alter the bacterial production of specific anticarcinogenic agents (Adlercreutz et al., 1982, Aldercreutz, 1984); and (b) via the effects of higher food intake on age at menarche (Frisch and McArthur, 1974), age of menopause (de Waard et al., 1964), and adipose tissue where androstenedione may be converted to estrogens (Grodin et al., 1973).

Conceptually attractive though many of these proposed mechanisms may be, the large number of them is itself a problem. Breast cancer, like most cancers, is undoubtedly of multifactorial origin, so that a list of potential pathways is not an insurmountable problem. Nonetheless, there is no clear understanding of the initiation, promotion, and progression of human breast cancer, no unequivocal precursor lesion, and no known biochemical marker. Therefore, it may be inappropriate to search for a mechanism in the absence both of data establishing that a high fat diet is indeed a risk factor for mammary tumorigenesis and of an understanding of the intermediate steps.

The dominant hypothesis for colon cancer derives from the relationship between dietary fat intake and bile acid metabolism. Fat intake, it is proposed, increases the amount or concentration of bile acids secreted into the small bowel; the normal bacterial flora of the large bowel metabolize the primary acids to secondary, and these, it is suggested, have toxic, cocarcinogenic, promotional, and trophic effects. There is a considerable amount of corroborative human metabolic and animal experimental evidence, which is, however, not totally coherent (McMichael and Potter, 1985, 1986). Other roles for fat have been proposed, including a direct toxic action on the bowel wall (Bruce, 1987).

McMichael (1981) cited data showing the gastrointestinal (GIT) hormones have both trophic and hyperplastic effects on the exocrine pancreas and could act as mediators of known or suspected dietary (and other) risk factors. Gastrin and cholecystokinin (CCK) are powerful stimulators of pancreatic hyperplasia (Johnson, 1981). CCK has been shown, in animal models, to be a significant promoter of pancreatic neoplasia (Howatson and Carter, 1985).

For the relationship between alcohol and breast cancer, there have been no major advances in relation to biologic mechanisms beyond that originally proposed by Williams (1976)—namely, stimulation of prolactin secretion. It is also possible, as a number of workers have argued, that, because alcohol is a significant energy source, the mechanism could be related to those postulated for obesity or caloric intake in general. For colorectal cancer, the evidence suggests that the effect of alcohol on bile acid metabolism is rather like that of fat (McMichael and Potter, 1985, 1986). A variety of mechanisms have been postulated to account for the causal association with cancers of larynx and esophagus including acting as a chronic irritant and inducing excess cell replication; acting as a solvent for direct-acting carcinogens, particularly those in cigarette smoke; being associated with specific nutrient deficiencies; and being a vehicle for other compounds present in alcoholic drinks (IARC, 1988). Spitz and colleagues (1988,1989) have begun to explore possible variability in susceptibility to the effects of alcohol and tobacco in upper aerodigestive cancers.

Mechanisms to explain the association between high grain consumption and increased risk of upper digestive tract cancers include traumatic effects of silicaceous fibers resulting in high epithelial cellular turnover and an associated reduction of intake of other plant foods that results in deficiencies either of micronutrients (van Rensberg, 1981) or specific nonnutrient substances.

Adaptation

The claim for the relevance of adaptation is more than a general affirmation of a human incapacity to handle a high fat intake, high alcohol intake, or a high intake of other nutrients or food components but remains speculative, and, as noted earlier, possibly circular.

The primary premise is that high fat, high alcohol, or high grain consumption were not dietary patterns to which humans in their original state were *regularly exposed*. An intermittent high intake (in a feast/fast environment) produced rapid adaptive responses—increased gut epithelial proliferation, increased bile acid and hormone secretion—both trophic and secretory-control hormones etc, which, as an energy-conserving mechanism then subsided when food became scare. High metabolic activity and cellular turnover is a cost to the organism that is not a good investment in the presence of reduced food availability. The capacity for rapid response becomes nonadaptive in the presence of consistent high intake leading not only to alcoholism and obesity but also to chronic high G.I.T. hormone levels and elevated epithelial proliferation rates. High intakes of abrasive fibers will result in elevated upper alimentary tract proliferation rates and increased risk of carcinogenesis.

There is a further aspect to the adaptive argument which is particularly related to the internal ecology of the colon. The large bowel can be considered a complex ecosystem in which the colonic contents act as a culture medium for bacterial and colonic cells (McMichael and Potter, 1986; Potter, 1989b). The culture medium, in turn, is influenced extensively by host conditions, including hormones, and by ingested foods and alcohol. This ecosystem may be one of the most flexible parts of the human-environment adaptation relationship; it is argued, however, that there are limits to its flexibility with consequences for carcinogenesis (McMichael and Potter, 1986; Potter, 1989b).

Specific Deficiencies (Nutrients and "Nonnutrients")

Evidence

Although the focus of this book and therefore this chapter is macronutrient consumption, any argument based on the idea of a diet to which we are adapted has to include some consideration of protective factors. One obvious "macronutrient" that has been proposed as protective is dietary fiber.

Fiber and cereals, as potentially protective agents particularly in colon cancer, have attracted considerable attention. Burkitt proposed in 1971 that the reason Africans were at low risk of colon cancer was not, as his mentor and colleague, Cleave, believed, because their diets were low in sugar but rather because their diets were high in fiber. This hypothesis is attractive but problematic, and the empirical evidence in its favor is debatable. I have elsewhere (Potter, 1989a) provided a detailed argument as to why I think the fiber–colon cancer link is unclear. In brief, there is a wide variety of substances all referred to as "fiber" that have never been subcategorized in epidemiologic studies largely because the dietary databases used in such studies are incomplete (and even inconsistent). Further these fibers vary extensively in their physico-chemical properties, solubility, bile acid–binding capacity, fermentability, and water-holding capacity. There is no reason to suppose that their effects are even unidirectional and some empirical data to show that they are not. Measurement problems compound the classification issue, and the problems of associated nutrients, associated dietary intake patterns, nutrient-nutrient and nutrient-host interactions have seldom been addressed (Potter, 1989a).

The association between "dietary fiber" as a composite variable and colon cancer, accordingly, has produced mixed findings (Potter, 1989a), and even the interpretations of the overall data are not consistent (Trock et al., 1990). However, there are data to show that a diet high in fiber may be relevant, not only in colon cancer, but also in pancreas (Howe et al., 1990) and other cancers. It may be that these effects are interpretable as consquences of the other less well-understood dietary constituents that are found in foods such as vegetables, fruit, and nuts for which "dietary fiber" as a nutrient may merely be a marker; however, other direct mechanisms are plausible (see below).

Van Rensberg (1981) has argued on ecologic grounds that specific cereals may be associated casually with higher risk of esophageal cancer—this, however, is an argument that relates to cereals as a food (with their intrinsic levels of micronutrients, and possibily the associated general dietary pattern in communities with different cereals as staples), not fiber as a nutrient. For colon cancer, too, some cereals (particularly rice) have been associated with increased, not decreased risk—despite the fact that, internationally, rice eating is associated with a reduced population risk of colon cancer.

The most obvious specific deficiencies after fiber (a specific deficiency of which is not a simple entity) are those of micronutrients. For β-carotene, retinol, and ascorbate, higher risks of particular cancers have been reported in individuals with lower intakes or blood levels, but these have largely been within the normal range (Wald et al., 1980; Kark et al., 1981; Peto et al., 1981). There are several cancers that have a probable relationship with micronutrient deficiencies—notably lung cancer and cervix cancer (Peto et al., 1981; Moon and Micozzi, 1989). Lower dietary ascorbate levels have been reported for rectal cancer (Bjelke, 1973; Potter and McMichael, 1986), and lower intakes of minerals such as calcium and trace elements such as selenium may be important (Willett et al., 1983; Bruce, 1987; Slattery et al., 1988b).

Not always clearly identified by epidemiologists as the most consistent finding in the dietary etiology of cancer is the more general relationship between a higher intake of vegetables and a lower risk of cancer of a wide variety of sites including mouth and pharynx, lung, stomach, pancreas, colon, and rectum (Micozzi et al., 1990). A comprehensive review of this area is currently in preparation by the author, but some existing review papers and specific individual studies are noted below.

For colorectal (Potter, 1989b) and pancreatic (Potter, 1989c) cancers, readers' attention is drawn to recent reviews. Of the 15 studies of colorectal cancer that have looked at the role of vegetables, 12 have reported a lower risk in association with higher consumption (see Table 3). Of the five studies of pancreas cancer, all have reported a lower risk in association with a higher intake of vegetables or fruit or both (Table 7). Recent studies of prostate (Oishi et al., 1988), mouth and pharynx (McLaughlin et al., 1988), lung (Byers et al., 1987; Koo, 1988) cervix (LaVecchia et al., 1988b; Brock et al., 1988), and stomach (LaVecchia et al., 1987; You et al., 1988) show similar findings for vegetables or fruit or both. In general, over 100 studies looking at the role of vegetable and fruit intake in relation to cancer reveal a very consistent picture of lower risk in association with higher consumption. This is unlikely to be due to publication bias, as the cost and time needed to undertake dietary studies, by and large, ensures a strong commitment to their publication.

The obvious question is whether these data, particularly given the apparent consistency at lest of the β-carotene/lung cancer story (Peto et al., 1981; Micozzi et al., 1990), are merely providing *less* specific support for the association between high intakes of defined micronutrients such as β-carotene and ascorbate and lower risk of cancers or whether additional factors are relevant. Some animal and in vitro studies suggest that this is a broader and more interesting phenomenon related to more than specific vitamins (but importantly not excluding them). Further, given the consistency of the vegetable intake data and the lower consistency of the cereal or fiber data, it seems worthwhile to consider this as more than merely the consequence of a low fiber or even a low carbohydrate diet. Indeed, again,

Table 7 Studies of Vegetables and Fruit in Relation to Pancreatic Cancer

Study type	Dietary variable	Relative risk		Ref.
Case-Control	Raw fruits and vegetables	H	P	Gold et al., 1985
	Ever vs. never	0.5	0.2	
	≥ 2 vs. < 2/week	0.5	0.7	
	≥ 5 vs. < 5/week	0.6	0.6	
Case-Control	Fresh fruits and vegetables	D	A	Mack et al., 1986
	≥ 5/wk vs. </wk	0.8	0.7	
		H	P	
Case-Control	Vegetables < 1/wk	1.0	1.0	Norell et al., 1986
	Every week	1.0	1.0	
	Almost daily	0.5	0.8	
	Raw vegetables < 1/wk	1.0	1.0	
	Every week	0.5	0.7	
	Almost daily	0.5	0.6	
	Citrus fruits < 1/wk	1.0	1.0	
	Every week	0.6	1.0	
	Almost daily	0.3	0.5	
	Fruit juices < 1/wk	1.0	1.0	
	Every week	0.9	0.6	
	Almost daily	0.6	0.6	
Case-Control	Fruits and juices	M	F	Falk et al., 1988
	< 25/month	1.0	1.0	
	25–63/month	0.6	0.6	
	≥ 64/month	0.4	0.5	
	Vitamin C			
	< 2000 mg/month	1.0	1.0	
	2000–4455 mg/month	0.5	0.8	
	≥ 4456 mg/month	0.4	0.6	
Cohort	Beans, lentils, peas			Mills et al., 1988
	< 1/wk	1.0		
	1–2/wk	0.5		
	≥ 3/wk	0.4		
	Dried fruits			
	< 1/wk	1.0		
	1–2/wk	0.5		
	≥ 3/wk	0.4		
	Green salad	> 1.0 (NS)		
	Cooked green vegetables	> 1.0 (NS)		

H = Hospital Controls; P = Population Controls; D = Directly Interviewed; A = All; M = Male; F = Female.

it is worth noting that Howe et al. (1990) found a higher risk for high carbohydrate intake in pancreatic cancer then for any other source of calories.

Rather than debate which nutrient (or even which food) is crucial, it may be worthwhile considering vegetables or plant foods as purpose-fitted packages of required intakes for humans (see below for a development of this argument).

Vegetables contain a wide variety of substances which have been shown to have anticarcinogenic properties—phenols, isothiocyanates, flavonoids, indoles, lignans, etc. (Wattenberg, 1985), as well as (possibly important for colon cancers at least) fermentable fiber with its effect on pH, bile acid–metabolizing enzymes, and short-chain fatty acid production, as well as vitamins and trace elements. A recent nested case-control study found serum lycopene levels to be markedly different between cases of pancreatic cancer and controls (RR low vs. high tertile =5.40). Lycopene is a carotenoid without retinoid activity (Burney et al., 1989).

It is not possible, at present, to provide a summary estimate of the intakes of most of the "nonnutrient" substances—food tables do not provide the data, most of the relevant food analyses have not been done, and it is likely that whole classes of these constituents, and certainly individual constituents, remain to be identified.

Mechanisms

Several roles have been identified (Wattenberg, 1985) for the known substances, including:

1. Inhibiting formation of direct-acting carcinogens. Ascorbate is effective in blocking the formation of N-nitrosamines in vivo (Mirvish, 1981; Bartsch et al., 1988).
2. Acting to prevent agents reacting with target tissues. There are a variety of ways in which this may occur (see Wattenberg, 1985). Agents include components, such as phenols, found in plant foods (Wood et al., 1982) that can react with active carcinogens.
3. Inducing enzymes that either detoxify or conjugate carcinogenic compounds. A variety of plant-related substances have been shown to be effective (Wattenberg, 1977,1983).
4. Acting to inhibit carcinogenesis even when delivered after known carcinogen exposure in animals. Wattenberg (1985) has included carotenoids and selenium in this category but the mechanisms are unclear.
5. Specific deficiencies of micronutrients have been shown to be associated with hyperplasia in a variety of epithelial tissues.

The original hypothesis for the role of fiber in colorectal cancer was as a bulking (diluting) agent that also reduced transit time and therefore epithelial exposure. More recently, it has become clear that fiber is extensively fermented, producing volatile fatty acids, which may be both a colonic cell fuel and anticarcinogenic. However, it is worth considering that an increase in fuel may also produce increased cell replication. There are animal experiments data to show that some fibers are associated with increased cell replication and carcinogenesis (Jacobs, 1983, 1984).

Plant foods, finally, are an important source of carcinogens in the diet also (Ames et al., 1987), including some of the compounds identified above as "anticarcinogens"; varying conditions and doses in animals experiments will alter the likely outcome—a yin/yang phenomenon.

Adaptation

This is where the adaptation argument has its most interesting implications (and perhaps significant testability). Some substances, including vitamins and trace elements, are known to be essential for the organism to grow, maintain integrity, and reproduce optimally. The consequences of low levels (dietary or tissue) of these substances *may* include carcinogenesis. The extension of the argument is that we are equally dependent on the environment to provide other substances that have specific anticarcinogenic properties. In the absence of these substances, organisms are at higher risk of cancers at a number of sites, particularly those where epithelial surfaces are exposed to environmental agents—lung, digestive tract, and cervix. These dietarily supplied compounds act to induce detoxifying enzymes, to block activation, etc., and organisms are reliant on them to do so, even if as Bresnick (personal communication) has pointed out, the real role of these enzymes is the conversion of hydrophobic to water-soluble compounds for easier transport and excretion. The defenses are multilayed (Ames et al., 1990), but can be enhanced by environmentally supplied nutrients that "tune" the system. In low doses (hence the yin/yang phenomenon) even carcinogens will be beneficial—tuning the system to handle high doses. In high doses, normally relatively benign compounds may overwhelm the systems and either produce toxic/carcinogenic effects themselves or allow other more potent compounds to do so.

Adaptation, as has been argued, relates to each of the dietary phenomena associated with increased cancer risk. There are more problems in the testability of the notion that humans are exposed to "unaccustomed levels" of total energy or specific nutrients than there are for specific deficiencies (or specific exposures). There is no way to modify unaccustomed levels (of energy or nutrients) in a controlled trial without also modifying others: e.g., any attempt to decrease fat will result in decreased calories or increases in other nutrients; similarly, attempts to reduce obesity or change body mass results in changes of nutient intakes, energy intake, energy expenditure, or all three. On the other hand, addition of either specific compounds to the diet or modification of vegetable intake provides a test of the protective effect (and perhaps of the "essential nutrient" hypothesis) *and* a test of possible public health strategies. There are also ways to test the adaptation argument with in vitro cellular studies.

There are areas of the world where cancer risk is related to reduced intakes of specific nutrients *and* to exposure to specific dietary carcinogens (e.g., China, where esophageal cancer is associated with N-nitroso compounds (Yang, 1980) and low intakes and blood levels of a variety of vitamins and trace elements (Thurnham et al., 1985)). Supplementation with the missing nutrients has been, to date, disappointingly ineffective in reducing risk (Munoz et al., 1985, Wahrendorf et al., 1988). It follows from the above adaptation argument that what may be missing are not the obvious micronutrients (these may be just markers for the real deficiencies) but specific compounds that keep the detoxifying enzymes "tuned." The essential experiments are obvious—either add a variety of vegetables and fruits or add some specific nonnutrient enzyme-inducers, blocking agents, etc. to the diet. The advantage of this strategy in this disease is that there is an identified precursor lesion. This allows rapid test of a variety of strategies on relatively small populations over short time periods.

Similar arguments apply to the testing of the role of vegetables in the prevention of recurrence of adenomatous polyps in addition to existing studies of single likely preventive agents (Bertram et al., 1987).

SUMMARY

There are a variety of ways in which diet may influence the development of human cancers. Previous reviews of this topic have largely been descriptive and mechanistic: Exposure to substance X is associated with increases in cancer A; increased intake of substance Y appears to reduce the risk of cancer B. What is proposed here is a theoretical framework and an argument that, while not yet fully developed, has the following features:

There is a dietary pattern to which humans are well adapted—an "original diet".

This original dietary pattern had specific features that included regular exposure to a variety of substances on which human metabolism is dependent but which have not, till now, been explicitly labeled as "essential nutrients." I would argue that this is now worthy of serious consideration.

The original dietary pattern was low in highly abrasive cereal products (consumption of large amounts of grains is a relatively recent phenomenon) with less resultant damage and less need for frequent cell repair particularly to the upper gastrointestinal tract.

The diet involved variablity in intake, which was accompanied by variability in cell-replication rates, particularly in the lower gastrointestinal tract, and little risk of obesity.

There was little intake of alcohol and therefore little capacity for its solvent and chronic cell-damage capacities.

Abandonment of each of these aspects of dietary adaptation has consequences for carcinogenesis. Most notable is the reduction of intake of vegetables and fruit with subsequent loss of enzyme "tuning," etc. and a generally increased rate of cancer at a number of sites. A high intake of fat, of grains, and of alcohol, and increased obesity are each associated with an identifiable pattern of cancers. Testable consequences follow. Increasing intake of vegetables and fruit should reduce the risk of colon cancer and perhaps of colonic adenomatous polyps even in the presence of a high fat intake, and of esophageal cancer even with exposure to specific carcinogenic compounds including those from cigarette smoke. Testing in vitro and in vivo will provide more definitive answers regarding the specific compounds and their sites and modes of action. In the meanwhile, the empirical data encourage us to eat more vegetables as well to reduce fat, alcohol, and obesity.

REFERENCES

Adlercreutz, H. Does fiber-rich food containing animal lignan precursors protect against both colon and breast cancer? An extension of the "fiber hypothesis." *Gastroenterology, 86*: 761–766 (1984).

Adlercreutz, H., Fotsis, T., Heikkinen, R., et al. Excretion of the lignans enterolactone and enterodiol and of equol in omnivorous and vegetarian postmenopausal women and in women with breast cancer. *Lancet 2*: 1295–1299 (1982).

Ames, B., Magaw, R., Gold, L. Ranking possible carcinogenic hazards. *Science 236*: 272–279 (1987).

Ballard-Barbash, R. M., Schatzkin, A., Carter, C. L., et al. Body fat distribution and breast cancer in the Framingham Study. *JNCI 82*: 286–290 (1990).

Bartsch, H. Castegnaro, M., O'Neill, I. K., Okada, M. *N-nitroso compounds: occurrence and biologic effects*. IARC Sci. Publications No. 41; IARC, Lyon, 1982.

Bartsch, H., Oshima, H., Pignatelli, B. Inhibitors of endogenous nitrosation. Mechanisms and implications in human cancer prevention. *Mutat. Res. 202*: 307–324 (1988).

Begg, C. B., Walker, A. M., Wessen, B., et al. Alcohol consumption and breast cancer. (letter). *Lancet 1*: 293–294 (1983).

Benito, E., Obrader, A., Bosch, X., et al. A population-based case-control study of colrectal cancer in Majorca. *Int. J. Cancer 45*:69–76 (1990).

Berta, J-L, Coste, T., Rautureau, J., Guilloud-Bataille, M., Pequinot, G. Alimentation et cancers rectocoliques. Resultats d'une etude "cas-temoin." *Gastroenterol. Clin Biol. 9*: 348–353 (1985).

Bertram, J. S., Kolonel, L. N., Meyskens, F. L. Rationale and strategies for chemoprevention of cancer in humans. *Cancer Res 47*: 3012–3031 (1987).

Bjelke, E. Epidemiological studies of cancer of the stomach, colon and rectum Vol. III, Case-control sudy of gastrointestinal cancer in Norway. Vol. IV, Case-control study of the digestive tract cancers in Minnesota. Ann Arbor, Univ. Microfilms, 1973.

Bristol, J. B., Emmett, P. M., Heaton, K. W., Williamson, R. C. N. Sugar, fat, and the risk of colorectal cancer. *Br. Med. J. 291*: 1467–1470 (1985).

Brock, K. E., Berry, G., Mock, P. A., et al. Nutrients in diet and plasma and risk of in situ cervical cancer. *JNCI 80*: 580–585 (1988).

Bruce, W. R. Recent hypotheses for the origin of colon cancer. *Cancer Res. 97*: 4237–4242 (1987).

Brukitt, D. P. Epidemiology of cancer of the colon and rectum. *Cancer 28*: 3–13 (1971).

Burney, P. G. J., Comstock, G. W., Morris, J. S. Serologic precursors of cancer: Serum micronutrients and the subsequent risk of pancreatic cancer. *Am. J. Clin. Nutr. 49*: 895–900 (1989).

Byers, T., Funch, D. P. Alcohol and breast cancer. (letter). *Lancet 1*: 799–800 (1982).

Byers, T. E., Graham, S., Haughey, B. P., et al. Diet and lung cancer risk: Findings from the western New York diet study. *Am. J. Epidemiol 125*: 351–363 (1987).

Chasseaud, L. F. The role of glutathione and glutathione S-transferases in the metabolism of chemical carcinogens and other electrophilic agents. *Adv. Cancer Res. 29*: 175–274 (1979).

Dales, L. G., Friedman, G. D., Ury, H. K., Grossman, S., Williams, S. R. A case-control study of the relationships of diets and other traits to colorectal cancer in American Blacks. *Am. J. Epidemiol 109*: 132–144 (1979).

de Waard, F., Baanders-van Halewijn, E. A., Huizinga, J. The bimodal age distribution of patients with mammary carcinoma: Evidence for the existence of 2 types of human breast cancer. *Cancer 17*: 141–151 (1964).

Donahue, R. B., Abbott, R. D., Bloom, F., et al. Central obesity and coronary heart disease in men. *Lancet 1*: 821–824 (1987).

Durbec, J. P., Chevillotte, G., Bidart, J. M., Berthezene, P., Sarles, H. Diet, alcohol, tobacco and risk of cancer of the pancreas: A case-control study. *Br. J. Cancer 47*: 463–470 (1983).

Eaton, B. S., Konner, M. Paleolithic nutrition. *N. Eng. J. Med. 312*: 283–289 (1985).

Elwood, J. M., Cole, P., Rothman, K. J., Kaplan, S. D. Epidemiology of endometrial cancer. *JNCI 59*: 1055–1060 (1977).

Falk, R. T., Pickle, L. W., Fontham, E. T., Correa, P., Fraumeni, J. F. Life-style risk factors for pancreatic cancer in Louisiana: A case-controlled study. *Am. J. Epidemiol. 128*: 324–336 (1988).

Feldman, R., Sender, A. J., Siegelaub, A. B. Difference in diabetic and non-diabetic fat distribution patterns by skinfold measurements. *Diabetes 18*: 478–486 (1969).

Folsom, A. R., Kaye, S. A., Potter, J. D., Prineas, R. J. Association of incident carcinoma of the endometrium with body weight and fat distribution in older women. Early findings of the Iowa Women's Study. *Cancer Res. 49*: 6828–6831 (1989).

Folsom, A. R., Kaye, S. A., Prineas, R. J., Potter, J. D., Gapstur, S. M., Wallace, R. B. Increased incidence of carcinoma of the breast associated with abdominal adiposity in post-menopausal women. *Am. J. Epidemiol 131*: 794–803 (1990).

Frisch, R. E., McArthur, J. W. Menstrual cycles: Fatness as a determinant of the minimum weight for height necessary for their maintenance or onset. *Science 185*: 949–951 (1974).

Frisch, R. E., Wyshak, G. Albright, N. L., et al. Lower prevalence of breast cancer and cancers of the reproductive system among former college athletes compared to nonathletes. *Br. J. Cancer 52*: 885–891 (1985).

Garabrant, D. H., Peters, J. M., Mack, T. M., Bernstein, L. Job activity and colon cancer risk. *Am. J. Epidemiol. 119*: 1005–1014 (1984).

Gerhardsson, M., Norell, S. E., Kiviranta, H., Pedersen, N. L., Ahlbom, A. Sedentary jobs and colon cancer. *Am J. Epidemiol 123*: 775–780 (1986).

Gold, E. B., Gordis, L., Diener, M. D., et al. Diet and other risk factors for cancer of the pancreas. *Cancer 55*: 469–467 (1985).

Gorbach, S. L. Estrogens breast cancer, and intestinal flora. *Rev. Infect. Dis. 6*(Suppl): 85–90 (1984).

Graham, S., Dayal, H., Swanson, M., Mittelman, A., Wilkinson, G. Diet in the epidemiology of cancer of the colon and rectum. *J. Natl. Cancer Inst. 61*: 709–714 (1978).

Graham, S., Marshall, J., Haughey, B., et al. Dietary epidemiology of cancer of the colon in western New York. *Am. J. Epidemiol. 128*: 490–503 (1988).

Graham, S., Marshall, J., Mettlin, C., et al. Diet in the epidemiology of breast cancer. *Am. J. Epidemiol. 116*: 68–75 (1982).

Greunke, L. D., Wrensch, M. R., Petrakis, N. H., et al. Breast fluid cholesterol and cholesterol epoxides: relationship to breast cancer risk factors and other characteristics. *Cancer Res 47*: 5483–5487 (1987).

Grodin, J. M., Siiteri, P. K., MacDonald, P. C. Source of estrogen production in postmenopausal women. *J. Clin. Endocrinol. Metab. 36*: 207–214 (1973).

Haenszel, W., Berg, J. W., Segi, M., Kurihara, M., and Locke, F. B. Large bowel cancer in Hawaiian Japanese. *JCNI 51*: 1765–1799 (1973).

Haenszel, W., Locke, F. B., and Segi, M. A case-controlled study of large bowel cancer in Japan. *JNCI 64*: 17–22 (1980).

Harris, R. E., Wynder, E. L. Breast cancer and alcohol consumption: a study in weak associations. *JAMA 259*: 2867–2871 (1988).

Harvey, E. B., Schairer, C., Brinton, L. A. et al. Alcohol consumption and breast cancer. *JNCI 78*: 657–661 (1987).

Hebert, J. R., Miller, D. R. Methodologic considerations for investigating the diet-cancer risk. *Am. J. Clin. Nutr. 47*: 1068–1077 (1988).

Heilbrun, L. K., Nomura, A., Hankin, J. H., Stemmermann, G. N. Diet and colorectal cancer with special reference to fiber intake. *Int. J. Cancer 44*: 1–6 (1989).

Helmrich, S. P., Shapiro, S., Rosenberg, L., et al. Risk factors for breast cancer. *Am. J. Epidemiol. 117*: 35–45 (1983).

Henderson, B. E., Casagrande, J. T., Pike, M. C., Mack, T., Rosario, I., Duke, A. The epidemiology of endometrial cancer in young women. *Br. J. Cancer 47*: 749–756 (1983).

Hiatt, R. A., Bawol, R. D. Alcoholhic beverage consumption and breast cancer incidence. *Am. J. Epidemiol 120*: 676–683 (1984).

Higginson, J. Etiological factors in gastrointestinal cancer in man. *JNCI 37*: 527–545 (1966).

Hill, P., Garbaczewski, L., Helman, P., et al. Diet, lifestyle, and menstrual activity. *Am. J. Clin. Nutr. 33*: 1192–1198 (1980).

Hill, M. J. Goddard, P., Williams, R. E. O. Gut bacteria and aetiology of cancer of the breast. *Lancet 2*: 472–473 (1971).

Hirayama, T. Epidemiology of breast cancer with special reference to the role of diet. *Prev. Med. 7*: 173–195 (1978).

Hirohata, T., Shigematsu, T., Nomura, A.M.Y., et al. Occurrence of breast cancer in relation to diet and reproductive history: a case-control study in Fukuoka, Japan. *Natl. Cancer Inst. Monogr. 67*: 187–190 (1985).

Howatson, A. G., Carter, D. C. Pancreatic carcinogenesis—enhancement by cholecystokinin in the hamster-nitrosamiane model. *Br. J. Cancer 51*: 107–114 (1985).
Howe, G. R. The use of polytomous dual response data to increase power in case-control studies: an application to the association between dietary fat and breast cancer. *J. Chronic Dis. 38*: 663–670 (1985).
Howe, G. R., Miller, A. B., Jain, M. Re "Total energy intake: implications for epidemiologic analyses." *Am. J. Epidemiol. 124*: 156–157 (1986).
Howe, G. R., Jain, M., Miller, A. B. Dietary factors and risk of pancreatic cancer: Results of a Canadian population-based case-control study. *Int. J. Cancer 45*: 604–608 (1990).
IARC (International Agency for Research on Cancer). *Alcohol Drinking*. IARC Monographs, Vol. 44; IARC, Lyon, 1988.
IARC (International Agency for Research on Cancer). *Some Naturally Occurring Substances*. IARC Monographs, Vol. 10; IARC, Lyon, 1976.
Jacobs, L. R. Enhancement of rat colon carcinogenesis by wheat bran consumption during the stage of 1,2-dimethylhydrazine administration. *Cancer Res. 43*: 4057-4061 (1983).
Jacobs, L. R. Stimulation of rat colonic crypt cell proliferative activity by wheat bran consumption during the stage of 1,2-dimethylhydrazine administration. *Cancer Res. 44*: 2458–2463 (1984).
Jacobsen, E. A., Newmark, H.L., McKeown-Eyssen, G., Bruce, W. R. Excretion of 3-methylhistidine in urine as an estimate of meat consumption. *Nutr. Rep. Int. 27*: 689-697 (1983).
Jain, M., Cook, G. M., Davis, F. G., Grace, M. G., Howe, G. R., Miller, A. B. A case-control study of diet and colo-rectal cancer. *Int. J. Cancer 26*: 757–768 (1980).
Johnson, L. R. Effects of gastrointestinal hormones on pancreatic growth. *Cancer 47*: 1640–1645 (1981).
Kark, J. D., Smith, A. H., Switzer, B. R., Hames, C. G. Serum vitamin A (retinol) and cancer incidence in Evans County, Georgia, *JNCI 66*: 7–16 (1981).
Katsouyanni, K., Trichopoulos, D., Boyle, P., et al. Diet and breast cancer: A case-control study in Greece. *Int. J. Cancer 38*: 815–820 (1986).
Kidwell, W. R., Knazek, R. A., Vonderhaar, B. K., et al. Effects of unsaturated fatty acids on the development and proliferation of normal and neoplastic breast epithelium. *Molecular Interrelations of Nutrition and Cancer*. Arndt, M. S., van Eys, J., Wang, Y. M., eds. New York, Raven Press, 1982, p. 219.
Kinlen, L. J. Meat and fat consumption and cancer mortality: A study of strict religious orders in Britain. *Lancet 1*: 946–949 (1982).
Kolonel, L. N., Hankin, J. H., Nomura, A. M., Chu, S. Y. Dietary fat intake and cancer incidence among five ethnic groups in Hawaii. *Cancer Res. 41*: 327–328 (1981).
Koo, L. C. Dietary habits and lung cancer risk among Chinese females in Hong Kong who never smoked. *Nutr. Cancer 11*: 155–172 (1988).
Larrson, B., Svarsudd, K., Welin, L. et al. Abdominal adipose tissue distribution, obesity, and risk of cardiovascular disease and death: 13 year follow-up of participants in the study of men born in1913. *Br. Med. J. 288*: 1401–1404 (1984).
La Vecchia, C., Decarli, A., Fasoli, M., et al. Dietary vitamin A and the risk of intraepithelial and invasive cervical neoplasia. *Gynecol. Oncol. 30*: 187–195 (1988b).

LaVecchia, C., Decarli, A., Franceschi, S., et al. Alcohol consumption and the risk of breast cancer in women. *JNCI 75*: 61-65 (1985).

LaVecchia, C., Franceschi, S., Decarli, A., Gallus, G., Tognoni, G. Risk factors for endometrial cancer at different areas. *JNCI 73*: 667-671 (1984).

LaVecchia, C., Negri, E., Decarli, A., et al. A case-control study of diet and colorectal cancer in northern Italy Int. J. Cancer 41: 492–498 (1988a).

LaVecchia, C., Negri, E., Decarli, A. et al. A case-control study of diet and gastric cancer in northern italy. *Int. J. Cancer 40*: 484-489 (1987).

Le, M. G., Hill, C., Kramer, A. et al. Alcoholic beverage consumption and breast cancer in a French case-control study. *Am. J. Epidemiol. 120*: 350–357 (1984).

Le, M. G., Moulton, L. H., Hill, C., et al. Consumption of dairy produce and alcohol in a case-control study of breast cancer. *JNCI 77*: 633-636 (1986).

Le Marchand, L., Kolonel, L. N., Earle, M. E., et al. Body size at different periods of life and breast cancer risk. *Am. J. Epidemiol. 128*: 137–152 (1988).

Lew, E. A., Garfinkel, L. Variations in mortality by weight among 750,000 men and women. *J. Chron. Dis. 32*: 563-576 (1979).

Lubin, F., Wax, Y., Modan, B. Role of fat, animal protein and dietary fiber in breast cancer etiology: A case-controlled study. *JNCI 77*: 605-612 (1986).

Lubin, J. H., Burns, P. E., Blot, W. J., et al. Dietary factors and breast cancer risk. *Int. J. Cancer 28*: 685-689 (1981).

Lyon, J. L., Gardner, J. W., West, D. W., Mahoney, A. M. Methodological issues in epidemiologic studies of diet and cancer. *Cancer Res. 43*(Suppl):2392-2396 (1983).

Lyon, J. L., Mahoney, A. W., West, D. W., Gardner, J. W., Smith, K. R., Sorenson, A. W., Stanish, W. Energy intake: Its relationship to colon cancer risk. *JNCI 78*: 853-861 (1987).

Mack, T. M., Paganini-Hill, A. Epidemiology of pancreas cancer in Los Angeles. *Cancer 47*: 1474-1483 (1981).

Macquart-Moulin, G., Riboli, E., Cornee, J., Charnay, B., Berthezene, P., Day, N. Case-control study on colorectal cancer and diet in Marseilles. *Int. J. Cancer 38*: 183–191 (1986).

Manousos, O., Day, N. E., Trichopoulos, D., Gerovassilis, F., Tzonou, A., Polychronopoulou, A. Diet and colorectal cancer: A case-control study in Greece. *Int. J. Cancer 32*: 1-5 (1983).

Martinez, I., Torres, R., Frias, Z., Colon, J. R., Fernandez, N. Factors associated with adenocarcinomas of the large bowel in Puerto Rico *Adv. Med. Oncol. Res. Ed. 3*: 45-52 (1979).

McLaughlin, J. K., Gridley, G., Block, G., et al. Dietary factors in oral and pharyngeal cancer. *JNCI 15*: 1237-1243 (1988).

McMichael, A. J., Potter, J. D. Diet and colon cancer: Integration of the descriptive, analytic, and metabolic epidemiology. *N.C.I. Monogr. 69*: 223-228 (1985).

McMichael, A. J., Potter, J. D. Dietary influences upon colon carcinogenesis. *Diet, Nutrition and Cancer* (Y. Hayashi et al., eds), Japan Sci. Soc. Press, Tokyo, pp. 275-290.

McMichael, A. J. Coffee, soya and pancreatic cancer. *Lancet 2*: 689-690 (1981).

McMurchie, E. J., Potter, J. D., Rohan, T. E., Hetzel, B. S. Human cheek cells: A non-invasive method for determining tissue lipid profiles in dietary and nutritional studies. *Nut Rep.Int. 29*: 519-526 (1984).

Micozzi, M. S. Nutrition, body size, and breast cancer. *Yearbook Phys. Antropol. 28*: 175-206 (1985).

Micozzi, M. S., Beecher, G. R. Taylor, P. R., Khachik, F. Carotenoid analysis of selected raw and cooked foods associated with a lower risk for cancer. *JNCI 82*: 282–285 (1990).

Miller, A. B., Howe, G. R., Jain, M., Craib, K. J. P., Harrison, L. Food items and food groups as risk factors in a case-control study of diet and colorectal cancer. *Int. J. Cancer 32*: 155-161 (1983).

Miller, A. B., Kelly, A., Choi, N. W., et al. A study of diet and breast cancer. *Am. J. Epidemiol. 1078*: 499–509 (1978).

Mills, P. K., Beeson, L., Abbey, D. E., Fraser, G. E., Phillips, R. L. Dietary habits and past medical history as related to fatal pancreas cancer risk among Adventists. *Cancer 61*: 2578–2585 (1988).

Mirvish, S. S. Ascorbic acid inhibition of N-nitroso compound formation in chemical, food and biological systems. In *Inhibition of Tumor Induction and Development* (M. S. Zedeck and M. Lipkin, eds.), Plenum, New York, 1981, pp. 101–126.

Modan, B., Barell, V., Lubin, F., Modan, M., Greenberg, R. A., Graham, S. Low-fiber intake as an etiologic fact in cancer of the colon. *JNCI 55*: 15–18 (1975).

Moon, T., and Micozzi, M. S. *Nutrition and Cancer Prevention: Investigating the Role of Micronutrients*, Marcel Dekker, New York, 1989.

Muñoz, N., Wahrendorf, J., Lu, J-B, et al. No effect of riboflavine, retinol and zinc on prevalence of pre-cancerous lesions of oesophagus. Randomized double-blind intervention study in high-risk population of China. *Lancet 2*: 111–114 (1985).

Neel, J. V. Current concepts of the genetic basis of diabetes mellitus and the biological significance of the diabetic predisposition. In *Diabetes* (J. Ostman and R. D. G. Milner, eds.), Excerpta Medica, Amsterdam, pp. 68–78.

Norell, S. E., Ahlbom, A., Erwald, R., et al. Diet and pancreatic cancer: A case-control study. *Am. J. Epidemiol. 124*: 894–902 (1986).

O'Connell, D. L., Hulka, B. S., Chambless, L. E., et al. Cigarette smoking, alcohol consumption, and breast cancer risk. *JNCI 78*: 229–234 (1987).

Oishi, K., Okada, K., Yoshida, O., et al. A case-controlled study of prostatic cancer with reference to dietary habits. *Prostate 12*: 179–190 (1988).

Paffenbarger, R. S., Hyde, R. T., Wing, A. L. Physicial activity and incidence of cancer in diverse populations: a preliminary report. *Am. J. Clin Nutr. 45*: 311–317 (1987).

Paffenbarger, R. S., Kampert, J. B., Chang, H-G. Characteristics that predict risk of breast cancer before and after the menopause. *Am. J. Epidemiol 112*: 258–268 (1980).

Paganini-Hill, A., Ross, R. K. Breast cancer and alcohol consumption. (letter) *Lancet 2*: 626–627 (1983).

Pariza, M. W., Simopoulos, A. P. Calories and energy expenditure in carcinogenesis. *Am. J. Clin. Nutr. 45*(Suppl): 149–272 (1986).

Peers, F., Bosch, X., Kaldor, J., et al. Aflatoxin exposure, hepatitis B virus infection, and liver cancer in Swaziland. *Int. J. Cancer 39*: 454–553 (1987).

Pernu, J. An epidemiological study on cancer of the digestive organs and respiratory system. A study based on 7078 cases. *Ann. Med. Intern. Fenn. 49*(Suppl. 3): 1–117 (1960).

Peto, R., Doll, R., Buckley, J. D., Sporn, M. B. Can dietary beta-carotene materially reduce human cancer rates? *Nature 290*: 201–208 (1981).

Petrakis, N. L., Mack, C. A., Lee, R. E., et al. Mutagenic activity in nipple aspirates of human breast fluid. *Cancer Res. 40*: 188–189 (1980).

Phillips, R. L. Role of life-style and dietary habits in risk of cancer among Seventh-day Adventists. *Cancer Res. 35*: 3513–3522 (1975).

Phillips, R. L., Garfinkel, L., Kuzma, J. W., et al. Mortality among California Seventh-day Adventists for selected cancer sites. *JNCI 65*: 1097–1107 (1980).

Phillips, R. L., Snowdon, D. A. Association of meat and coffee use with cancers of the large bowel, breast and prostate among Seventh-day Adventists: Preliminary results. *Cancer Res. 43*(Suppl):2403–2408 (1983).

Pitot, H. C. *Fundamentals of Oncology*, 3rd ed. Marcel Dekker, New York, 1986.

Potter, J. D. The epidemiology of fiber and colorectal cancer: Why don't the analytic epidemiology make better sense? In *Dietary Fiber: Chemistry, Physiology, and Health Effects* (D. Kritchersky et al., ed.), Plenum Press (1989a).

Potter, J. D. Large bowel cancer: Epidemiology and biology. *Verh. Bd. 24*: 137–140 (1989b).

Potter, J. D. The epidemiology and prevention of pancreas cancer. In *Cancer Prevention Vital Statistics to Intervention* (W. Zatonski et al., eds.), Interpress, Warsaw, PA (1990).

Potter, J.D., Graves K.L. Diet and cancer: evidence and mechanisms—an adaptation argument. In *Nutrition Toxicity and Cancer* (I. Rowland, ed.), CRC Press (1991).

Potter, J. D., McMichael, A. J. Diet and cancer of the colon and rectum A case-control study. *JNCI 76*: 557–569 (1986).

Potter, J. D., McMichael, A.J., Hartshorne, J. M. Alcohol and beer consumption in relation to cancer of bowel and lung: An extended correlation analysis. *J. Chronic Dis. 35*: 823–824 (1982).

Rohan, T. E., Bain, C. J. Diet in the etiology of breast cancer. *Epidemiol. Rev. 9*: 120–145 (1987).

Rohan, T. E., McMichael, a. J. Alcohol consumption and risk of breast cancer. *Int. J. Cancer 41*: 695–699 (1988).

Rohan, T. E., Potter, J. D. Retrospective assessment of dietary intake. *Am. J. Epidemiol. 120*: 876–887 (1984).

Rosenberg, L., Slone, D., Shaprio, S., et al. Breast cancer and alcoholic-beverage consumption. *Lancet 1*: 267–271 (1982).

Schatazkin, A., Carter, C. L., Green, S. B. et al. Is alcohol consumption related to breast cancer? Results from the Framingham Heart Study. *JNCI 81*: 31–35 (1989).

Schatzkin, A., Jones,Y., Hoover, R. N., et al. Alcohol consumption and breast cancer in the epidemiologic follow-up study of the first National Health and Nutrition Examination Survey. *N. Engl. J. Med 316*: 1169–1137 (1987).

Selby, J. V., Friedman, G. D., Quesenberry, C. P. Precursors of essential hypertension. The role of body fat distribution pattern. *Am. J. Epidemiol. 129*: 43–53 (1989).

Shun-Zhang, Y. Rui-Fang, L., Da-Dao, X. Howe, G. R. A case-control study of dietary and nondietary risk factors for breast cancer in Shanghai. *Cancer Res. 50*: 5017–5021 (1990).

Slattery, M. L., Schumacher, M. C., Smith, K. R., West, D. W. Abd-Elghany, N. Physical activity, diet and risk of colon cancer in Utah. *Am. J. Epidemiol 128*: 989–999 (1988a).

Slattery, M. L., Sorenson, A. W., Ford, M.H. Dietary calcium intake as a mitigating factor in colon cancer. *Am. J. Epidemiol. 128*: 504–514 (1988b).

Spitz, M. R., Fueger, J.J., Beddingfield, N. A., Annegers, J. F., Hsu, T. C., Newell, G. R. Chromosome sensitivity to bleomycin-induced mutagenesis, an independent risk factor for upper aerodigestive tract cancers. *Cancer Res.49*: 4626–4628 (1989).

Spitz, M. R., Fueger, J. J., Goepfert, H., Hong, W. K., Newell, G. R. Squamous cell carcinoma of the upper aerodigestive tract: a case comparison analysis. *Cancer 61*: 203–208 (1988).

Stacewicz-Sapuntzakis, M., Bowen, P. E., Kikendall, J. W., Buress, M. Simultaneous determination of serum retinol and various carotenoids: Their distribution in middle-aged men and women. *J. Micro. Analysis. 3*: 27–45 (1987).

Stocks, P. Breast cancer anomalies *Br. J. Cancer 24*: 633-643 (1970).

Stocks, P. Cancer incidence in North Wales and Liverpool region in relation to habits and environment. Brit. Emp. Cancer Campaign 35th Annual Report Suppl. to Part 2, London, 1957, pp. 1–127.

Stragand, J. J., Hagemann, R. F. Effect of lumenal contents on colonic cell replacement. *Am. J. Physiol 233*: E208-E211 (1977).

Talamini, R., LaVecchia, C., Decarli, A., et al. Social factors, diet and breast cancer in a northern Italian population. *Br.J. Cancer 49*: 723–729 (1984).

Thurnham, D. I., Zheng, S-F, Munoz, N. et al. Comparison of riboflavin, vitamin A, and zinc status of Chinese populations at high and low risk for esophageal cancer. *Nutr. Cancer 7*: 131–143 (1985).

Trock, B., Lanza, E., Greenwald, P. Dietary fiber, vegetables and colon cancer: Critical review and meta-analysis of the epidemiologic evidence. *JNCI 82*: 650–661 (1990).

Tuyns, A. J., Kaaks, R., Haelterman, M. Colorectal cancer and the consumption of foods: A case-control study in Belgium. *Nutr. Cancer 11*: 189–204 (1988).

Vague, J. The degree of masculine differentiation of obesities: A factor determining predisposition to diabetes, atherosclerosis, gout and uric calculous disease. *Am. J. Clin. Nutr. 4*: 20–34 (1956).

van Rensburg, S. J. Epidemiologic and dietary evidence for a specific nutritinal predisposition to esophageal cancer. *JNCI 67*: 243–251 (1981).

Velema, J. P., Walker, A. M., Gold, E. B. Alcohol and pancreatic cancer: Insufficient epidemiological evidence for a causal relationship. *Epidemiologic Reviews 8*: 28–41 (1986).

Vena, J. E., Graham, S., Zielezny, M., Swanson, M. K., Barnes, R. E., and Nolan, J. Lifetime occupational exercise and colon cancer. *Am. J. Epidemiol 122*: 357–365 (1985).

Vitale, J. J., Broitman, S. A. Lipids and immune function. *Cancer Res. 41*: 3706–3710 (1981).

Wahrendorf, J., Munoz, N., Lu, J-B, et al. Blood retinol, zinc, riboflavin status in relation to pre-cancerous lesions of the eosphagus: Findings for a vitamin intervention trial in the People's Republic of China. *Cancer Res. 48*: 2280–2283 (1988).

Wald, N., Idle, M., Boreham, J., Bailey, A. Low serum-vitamin A and subsequent risk of cancer. Preliminary results of a prospective study. *Lancet 2*: 813–815 (1980).

Wattenberg, L. W. Chemoprevention of cancer. *Cancer Res. 45*: 1-8 (1985).

Wattenberg, L. W. Inhibition of carcinogenic effects of polycyclid hydrocarbons by benzyl isothiocyanate and related compounds. *JNCI 58*: 395–398 (1977).

Wattenberg, L. W. Inhibition of neoplasia by minor dietary constituents. *Cancer Res. 43* (Suppl):2448s–2453s (1983).

Webster, L. A., Layde, P. M., Wingo, P. A., et al. Alcohol consumption and risk of breast cancer. *Lancet* 2: 724–726 (1983).

Welsch, C. W., Aylsworth, C. F. Enhancement of murine mammary tumorigenesis by feeding high levels of dietary fat: A hormonal mechanism. *JNCI 70*: 215–221 (1983).

Willett, W. C. *Dietary Epidemiology*. Oxford University Press, New York, 1989.

Willett, W. C., Browne, M. L., Bain, C. et al. Relative weight and risk of breast cancer among premenopausal women. *Am. J. Epidemiol. 122*: 731–740 (1985).

Willett, W. C., Polk, B. F., Morris, J. S. et al. Prediagnostic serum selenium and risk of cancer. *Lancet* 2: 130–134 (1983).

Willett, W. C., Stampfer, M. J. Total energy intake: Implications for epidemiologic analyses. *Am. J. Epidemiol 124*: 17–27 (1986).

Willett, W. C., Stampfer, M. J., Colditz, G. A., et al. Dietary fat and risk of breast cancer. *N. Engl. J. Med. 316*: 22–28 (1987a).

Willet, W. C., Stampfer, M.J., Colditz, G. A., et al. Moderate alcohol consumption and the risk of breast cancer. *N. Engl. J. Med. 316*: 1174–1180 (1987b).

Willett, W. C., Stampfer, M. J., Colditz, G. A. et al. Relation of meat, fat, and fiber intake to the risk of colon cancer in a prospective study among women. *N. Engl. J. Med. 323*: 1664–1672 (1990).

Williams, R. R. Breast and thyroid cancer and malignant melanoma promoted by alcohol-induced pituitary secretion of prolactin, TSH, and MSH. *Lancet 1*: 996–999 (1976).

Williams, R. R., Horm, J. W. Association of cancer sites with tobacco and alcohol consumption and socioeconomic status of patients: interview study from the Third National Cancer Survey. *JNCI 58*: 525–547 (1977).

Wood, A. W., Huang, M. T., Chang, R. L. et al. Inhibition of the mutagenicity of bay-region diol epoxides of polycyclic hydrocarbons by naturally occurring plant phenols: exceptional activity of ellagic acid. *Proc. Nat. Acad. Sci. 79*: 5513–5517 (1982).

Wu, A.H., Paganini-Hill, A., Ross, R. K., Henderson, B. E. Alcohol, physical activity and to her risk factors for colorectal cancer: a prospective study. *Br. J. Cancer 55*: 687–694 (1987).

Wynder, E. L., Kajitani, T., Ishikana, S., Dodo, H., Tako, A. Environmental factors of cancer of the colon and rectum II. Japanese epidemiological data. *Cancer 23*: 1210–1220 (1969).

Wynder, E. L., Shigematsu, T. Environmental factors of cancer of the colon and rectum. *Cancer 20*: 1520–1561 (1967).

Yang, C. S. Research on esophageal cancer in China: A review. *Cancer Res. 40*: 2633–2644 (1980).

You, W-C., Blot, W. J., Chang, Y-S, et al. Diet and high-risk of stomach cancer in Shandong, China. *Cancer Res. 48*: 3518–3523 (1988).

Young, T. B. A case-control study of breast cancer and alcohol consumption habits. *Cancer 64*: 552–558 (1989).

Young, T. B., Wolf, D. A. Case-control study of proximal and distal colon cancer and diet in Wisconsin. *Int. J. Cancer 42*: 167–175 (1988).

part two

METHODS FOR INVESTIGATING THE ROLE OF MACRONUTRIENTS

4

Dietary Assessment Methods for Macronutrients

Anne M. Hartman and Gladys Block*
National Cancer Institute
National Institutes of Health
Bethesda, Maryland

The ability to examine associations between diet and disease, to monitor diet change in prevention studies, and to control for dietary factors in studies of other risk factors all depend on the adequacy of the dietary assessment methods. This chapter will discuss the dietary methods, their validity, and the limitations and appropriate uses of the types of data they produce, including adjustment for energy intake and measurement error, and implications for sample size. Before turning to the specific methods, however, two overriding issues must be considered—the nutrients to be assessed and the need for data representative of the usual diets of individuals.

SELECTED DIETARY COMPONENTS OR THE WHOLE DIET?

Collecting information on one or a few nutrients may be justified in some situations. However, for etiologic research, control of confounding, or examination of effect modification, it is usually unwise and poor economy to restrict data collection to a limited list of a few nutrients. Current laboratory or epidemiologic data suggest that relationships exist between cancer and a number of macronutrients and related dietary components including total calories, total fat, percent of calories derived from fat, specific fat fractions, cholesterol, dietary fiber and fiber fractions, alcohol, and others (see other chapters in this volume). In addition, there is strong evidence of a relationship between cancer and micronutrients and food

**Current affiliation*: University of California, Berkeley, California

groups, such as fruits and vegetables and cruciferous vegetables (1–4). Studies that do not attempt to assess the whole diet may, at worst, result in erroneous conclusions. Foods contain many nutrients simultaneously. If we only ask about a specific macronutrient, we may conclude that an observed effect is due to the specific macronutrient, when instead it may simply be that it is positively (or negatively) associated with the true etiologic factor. A great deal of effort, expense, and public credibility may then be wasted conducting interventions on the wrong dietary factor.

For example, to assess the importance of fat in cancer prevention, it is essential to simultaneously consider the role of total energy (calories), necessitating the inclusion of a wider range of food intake than simply those foods that are major contributors of fat. Willett and Stampfer (5) have emphasized the importance of considering total calorie consumption when investigating fat as well as the relation of any other dietary component to disease. We will return to the issue of energy adjustment later in this chapter.

At best, studies collecting data on only a few elements of the diet leave a great many questions unanswered. Is a high polyunsaturated fat intake only harmful in the presence of a low intake of vitamin E, a lipid antioxidant? (In processed foods, some of the vitamin E normally associated with polyunsaturates may be destroyed.) Is it dietary fiber or something else like vitamin C, folacin, or carotenoids contributed by the vegetable kingdom that is protective against colon cancer? Only by capturing the whole multidimensional diet can we begin to examine dietary associations and interactions such as those noted above and others related to food patterns (6), an area where our understanding is minimal at best (7).

AN INDIVIDUAL'S USUAL DIET

It is necessary to consider the purposes of the dietary data when choosing assessment methods, because the methods vary in their ability to measure validly the usual intake of an individual. It is the latter that is needed for studies of diet-disease relationships. For some purposes, data on the mean intake of groups may be useful. Group means may be used to compare the progress of two randomized diet groups, for example, or to examine the balance on baseline dietary characteristics. They may also be used to assess whether the mean intake of a population subgroup meets the Recommended Dietary Allowances (RDA) for a given nutrient, in which case the nutrient estimate is needed with accuracy and precision, but at the group mean level. Even in those cases, however, more useful information would be obtained by describing the *distribution* of intakes, such as what proportion is below a certain level, something for which the mean alone is useless (8–10).

To study the relationship between diet and disease or other physiologic characteristics with adequate statistical power, data are needed, not at the group level, but at the individual level. International correlations between cancer mortality and food disappearance data, or other comparisons of groups, provide "clues" but not direct answers to etiologic hypotheses (11). It may be thought that epidemiologists and other medical researchers study groups—cases and controls, for example—and consequently that methods appropriate for group data may be used. However, analytic epidemiologic studies, including *case-control studies* and *prospective studies*, involve not the examination of group means but the *categorization* of *individuals* into exposed or nonexposed. Dietary methods that cannot at least place individuals into approximately the correct quantile of the distribution of intake of a nutrient will not permit studies of this sort with any statistical power or precision of risk estimates.

Prevention studies or clinical trials may use group means for the purpose of monitoring whether study groups are adhering to a prescribed diet or evaluating balance between the groups with respect to group means. However, to investigate whether the effect of the intervention may be different in subsets with high or low dietary intake (effect modification), or for managing individual noncompliance with the prescribed diet, individually valid data are needed.

DIETARY ASSESSMENT METHODS: DESCRIPTION AND VALIDITY

This has been reviewed extensively elsewhere (10,12–18). Thus, we will only briefly describe methods and highlight a few studies and issues.

24-Hour Recalls

In this method, the respondent reports his or her complete dietary intake of all foods and beverages consumed over the past 24 hours. Its strength lies in the fact that, if properly performed, it can provide information detailed enough to permit extremely precise coding of the foods consumed, and thus of the nutrients consumed during that 24-hour period. This accuracy is, however, dependent on a number of factors. First, portion size must be obtained accurately, ideally with three-dimensional models or picture booklets, since research indicates that individuals of all ages are poor estimators of their portion sizes (19). Second, precision in coding requires careful probing and interviewers with nutrition experience. Finally, a detailed database for exact food type and preparation method is needed to minimize use of "Not Further Specified" codes, an important source of imprecision in group as well as individual estimates. Values for "Not Futher Specified" codes should be assigned based on foods that are most commonly eaten rather than by the so-called "conservative" approach, which uses the most extreme value in the database (the fattiest cuts of meat, for example), regardless of its frequency of consumption.

The 24-hour-recall method thus requires a highly trained interviewer and usually takes 20–30 minutes to perform. The coding of the completed interview also requires considerable time and well-trained coders. Some investigators have used it with telephone interviews, and Posner et al. (20) have developed two-dimensional models and pictures, which are sent to the respondent ahead of time to enhance portion size accuracy.

The method has been validated by comparing the mean nutrient estimates with estimates produced by collecting and weighing duplicate meals or by direct observation (21–24), or by detailed food diaries (25,26). It generally produces estimates of the mean nutrient intake of a group that are similar to those of a reference method. However, there is also evidence that forgetting may produce underestimation of nutrient intake (13,17,21).

The chief drawback of the 24-hour recall for research on the relationship between diet and disease or diet and serum levels is that it does not provide precise estimates of the *usual* diet of *individuals* (26–28). This is a result of the day-to-day variability in ordinary diets. Thus, a single 24-hour recall is primarily useful only to measure the *mean* intake of groups. If used to obtain multiple recalls per person taken on nonconsecutive days, however, it can be used to assess individual "usual" intake (29). Day-to-day variability and number of days required are discussed below under "Errors in Dietary Assessment: Impact and Adjustment."

Diet Records

In this method respondents are asked to record their diet as they are consuming it, thus minimizing errors of memory. When a diet record is performed carefully, it can capture components of diet which might be overlooked by a recall, and affords the opportunity to obtain more accurate portion size estimation through measuring or weighing. It requires that respondents be reasonably literate and comfortable with the idea of careful record keeping and be sufficiently committed to the goals of the study to perform the record keeping conscientiously and *not* change eating habits as a result of food recording.

Using direct observation of an elderly congregate meal site as a reference method, Gersovitz et al. (22) found that a 7-day record reasonably represented group means for most nutrients studied, but accuracy of the recorded values declined after the first 2 days. Because of this decline, and because consecutive days have been shown to provide less information about usual diet than the same number of nonconsecutive days, multiple-day food records should be in the form of 1- or at the most 2-day units scattered over a longer period of time (30,31).

Multiple-day records demand the time and cooperation of the respondents. Thus, they are of limited use in large-scale population studies, in which the cost would be extremely high, and the sample that could be induced to participate might be unrepresentative. They also require careful instruction beforehand by a nutritionist, careful review afterwards, and are extremely demanding of expert time in the coding process (in 1990, coding alone costs nearly $100 per person per 4-day record). For studies that can afford them, 1- to 2-day records, like 24-hour recalls, can provide reasonably valid data on the mean intake of groups; however, to assess the usual intake of individuals, multiple food records, like multiple 24-hour recalls, are necessary.

Diet History and Food Frequency Questionnaires

Historically, the diet history as proposed by Burke and Stuart (32,33) required a detailed interview with a trained nutritionist, 1–1.5 hours in length, asking about a typical day's consumption pattern utilizing a 24-hour recall. The interviewer asked about deviations from this pattern, and also used a list of foods for cross-checking. The respondent was also required to complete a 3-day food record. Utilizing all of these components, overall subjective estimates of nutrient intakes were made. Thus, because the traditional diet history (composite) included a 24-hour recall and a 3-day food record, it may have been heavily influenced by the individual's diet of the last few days (34).

Since then, simplified and more objective questionnaires, primarily list-based and structured, have been developed requiring a shorter time to complete and less dependent on the diet of the last few days. They may be administered by nonnutritionist interviewers or may be self-administered. It is thus possible to use them in large population studies in which the purpose is to categorize individuals broadly with respect to usual intake. Coding of such questionnaires is usually relatively fast and does not require nutritional expertise, and can even be made machine-readable (35,36). These questionnaires may ask the respondent to report his usual frequency of consumption of single food items or groups of food to assess intake of single nutrients, or their compostion may be more varied in order to capture the "whole" diet. To estimate the nutrients, the food list must reflect the population's major sources of those nutrients, influenced by frequency of consumption, portion size, and nutrient content of food items (37–41). It is also necessary for the food items to be distinct.

If information is sought on portion size, either through use of household measures or food models (29,34,42), photographs (40,41,43,44), or a small-medium-large approach (45,46), the questionnaire is termed a diet history; if no portion size information is asked of the respondent, the questionnaire is termed a food frequency. Nutrient estimates are obtained by multiplying the frequency of consumption by the nutrient content of the reported portion size (or nutrient content in a standard portion size if individual portion size information is not asked).

Portion Size

There is controversy about the need for portion size information in epidemiologic studies (16). In some studies, there is evidence that portion size assessment yields higher correlations between the questionnaire and food records (46–50); in other studies there is little or no advantage with respect to correlations with food records (16,51) or, for vitamin A, with respect to ranking or relative risk (52,53). Other studies have suggested that self-reporting portion sizes without any aids is not accurate (19,54,55) or have indicated a bias in reporting for obese persons (56) or a "flattened slope syndrome," where there is a tendency for the instrument to overestimate small intakes and underestimate larger intakes (21,22); still others have found no problem with self-reported portion size (23,41). Hunter et al. (57) found that within-person variability of portion size estimates is much greater than between-person variability, suggesting that a respondent might have difficulty identifying a "typical" portion size. While there is controversy over portion size, the evidence suggests that simple methods (photos and small-medium-large approach) have improved some correlations with little extra time and expense. Even small improvements in accuracy may be useful, especially if the extra time and expense are trivial. In addition, better estimates of the *absolute level* of nutrient intake have been found with inclusion of portion size information (45,46,48–50,58). For purposes of monitoring nutrient status or for interpreting biochemical, clinical, and epidemiologic findings in a public health framework, portion size information is likely to be beneficial.

Pattern of Intake Vesus Exact Memory

Diet history or food frequency questionnaires attempt to elicit information about the respondents' customary dietary intake at the present time in their lives, or in case-control studies sometime in the recent past, for example, just before diagnosis of cancer. For cohort and intervention studies, the time frame often specified is the past year, a period long enough to encompass normal seasonal variation and to smooth out shorter-term aberrations. Sometimes diet histories focus the respondent on a shorter time period, such as the past month, in the belief that recall over a shorter, more recent time may be more accurate. While this has not been definitively studied, a shorter time frame runs the danger of reflecting an unrepresentative seasonal peak or trough, or a time when a certain food was eaten with atypical frequency. Furthermore, restricting the reported period to a shorter time may lead the respondent to attempt to *remember exactly* (specific memory) rather than report a usual pattern of frequency (generic memory). Requiring subjects to "remember" exactly what they eat is not a good practice because recent reports investigating cognitive skills suggest that actual memory of food consumption rapidly declines with time and is affected by frame of reference (54,55,59–62).

One often hears the objection, "I can't remember what I ate yesterday; how could anyone remember what they ate in the past year?" However, this reflects a misunderstanding of the cognitive process involved. Unlike the 24-hour recall, responses to frequency questionnaires or diet histories asking about "usual diet" over a larger period of time ($\geq$ one month) do not invoke *memory* and do not involve the remembering of specific instances or events. Rather, they involve the recognition and reporting of a *pattern* of behavior. When asked, "How often do you eat eggs?," the respondent does not attempt to remember each instance of egg-eating over the past year. Rather, he reports a pattern: "I eat eggs about twice a week."

Retrospective Diet

Sometimes there is interest in past diet, much further back than one year, particularly with respect to macronutrients and alcohol intake. Some diet components may actually have an effect during adolescence or childhood. Little is known about the validity of an adult's retrospective diet assessment from a questionnaire that far back in time. Various studies have evaluated the validity of retrospective diet assessment back as far as about 20 years ago (49,63–70). Results indicate that diet assessed retrospectively agrees moderately well with past diet, and generally is correlated with present diet.

Validity

It is actually meangingless to speak of the validity of *the* diet history or *the* food frequency questionnaire. Validity is profoundly dependent on the particular food list, its format, quality control, and the particular quantitation method of each instrument. Observed correlations may be as much a function of imperfect portion size assumptions made by the investigators, for example, as a function of the respondent's ability to report his usual diet (71). Further, the appropriateness of the reference method must be carefully examined. Because of day-to-day variability, it is likely that even a 7-day record may not be an appropriate "truth" measure for long-term usual diet for many nutrients, against which a test instrument is to be judged (see "Errors in Dietary Assessment: Impact and Adjustment," later in this chapter). Low correlations found in some validation studies may be in part a reflection of unrepresentative reference periods rather than unreliable questionnaires. In Beaton's data (27), for example, only percent of calories from carbohydrate and fat (but not calories or grams of fat or carbohydrate) could be obtained from both men and women in 7 days to an accuracy of $\pm$ 20% of the individual's true long-term intake.

Those investigators using reasonably *adequate* reference data have generally found correlations in the range of 0.5–0.8 (10,29,34,40,43,46,47,72) between the reference data and more extensive questionnaires, usually having some assessment of portion size by one of the methods described earlier. Much shorter list-based questionnaires, especially without portion size, tended to have somewhat lower correlations (35,73). These figures are for estimates excluding vitamin supplements; since populations vary in the extent to which they use vitamin supplements, it is important to evaluate the performance of diet instruments for the assessment of diet alone, as well as with vitamin supplementation.

ENERGY-ADJUSTMENT: RATIONALE AND METHODS

Rationale

Macronutrient associations with cancer are always potentially confounded by energy intake, because by definition they represent the only sources of energy. Larger, more active, or less metabolically efficient persons tend to consume more food (see Chapter 5) and thus simultaneously more energy and more nutrients, especially energy-providing ones. It is critical to *try* to distinguish between the unique association of a macronutrient (such as fat) with cancer and the association of total energy with cancer. (Evidence for the possible role of energy intake in cancer incidence is described in Chapter 8.) Even if a nutrient is not highly correlated with energy intake, omitting energy from a model of cancer's association with that nutrient could alter the estimates of association, if energy is an important risk factor to cancer ("omitted covariate effect") (74,75). Energy may also be needed in a model together wtih an interaction term, if there is interest in examining effect modification (interactions), i.e., whether or not level of energy intake changes the relationship between the macronutrient and cancer.

Table 1 illustrates the extent of some of the nutrient-energy and nutrient-nutrient correlations, with examples from three different studies (16,46,76). The highest correlations are those between monounsaturated fat and saturated fat (0.89–0.94), energy and fat (0.83–0.92), and energy and carbohydrate (0.80–0.89) among the three studies. Both crude and dietary fiber correlate quite highly with the micronutrients vitamin C, carotene, and vitamin A; these micronutrients in turn (expressed as nutrient densities) have moderate *negative* correlations with percent of calories from fat. Because of these considerable correlations between fiber and micronutrients commonly available in fruits and vegetables (major sources of fiber), it has often been difficult to separate out the relative importance of each diet factor in determining cancer risk.

Moderately high correlations such as those just described create problems when trying to model several risk factors' associations with disease (77,78). These interrelations between the various dietary factors, where one or more factors are linear combinations of two or *more* other factors, are termed multicollinearity. Thus, examining correlations between pairs of factors is only a start of the examination of a possible multicollinearity problem if more than two factors are in a model. The impact of multicollinearity is to destablize the estimates of the regression coefficients and to increase their standard errors. Although an overall model may be effective in predicting disease, none of the variables may be statistically significant. In extreme cases, multicollinearity may make it impossible to distinguish among risk factors or measure their effects of disease (computational errors). In an attempt to solve the problem of multicollinearity between energy and nutrient intakes, in particular macronutrients, several methods of adjusting nutrient intake for caloric intake have been explored. These methods will be described below and their equivalent factors will be highlighted. However, it should be noted at the onset that although these approaches *appear* to remove multicollinearity by putting independent diet factors into the model, they do not in fact do so. This is discussed further below.

Methods and Equivalences

Methods of calorie adjustment fall into two main categories: (a) use of nutrient densities (dividing nutrient intake by total calorie intake) or its equivalent for energy-providing nutrients, percent of total calorie intake, and (b) stratified analyses or regression models.

Nutrient Densities

While it would seem to do so, adjusting for calories by using nutrient densities does not always remove the association between the nutrient and calories for the following reason. Between-person variability of the nutrient density measure depends on the ratio of variability of nutrient to variability of calories. Thus, as between-person variability in nutrient intake decreases, nutrient density approaches the inverse of calorie intake times a constant. This is a variable that is obviously still related to calories. Nutrient density measures *may* greatly reduce correlation with energy, particularly for energy-providing nutrients highly correlated with calories, such as fat. For example, the correlation of fat nutrient density with calorie intake was 0.05 among nurses (16) and 0.04 among men in the Irish-Boston Heart Study (79). On the other hand, nutrient density may do nothing to remove the confounding by calorie intake but change the direction of the relationship, especially with nutrients originally weakly correlated with total energy or having low variability, such as micronutrients and protein, respectively. Vitamin C without supplements correlated with calories at 0.28, while the vitamin C nutrient density measure correlated with calories at −0.20 among nurses (16). Similarly, protein correlated with calories at 0.60, while protein nutrient density correlated with calories at −0.57 among nurses. If energy intake is related to disease, a nutrient density measure tends to be related to disease in the opposite direction to that of energy, even in the absence of a nutrient effect. Thus, it is generally inappropriate to use only a nutrient density term in a model of a nutrient's association with disease, unless the correlation between nutrient density and total energy is close to zero, and energy is not strongly related to disease in that dataset (i.e., there is no "omitted covariate effect").

Table 1 Correlations Between Intakes of Specific Diet Components

Diet component	Boston Nurses[a] Records	Colorectal Study[b] Questionnaire	Women's Health Trial[c] Records	Women's Health Trial[c] Questionnaire
Energy and total fat	0.86	0.92	0.83	0.87
Energy and polyunsaturated fat	0.59	0.57	0.67	0.77
Energy and cholesterol	0.47	0.71	0.53	0.68
Energy and carbohydrate	0.82		0.80	0.89
Energy and protein	0.59	0.86	0.68	0.85
Energy and crude/dietary fiber	0.24	0.54	0.40	0.64
Fat and vitamin C	0.002	0.13	0.12	0.24
Nutrient densities	−0.47		−0.42	−0.51
Calorie-adjusted	−0.45			
Fat and vitamin A	0.08			
Nutrient densities	0.33			
Calorie-adjusted	−0.32			
Fat and protein	0.44	0.83	0.46	0.63
Nutrient densities	−0.13		−0.30	−0.54
Calorie-adjusted	−0.14			

Fat and crude/dietary fiber	0.01	0.41	0.09	0.32
Nutrient densities	−0.44		−0.51	−0.69
Calorie-adjusted	−0.45			
Monounsaturated fat and saturated fat		0.89	0.91	0.94
Cholesterol and saturated fat	0.55	0.77	0.61	0.76
Nutrient densities	0.22		0.30	0.36
Calorie-adjusted	0.26			
Vitamin C and crude/dietary fiber	0.61	0.49	0.66	0.58
Nutrient densities	0.62		0.63	0.45
Calorie-adjusted	0.59			
Vitamin A and crude fiber	0.66			
Nutrient densities	0.64			
Calorie-adjusted	0.61			
Carotene and dietary fiber				0.66

[a] Data from Ref. 16 based on individual means of 28 days of diet recording by each of 194 women. Fiber data is expressed as *crude* fiber.
[b] Data from Ref. 76 based on individual means of diet history questionnaire by each of 832 male cases and controls. Data from women (not presented here) were generally similar. Fiber data is expressed as *crude* fiber.
[c] Data from Women's Health Trial Feasibility Study, unpublished information. Based on one diet history questionnaire (46) and individual means of three 4-day records for 102 women in the "usual-diet" group. Fiber data is expressed as *dietary* fiber.

Stratified Analyses

If the intention is to examine the risk associated with discrete categories of intake, one may consider stratified analyses. In this approach, relative risk estimates for a given nutrient, controlling for total calorie consumption, are obtained by a Mantel-Haenszel pooled stratified analysis (80). However, this method can only be used when the total number of strata (number of other variables and levels of each variable) is not too large with respect to the number of cases or outcome events reported, and when the risk estimates are more or less homogeneous over the strata, i.e., no interactions are present. In addition, when nutrients are highly correlated, it will often be difficult to find people in the extreme opposite quantiles of intake (e.g., high total fat and low total calorie intake) causing small cell size and problems with the stratified analysis. Typically, regression models will ultimately be needed to control for other diet and nondiet factors and to examine interaction, as well as to examine nutrient and nondiet variables on a continuous scale.

Regression Models

Various regression models have been proposed to examine the effects of calories and one or more nutrients of interest. For illustration, we will consider here and in Table 2 fat intake and calorie intake. The first model is the classic multiple regression model, in which the nutrient and calories variables are simultaneously in the model, with the usual interpretation that each variable's coefficient is controlled for the effect of the other variables.

$$E(Y_i) = a_0 + a_1 \text{ Calories}_i + a_2 \text{ Fat}_i \qquad (1)$$

where $E(Y_i)$ is the expected value of the dependent variable under the specified model for an individual with intakes i, a_o is the y-intercept, and a_1 and a_2 are the calories and fat coefficients, respectively. Here $E(Y_i)$ may be the probability of disease for an individual with intakes i, or some function of this probability (such as the logistic), or serum or blood levels (e.g., serum cholesterol). Remember that the problem with this model is one of multicollinearity; calories and fat are highly correlated with each other. The next two models (Eqs. (2) and (3)) use a technique popularized by Willett and Stampfer (5,16), called the calorie-adjusted nutrient residual approach.

$$E(Y_i) = b_0 + b_2 \text{ Fat Residual}_i \qquad (2)$$

$$E(Y_i) = c_0 + c_1 \text{ Calories}_i + c_2 \text{ Fat Residual}_i \qquad (3)$$

The "fat residual" is derived by regressing nutrient intake (e.g., fat) as the dependent variable (Y) on calorie intake as the independent variable (X) in a simple linear regression; the residuals from this regression (predicted fat intake minus observed fat intake) are then used as the nutrient variable (calorie-adjusted fat)

Table 2 Mathematical Models for Energy Adjustment and Their Equivalences[a]

Model 1	Disease[b] $= a_0 + a_1$ Total Calories $+ a_2$ Fat
Model 2	Disease $= b_0 + b_2$ Fat Residual
Model 3	Disease $= c_0 + c_1$ Total Calories $+ c_2$ Fat Residual
Model 4	Disease $= d_0 + d_1$ Other Calories $+ d_2$ Calories From Fat
Model 5	Disease $= e_0 + e_1$ Total Calories $+ e_2$ Fat Density

If "total calories" is strongly related to disease:

Coefficients and their standard errors: $a_2 = c_2 = d_2 - d_1$[c]; $a_1 = d_1$; $d_2 = a_2 + a_1$

If "total calories" is weakly or not related to disease:

Coefficients and their standard errors: $a_2 = b_2 = c_2 = d_2 - d_1$; $a_1 = d_1$; $d_2 = a_2 + a_1$

[a] For simplicity, we assume "Fat" and "Fat Residual" are expressed in calories (1 g fat = 9 cal.). If "grams of fat" is used in models (1), (2), and (3), then coefficients $a_2 = b_2 = c_2 = (d_2 - d_1)w$, where $w = 9$.
[b] "Disease" represents the probability of disease or some function of this probability, or the expected value of a continuous variable such as serum or blood levels.
[c] The coefficient b_2, but not its standard error, is also equal to a_2, c_2 and $d_2 - d_1$ in a linear model (e.g., modeling serum cholesterol), but not in a logistic model.

in Eqs. (2) or (3). This nutrient variable is, by definition, independent of calorie intake.

The fourth model, energy decomposition, popularized by Howe for macronutrients (81,82), consists of dividing up the major sources of energy into separate variables. Here for simplicity we illustrate with two variables, fat calories versus other calories.

$$E(Y_i) = d_0 + d_1 \text{ Other Calories}_i + d_2 \text{ Calories from Fat}_i \quad (4)$$

Finally, a fifth model, multivariable nutrient density, includes total calories as well as one or more nutrient density variables.

$$E(Y_i) = e_0 + e_1 \text{ Total Calories}_i + e_2 \text{ Fat Density}_i \quad (5)$$

This model considers association between disease and the fat *composition* of *diet* holding total energy constant. It overcomes the original problem with nutrient density alone in the model, i.e., controlling for residual confounding, which might have been generated by the inverse of the calorie factor, as well as examining diet composition relative to total energy intake directly, if this variable is the relevant factor related to disease.

The latter four models appear to have eliminated multicollinearity by placing two independent or nearly independent variables in the model to substitute for the nutrient and total calories variables in Eq (1). In the second and third models, the fat residual is the part not related to total calorie intake and thus independent of total calories; in the fourth model, "other calorie sources" is less related to "fat calories" than is total calories; and in the fifth model, fat density is generally not highly correlated with total calories.

However, as we mentioned earlier, the *impact* of multicollinearity still remains; we cannot abolish the fact that nutrients and calories come along in the same foods. We can see that multicollinearity remains by observing that there are equivalences of regression coefficients and standard errors among the models. Coefficients a_2, c_2, $d_2 - d_1$ are all equal (83). In a linear model, where disease is replaced with a continuous variable such as serum cholesterol or a biochemical marker of disease, b_2 is also equal to a_2, c_2, and $d_2 - d_1$. In a logistic regression model, providing that there is an unimportant relation between total calories and disease, b_2 will also be nearly equal to those above. The standard errors of the above coefficients are also equivalent. When total calories are strongly related to disease, however, the standard error for the b_2 coefficient is not equal to the standard errors of a_2, c_2 and $d_2 - d_1$ because of omitting an important covariate. Also, $a_1 = d_1$, each interpreted as the effect of "other sources of calories" after controlling for the effect of fat. The various coefficients have different interpretations. Thus, care must be taken in interpretation when different models are used.

Questions of Interest

Most questions can be answered by one of these models. Questions of interest include, "Is the effect of fat intake on disease *different* from the effect of other calorie sources, i.e., is the effect of a fat calorie equivalent to the effect of a calorie from other sources?" This question can be answered by examining a_2, c_2, or $d_2 - d_1$. Willett (16) has pointed out that simply looking for d_2 significance and d_1 nonsignificance is inappropriate to answer this question because d_1 may not have a sufficient degree of variation to be significant; one must look at the difference between d_2 and d_1. Howe (82) cautions that this type of examination only allows us to conclude that there is a *difference* in effect, *but not* that fat intake is associated with disease. For example, if carbohydrate, protein, or alcohol has a negative association with disease (d_1 is negative) and fat has no association with disease ($d_2 = 0$), a_2 in model (1) and c_2 in model (3) will be positive, indicating a difference between the various sources of calories but not that fat is positively associated with disease. To answer the question "Is there an association between absolute fat intake and disease risk?", then d_2 in model (4) (or its equivalent, $a_2 + a_1$ from model (1)) is examined. The model (4) fat coefficient, d_2, relates to the absolute fat intake in contrast to the relative diet composition, e.g., if the proportion of calories derived from fat is decreased by increasing other calories through consumption of more beer, or vice versa, and fat calories are unchanged, there will be no effect on disease risk if the absolute amount of fat is what is related to disease (d_2 is positive or negative).

Finally, to investigate the association between total calories and disease, c_1 from model (3) is relevant. If the fat effect is weak or nonexistent, then a model with only total calories will have a similar coefficient and standard error to those for c_1.

More Complex Model and Issues

The preceding models can be used in more complex analyses with more than one nutrient. However, if model (1) or (3) is used, all of the energy-providing nutrients may not be included simultaneously, because one variable, total calories, would be exactly equal to a linear combination of the calorie source variables (redundancy). Model (4) may also be extended to use all nutrient sources of energy as separate variables, providing there is sufficient independent variation to produce stable estimates. Likewise, these approaches can be used to analyze subcategories of the macronutrients, e.g., saturated, monounsaturated, and polyunsaturated fats, with the same restrictions.

Effect modification among nutrients should be examined, by incorporating interaction terms in models. For example, is a high calorie or fat intake only harmful in the presence of a low intake of fruits and vegetables (or antioxidants such as vitamin C, E, or carotenoids)? Effect modification can also be examined by analyzing the effect of one nutrient (e.g., fat intake) within separate strata of another factor (e.g., high or low fruit/vegetable intake).

As models become more complicated with more variables and possibly interaction terms, the chance of multicollinearity increases and diagnostic procedures for this must be evaluated (84). Multicollinearity among linear combinations of more than two variables may be stronger than correlations between any two variables.

In considering the preceding discussion of models, coefficients and equivalences, several cautions should be borne in mind. First, diet variables were modeled as continuous variables. However, in epidemiologic studies diet variables are often treated as categorical and expressed as quantiles of intake. To the author's knowledge, no statistical theory has been developed for this situation, and future research is needed to look at the previous models and their equivalence or lack of equivalence when nutrients are analyzed as quantiles of intake.

It is often helpful to work with distributions of dietary variables that are normally distributed or at least less skewed than is typical of most diet variables. It will often be useful to transform diet variables (such as in Eqs. (1) to (5)) to reduce skewness and, thus, to avoid undue influence of individual observations and minimize the effects of outliers. In addition, the nutrient variable, the dependent variable in the first step of Willett's calorie-adjusted residual approach, may require transformation to help fulfill assumptions of normality of error terms and equality of variances. If these transformed diet variables are used in the models above, and if they are transformed in the same way for each model (e.g., log fat intake is used whenever fat intake was indicated before) equivalences should hold between a_2 and c_2, but interpretation of "log other calorie sources" will not be equal to "log total calories" minus "log fat calories," thus a_1 will not equal d_1. Thus, care must be taken when interpreting transformed data.

A third consideration is that the previous discussion has placed an emphasis on dichotomous disease states, where a logistic regression model is generally appropriate. If instead of a dichotomous variable for disease, a continuous dependent variable such as a biochemical marker of cancer is being modelled, and there are repeated measures on all other relevant variables, Leigh (85) has suggested yet another model often used by econometricians to reduce multicollinearity.

Other considerations include the effect of measurement error of the diet variables, as reflected in validity studies. Measurement error causes adjustment for calorie intake and other comfounders to be incomplete (see next section). Willett (16) has suggested that the calorie-adjusted nutrient residual approach will reduce errors in measuring diet (from questionnaires) and disease relations, but Flegal and Larkin (86) indicate that considerable misclassification of the diet variable still exists after calorie adjustment.

In conclusion, because of the equivalences between the various approaches to energy adjustment, one may choose the approach(es) that is (are) most convenient for asking the salient questions, but the impact of the original problem of multicollinearity still remains. This can be seen by the equivalence of the coefficients and stardard errors discussed above and in Table 2. The impact of multicollinearity is to destabilize the estimates of the regression coefficients and to increase their standard errors. Thus, it may not always be possible to separate the effects of certain macronutrients and calorie consumption and/or other diet components. In some cases this problem may be partially overcome by increasing the sample size to reduce the coefficent variances and by increasing the heterogeneity of the population with respect to total calorie consumption and nutrient intake. The International Agency for Research in Cancer (IARC) is attempting to do just this. They are planning a large inter-European prospective study of diet and cancer with larger sample sizes and a greater degree of diet heterogeneity than most other studies. This may still be inadequate for the study of some diet factors. The final recourse is to separate the diet component(s) of interest experimentally through a randomized clinical trial, such as the Women's Health Trial (87,88), originally proposed to examine the impact of a 20% versus 40% fat diet. Even within a clinical trial setting, heterogeneity among other nutrients may need to be increased within each arm in order to explore disease association with other diet components not targeted by the intervention.

ERRORS IN DIETARY ASSESSMENT: IMPACT AND ADJUSTMENT

Importance

All dietary assessment methods entail *imprecision* in the estimate of an individual's usual dietary intake and entail *misclassification* of individuals with respect to their place along the distribution of long-term dietary intake. Misclassification and some types of imprecision have a profound impact on the ability to detect and estimate true relationships if they exist, and on the power of a study and the sample size needed. It is an aspect of dietary research which cannot be overlooked and which must be included in all considerations of study design and selection of dietary assessment methods. Methods have been developed to evaluate the impacts and to adjust the observed risk estimates and standard errors, and these will be discussed in this section. In addition to this basic effect, measurement error in dietary reference data affects evaluation of another instrument's validity, while measurement error in any diet data affects the impact of calorie or other dietary component adjustment for controlling confounding. In the following section we will discuss the distinctions between and implications of imprecision and misclassification, and random and systematic errors; the number of days required to estimate an individual's usual intake with a desired precision, to estimate correlations, to evaluate the ability to categorize individuals along distributions of intakes and subsequent effect on relative risk estimates; model-based adjustments in risk estimates to compensate for measurement error; and finally, sample size requirements (number of individuals and number of days of reference data per individual) for various kinds of studies.

Types and Sources of Error

In our context imprecision means that the absolute value of the nutrient estimate (of fat, for example) differs from the true nutrient intake of the individual to some degree. Imprecision is undesirable if one wishes to counsel individuals regarding their dietary intake or identify persons at risk because of nutrient deficiency or excess; it may be less serious in a study of diet-disease relationships *unless combined with misclassification*. Misclassification means that individuals are not categorized correctly along the distribution of intake. A dietary assessment method may be imprecise in the estimates it produces but still be satisfactory at ranking or categorizing individuals correctly, as reflected in the correlation between that method and a reference method. For example, a food use questionnaire among 158 older middle-aged Finnish men (43) estimated the group mean dietary fiber intake at 26.4 g, while their group mean from 12 2-day food records yielded an estimate of 20.4 g; however, the correlation between these two estimates was high, $\hat{\varrho} = 0.71$. Conversely, two methods may produce similar group means, but nevertheless one method may have much poorer ability to classify individuals.

For example, Stuff et al. (89) estimated similar mean intakes of fat among 40 lactating women with comparing 7-day records to a food frequency questionnaire (86.5 g vs. 88.7 g, respectively), but there was no relationship between the rankings produced by the two methods ($\hat{\varrho}$ = 0.04). Others have observed a similar result (49,73).

All methods entail imprecision and misclassification, but the sources of these errors are different for the various methods, and the available remedies are different. Errors are considered *random* (unbiased), resulting in fluctuations around a true mean, or *systematic* (biased), resulting in consistently over- or underestimating true mean intake. Random errors result in unbiased estimates of the true mean but exaggerated standard errors. If systematic errors were *equal* for all persons, mean intakes would be biased, but standard errors and the ability to rank or classify individuals would be unaffected. Errors can be within an individual or between-individual (among a group of individuals). Within-person *random* error is most typical of 1-day or multiple-day methods as measures of an individual's long-term *usual* intake, due to dietary variability from day to day. Within-person *systematic* error is more typical of food frequency questionnaires, some of which over- or underestimate intake; random errors can occur, as well.

These errors make it difficult to detect differences between groups or individuals and to categorize persons accurately, because they introduce noise into the system, When a diet exposure variable is examined singly, random errors in it usually result in attenuation of measures of association such as correlations, regression coefficients, and relative risk. When multiple exposures (diet and others) are evaluated together in a model, the effect of error is more complex, and *could be in either direction*.

A remedy for random error due to day-to-day variability is increasing the number of days of assessment on each individual (27,90). Since 1 day provides inadequate characterization of an individual's usual intake, numerous investigators have used 3 or more consecutive days of diet, either by record or a combination of record and recall, in an attempt to achieve both quantitative precision and greater representativeness of usual diet. How many days, then, are required to obtain adequate representation of an individual's usual diet?

Number of Days Required to Estimate an Individual's Usual Intake

How many days are required to provide an estimate that is "close to" the actual level of the individual's usual intake (precision). Although first studied by Chalmers in 1952 (91), this question has been studied intensively in the last decade by those indicated in Table 3, as well as others (13,26,30,90,92–94). The data all indicate that a small number of days of diet information does not represent an individual's longer-term usual intake with any precision.

Table 3 Number of Days Required to Produce Nutrient Estimate that is ±20% of an Individual's True Long-Term Usual Intake[a]

	Beaton[b]		Balogh[c]	McGee[d]	Helsinki[e]	Basiotis[f]		Marr[g]
Nutrient	Male	Female	Male	Male	Male	Male	Female	Mate
Energy	7	10	4	5	6	7	9	3
Protein	13	10	11,7	9	9	9	12	—
Fat	10	16	8	12	11	15	18	5
Fat as % of energy	4	5	—	5	4	—	—	2
Cholesterol	28	30	20	23	24	35	50	28
Carbohydrate	9	13	5	6	8	10	11	4
Fiber	25	25	—	—	12	21	22	10

[a]Calculated using the following formula from Ref. 27: $N = 4\,CV_w^2/D_w^2$, where N is the number of days, CV_w is the within-person coefficient of variation, and D_w is the percent deviation of an individual's observed intake from his usual mean intake.
[b]Data based on six nonconsecutive days from 30 males and 30 females, aged 25–44 years. Fiber data as "crude" fiber. From Refs. 27,28.
[c]Data based on 2–11 random days over one year from 100 Israeli males. Protein expressed as animal, vegetable, respectively. From Ref. 29.
[d]Data based on 7-day records from 329 males. From Ref. 124.
[e]Data based on 12 2-day records from 162 Finnish males, aged 55–69 years. Fiber data as "dietary" fiber. From Ref. 31.
[f]Data based on 365-day records from 13 males and 16 females, aged 20–53 years. Fiber data as "crude" fiber. From Ref. 125.
[g]Data based on 7-day records from 68 British male civil servants, aged 40–49 years. Fiber data as "dietary" fiber. From Ref. 95.

Chalmers et al. (91) calculated that to have a 95% confidence interval equal to ±15% of the then-RDA for calories and other nutrients (excluding vitamins A and C), one would need 14 days for men and 11 for women. Beaton et al (27) found that to be 95% confident of producing an estimate within ±20% of the true usual fat intake (a rather generous criterion representing, e.g., being between 80 and 120 g), it would require on average 10 days for males and 16 days for females, while Balogh et al. (29) found it would require 23 days for 90% of the population and more days for the most variable 10% of the population. The general pattern of results is extremely consistent across all of these investigators and their different study populations. Cholesterol and fiber required the greatest number of days among those indicated in Table 3, while fat as percent of calories required the fewest days. The number of days required to estimate dietary fiber among the Finnish and British men was considerably lower than crude fiber among the Canadian and U.S. populations. Note some micronutrients, such as vitamins A and C, require at least as many days as cholesterol and sometimes more.

This inability of one or a few day's intake to represent usual diet is only somewhat relieved by restricting analysis to nutrients as a percent of calories. Beaton et al.(27) indicated that "the relatively high intraindividual variability (of nutrients expressed per 1000 kilocalories) suggests wide variation, day by day, in the *composition* [emphasis added] of self-selected diet." James et al. (13) also concluded that "an individual's variable intake of protein and energy is sufficient from day to day to limit the possibility of using nutrient density rather than absolute intakes as discriminators between individuals" (on usual intake).

If the within-person variance is known, the number of days of dietary data required for a given precision for an individual (or the precision provided by a given number of days) can be calculated (27). See Table 3 footnote for formula.

Number of Days Required for Accurate Classification and Correlation Between Individuals

Often, researchers do not require precision in the individual's nutrient estimate, but the ability to rank individuals with some accuracy. Liu et al. (90) examined the ability to classify individuals into quintiles of the distribution of cholesterol intake. In order to have less than a 5% chance of grossly misclassifying someone from the first to the fifth quintile, again a rather generous criterion, it would require 7 days of diet information. In order to avoid misclassifying someone from the first to the third quintile or vice versa, it would require 11 days. James et al. (13) in England found that to correctly classify 80% of men into the correct third of the distribution would require 5 days for calories, 9 days for fat, and 18 days for percent of calories from fat. Marr and Heady (95) found similar results, except that percent of calories from fat required only 6–9 days among their population.

Sempos et al. (94) used a somewhat different criterion. Suppose one wanted to ensure that an observed correlation between a dietary factor and a physiologic factor such as serum cholesterol was at least as much as 90% of the real correlation. Then it would take 7 days for calories, 9 for protein, 6 for calcium, and at least 15 for micronutrients, such as the B vitamins.

Linking Classification and Correlation with Relative Risk

When the diet method involves diet records or recalls, the ratio of within to between-person variability of intake is key to determining how accurately the method can estimate correlations with physiologic factors, or can classify individuals into categories of intake, and thus how accurately it can estimate measures of association such as relative risk of cancer. Most of the investigators mentioned in Table 3 have measured this ratio. For most nutrients and food components this ratio is greater than one, generally in the range of 1.1–3.5 (16,27,28,31, 94,96). For some micronutrients, such as vitamin A, selenium, and cholesterol, and some food groups this ratio is even higher, 4.0–10.0 (31,96,97).

Figure 1 illustrates the effects of the within to between-person variance ratio on the observed correlation between "true" usual intake and an estimate based on n days of food recording. An infinite number of days of diet recording is assumed to correlate with "true" intake at 1.0 (27,31,90). The smaller the ratio of within-subject to between-subject variation, the closer to unity will be the correlation between diet records and "true" intakes. If the variance ratio for a population is known, Fig. 1 can be used to estimate the number of independent days of diet information required for a given degree of correlation with "truth."

For multiple days of diet recording, variance ratios are used to estimate the correlation of n days of records with true usual intake. For this purpose, days must be independent, not consecutive (30,31). For questionnaires, the correlation with truth is usually estimated from a validation study comparing the questionnaire with a (hopefully) more valid method. Whichever way that estimated correlation with truth is obtained, it represents an estimate of measurement error and can be used to calculate the probable degree of attentuation of risk estimates. A given level of correlation with "truth" implies a given level of misclassification—that is, individuals will be placed in the wrong quintile—and this level of misclassification can be estimated (98). As noted earlier, in a single-variable situation misclassification due to random error generally results in a biasing of relative risk estimates toward the no-effect level, relative risk = 1.0. Figure 2 shows the resulting attenuation in risk estimates for varying levels of correlation of a questionnaire, or n days of food recording with "truth" at various levels of "true" relative risk. Taken together, Figs. 1 and 2 show that there is greater attentuation in risk estimates with increasing within to between-variance ratio, and less attenuation with increasing days of diet data, as well as greater attentuation at higher

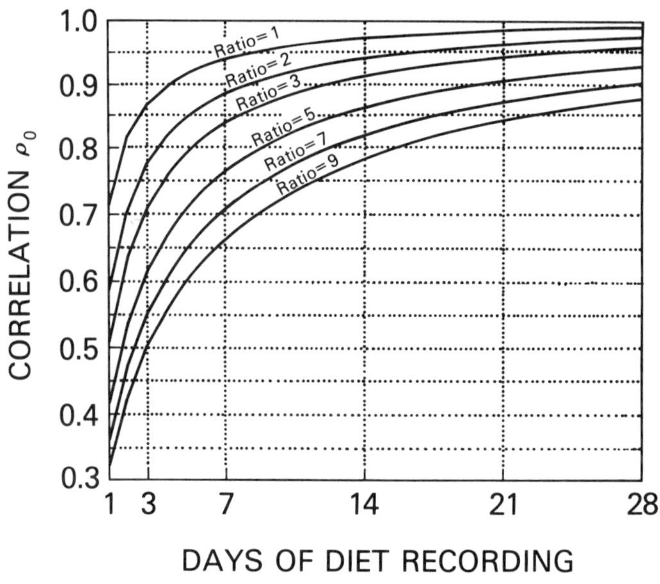

Figure 1 Correlation (ϱ_0) between "true" usual daily dietary intake and estimated usual intake based on a sample of n independent days of diet recording for various within-to between-person variance ratios. (Reproduced with permission from the American Journal of Epidemiology, Hartman et al., 1990 (31).)

true relative risks. For example, one day of diet recording correlates with "true" usual intake between 0.3 and 0.7 (Fig. 1) resulting in attenuations of 50–83% for a true relative risk of 3.0 (Fig. 2). Increasing the number of sampling days to 7 increases the correlation to 0.66–0.93 and decreases the attenuation to 16–55% for a true relative risk of 3.0. Additional days of diet recording will continue to decrease the relative risk attenuation but at a diminishing rate. Figure 1 shows that the largest increases in the correlation ϱ_0, and thus reductions in attenuation, have already occurred by 7–14 independenet days of diet recording.

Figure 2 can also be used to evaluate a questionnaire's ability to correctly estimate relative disease risk for lowest versus highest quintiles of dietary intake (the relative risk curves in Fig. 2 represent the risk for lowest versus highest quintile). Walker and Blettner (98) have shown that the estimated correlation between a questionnaire and "truth" can be used to calculate the agreement between the two methods when classified into quintiles. Data from three large validation studies with multiple food records and questionnaire-derived nutrient intakes (35,43,46) have generally shown very good correspondence between the degree

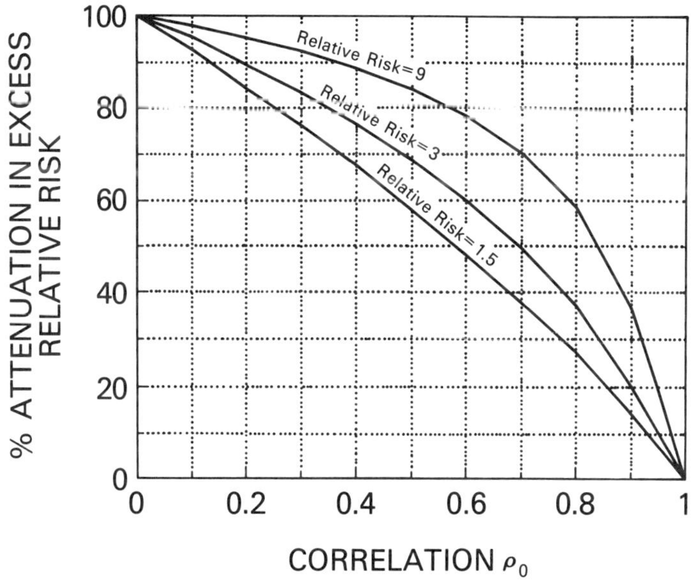

Figure 2 Percentage of attenuation in excess relative risk as a function of the correlation (ϱ_0) between "true" and estimated usual intake for different levels of true relative risk. The percentage of attenuation in excess relative risk is equal to $1-((\text{obsRR} - 1)/(\text{true RR} - 1))$, where obsRR denotes the observed, attenuated relative risk and trueRR denotes the true relative risk. Because many studies of the association between lung cancer and diet have resulted in attenuated estimates of 1.3–2.4 (1–4), a true relative risk of 3.0 is thought to represent a reasonable level for a "true" diet-disease relation. True relative risks of 1.5 and 9.0 are used to illustrate the effects of less and more extreme cases. (Reproduced with permission from the American Journal of Epidemiology, Hartman et al., 1990 (31).)

of correct classification predicted by the correlation ϱ_0 and actual observed joint classification of food record and questionnaire estimates.

Adjusting Observed Correlations with Imperfect Reference Data

The preceding section has shown that it is possible to estimate the degree of attenuation in correlations. It is also possible to proceed in the opposite direction, to start with an observed correlation and estimate what the true correlation may be if random measurement error is taken into account. This would be useful for correcting correlations from a validation study which used less than optimum reference data or correcting correlations between a serum measure and a diet measure based on multiple days.

Since the reference data are usually multiple-day diet records, the correlation adjustment makes use of the ratio of within- to between-individual variance seen in the records (90,99). The "true" correlation between questionnaire and true usual diet is estimated as $\varrho_t = \varrho_0 (1 + (\text{variance ratio/n days}))^{1/2}$, where ϱ_t = true correlation, ϱ_0 = observed correlation between the questionnaire estimate and the mean estimate from the food records, and n days = number of *independent* observations per person on which ϱ_0 is based. It is possible to correct for random error in both diet measures if more than one questionnaire is to be administered (90). In addition, Rosner and Willett (99) describe a method for constructing a confidence interval around such an adjusted estimate of the "true" correlation between questionnaire (or a serum value) and usual intake (such as estimated from food records).

Such adjusted correlations are useful in estimating the adequacy of a questionnaire, and can be used with Fig. 2 to estimate how attenuated the resulting risk estimates would be and how much the sample size must be increased (98). However, such adjusted correlations must always be viewed with great caution. A very poor questionnaire estimate can be inflated to appear excellent merely because the variance ratio is large. The most that can be said with confidence is that the true correlation is probably larger than the observed, but the extent of improvement is unclear, and the degree of uncertainty will be revealed by the width of the adjusted confidence interval.

Model Based Relative Risk Adjustment for Measurement Error

Earlier discussion has focused on the attenuation of relative risk estimates for discrete categories such as quintiles. However, we often *model* diet and disease associations, as mentioned earlier in this chapter, with a logistic regression model in which other variables can be controlled and which can also accommodate intake on a continuous scale. For such models, statistical methods have been developed which permit an adjustment of the risk estimates and confidence intervals around them, to account for systematic and random measurement error. The observed risk of disease from a logistic regression model can be adjusted to estimate the true risk, if a validation study has been conducted.

The validation study produces a correlation between questionnaire and reference data, and standard deviations of questionnaire and of reference data. A correction in the risk estimate is then possible. The relative risk (odds ratio) is calculated from the exponentiation (antilog) of the beta coefficient of the dietary variable in a logistic regression. The correction factor is the product of the correlation between "true" and questionnaire intake and the ratio of their standard deviations. The true beta coefficient is obtained by dividing the beta estimated from the logistic regression by this correction factor.

The following formulas describe the relationship between the logistic regression estimate of disease risk and the error in the dietary measure:

Logistic Regression Model Relating "True" Exposure of Disease Risk

Log odds of disease for an individual i, given a certain true dietary intake, X_i, is:

$$\ln [\text{Prob } (D | X_i)/\text{Prob } (\overline{D} | X_i)] = \alpha + \beta_t X_i \quad (6)$$

where α is the y-intercept, D is with disease, $\overline{D}$ is without disease, and β_t is the "true" coefficient of the dietary factor.

Logistic Regression Model Relating Surrogate Exposure to Disease Risk

Log odds of disease for an individual i, given an imperfectly estimated dietary intake, Z_i, is:

$$\ln [\text{Prob } (D | Z_i)/\text{Prob } (\overline{D} | Z_i)] = \alpha' + \beta_o Z_i \quad (7)$$

where α' is the y-intercept, and β_o is the observed coefficient of the dietary factor. Before we can make the correction of β_o, we need a way of relating β_t to β_o. This can be seen in Eqs. (8) and (9).

Linear Regression Model Relating "True" Exposure to Surrogate Exposure

True dietary intake, X, is related to a surrogate measure of intake, Z:

$$E(X | Z_i) = \alpha'' + \gamma Z_i \quad (8)$$

where $E(X | Z_i)$ is the expected value for the true intake X given Z_i, Z_i is the questionnaire estimate, and γ is its coefficient. Several authors have shown (16,88,100) that the coefficient γ is the product of the correlation ϱ_{xz} between X and Z, and the ratio of their standard deviations (σ_x/σ_z). These may be estimated from the validation study. Therefore, an adjustment of the disease risk estimated from the beta coefficient is as follows:

$$\beta_t = \beta_o/\gamma$$

or equivalently (9)

$$\beta_t = \beta_o/((\varrho_{xz})\ (\sigma_x/\sigma_z))$$

Rosner et al. (100) describe methods for constructing confidence intervals around the resulting adjusted odds ratios to reflect the uncertainty in the measure of γ from the validation study.

The preceding discussion has assured that we have a "true" measure of usual intake or, for example, at least a large number of days of diet recording to approximate truth in the questionnaire (Z) validation study. However, 21–28 days of diet recording is often not feasible, and the number of days of diet recording available from a validation study may be far fewer. If the mean of fewer days of diet recording is an unbiased estimate of "true" intake, then it turns out that the point estimate of gamma in Eq. (8) will be the same on average as that estimate obtained using many more days of diet recording. This equality of the γs occurs despite that decrease in ϱ_{xz} because the standard deviation of the mean of fewer days of diet recording increases [Eq. (9)] in a compensating manner. However, the precision of the γ estimate will be poorer (larger variance), therefore the precision of the adjusted beta coefficient in the logistic regression model (9) will also be worse, resulting in a wider confidence interval around the relative risk estimate. Although it may be tempting to greatly reduce the number of records in a validation study, one must be careful to not make the confidence interval so wide to be meaningless.

Although modeled on a continuous scale, the formulas of Rosner et al. can be used to calculate risk estimates which are interpretable as the equivalent risk of the highest compared with the lowest quintile. This is achieved by calculating the difference between the median of the highest and median of the lowest quintiles, multiplying that times the β_t obtained in Eq. (9), and applying the exponential function. Rosner et al. provides a table relating γ in Eq. (8) to observed relative risk for different values of "true" relative risk (assuming that the diet variables and risk estimates are defined above as the quintile distance). If the standard deviations for X and Z are equal, Fig. 2 can be used to *approximate* these relative risks since γ reduces to ϱ_{xz} (ϱ_0 in Fig. 2) as indicated by Eq. (9).

The Real World: Problems Beyond Simple Measurement Error

Up until this point we have discussed how random measurement error of one dietary exposure attenuates measures of association (such as correlation, regression coefficient, and relative risk). Generally, analysis of epidemiologic studies and cancer prevention trials consists of modeling multiple dietary factors as well as other nondietary factors. This situation worsens the problem of measurement error or misclassification, because in the presence of other covariates measured with error, the errors in estimating relative risks may be in either direction, *even for variables measured without error* (101–105). Rosner et al. (106) have developed a procedure to adjust multiple covariate relative risk estimates and confidence intervals for measurement error. This procedure makes use of covariances among the variables of interest, those with and without measurement error. The method allows one or more continuous variables to be measured with error and one or more variables, either continuous or discrete, to be error-free. They used the Nurses' Health Study data relating breast cancer to age and intakes of alcohol, calories, and saturated fat to illustrate the unpredictability of the direction of adjustment for the various factors. The effect of age, which was assumed to be error-free, was overestimated before adjustment, and the other variables, including alcohol measured with little error, were attenuated before adjustment.

Armstrong et al. (107) proposed a method for adjusting case-control studies for both nondifferential systematic error and differential systematic error (that is, error which may be different for cases and controls due to recall bias), including construction of confidence intervals and significance test corrections. Their method was applied to a logistic regression of case-control data from a study of colon cancer and diet. They found substantial correlation among measurement errors and among true intakes for fiber and calories in one model and, among calories, fat and protein in a second model. Correction for measurement error made the associations more pronounced but attenuated levels of statistical significance. Additional correction for recall bias slightly enhanced associations and made them more significant. Odds ratios adjusted for error were stronger and the significance levels were changed only slightly. Their results illustrate the combined effect of multicollinearity (discussed earlier in this chapter) and measurement error.

Other investigators have examined approaches for adjusting for measurement error in other types of epidemiologic analyses (108–111). Pepe et al.(112), building on the work of Prentice (113), describe issues related to covariate measurement errors in cohort studies with time-to-response data. They make special note of the sensitivity of various parametric models to modeling assumptions and caution us to consider various models and try to examine the behavior of these models and, perhaps more appropriately, to develop nonparametric models with fewer assumptions. In response to this plea, Carroll and others (114–116) describe some semiparametric and nonparametric alternatives to assessing and adjusting for measurement error for logistic models.

Use of Dual Measurements to Reduce the Effects of Measurement Error

An alternative to directly adjusting for measurement error, as discussed in the last few sections, is to make use of dual measurements with independent errors. For example, Marshall and Graham (117) examined this approach with a dichotomous exposure variable. In a case-control setting, they showed that if analysis is restricted to those subjects whose exposure status is concordant by both measures, the relative risk estimate is less biased (attenuated) than the estimate based on the subjects' classification by only one set of measures. Similar results were found by Bjelke (118), who observed stronger and more significant relative risks among subjects whose spouses' estimates of the subjects' dietary intake agreed with the subjects' estimates. Likewise, Howe (119) found that dual response data can increase power in case-control studies, but found it useful to include rather than exclude those discordant on exposure category.

Sample Size Requirements to Compensate for Measurement Errors

As we have seen, the effect of measurement error in an exposure variable is usually to attenuate measures of association such as correlation and relative risk. This attenuation leads to decreases in the power to detect diet and cancer associations. Several investigators have considered methods to determine appropriate sample sizes to overcome the effects of measurement error. In addition to adjusting the sample size of the main study, it is possible to calculate the appropriate size and number of replicates for a validation study, so that the correlation between questionnaire and reference data and its precision are not artificially reduced by measurement error in the reference data. It is important that observed correlations in validation studies be adjusted for measurement error in the reference data before the resulting correlations are used to calculate sample sizes for the main study.

For a validation study, Rosner and Willett (99) provide information on the optimal reference data (number of days of diet data and number of persons) required to minimize the confidence interval around the *adjusted* correlation (adjusted for measurement error) between "true" usual intake, as measured by multiple diet records, and a surrogate measure of intake, such as a diet questionnaire. Table 4, adapted from Rosner and Willett, shows these calculations for correlations of 0.3–0.9 and for their corresponding within to between-person variance ratios (1.0–9.0). Since usual correlations are between 0.4 and 0.7 and common variance ratios are between 1.0 and 3.0, this table suggests that for any *fixed number* of *observations* (person × replicates) collection of 3 nonconsecutive day replicates is generally optimum. This implies that it is generally better to increase the number of individuals studied rather than increasing the number of replicates above three. However, in view of the advisability of considering the "whole diet," as discussed earlier in this chapter, it is prudent to consider the less well-behaved nutrients and food groups. Alcohol, for example, with a high correlation of approximately 0.9 (43,120) and a within- to between-person variabilty ratio of 2.4 (31), requires 5–9 days of diet recording; the beef, pork, and poultry subgroup and vitamin A probably need at least 5 days of recording. Thus it appears that the earlier recommendation to use 7–14 days (for some diet components may need up to 28 days) of intake for estimating correlations from Fig. 1 may be reduced somewhat to 5–10 days, if one calculates an *adjusted* correlation and compensates by increasing the number of persons being studied.

As with correlations, attenuations in relative risk due to measurement error also affect the sample size needed to detect as statistically significant a true

Table 4 Required Number of Replicates Per Subject for Fixed Total Sample Size to Minimize Correlation Variance, according to "True" Correlation (ϱ_t), Intraclass Correlation (ϱ_I) and Within- to Between-Person Variance Ratio (σ_W^2/σ_B^2)[a]

ϱ_t	ϱ_I	$\frac{\sigma_W^2}{\sigma_B^2}$	No. replicates per subject
	0.1	9.0	3
0.3	0.3	2.3	2
	0.5	1.0	2
	0.1	9.0	5
0.5	0.3	2.3	2
	0.5	1.0	2
	0.1	9.0	8–10[b]
0.7	0.3	2.3	3
	0.5	1.0	2
	0.1	9.0	10
0.9	0.3	2.3	5–9[c]
	0.5	1.0	2–5[d]

[a] Adapted from Table 2 of B. Rosner and W. C. Willett, 1988 (99), with permission from the *American Journal of Epidemiology*.
[b] 10 minimized variance, but 8–10 replicates only ranged from 12.7 to 12.9.
[c] 9 minimized variance, but 5–9 replicates only ranged from 1.7 to 2.0.
[d] 5 minimized variance, but 2–5 replicates only ranged from 0.7 to 1.0.

dose-response trend across diet exposure categories. If there were a linear trend in risk, and true relative risk = 3 from top to bottom quintile, a diet instrument which correlated at 0.7 with the truth would attenuate the relative risk estimate to 1.96 and require a 2.4-fold increase in sample size (according to Mantel-Haenszel test for linear trend (98,121)) above the sample size estimated in the standard calculations which assume no error in the measurement of the exposure variable. For an instrument which correlated at 0.4 with true long-term diet, the relative risk estimate would be attenuated to 1.47, and one would need almost an eightfold increase in sample size. Tables for estimating the required increase in sample size may be found in Walker and Blettner (98).

Freedman et al. (122) consider calculating the required sample size of a cohort study in which the risk associated with a nutrient will be expressed in terms of the absolute level of intake (e.g., > 100 g of fat) and the distribution of intake in the population is estimated in the planning phase using the same instrument to be used in the study. The calculations take into account both measurement error and the narrower distribution (greater homogeneity) of "true" intake compared to the distribution estimated from some dietary instruments. Walker and Blettner accounted only for the misclassification of exposures into quintiles, and assumed that the relative risk between upper and lower quintiles can be specified. In practice this specification would usually require some assessment of the true usual intake distribution of the nutrient. Considering a linear trend across their five categories, Freedman et al., like Walker and Blettner, calculate sample size for a given power. Their results show that if the intake distribution is estimated from the same dietary instrument, then accounting for the narrower distribution in addition to misclassification when the instrument is correlated with truth at 0.65, increases the required sample size sixfold over that required when the correlation is one. This is two times the sample size that would have been calculated only accounting for misclassification (98). Freedman et al. also note that if there is systematic bias, the increase in sample size may not be as great, so that assuming a random error model may be conservative.

Spiegelman and Gray (123) consider three alternatives for the purpose of choosing a cost-efficient cohort study and accompanying validation study (the latter conducted to estimate measurement error and then adjust the relative risk estimate and its confidence interval). The results show that the proportion of overall study resources that should be allocated to the validation study increases with increasing disease incidence, increasing magnitude of the "true" relative risk, and in a nonlinear way depends on extent of measurement error, as well as other factors. An internal validity study is preferred for generalizability.

Such sample size estimates, derived from the methods described above, are invariably several times the sample size calculated under the usual assumption of perfect measurement. Researchers must bear in mind when using food records or recalls as the measure of dietary intake in an epidemiologic study, or as a reference measure in a questionnaire validity study, that the ideal goal is to use as many food records/recalls as necessary, as indicated by Table 2 and Figs. 1 and 2 (and corresponding formulas); this will ensure the least possible attenuations in correlations and relative risks, little loss of power, and more precise estimates of individual intake. If fewer days of diet intakes and/or poorer questionnaires are used, then adjustment methods appropriate for the data at hand can be used, *but* researchers will still pay the price in (a) loss of power, (b) wider confidence intervals for correlations, regression coefficients, and relative risk estimates, and (c) loss of precision of individual intake estimates. Only the former two can be compensated for by increasing the sample size (study participants). Thus, investigators need to make their sample size estimates, and to balance requirements, in terms of research goals and desired precision, against the cost in dollars and human resources. Investigators must also bear in mind that the choice of variables to include in a model (involving issues such as confounding by unexamined dietary variables, calorie adjustment, etc.), or the form or type of the model (e.g., logistic, linear, discriminant, nonparametric) are at least as critical as measurement error. The model and adjustments must be appropriate for the data at hand; it is wise to check the fit of the various models, otherwise wrong conclusions may be obtained. Progress in our understanding of the relationship between diet and disease requires that we have an accurate reflection of the strength of our conclusions.

REFERENCES

1. G. Block, Vitamin C and cancer prevention: The epidemiologic evidence, *Am. J. Clin. Nutr., 53*, 270S (1991).
2. R. G. Ziegler, A review of epidemiologic evidence that carotenoids reduce the risk of cancer, *J Nutr., 119*, 116 (1989).
3. M. S. Micozzi, G. R. Beecher, P. R. Taylor, and F. Khachik, Carotenoid analyses of selected raw adn cooked foods associated with a lower risk of cancer, *JNCI, 82*, 282 (1990).
4. G. Block, B. Patterson, and A. Subar, Fruits, vegetables and cancer prevention: The epidemiologic evidence, *Nutr. Cancer.* (In press).
5. W. Willett and M.J. Stampfer, Total energy intake: Implications for epidemiologic analyses, *Am. J. Epidemiol., 124*, 17 (1986).
6. H. N. Jacobson, and J. L. Stanton, Pattern analysis in nutrition, *Clinical Nutrition, 5*, 249 (1986).
7. E. Randall, J. Marshall, S. Graham, and J. Brasure, Frequency of food use data and the multidimensionality of diet. *J. Am. Diet. Assoc. 89*, 1070 (1989).
8. National Research Council, *Nutrient Adequacy. Assessment Using Food Consumption Surveys*, National Academy Press, Washington, DC, 1986.
9. United States Department of Agriculture, Human Nutrition Information Service, *Nutrient Intakes: Individuals in 48 States, Year 1977–78. Nationwide Food Consumption Survey 1977–78. Report I-2*, United States Department of Argriculture, Hyattsville, MD, 1984.
10. G. Block and A. M. Hartman, Dietary assessment methods, In *Nutrition and Cancer Prevention. Investigating the Role of Micronutrients* (T. E. Moon and M. S. Micozzi, eds.), Marcel Dekker, New York, 1989, p. 159.
11. A. M. Lilienfeld and D. E. Lilienfeld, *Foundations of Epidemiology*, Oxford University Press, New York, 1980, pp. 14, 291.
12. M. C. Burk and E. M. Pao, *Methodology for Large-Scale Surveys of Household and Individual Diets*, United States Department of Agriculture, Washington, DC, 1976.
13. W. P. T. James, S. A. Bingham, and T. J. Cole, Epidemiological assessment of dietary intake, *Nutr. Cancer, 2*, 203 (1981).
14. G. Block, A review of validations of dietary assessment methods, *Am. J. Epidemiol, 115*, 492 (1982).
15. C. Medlin and J. D. Skinner, Individual dietary intake methodology: A 50-year review of progress, *J. Am. Diet. Assoc., 88*, 1250 (1988).
16. W. Willett, *Nutritional Epidemiology*, Oxford University Press, New York, 1990.
17. S. A. Bingham, The dietary assessment of individuals; methods, accuracy, new techniques and recommendations, *Nutr. Abst. Rev. (Series A), 57*, 705 (1987).

18. H. Lee-Han, V. McGuire, and N. F. Boyd, A review of the methods used by studies of dietary measurement, *J. Clin. Epidemiol., 42*, 269 (1989).
19. H. A. Guthrie, Selection and quantification of typical food portions by young adults, *J. Am. Diet. Assoc., 84*, 1440 (1984).
20. B. M. Posner, C. L. Borman, J. L. Morgan, W. S. Borden, and J. C. Ohls, The validity of a telephone-administered 24-hour dietary rcall methodology, *Am. J. Clin. Nutr., 36*, 546 (1982).
21. J. P. Madden, S. J. Goodman, and H. A. Guthrie, Validity of the 24-hr. recall: Analysis of data obtained from elderly subjects, *J. Am. Diet. Assoc., 68*, 143 (1976).
22. M. Gersovitz, J. P. Madden, and H. Smiciklas-Wright, Validity of the 24-hr. dietary recall and seven-day record for group comparisons, *J. Am. Diet. Assoc., 73*, 48 (1978).
23. A. J. Stunkard and M. Waxman, Accuracy of self-reports of food intake, *J. Am. Diet. Assoc., 79*, 547 (1981).
24. R. Karvetti and L. Knuts, Validity of the 24-hour recall, *J. Am. Diet. Assoc. 85*, 1437 (1985).
25. C. M. Young, G. C. Hagan, R. E. Tucker, and W. D. Foster, A comparison of dietary study methods. II. Dietary history vs. seven-day record vs. 24-hr. recall, *J. Am. Diet. Assoc., 28*, 218 (1952).
26. K. S. Todd, M. Hudes, and D. H. Calloway, Food intake measurement: Problems and approaches, *Am. J. Clin. Nutr., 37*, 139 (1983).
27. G. H. Beaton, J. Milner, P. Corey, V. McGuire, M. Cousins, E. Stewart, M. de Ramos, D. Hewitt, P. V. Grambsch, N. Kassim, and J. A. Little, Sources of variance in 24-hour dietary recall data: implications for nutrition study design and intepretation, *Am J. Clin. Nutr., 32*, 2546 (1979).
28. G. H. Beaton, J. Milner, V. McGuire, T. E. Feather, and J. A. Little, Source of variance in 24-hour dietary recall data: Implications for nutrition study design and interpretation. Carbohydrate sources, vitamins, and minerals, *Am. J. Clin. Nutr., 37*, 986 (1983).
29. M. Balogh, H. A. Kahn, and J. H. Medalie, Random repeat 24-hour dietary recalls, *Am. J. Clin Nutr., 24*, 304 (1971).
30. K. J. Morgan, S. R. Johnson, and B. Goungetas, Variability of food intakes, An analysis of a 12-day data series using persistance measures, *Am. J. Epidemiol. 126*, 326 (1987).
31. A. M. Hartman, C. C. Brown, J. Palmgren, P. Pietinen, M. Verkasalo, D. Myer, and J. Virtamo, Variability in nutrient and food intakes among older middle-aged men: Implications for design of epidemiologic and validation studies using food recording, *Am. J. Epidemiol., 132*, 999 (1990).
32. B. S. Burke and H. C. Stuart, A method of diet analysis: Applications in research and pediatric practice, *The Journal of Pediatrics, 12*, 493 (1938).
33. B. S. Burke, The dietary history as a tool in research, *J. Am. Diet. Assoc., 23*, 1041 (1947).
34. M. Balogh, J. H. Medalie, H. Smith, and J. J. Groen, The development of a dietary questionnaire for an ischemic heart disease survey. *Isr. J. Med. Sci., 4*, 195 (1968).
35. W. C. Willett, L. Sampson, M.J. Stampfer, B. Rosner, C. Bain, J. Witschi, C. H. Hennekens, and F. E. Speizer, Reproducibility and validity of a semiquantitative food frequency questionnaire, *Am. J. Epidemiol., 122*, 51 (1985).

36. R. Smucker, G. Block, L. Coyle, A. Harvin, and L. Kessler, A dietary and risk factor questionnaire and analysis system for personal computers, *Am. J. Epidemiol.*, *129*, 445 (1989).
37. L. W. Pickle and A. M. Hartman, Indicator foods for vitamin A assessment, *Nutr. Cancer*, *7*, 3 (1985).
38. G. Block, C. M. Dresser, A. M. Hartman, and M. D. Carroll, Nutrient sources in the Ameircan diet: Quantitative data from the NHANES II survey. I. Vitamins and minerals, *Am. J. Epidemiol.*, *122*, 13 (1985).
39. G. Block, C. M. Dresser, A. M. Hartman, and M. D. Carroll, Nutrient sources in the American diet: Quantitative data from the NHANES II survey. II. Macronutrients and fats, *Am. J. Epidemiol*, *122*, 27 (1985).
40. J. H. Hankin, 23rd Lenna Frances Cooper Memorial Lecture: A diet history method for research, clinical, and community use. *J. Am. Diet. Assoc.*, *86*, 868 (1986).
41. J. H. Hankin, Development of a diet history questionnaire for studies of older persons, *Am. J. Clin. Nutr.*, *50*, 1121 (1989).
42. T. Byers, J. Marshall, R. Fiedler, M. Zielezny, and S. Graham, Assessing nutrient intake with an abbreviated dietary interview, *Am. J. Epidemiol.* *122*, 41 (1985).
43. P. Pietinen, A. M. Hartman, E. Haapa, L. Rasanen, J. Haapakoski, J. Palmgren, D. Albanes, J. Virtamo, and J. K. Huttunen, Reproducibility and validity of dietary assessment instruments: I. A self-administered food use questionnaire with a portion size picture booklet, *Am. J. Epidemiol.*, *128*, 655 (1988).
44. M. G. Jain, L. Harrison, G. R. Howe, and A. B. Miller, Evaluation of a self-administered dietary questionnaire for use in a cohort study, *Am. J. Clin. Nutr.*, *36*, 931 (1982).
45. G. Block, A. M. Hartman, C. M. Dresser, M. D. Carroll, J. Gannon, and L. Gardner, A data-based approach to diet questionnaire design and testing. *Am. J. Epidemiol.*, *124*, 453 (1986).
46. G. Block, M. Woods, A. Potosky, and C. Clifford, Validation of a self-administered diet history questionnaire using multiple diet records, *J. Clin. Epidemiol.*, *43*, 1327 (1990).
47. J. H. Hankin, G. G. Rhoads, and G. A. Glober, A dietary method for an epidemiologic study of gastrointestinal cancer, *Am. J. Clin. Nutr.*, *28*, 1055 (1975).
48. S. R. Cummings, G. Block, K. McHenry, and R. B. Baron, Evaluation of two food frequency methods of measuring dietary calcium intake, *Am. J. Epidemiol.*, *126*, 796 (1987).
49. J. Sobell, G. Block, P. Koslowe, J. Tobin, and R. Andres, Validation of a retrospective questionnaire assessing diet 10–15 years ago, *Am. J. Epidemiol*, *130*, 173 (1989).
50. G. Block, F. E. Thompson, A. M. Hartman, F. A. Larkin, and K. E. Guire, A. comparison of two diet questionnaires validated against multiple diet records colleced over one year, *J. Am. Diet. Assoc.*. (In Press).
51. M. Hernandez-Avila, C. Master, D. J. Hunter, J. Buring, J. Phillips, W. C. Willett, and C. H. Hennekens, Influence of additional portion size data on the validity of a semi-quantitative food frequency questionnaire, *Am. J. Epidemiol.*, *128*, 891 (1988). (Abstract)
52. J. M. Samet, C. G. Humble, and B. E. Skipper, Alternatives in the collection and analysis of food frequency interview data, *Am. J. Epidemiol.*, *120*, 572 (1984).

53. C. G. Humble, J. M. Samet, and B E. Skipper, Use of quantified and frequency indices of vitamin A intake in a case-control study of lung cancer, *Int. J. Epidemiol.*, *16*, 341 (1987).
54. J. T. Dwyer, E. A. Krall,, and K. A. Coleman, The problem of memory in nutritional epidemiology research, *J. Am. Diet. Assoc.*, *87*, 1509 (1987).
55. A. F. Smith, J. B. Jobe, and D. J. Mingay, Question-induced cognitive biases in reports of dietary intake by college men and women, *Health Psychology, 10*, 244 (1991).
56. D. Lansky, and K. D. Brownell, Estimates of food quantity and calories: errors in self-report among obese patents, *Am. J. Clin. Nutr.*, *35*, 727 (1982).
57. D. J. Hunter, L. Sampson, M.J. Stampfer G. A. Golditz, B. Rosner, and W. C. Willett, Variability in portion sizes of commonly consumed foods among a population of women in the United States, *Am. J. Epidemiol.*, *127*, 1240 (1988).
58. S. Y. Chu, L. N. Kolonel, J. H. Hankin, and J. Lee, A comparison of frequency and quantitative dietary methods for epidemiologic studies of diet and disease, *Am. J. Epidemiol. 119*, 323 (1984).
59. A. F. Smith, J. B. Jobe, and D. J. Mingay, Concerning the suitability of diarykeeping to validate recall of dietary information, Manuscript submitted for publication.
60. A. F. Smith, J. B. Jobe, and D. J. Mingay, Retrieval from memory of dietary information, *Applied Cognitive Psychology, 5*, 269 (1991).
61. E. A. Krall, J. T. Dwyer, and K. A. Coleman, Factors influencing accuracy of dietary recall, *Nutr. Res.*, *8*, 829 (1988).
62. A. F. Smith, J. B. Jobe, and D. J. Mingay, A cognitive investigation of responses to dietary surveys, In *Proceedings on the Section of Survey Methods Research*, Alexandria, VA (eds.), American Statistical Association, 407, 1989.
63. F. E. Van Leeuwen, H. C. W. De Vet, R. B. Hayes, W. A. van Staveren, C. E. West, and J. G. A. J. Hautvast, An assessment of the relative validity of retrospective interviewing for measuring dietary intake, *Am. J. Epidemiol.*, *118*, 752 (1983).
64. O. M. Jensen, J. Wahrendorf, A. Rosenqvist, and A. Geser, The reliability of questionnaire-derived historical dietary information and temporal stability of food habits in individuals, *Am. J. Epidemiol.*, *120*, 281 (1984).
65. T. E. Rohan and J. D. Potter, Retrospective assessment of dietary intake, *Am. J. Epidemiol 120*, 876 (1984).
66. W. A. van Staveren, C. E. West, M. D. A. F. Hoffmans, P. Bos, A. F. M. Kardinaal, G. A. F. C. Van Poppel, H. Jan-Aart Schipper, J. G. A. J. Hautvast, and R. B. Hayes, Comparison of contemporaneous and retrospective estimates of food consumption made by a dietary history method. *Am. J. Epidemiol.*, *123*, 884 (1986).
67. F. E. Thompson, D. E. Lamphiear, H. L. Metzner, V. M. Hawthorne and M. S. Oh, Reproducibility of reports of frequency of food use in the Tecumseh diet methodology study, *Epidemiol.*, *125*, 658 (1987).
68. T. Byers, J. Marshall, E. Anthony, R. Fiedler, and M. Zielezny, The reliability of dietary history from the distant past, *Am. J. Epidemiol.*, *125*, 999 (1987).
69. M. L. Wu, A. S. Whittemore, and D. L. Jung, Errors in reported dietary intakes II. Long-term recall, *Am. J. Epidemiol.*, *128*, 1137 (1988).

70. W. C. Willett, L. Sampson, M. L. Browne, M. J. Stampfer, B. Rosner, C. H. Hennekens, and F. E. Speizer, The use of a self-administered questionnaire to assess diet four years in the past, *Am. J. Epidemiol.*, *127*, 188 (1988).
71. G. Block and A. M. Hartman, Issues in reproducibility and validity of dietary studies, *Am. J. Clln. Nutr.*, *50*, 1133 (1989).
72. W. C. Willett, R. D. Reynolds, S. Cottrell-Hoehner, L. Sampson, and M. L. Browne, Validation of a semi-quantitative food frequency questionnaire: comparison with a one-year diet record, *J. Am. Diet. Assoc.*, *87*, 43 (1987).
73. P. Pietinen, A. M. Hartman, E. Haapa, L. Rasanen, J. Haapakoski, J. Palmgren, D. Albanes, J. Virtamo, and J. K. Huttunen, Reproducibility and validity of dietary assessment instruments: II. A qualitative food frequency questionnaire, *Am. J. Epidemiol.* *128*, 667 (1988).
74. M. H. Gail, S. Wieand, and S. Piantadosi, Biased estimates of treatment effect in randomized experiments with nonlinear regressions and omitted covariets, *Biometrika*, *71*, 431 (1984).
75. S. L. Zeger, K. Y. Liang, and P. S. Albert, Models for longitudinal data: a generalized estimating equations approach, *Biometrics*, *44*, 1049 (1988).
76. M. Jain, G. M. Cook, F. G. Davis, M. G. Grace, G. R. Howe, and A. B. Miller, A case-control study of diet and colo-rectal cancer, *Int. J. Cancer*, *26*, 757 (1980).
77. D. McGree, D. Reed, and K. Yano, The results of logistic analyses when the variables are highly correlated: An empirical example using diet and CHD incidence, *J. Chron. Dis.*, *37*, 713 (1984).
78. T. Gordon, M. Fisher, and B. M. Rifkind, Some difficulties inherent in the intepretation of dietary data from free-living populations, *Am. J. Clin. Nutr.*, *39*, 152 (1984).
79. L. H. Kushi, Re: "Total energy intake: implications for epidemiologic analysis" (letter), *Am. J. Epidemiol.*, *126*, 981 (1987).
80. N. Mantel and W. Haenszel, Statistical aspects of the analysis of data from retrospective studies of disease, *JNCI*, *22*, 719 (1959).
81. G. R. Howe, A. B. Miller, and M. Jain, Re: "Total energy intake: implications for epidemiologic analysis" (letter), *Am. J. Epidemiol.*, *124*, 157 (1986).
82. G. R. Howe, Re: "Total energy intake: implications for epidemiologic analyses" (letter), *Am. J. Epidemiol.*, *129*, 1314 (1989).
83. M. C. Pike, L. Bernstein, and R. K. Peters, Re: "Total energy intake: implications for epidemiologic analyses" (letter), *Am. J. Epidemiol.*, *129*, 1312 (1989).
84. D. A. Belsely, E. Kuh, and R. E. Welsch, *Regression Diagnosis*, Wiley, New York, 1980.
85. J. P. Leigh, Highly correlated variables in logistic analyses: Comment (letter), *J. Chron. Dis.*, *39*, 151 (1986).
86. K. M. Flegal and F. A. Larkin, Partitioning macronutrient intake estimates from a food frequency questionnaire, *Am. J. Epidemiol.*, *131*, 1046 (1990).
87. R. L. Prentice, F. Kakar, S. H. Moolgavkar, S. Hursting, L. Sheppard, R. Klein, and L. H. Kushi, Aspects of the rationale for a Women's Health Trial, *JNCI*, *80*, 802 (1988).
88. D. P. Byar and L. S. Freedman, Clinical trials in diet and cancer, *Prev. Med.* *18*, 203 (1989).

89. J. E. Stuff, C. Garza, E. O'Brien Smith, B. L. Nichols, and C. M. Montandon, A comparison of dietary methods in nutritional studies, *Am. J. Clin. Nutr.*, *37*, 300 (1983).
90. K. Liu, J. Stamler, A. Dyer, J. McKeever, and P. McKeever, Statistical methods to assess and minimize the role of intra-individual variability in obscuring the relationship between dietary lipids and serum cholesterol, *J. Chron. Dis.*, *31*, 399 (1978).
91. F. W. Chalmers, M. M. Clayton, L. O. Gates, R. E. Tucker, A. W. Wertz, C. M. Young, and W. D. Foster, The dietary record—How many and which days? *J. Am. Diet. Assoc.*, *28*, 711 (1952).
92. J. H. Hankin, W. E. Reynolds, and S. Margen, A short dietary method for epidemiologic studies. II Variability of measured nutrient intakes, *Am. J. Clin. Nutr. 20*, 935 (1967).
93. W. C. Hunt, A. G. Leonard, P. J. Garry, and J. S. Goodwin, Components of variance in dietary data for an elderly population, *Nutr. Res.*, *3*, 433 (1983).
94. C. T. Sempos, N. E. Johnson, E. L. Smith, and C. Gilligan, Effects of intraindividual and interindividual variation in repeated dietary records, *Am. J. Epidemiol.*, *121*, 120 (1985).
95. J. W. Marr and J. A. Heady, Within- and between-person variation in dietary surveys: number of days needed to classify individuals, *Hum. Nutr. Appl. Nutr. 40A*, 347 (1986).
96. C. T. Sempos, N. E. Johnson, C. Gilligan, and E. L. Smith, Estimated ratios of within-person to between-person variation in selected food groups, *Nutrition Reports International*, *34*, 1121 (1986).
97. S. Salvini, D. J. Hunter, L. Sampson, M. J. Stampfer, G. A. Colditz, B. Rosner, and W. C. Willett, Food based validation of a dietary questionnaire: The effects of week-to-week variation in food consumption, *Int. J. Epidemiol.*, *18*, 858 (1989).
98. A. M. Walker and M. Blettner, Comparing imperfect measures of exposure, *Am. J. Epidemiol.*, *121*, 783 (1985).
99. B. Rosner and W. C. Willett, Interval estimates for correlation coefficients corrected for within-person variation: Implications for study design and hypothesis testing, *Am. J. Epidemiol.*, *127*, 377 (1988).
100. B. Rosner, W. C. Willett, and D. Spiegelman, Correction of logistic regression relative risk estimates and confidence intervals for systematic within-person measurement error, *Stat. Med. 8*, 1051 (1989).
101. K. Liu, Measurement error and its impact on partial correlation and multiple linear regression analyses, *Am. J. Epidemiol. 127*, 864 (1988).
102. T. M. Morgan and R. M. Elashoff, Effect of covariate measurement error in randomized clinical trials, *Stat. Med.*, *6*, 31 (1987).
103. L. L. Kupper, Effects of the use of unreliable surrogate variables on the validity of epidemiologic research studies, *Am. J. Epidemiol.*, *120*, 643 (1984).
104. S. Greenland and J. M. Robins, Confounding and misclassification, *Am. J. Epidemiol.*, *122*, 495 (1985).
105. D. A. Savitz and A. E. Baron, Estimating and correcting for confounder misclassification, *Am. J. Epidemiol.*, *129*, 1062 (1989).

106. B. Rosner, D. Spiegelman, and W. C. Willett, Correction of logistic regression relative risk estimates and confidence intervals for measurement error: the case of multiple covariates measured with error, *Am. J. Epidemiol.*, *132*, 734 (1990).
107. B. G. Armstrong, A. S. Whittemore, and G. R. Howe, Analysis of case-control data with covariate measurement error: Application to diet and colon cancer, *Stat. Med.*, *8*, 1151 (1989).
108. R. J. Carroll, Covariance analysis in generalized linear measurement error models, *Stat. Med.*, *8*, 1075 (1989).
109. T. T. Chen, A review of methods for misclassified categorical data in epidemiology, *Stat. Med.*, *8*, 1095 (1989).
110. N. A. Hasabelnaby, J. H. Ware, and W. A. Fuller, Indoor air pollution and pulmonary performance: investigating errors in exposure assessment, *Stat. Med.* *8*, 1109 (1989).
111. T. D. Tosteson, L. A. Stefanski, and D. W. Schafer, A measurement-error model for binary and ordinal regression, *Stat. Med.*, *8*, 1139 (1989).
112. M. S. Pepe, S. G. Self, and R. L. Prentice, Further results on covariate measurement errors in cohort studies with time to response data, *Stat. Med.* *8*, 1167 (1989).
113. R. L. Prentice, Covariate measurement errors and parameter estimation in failure time regression model, *Biometrika*, *69*, 331 (1982).
114. L. A. Stefanski and R. J. Carroll, Structural logistic regression measurement error models, In *Proceedings of the AMS-IMS-SIAM Joint Summer Research Conference on Statistical Measurement Error Models* (P. J. Brown and W. A. Fuller, eds.), American Mathematical Society, Providence, RI, 1990.
115. R. J. Carroll and L. A. Stefanski, Approximate quasilikelihood estimation in measurement error models, *J. Am. Stat. Assoc.*, *85*, 652 (1990).
116. R. J. Carroll and M. P. Wand, Semiparametric estimation in logistic measurement error models, *J. R. Stat. Soc.*, *Ser. B*, *53*, (1991). (In Press).
117. J. Marshall and S. Graham, Use of dual responses to increase validity of case-control studies, *J. Chron. Dis.*, *37*, 125 (1984).
118. E. Bjelke, *Epidemiologic Studies of Cancer of the Stomach, Colon, and Rectum: With Special Emphasis on the Role of Diet. Vols I–IV. Doctoral dissertation, 1973*, University Microfilms International, Ann Arbor, MI, 1973.
119. G. R. Howe, The use of polytomous dual reponse data to increase power in case-control studies: An application to the association between dietary fat and breast cancer, *J. Chron. Dis.*, *38*, 663 (1985).
120. W. C. Willett, M. J. Stampfer, G. A. Colditz, B. A. Rosner, C. H. Hennekens, and F. E. Speizer, Moderate alcohol consumption and the risk of breast cancer, *N. Engl. J. Med.*, *316*, 1174 (1987).
121. N. Mantel, Chi-square tests with one degree of freedom; extensions of the Mantel-Haenszel procedure, *J. Am. Stat. Assoc.*, *60*, 690 (1963).
122. L. S. Freedman, A. Schatzkin, and Y. Wax, The impact of dietary measurement error on planning sample size required in a cohort study, *Am. J. Epidemiol.*, *132*, 1185 (1990).
123. D. Spiegelman and R. Gray, Cost efficient study designs for binary response data with generalized Gaussian measurement error in the covariate, *Biometrics*, (1991). (In Press)

124. D. McGee, G.Rhoads, J. Hankin, K. Yano, and J. Tillotson, Within-person variability of nutrient intake in a group of Hawaiian men of Japanese ancestry, *Am. J. Clin. Nutr.*, *36*, 657 (1982).
125. P. P. Basiotis, S. O. Welsh, F. J. Cronin, J. L. Kelsay, and W. Mertz, Number of days of food intake records required to estimate individual and group nutrient intakes with defined confidence, *J. Nutr. 117*, 1638 (1987).

5

Assessment of Energy Intake and Expenditure

Johanna T. Dwyer
Tufts University Medical School and
New England Medical Center Hospitals
Boston, Massachusetts

INTRODUCTION

Rationale and Reasons for Concern

Energy intake and output deserve attention because they may be the primary causes of diseases including cancer. The dependence of tumor formation on calorie intake has long been known, although the mechanisms involved are still poorly understood (Shils, 1988). Energy intakes may also be secondarily associated with cancer development. Actual effects may be due to total energy intake or energy balance, to one of the energy-providing nutrients, or to other lifestyle factors associated with energy output (Willett, 1990). Variations in intakes of energy-providing and other nutrients arise not only from differences in dietary patterns, but also because an individual's overall energy intakes vary. By measuring and correcting for total energy intakes, extraneous sources of error due simply to level of energy intake can be eliminated.

Also such measurements of energy intake and output provide useful crosschecks against other variables. By measurement of energy intakes and outputs rather than solely of variables such as fatness or weight, which represent the balance of calorie intake and energy expenditure, clearer interpretations of the effects of these factors on cancer risks may be possible in the future. Finally, when energy intakes or outputs are consistently above or below a person's energy needs, changes in body composition including but not limited to fat stores will eventually be affected, and these changes in turn may influence human disease. Measurements of energy intake or output may permit earlier detection of these trends.

Definitions

Some basic definitions are provided below. The reader is referred to several comprehensive reviews for further details (Gallow, 1978; Committee on Diet and Health, 1989).

Kilocalories and Kilojoules

A kilocalorie is the amount of heat needed to raise 1 kg water from 15 to 16°C. The accepted international unit of energy is the joule (J). However, in American literature, calories or kilocalories are still often used. To convert energy expressions such as kilocalories to kilojoules (kJ), a factor of 4.2 is used, that is, a Kcal = 4.184 kJ. Because energy inputs and outputs are usually greater than 1000 kJ, the preferred unit is the megajoule (MJ) or 1000 kJ.

Recommended Allowances for Energy

Recommended allowances for energy have been calculated by the Food and Nutrition Board and other bodies (World Heath Organization, 1985; Subcommittee on Tenth Edition of RDA, 1989).

These recommendations represent minimum average energy allowances for hypothetical reference individuals, given certain assumptions about physical activity, physiological conditions, resting metabolism, ambient temperature and pressure, climate, thermogenesis, and other factors. Unlike recommendations for most nutrients, energy recommendations are not set high enough to meet upper levels of variability in requirements. Rather, they are set to be minimal average requirements for the reference individual. They should not be assumed to represent the actual needs of populations or individuals under study without adjustments in the above assumptions, which may be incorrect for particular target groups of interest. For example, actual populations under study may be much more sedentary than the reference populations.

Energy allowances are stated in terms of the amount of potential food energy that can be absorbed and utilized from the food, or physiologically available energy. These estimates in turn are based on digestibility trials performed on healthy individuals using various foods (Merrill and Watt, 1955). Under most circumstances, the general energy conversion factors of 4 Kcal/g for protein or carbohydrate, 9 Kcal/g of fat, and 7 Kcal/g (or 5.6 Kcal/ml) of alcohol are appropriate. When diets consist largely of single foods, especially when these are high in dietary fiber or in other factors that hinder absorption, more specific energy conversion factors may be necessary to account for decreased absorption. On very high fiber diets, energy intakes may be 2–3% less than expected, due to lessened absorption (World Health Organization, 1985).

In healthy individuals the proportion of food energy absorbed and utilized does not appear to vary by body weight. However, in ill health, especially when the individual is underweight, the amount of physiologically available energy may also be decreased, owing to malabsorption. Moreover, the tissue constituting weight gain varies depending on stage in the life cycle and during rehabilitation, making it difficult to predict weight gain without taking account of these variables.

The conversion of fats in food to body fat is theoretically more efficient than the conversion of carbohydrates or protein in food to body fat, actually being 9 for fat compared to approximately 3.27 or less for carbohydrate in growing rats (Donato and Hegsted, 1985; Bursey et al., 1987). The conversion of alcohol to body fat has not been studied, but at moderate levels of intake it may also be more efficient than carbohydrate or protein. While these issues are of considerable theoretical biological significance, they remain unconfirmed by direct experiment in humans.

Importance of Assessing Both Calorie Intakes and Output

Both intakes and outputs of energy are of interest because energy intakes, energy outputs, and weight (or body mass index) appear to have different and conflicting influences upon the risks of developing certain cancers and other diseases, such as coronary artery disease (Paffenbarger, et al. 1987). For example, there is a positive association between calorie intake and later colon cancer development (Lyon et al., 1987) and a negative association between energy output and this same disease (Garabrant et al., 1984; Vera et al., 1985; Gerhardsson et al., 1986). Many complex, recursive relationships exist, with intakes and physical activity modifying diet, weight, and risk in different ways.

Other mechanisms for colon cancer development that have been linked more tightly to diet than to energy output are several. They include dietary fat, increased bile acid secretion, production of degradation products that are colon cancer promoters, and the formation of carcinogens by bacterial degradation of substances in food.

Another reason it is important to assess both intakes and outputs is that they may furnish clues to the underlying mechanisms involved in cancer development. For example,increased energy intakes might signal the presence of a metabolic factor that not only increased energy needs but also stimulated cancer development (Willett and Stampfer, 1985). Others have hypothesized that increased energy outputs might alter gastrointestinal transit times or some other factor affecting colon cancer risk (Holdstock et al., 1970).

Finally, the errors in measurement of both energy intake and output are considerable (Berlin and Colditz, 1990; Gibson, 1990). By using measurements of energy intakes and outputs, somewhat greater precision may be obtained.

Thus, the pathogenetic mechanisms involved in obesity, leanness, cancer, and coronary artery disease may be clarified by assessing associations between factors which, like body weight, are influenced by energy balance (Manson et al., 1987; Garfinkel and Stillman, 1988). Without such assessments, these intake and output variables may confound or obscure actual causative relationships. For example, effects of obesity on reproductive function may influence breast or colon cancer risks (McMichael and Potter, 1980; Wu et al., 1987). Also, alcohol and fat use may be involved via lipid metabolism (Wu et al., 1987).

Validity, Reliability, and Representatives of Measurements of Energy Input and Output

Validity is the degree to which a tool measures what it purports to measure. Reproducibility is the extent to which results are repeatable; the terms repeatability, replicability, and precision are also often used. Accuracy refers to both validity and reproducibility. Representativeness refers to how similar the distributions of subjects under study or the observation periods are to the larger group they are supposed to represent.

Sources of Error

Measurements of energy intakes and outputs are subject to various sources of error. The greatest threats to validity are systematic, nonrandom errors, or biases. Systematic defects in information may be due to the technique chosen or to response bias. Reliability is damaged the most by random errors either due to random response errors or to errors owing to biological variation within the individuals being measured. Lack of representativeness of the subjects under study, or of measurement periods within subjects, also affects validity. Common threats to representativeness include failures to account for within-person biological variation in energy inputs and outputs and misinterpretation due to sample selection or selection of study days.

In general, group data are easier to validate than individual data. When individuals are the focus of analysis, reproducibility is of special concern. The smaller the within-person variation, the greater the reproducibility. Unfortunately, energy intakes tend to have a rather large level of intraindividual variation, so that sampling of sufficiently long periods of observation is essential if energy intakes of individuals are to be characterized.

Repeatability is not synonymous with validity. Systematic response errors or systematic imperfection of the underlying information may still exist, even when data are reproducible.

MEASUREMENT OF ENERGY INTAKE

Factors Influencing Energy Intake

Among the factors influencing requirements for energy and energy intake are age, sex, environmental temperature, energy output, growth, hormonal status, and dieting behaviors (Committee on Diet and Health, 1989, p. 6–3). Of particular concern for present purposes is the fact that individuals in good health and at optimal levels of physical activity normally have physiological mechanisms that feed back to influence energy intake so that a steady-state energy balance may exist at many different levels of energy output. Positive energy states occur in growth, pregnancy, lactation, and rehabilitation from illness, when stores of energy-providing nutrients are laid down in body tissues, in milk, or in fetal tissues and other products of conception. Negative energy states occur in many diseases either because resting metabolism rises due to fever or other catabolic processes or because energy intake falls.

Athletes and others who are very physically active usually have high energy intakes. At more moderate levels of physical activity, energy intakes may increase in lean, but not obese individuals as energy outputs rise, so that the obese may benefit particularly from moderate increases in physical activity (Woo et al.,1985). And, at very sedentary levels of physical activity, the obese may increase their energy intakes to a greater extent than the nonobese, with the result that they are in a positive energy state, and gain adipose tissue.

Purpose of Measurement

The choice of the method for assessing energy intake depends first and foremost on the purpose of the study.

The types of information on energy intake that may need to be obtained involve either data on individuals or groups. Absolute amounts as opposed to rank-ordered or relative energy intakes in tertiles or quartiles may be required for some study purposes on individuals. For groups, means, means and distributions of food consumption, or relative rankings of intakes may be required.

Data collection at the individual level has been extensively reviewed (Bingham, 1987; Bingham et al., 1988). Methods suitable for collection at the household or institutional level have also been well described (Burk and Pao, 1976; Food and Nutrition Board 1981, 1984, 1986; Anderson, 1986; Flores and Nelson, 1988; Pao and Cypel, 1990).

Methods

Two major methods are available: prospective (recorded at or shortly after eating) and retrospecive (in the recent or more distant past).

The basic problem with both of these methods for assessing energy intake in individuals is that the information provided is under the subject's control to at least some degree, and there is often no independent biochemical or other method for validating the information so obtained. For some nutrients simultaneous biochemical measures can be used to check food intakes, but for energy intake, as yet no absolute "gold standard" exists. If an individual is in energy balance, doubly labeled water can be used to estimate energy output, and energy intakes can be derived from that. But when energy balance cannot be assumed, this independent validity check is not possible (Prentice et al., 1980).

Increased energy intakes do not appear to be the cause of positive energy balance observed in most adults; probably reductions in physical activity are also involved. Thus, overweight people frequently eat the same amount of food or less than do normal-weight individuals, but their physical activity and exercise are less (Kromhaut, 1983; Committee on Diet and Health, 1989, pp. 6–10).

Errors in Assessing Energy Intakes

The most common threats to validity in energy assessment methods are summarized in Table 1. Both systematic and random errors are involved.

Many sources of error may arise in assessing energy intake. These are summarized in Table 2 and described in detail in the monographs mentioned above (Bingham, 1987; Bingham et al., 1988).

Most methods commonly used to assess individual under- rather than overestimate energy needs. Underestimates of energy intake are common for at least three reasons (Durnin, 1990): faulty methodology, inadequate sample size and sampling of days on which intakes of food are artificially low or are low due to a seasonal shortage (Durnin, 1990). Systematic errors in estimates may also exist for certain individuals (Schoeller, 1990).

Faulty Methodology

Absolute energy intake estimates usually differ by method, generally being higher by dietary history than by prospective records of weighed or measured values. Relative ranked intakes tend to be more consistent, with between a third and a half of all individuals classified in the same third by energy intake. However, 5–10% may be grossly misclassified (Block, 1981; Marr, 1981; Block, 1982). The result of such misclassification of energy intakes is that estimates of relative risk are reduced (Marshall et al., 1981; Walker and Blettner, 1985).

Table 3 summarizes the validity and reliability of various measures of energy intake. There is no single, perfect method. Each has its strengths and limitations.

Table 1 Common Threats to Validity in Energy Intake Assessment Methods

	Validity threats		Reproducibility threats		Representativeness threats	
	Systematic imperfection of information	Systematic response error	Random response error	Biological within-person variation	Biological between-person variation	Misinterpretation by selection of sample or/and by selection of study days
Weighed food records	X	X		X		X
Household measure food records				X		X
Duplicate portions of food samples	X	X (collection)		X		X
24-hour recalls		X	X	X	X	
Diet history		X	X			? Probably reflects recent intake
Semiquantitative food frequency questionnaire		X	X			? Probably reflects recent intake

Source: Adapted from Bingham, 1987; Bingham et al., 1988.

Table 2 Sources of Error in Methods For Estimating Food Consumption and Energy Intake

	Duplicate portion	Weighed record	Estimated (household) measure record	24-hour recall	Diet history	Semiquantitative food frequency
Response errors						
Omit food	−	±	±	+	+	+
Add food	−	−	−	+	+	+
Estimate of weight or portion size of food	−	−	+	+	+	+
Estimate of frequency/ consumption	−	−	−	−	+	+
Day-to-day variation	+	+	+	+	−	−
Changes in diet	+	+	±	−	−	−
Coding errors	−	+	+	+	+	+
Errors in conversion to nutrients						
Food composition tables	−	+	+	+	+	+
Sampling errors	+	−	−	−	−	−
Direct analysis	+	−	−	−	−	−

Source: Adapted and modified from Bingham, 1987; Bingham et al., 1988.

Table 3 Validity and Reliability of Various Measures of Energy Intake

Weighed Records, Groups

Validity

Weighed records compare well to group means of energy output on normal-weight people obtained using doubly labeled water technique (Prentice et al., 1986; Prentice and Coward, 1986).

Weighed records lower than energy expenditure in obese women using urinary nitrogen excretion or other means (Steen et al., 1978; Warnold et al., 1978).

Energy intakes of 1.3–1.4 times calculated BMR in groups of females and 1.3–1.8 in men are usual, using newer tables for estimating RMR (Schofield et al., 1985; Bingham et al., 1981; Bingham et al., 1982, IARC, 1982, Thompson et al., 1982; Widdowson and McCance, 1936a,b).

Weighed records for groups can be indirectly validated by using 24-hour urinary nitrogen appearance to provide validation of nitrogen intakes and indirect information on validity of energy intakes, but many samples are needed (Isaksson, 1980; Bingham and Cummins, 1983; Bingham and Cummings, 1985).

Weighed Records, Individuals

Predicted BMR varies by at least 12%, and energy expenditures are often double RMR, so tables cannot be used to predict intakes (Willett and Sampson et al., 1985). However, energy intakes ± 3 SD from predicted RMR times an activity factor of 1.2 are probably incorrect (Bingham et al., 1988).

Weighed Records, Groups

Reliability

For sample sizes of 500, the % detectable difference in means is 6% for one-day weighed records, 5% for 3-day weighed records, and 4% for 7-day weighed records (Bingham et al., 1982) at alpha errors 95, beta error 0.20.

Weighed Records, Individuals

For energy, to determine mean energy intake of idividuals with ± 10% SE or less in 90% of population, 13 days needed, 7 days for 70% of population, and 5 days for 50% of population (Bingham et al., 1981). Within-person variation average is 23%, with range of 4–45% in most studies of energy intake (Bingham, 1988). Many more observations are needed for individuals because of intraindividual variation. For example, average number of records to be ± 10% of energy intakes was 5 days, and the average % standard error for energy was 9%, using Balough's data for 24-hour recalls (Bingham et al., 1988; Balough et al., 1971).

continued

Table 3 *Continued*

Weighed Records, Individuals

To classify 80% of male subjects in various studies by correct tertiles by energy, 5–7 days of recording using weighed records are necessary (Bingham et al., 1988, p. 64).

Because reproducibility is poor and intraindividual variation great, (e.g., greater or less than 10% for most nutrients) even with 5+ days' intakes, correlations between diet and other biological variables are low (Sempos et al., 1985).

Estimated (Household Measure) Records, Groups

Validity

Compared to weighed records, differences between them and household measures ranges from 2 to 12% depending on the nutrient and the population studied (Black et al., 1984; Bransby et al., 1948; Eppright et al., 1952; Hackett et al., 1983; Huenemann et al., 1942; Young et al., 1953; Wilson et al., 1980). Possibly, use of prepackaged foods can reduce errors to 2–5% or less (Nettleton, 1980).

Estimated (Household Measure) Records, Individuals

Errors are large for individuals, especially when absolute magnitude of intakes is of interest (Bingham et al., 1988). The percent of individual intakes within 10% of values based on weighed estimates ranged for energy from 33% for children (Eppright, 1953) to 71% among women (Bransby, 1948) to 92% for recent studies, using many prepacked foods (Nettleton, 1980).

When ranking is of interest, errors will lead to 15–20% subjects being classified in adjacent thirds, and only 1% in opposite thirds, compared to weighed records (Bingham et al., 1988).

Estimated Records, (Household Measure) Groups

Reliability

Between- and within-person variations are increased because of inaccuracy of household measures and estimates, as opposed to weighed measures. Differences are less apparent in ranking individuals than in absolute magnitudes of individual intakes (Bingham et al., 1988).

continued

Table 3 *Continued*

Estimated Records, (Household Measure) Individuals

Validity

Relative rankings of individuals using weighed and estimated intakes may remain same in spite of greater inaccuracies in actual magnitude of intakes (Black et al., 1983, Bransby et al., 1948, Eppright et al., 1952, Hackett et al., 1983, Nettleton et al., 1980, Todd et al., 1983, Young et al., 1953).

24-Hour Recall, Groups and Individuals

Validity

Means are either acceptable or underestimates of energy intakes. Results are most valid among middle-aged women (Campbell and Dodds, 1967; Karvetti and Kuuts, 1985). However, direct validations of 24-hour recalls of total intakes of individuals living in their own homes have not been done.

Group means usually agree well with intakes obtained from weighed or estimated food records. Means are lower and variances wider for 24-hour recalls than for diet history, and vary with nutrient or intake under consideration (Bazarre and Myers, 1978).

Reliability

Single recalls are unreliable for estimates of individual intakes, although they are satisfactory for group intakes. For estimating actual intakes of individuals, serial 24-hour recalls are needed (Beaton et al., 1979).

For reasonable energy precision, food patterns of the population under study and their inherent variability are helpful. Correlations between energy intake and weight or other measures of body composition rise with increased numbers of recalls or records.

Dietary History

Validity

Inability to provide correct information on frequencies and/or portion size estimates or to remember intakes hobbles recall. Discrepancies between absolute intakes using different food recall methods are common, and vary in their direction (Bingham et al., 1988). Discrepancies between relative intakes as assessed by ranking are less. 33–50% of subjects are classified in same tertiles, and 5–10% grossly misclassified in opposite tertiles, using energy intakes and rankings (Black, 1981, 1982; Marr, 1971). These may be so great as to reduce observable relative risks greatly (Marshall et al., 1981; Walker and Blettner, 1985). The implication is that sample size estimates must be greatly increased.

continued

Table 3 *Continued*

Dietary History

Reliability

Generally good for energy, but depends on population time of reference (Bingham et al., 1988).

Semi-Quantitiative Food Frequency Questionnaire, Group

Validity

Questionnaires vary, but in general those focusing on specific nutrients are better than those tapping total diet. Short questionnaires have not been successful in quantifying individual energy intakes with precision.

Reliability

Now being determined.

Source: Adapted from Bingham (1987).

Inadequate Sample Size

Studies of energy intake often are based on too few individuals to truly detect differences when they are present. Because energy intakes are so variable from day to day within individuals, sample sizes must be very large to find associations between energy intake, body weight, and obesity, for example.

However, when sample sizes are adequate, total weight gain can be predicted for groups from the degree of excess calorie ingestion (Forbes, 1987). Also, with adequate sample, sizes, and observation periods, energy outputs correlate well with body weight and physical activity levels (Garrow,1978).

Inadequate or Distorted Sampling of Days

In studies of energy intake, sampling issues often account for low intakes observed. Subjects may inadvertently alter their food intakes on recording days, or they may deliberately misreport their intakes for other reasons when prospective methods are used, and with retrospective methods reporting errors are common. Also, energy intakes are highly variable from day to day within individuals. For example, correlations between energy intakes and expenditures within individuals only become significant after 7 or more days of observation (Edholm et al., 1970).

Energy Intake and Cancer

The associations of total energy intakes with human cancer risk have not been extensively studied, but existing data have been well summarized (Committee on

Diet, Nutrition and Cancer, 1982; Committee on Diet and Health, 1989). Some evidence exists for an association between high energy intakes and colorectal and breast cancers; but studies are few, and interpretatiaon is confounded by possible effects of deficiencies of fiber and micronutrients or excesses of fat in the diet. Animal experiments permit more elegant studies to be carried out. Clear effects on the development of certain cancers appeared to be present in animal models, particularly in the tumor-promotional stages in both colon and breast cancers. But the applicability of these animal models to human cancers remains in dispute.

Adjustments for Energy Intake in Analysis

The rationale for making statistical adjustments in energy intake is that the biological effects of energy intake upon health probably vary. For analytical purposes it is sometimes important to separate out the effects of total energy intake from absolute amounts of nutrients, which usually increase as energy intakes rise, or the proportion a nutrient contributes to total energy intake. When making dietary recommendations, it is important to determine if changes in calorie intake or changes in deitary composition at existing levels of energy intake are necessary to bring about desired health effects.

Body size, physical activity, metabolic efficiency, disease, and the specific nutrients providing energy may all be responsible for the associations observed between total energy intakes and diseases such as cancer. Before it is possible to attribute effects observed to specific nutrients, the effects of these other factors on total energy intake must be removed. However, because energy intakes or outputs may also be associated with disease themselves, it is important to measure total intakes of energy as well as intakes of specific nutrients.

This section reviews some of the major methods used to study the complex associations between these various dietary factors and diseases and briefly addresses the biological implications of the different analytical approaches. These methods have been well described by Willett (1990) and by Willett and Stampfer (1986). The reader is referred to these sources for details.

Methods of adjustment to control for the effects of total calorie intake in investigating diet/disease relationships are several. Intakes are often expressed per kilogram to control for body size. Nutrient densities (nutrient values divided by total calorie intake) or expressions of energy-yielding nutrients as a percent of total calories are also frequently employed. However, dividing by calories does not necessarily remove the effect of calories, and it may lead to confusion in interpretation (Willett, 1990).

In order to employ a measure of nutrient intake that is independent of total calorie intake in situations in which it is suspected that calorie intake is associated with disease, new analytical strategies have been proposed. First is the energy-adjusted nutrient intake method, which computes intakes as residuals from the regression model, when total calories are the independent variable and absolute nutrient intake is the dependent variable. Usually a constant such as expected nutrient intake for mean intakes in the population is added to provide an intuitive sense of actual nutrient intakes. If total energy intakes are thought to be predictors of disease, total calorie intake is included in the model with the nutrient-adjusted calorie term (Willett and Stampfer, 1986; and Willett et al., 1987).

A second method of control is the standard multivariate method, using both calorie intakes and absolute nutrient intakes in a multiple regression model, with disease outcome as the dependent variable (Willett, 1990).

A third method, the energy decomposition method, is a multiple logistic regression model in which separate terms are entered for energy from some specific macronutrient and for energy from other macronutrients (Howe et al., 1986).

Finally, there are multivariate nutrient-density models that involve the computation of nutrient density, which is then entered along with total energy in a multiple logistic regression model to control for confounding by energy intake (Jain et al., 1980). Alternatives include an "energy determinant method", which includes the major determinants of energy intake such as body size, physical activity, and metabolic efficiency as separate variables in the multivariate model (Willett, 1990). Other, more complex models, which include several macronutrients simultaneously, can also be considered.

MEASUREMENT OF ENERGY OUTPUT

Factors Affecting Energy Output

The major components of energy output are resting metabolic rate (RMR), the thermic effects of food (TEF), physical activity, and growth in healthy individuals. In ill health, endocrine disturbances, fever, and shivering thermogenesis may also increase energy expenditures in a pathologic fashion, owing to changes in thyroxin, catecholamines, and insulin, among other hormonal factors.

RMR is usually at least 60–65% of total energy expenditure in healthy individuals, and an even higher percentage of total energy needs in very sedentary or bed-bound people. The major factors affecting resting energy expenditure (RMR) in health persons are age, sex, body weight, hormone status, and growth. RMR declines with age, owing largely to decreases in lean body mass, the actively metabolizing tissue of the body. Sex differences in RMR are also present. They are attributable to differences between males and females in lean body mass, with males having a higher RMR due to their correspondingly higher lean body mass. Body weight and lean body mass are also positively correlated with RMR, people with high body weights having high RMR. Because of their usually higher lean body mass, obese individuals have higher RMRs than do the lean.

Physical activity is the second major component of energy output. Both obligatory (required for the lifestyle) and discretionary (or recreational) physical activity must be considered, especially in populations in which the use of labor-saving devices has decreased difference due to occupation. Those with large bodies require more energy for activities that require moving mass over distance. Efficiency and duration as well as the pace of work performed may also influence energy expenditures in physical activity. When weight is lost, as in weight reduction, in addition to declines in RMR due to loss of some lean body mass, less energy is required for moving the lighter body, and therefore total energy needs fall.

The metabolic response of food, or TEF, is a smaller but also significant contributor to overall energy output, which accounts for 5–10% of energy ingested. Depending on the size and composition of the meal, metabolic rate increases, reaches a maximum about an hour after consumption, and declines to usual levels by about 4 hours later (Garrow, 1978). Some genetic effects may be present in the size of TEF, but as yet these are poorly defined (Poehlman and Horton, 1989). On usual mixed diets, differences in diet composition on TEF are thought to be inconsequential, but more data are needed.

Growth requires energy for deposition of protein, fat, and carbohydrate in body tissue, in addition to the costs of synthesizing tissue. Average energy costs are about 5 kcal/g of tissue during infant growth, but these costs vary depending upon the type of tissue being laid down (Forbes, 1987b; Roberts and Young, 1988). The energy costs of growth at other times of life depend on the tissue being deposited.

Prolonged environmental exposure to cold or heat can also influence energy outputs via alterations in metabolic rate. This is referred to as adaptive thermogenesis (AT). Below 14 °C and above 37 °C, energy requirements may be increased to maintain thermal balance (Johnson, 1963). However, under usual circumstances, between 20 and 30 °C (68–86 °F), or when the individual is insulated from exposures to the environment, these influences on energy output are of little practical significance. Even under extreme circumstances they rarely account for more than 10–15% of total energy outputs.

Alterations in energy intake of a chronic nature lead to adaptations in energy output, that is, overall RMR decreases during food restriction, and increases with overfeeding (Woo, 1985; Forbes, 1987). New work indicates that in addition to RMR, TEF may also be affected by under- and over-feeding as well as by exercise (Poehlman and Horton, 1989).

Methods

Direct Estimates of Energy Output

The estimation of energy output has been a major preoccupation of physiologists and nutritionists for over two centuries. A comprehensive review of the many techniques that can be utilized in the direct measurement of energy output is beyond the scope of this chapter. However, excellent treatises exist that describe these techniques in great depth (Kleiber, 1975; Garrow, 1978; Kinney, 1988; Pi-Sunyer, 1988; Hoffer, 1988; Hultman et al., 1988; McLean and Tobin, 1988; Gibson, 1990).

The measurement of total energy output by direct calorimetry (Snellen et al., 1983) and indirect calorimetry using room respiration chambers has been well described elsewhere (Ravussin et al., 1982; Bessard et al., 1983; deBoer et al., 1986; Ravussin et al., 1985; Geissler et al., 1987). Additional discussion of various methods for estimating energy output is provided in McArdle's text (McArdle et al., 1986).

The advantage of such measurements, especially those that involve constant observation of the subject is that, with additional devices and measurements, both the energy cost and amount of physical activity can be estimated. The disadvantage of direct estimates of energy output is that subjects are confined, and they cannot go about their daily activities in their usual ways. Direct and indirect calorimetry in room respiration chambers, or by use of respiration apparatuses, involve confinement of the subject, decreased or altered physical activity, and thus generally result in lower estimates of energy expenditure than do energy balance, heart rate; doubly labeled water, or weight stabilization and exogenous weight replacement techniques.

Indirect Estimates of Energy Output

Several indirect methods for estimating energy output exist. A factorial approach is usually utilized clinically in estimating energy outputs, with different assumptions or measurements being used for calculating the likely effect of each component of energy output. Such a method is suggested in the 1989 Recommended Dietary Allowances for energy, which are calculated from RMR and an activity factor (Committee on Dietary Allowances, 1989).

Currently it is thought that activity patterns most likely to be typical of the U.S. population are in the light (1.5–1.6 × REE) and moderate categories (1.6–1.7 × REE). Although actual activity levels in the population are probably lower, levels of less than 1.3 × REE are thought to be incompatible with cardiovascular fitness. Therefore, the 1989 RDA employs multiples of 1.5–1.7 × REE in providing recommendations for energy intakes (Subcommittee on Dietary Allowances, 1989).

Factorial Method: Estimates of Components of Energy Output.

1. Resting metabolic rate: The estimations of resting metabolism by direct calorimetry (Snellen et al., 1983) and indirect calorimetry (Barzstein et al., 1977) are described at length elsewhere. These methods provide the most valid measurements of RMR, but they are costly and time consuming. Usually RMR

is estimated and not measured in clinical practice, unless very precise estimates of RMR are needed. Basal energy outputs are positively related to fat-free mass, body surface area, and body weight (Kleiber, 1975; Garrow, 1978). Because body weight is the most easily obtained measurement, RMR is most frequently estimated from it. Recently, updated formulas have been published that permit this to be done (Owen, 1986, 1987):

$$\text{RMR for mean} = 900 - 10 \text{ (body weight, kg)}$$

$$\text{RMR for women} = 800 + 7 \text{ (body weight, kg)}$$

Several other equations for specific age groups are also available (WHO, 1985) which provide more precise estimates. None of these equations are accurate for individuals, but they suffice for dietary planning purposes for groups and provide rough estimates for individuals.

2. Usual overall activity level: The Committee on Diet and Health (1989) suggested multipliers for usual levels of physical activity to roughly estimate total energy needs. Total energy need is estimated by calculating RMR using the equations of Owen (1986,1987) and then applying activity factors of 1.2 × REE for sedentary levels of activity, 1.4 for moderate activity, and 1.6 for high levels of activity such as those involving regular exercise or manual labor, a method similar to that suggested in the RDA.

3. Time and activity estimates: Another approach that permits somewhat more precise activity level estimates involves the use of representatives values for specific activities. These values are derived from the work of Durnin and Passmore (1967) and others (WHO, 1985). Some commonly used activity factors for these specific activities are provided in Table 4. Representative values for the activity factor are multiplied by the time spent in each activity, and these are summed to provide an estimate of total energy output. But coefficients of variation are high, probably at least 20% for light and moderate activity levels. Therefore, such calculations are simply approximations. Reports of physicial activity by subjects have been used in several studies as proxies for physical activity. These are highly subjective, but may be useful under certain circumstances (Garfinkel and Stellman, 1988).

4. Activity diaries: Rather than relying solely on subjective estimates of time spent in different activities in order to obtain greater precision, diaries of physical activity are frequently used in epidemiologic studies of energy expenditure. The various types of activity diaries and other survey instruments have been described in several monographs (Durnin and Passmore, 1967; Garrow, 1978; LaPorte et al., 1985).

5. Occupational or job classifications: In the days when occupations or jobs varied greatly in the mandatory levels of physical activity which were required, such classifications were useful in obtaining rough measures of this component of physical activity. However, the differences between jobs today in the physical

Table 4 Suggested Activity Factors for Estimating Energy Expenditure in Various Activities

Activity	Activity factor per unit time
Resting (sleep, reclining)	1.0 × REE
"Sedentary" activity	1.2 × REE
Very light activity: Seated and standing activities, painting trades, driving, laboratory work, typing, sewing, ironing, walking, playing cards, or a musical instrument	1.5 × REE
"Light activity: Walking on level surface at 2.5–3 mph, garage work, electrical trades, carpentry, restaurant trades, housecleaning, child care, golf, sailing, ping pong	2.5 × REE
"Moderate" activity: Walking 3.5–4 mph, weeding, hoeing, carrying a load, cycling, skiing, tennis, dancing	5.0 × REE
"Heavy" activity: Walking with load uphill, tree felling, heavy manual digging, basketball, climbing, football, soccer	7.0 × REE

activity they require are less than they were years ago. Therefore, these indicators are no longer useful in and of themselves for most investigational purposes.

6. Other Factors: Further adjustments in estimates of energy output are made for pregnancy, lactation, and growth. Other factors, such as the thermic effect of food, are small, and adjustments are not usually made to account for them. However, in research studies these may be important.

Indirect measurement of energy output using doubly labeled water. Doubly labeled water ($^2H_2O^{18}$ or D_2O^{18}) is employed in a new technique for measuring energy output in free living individuals (Schoeller, 1986). A tracer dose is given. The oxygen is incorporated into body water and bicarbonate, and is eventually excreted as either carbon dioxide or water, and the stable isotope of oxygen can be measured by taking samples of expired air and urine. The deuterium mixes with body water, and a small amount (probably 2–3%) also exchanges with labile body hydrogen in protein and other constituents. An indirect measurement of metabolic rate can be derived by comparing the rate at which the heavy oxygen declines vs. the decline in deuterium, as body water is continually diluted with newly inspired oxygen uptake and carbon dioxide output in respiration. Thus the disappearance of deuterated hydrogen in heavy water is due to turnover of body water, and the disappearance of O^{18} in the doubly labeled water is due to *both* the turnover of body water and carbon dioxide production. The end result is that both average carbon dioxide production and total energy expenditure can be determined from the differential disappearance rate of the isotopes over about 2 weeks (Matthews and Bier, 1983). Its use in validating energy intakes has recently been reviewed by Schoeller (1990). The technique has proven useful in identifying underestimates of energy intake, which are common when dietary records are used (Livingstone et al., 1990). The method offers much promise, but it is still experimental and costly, and presently the availability of doubly labeled water is limited (LaPorte et al., 1985).

Heart rate. Because heart rate varies directly with physical activity level, it has been proposed as a measure of energy output. However, heart rate is not a good index of energy output at rest, and therefore the errors in this type of measurement are considerable (LaPorte et al., 1985).

Weight stabilization and exogenous weight replacement: A new energy balance technique. The weight stabilization technique places subjects on a precisely known energy intake using a completely metabolizable formula diet. Intakes are adjusted until weight stability is achieved. Metabolizable energy intake is then assumed to equal energy output (Weigle and Brunzell, 1990). Exogenous weight replacement (using divers' weights or similar weights) is used to fractionate decreases in energy intake during dieting. A vest, into which weights are inserted to compensate for weight loss on a reducing diet, is worn by the subject. When coupled with weight stabilization and estimates of resting metabolism, the thermic effect of exercise can be estimated by making comparisons between individuals who lose weight and have exogenous weight replacement, and those who do not (Weigle, 1988; Weigle et al., 1988). These techniques are useful, since they permit subjects to engage in more usual levels of physical activity than is the case with direct or indirect calorimetry in chambers or with bulky apparatus. When subjects are not confined, estimates of energy expenditure are generally higher, probably because they engage in more physical activity. Energy expenditure is reduced after weight loss has occurred, and much of this is due to decreased costs or amount of physical activity; a smaller component is associated with decreased resting metabolism due to lessened lean body mass. In weight loss situations this technique is especially useful.

The major disadvantage of this technique is that body composition must be presumed to be constant if weight is constant and no other measures are employed, but this may not be so. Methods for estimating body composition can overcome this problem. Another difficulty is that compliance may be imperfect, both in adhering to formula diets and in wearing weights if the weight replacement technique is used. These problems can be overcome by confining the subjects or by monitoring them, but such procedures may alter usual activity levels.

Energy balance techniques. If energy intake can be measured accurately and body composition is assumed to be constant, total energy output should equal energy intake. The energy balance technique for estimating energy output has been used in many studies (Calloway and Zanni, 1980; Webb and Abrams, 1983; Borel et al., 1984; Leibel and Hirsch, 1984). Its advantage is that the method is applicable to unconfined individuals, and thus more normal estimates of physical activity can be obtained than when direct calorimetry or indirect calorimetry, which confines or otherwise restricts activity, are employed.

The major problems are that energy intakes only reflect output over a period of many weeks, errors in estimating energy intake are large and tend to be underestimates, and techniques for determining small changes in body composition are cumbersome.

Other Measurements. Other methods for assessing energy output include calorimetry, behavioral observation, survey procedures, physiologic markers, mechanical and electronic markers. These have recently been reviewed by LaPorte et al. (1985).

Exercise reports or reports of physical activity have been used in several studies as proxies for physical activity (Garfinkel and Stellman, 1988). These are highly subjective, but under certain circumstances they may be useful.

Errors in Assessing Energy Expenditure

Some of the major threats to validity from measures of energy output are summarized below.

Use of calorie expenditure estimates for various activities is imprecise. For many common activities involved in daily living, energy outputs have been measured by the use of indirect calorimetry, and values have been published. From such tables for a given intensity of the activity, if calorie expenditures and duration are estimated, energy output estimates can be calculated (Taylor et al., 1978). However, this procedure is at best a semiquantitative one, since such factors as skill and dexterity as well as weight (for activities involved in moving the body) are usually not totally accounted for.

Use of occupational classifications. Jobs are often classified by their levels of energy output. However, for a variety of reasons such as seniority and union work rules, jobs vary, even within categories. Also, people's jobs change, and so periodic adjustments may be needed (Paffenbarger et al., 1987). Finally, as jobs have become more sedentary, most occupations are more similar to each other than they used to be. Thus, traditional estimates based on occupation are no longer accurate measures of energy output.

High and low numbers of hours of vigorous physical activity at some prior point in life. Often, vigorous participation in sports has been used to categorize people by their physical activity levels. It is often assumed that the active will stay active in later life, and that differences in later outcomes are due to differences in physical activity. In fact, this assumption may not be valid. More complete descriptions of life-long physical activity need to be developed.

Energy requirements from estimates of energy output. Underestimates of energy requirements may result from estimates of energy output based on a constant fixed multiplicative relationship between resting metabolic rate and the energy cost of activities not requiring locomotion. That is, when the energy cost of activity is stated as a certain increment in calories over basal levels, those whose RMR is depressed or low owing to undernutrition may be penalized.

To illustrate this point, consider a 50-kg woman with a RMR of 1260 kcal/day. According to current WHO standards (World Health Organization, 1985), she has a calorie cost of 2.5 kcal/min for housework (or 1.4 kcal over RMR), but a heavier woman with a RMR of 1440 kcal/day has a cost of 1.5 kcal over baseline (Gopalan, 1990), which is surely not correct. Moreover, there is *no* reason to suspect that the energy cost is in fact any less among people with lower body weights for activities not requiring locomotion. These observations have led Durnin to suggest that the new procedures for estimating energy needs that have been adopted by World Health Organization and the Food and Nutrition Board need examination (Durnin, 1990).

Contemporary physical activity levels as estimates of long-term status. In this case, the assumption that contemporary activity reflects longstanding activity may be erroneous.

Comparisons with Standards: Potential Problems

It is well known that reported energy intakes are substantially below the 1980 RDA for women after early adolescence and also among adult men (Committee on Diet and Health, 1989). In 1989 the RDAs were raised to ideal levels, and it is likely that now even more groups will have intakes and outputs that are substantially below the RDA (Subcommittee on Tenth Edition of RDA's, 1989). Underestimates of food intake are especially common for fat and alcohol (National Research Council, 1986; Caliendo, 1989). The latest data from the National Nutrition Monitoring System shows that reported energy intakes are lower than recommended intakes, but that the prevalance of overweight is also considerable among adult Americans (Life Sciences Research Office, 1989, p. 50). Additional information on both energy intakes and expenditures is needed to evaluate the relative impact of these factors on the occurrence of obesity.

The fact that most reported energy intakes are not valid is obvious when diaries of energy outputs are compared with reported energy intakes. For most individuals in developing countries, activity diaries suggest that at least 1.5 times basal metabolic rates are needed for reported activities (Durnin, 1990). Yet reported energy intakes are often extremely low, much lower than this, suggesting that methodological errors are present which lead to underreporting of energy intakes.

Table 5 Studies on Physical Activity and Cancer in Humans

Energy output	Energy intake	Other variables	Outcome	Conclusions	Ref.
Occupational category and physical activity by questionnaire on multiphasic health questionnaire (w/job classification).	None	Adjusted for age, not smoking or obsesity status.	Morbidity, total and cause-specific mortality.	Physical activity delays all cause mortality. Also at least in some studies, vigorous activity in college decreases rectal cancer incidence and increases prostate cancer incidence.	Paffenbarger et al., 1987
In one study, participation in sports hr/week also obtained by questionnaire	None		No association w/breast cancer of physical activity in females; possible protective effect of activity on colon and rectal cancer.		
In a study of college alumni, number of city blocks walked, stairs climbed, and types and times of sports-related activities assessed, and then assigned calorie values and totalled into a physical activity index in calories/week.	Not assessed	Adjusted for age, smoking, body mass index	Cause-specific and total mortality.	Among stevedores and longshoremen, more active had slightly higher (nonsignif) risks of death fr pancreatic or colorectal cancer.	Paffenbarger et al., 1984, 1986

Sports participation as assessed by questionnaire in former college athletes.					Frisch et al., 1985
Questionnaire on exercise and amount/time spent/day on physical activities (did not include housework, so may have missed associations in women).	Semiquantitative food frequency questionnaire on 56 items to estimate intakes of vitamin A, C, D, β-carotene, and dietary fiber.	Alcohol, smoking, intakes/vitamins number/children	Neither alcohol, smoking, Quetelet index, nor physical activity had a significant and independent effect on colon cancer in females although all did in males.	Among 11,888 elderly people at 4.5 yr of follow-up, alcohol intakes, Quetelet's index. positively and leisure time physical activity negatively associated w/colorectal cancer in males (signif) and females (nsd).	Wu et al., 1987
Occupation (physically active) used.	Not measured	Asbestos, organic solvents, trichlorethylene all increased risks in exposed occupations	Morbidity	In 329 cases and 658 controls, physically active occupations had decreased risks of colon cancer, esp. in descending and sigmoid colon.	Fredriksson et al., 1989
Exercise patterns by question on amount of exercise at work or play (single question).	Not measured	Controls for smoking and body wt.	Cancer-related mortality.	Among 868,620 respondents in year 2 of study, inverse association between exercise and mortality; even after control for smoking.	Garfinkel and Stillman, 1988

(continued)

Table 5 *Continued*

Energy output	Energy intake	Other variables	Outcome	Conclusions	Ref.
2-yr retrospective questionnaire on leisure time and occupation by level of intensity of physical activity, converted to caloric output per wk. Both time at leisure (light, moderate, high-intensity activities) and job-related activities (as assessed by open-ended questionnaires obtained and converted to total activity.	2-yr retrospective quantitative food frequency questionnaire	Controls for age and body mass index by multiple logistic regression analysis.	Colon cancer	Among 384 population based controls and 229 cases, total physical activity protected against colon cancer development when highest and lowest levels of physical activity compared (OR 0.70 males OR 0.48 females). The greatest effects were from intense physical activity. Effects remained after adjusting diet calories. Also, even after adjusting for physical activity there was a positive association between diet and colon cancer. Conclusion: Physical activity modifies colon cancer dietary risk.	Slattery et al., 1988

Job type or workload	N.A.	Large bowel cancer risk is elevated in those with sedentary jobs or light workloads, but no association with rectal cancer in case-control study.	Garabrant et al., 1984
Job type or workload	N.A.	Large bowel cancer risk is elevated in those with sedentary jobs or light workloads, but no association with rectal cancer in case-control study.	Vera et al., 1985
Job type or workload	N.A.	Large bowel cancer risk is elevated in those with sedentary jobs or light workloads, but no association with rectal cancer in case-control study.	Gerhardsson et al., 1986

Energy Expenditures and Cancer

Human studies of energy output and cancer risk are few, but the limited evidence available is of interest. These studies are summarized in Table 5 for colon cancer. Findings are inconsistent and do not permit conclusions to be reached about the effects of physical activity on cancer risk. However, they do suggest that additional work may be fruitful.

Animal studies on the relationship between energy expenditures and cancer have been well reviewed in a recent monograph (Committee on Diet and Health, 1989). Both calorie restriction and physical activity, both of which lead to depletion of energy stores, seem to alter tumorigenesis. Endocrine, paracrine, or neurohormonal responses may be involved, but at present the role of energy output on cancer development remains obscure in humans and in animal models.

CONCLUSIONS AND FUTURE RESEARCH NEEDS

Quantitative and qualitative aspects of food energy intake may be associated with cancer development. At present, our understanding of the mechanisms whereby these effects are exerted is obscure. The assessment of energy intakes is still imprecise and fraught with difficulties.

The type, timing, frequency, duration, intensity, intermittance, and seasonality of physical energy expenditure may be involved in the initiation, promotion, or suppression of certain forms of cancer. The mechanisms whereby these effects occur is unclear. We need to better measure the associations between different types of energy expenditure and cancer-related outcomes in the future.

No single method for assessing energy output is valid, reliable, and practical, while not affecting behavior (LaPorte, 1985). The methods that are most precise are impractical for large-scale studies. Nevertheless, even with imperfect methods of measuring energy intakes and outputs, some useful associations with health have been found. With further developments in assessment techniques, these associations may become stronger.

REFERENCES

Anderson, S. A. (ed.). *Guidelines for Use of Dietary Intake Data*, Life Science Research Office, Federation of American Societies for Experimental Biology, Bethesda, MD, 1986.

Balough, M., Kahn, H. A., Medalie, J. H. Random Repeat 24-hour dietary recalls. *Am. J. Clin. Nutr. 24*:304–310 (1971).

Bazarre, T., Myers, M. The collection of food intake data in cancer epidemiology studies. *Nutrition Cancer 1*: 22–45 (1978).

Beaton, G. H., Milner, J., Corey, P., et al. Sources of variance in 24-hour dietary recall data: Implications for nutrition study design an interpretation. *Am. J. Clin. Nutr. 32*: 2546–2559 (1979).

Berlin, J. A., Colditz, G. A. A meta-analysis of physical activity in the prvention of coronary heart disease. *Am. J. Epidemiol. 132*: 612–628 (1990).

Bessard, T., Schutz, Y., Jequier, E. energy Expenditure and postprondial thermogenesis in obese women before and after weight loss. *Am. J. Clin. Nutr. 38*: 680–632 (1983).

Bingham, S. The dietary assessment of individuals: Methods, accuracy, new techniques, and recommendations. *Nutrition Abstracts and Reviews* (Series A) *57*: 705–742 (1987).

Bingham, S., Cummings, J. H. Urine nitrogen as an indpeendent validity measurement of dietary intake. *Am. J. Clin. Nutr. 42*: 1276–1289 (1985).

Bingham, S., Cummings, J. H. The use of 4 amino benzoic acid as a worker to validate the completeness of 24-hour urine collections in men. *Clin. Sci. 64*: 629–635 (1983).

Bingham, S. McNeil, N. I., Cummings, J. H. The diet of individuals: A study of a randomly-chosen cross section of British adults in a Cambridgeshire village. *British J. Nutr. 45*: 23–25 (1981).

Bingham, S. A., Nelson, M. Paul, A. A., Haraldsdottir, J., Bjorge-Loken, E., and Van Staveren, W. A. Methods for data collection at an individual level. In *Manual on Methodology for Food Consumption Studies* (M. E. Cameron and W. A. Van Staveren, eds.), Oxford Medical Publications, 1988, pp. 53–106.

Bingham, S., Wigigns, H. S., Evelyst, H., et al. Methods and validity of dietary assessments in four Scandinavian populations. *Nutrition and Cancer 4*: 23–33 (1982).

Black, A. E. In *Pitfalls in Dietary Assessment in Recent Advances in Clinical Nutrition* (A. N. Howard and I. McClean Baird, eds.), John Libbey, London, 1981, pp. 11–18.

Black, A. E., Cole, T. J., Wiles, S. J., White, F. Daily variation in food intake of infants from 2 to 18 months. *Human Nutrition, Applied Nutrition 37A*: 448–458 (1983).

Black, A. E., Ravenscroft, C., Sims, A. J. The NACNE Report: Are dietary goals realistic? Comparisons with the dietary patterns of dietitians. *Human Nutrition, Applied Nutrition 38*A:165–179 (1984).

Blair, S. N., Jacobs, D. R., Powell, K. E. Relationship between exercise or physical ac tivity and other health behaviors. *Public Health Reprint 100*: 172–179 (1987).

Block, G. A review of validations of dietary assessment methods. *Am. J. Epidemiol. 115*: 492–505 (1982).

Block, G., Hartman, A. M. Dietary assessment methods, In *Nutrition and Cancer Prevention: Investigating the Role of Micronutrients* (T. E. Moon and M. S. Micozzi, eds)., Marcel Dekker, New York 1989, pp. 159–180.

Bogardus, C. Commentary on: Assessment of energy expenditure in ambulatory reduced obese subjects by the techniques of weight stabilization and exogenous weight replacement. *Int. J. Obesity 14* (Suppl 1): 77–78 (1990).

Borel, M. J., Riley, R. E., Snook, J. T. Estimation of energy expenditure and maintenance energy requirements of college age men and women. *Am. J. Clin. Nutr. 40*: 1264–1272 (1984).

Bransby, E. R., Daubney, C. G. King, J. Comparison of results obtained by different methods of individual dietary survey. *Br. J. Nutr. 2*: 89–110 (1948).

Burema, J., Van Staveren, W. A., Van Den Brandt, P. A. Validity and reproducibility, *Manual on Methodology for Food Consumption Studies*, (M. E. Cameron and W. A. Van Staveren, eds.), Oxford University Press, 1988, pp. 171–181.

Burk, M. C., Pao, E. M. *Methodology for Large-Scale Surveys of Household and Individual Diets*, Home Economics Research Report No. 40. U. S. Government Printing Office, Washington, DC, 1976.

Bursey, R., Huth, P., Hunt, C., Olson, R. Efficiency of energy deposition from sucrose, starch, dextrose, and corn oil in growing rats. *Proc. Nat. Acad. Sci.* (1987).

Burzstein, S., Saphar, P., Glaser, P., Taitelman, U., deMyttenaere, S., Nedley, R. Determination of energy metabolism from respiratory functions alone. *J. Appl. Physiol. Respirat. Environ. Exercise Physiol. 42*: 117–119 (1977).

Caliendo, M. A. Study of food intake by mean *Methodological Research for Large-Scale Dietary Intake Surveys 1975–88.* (E. M. Pao, K. E. Sykes, and Y. S. Cypel, eds.), U. S. Department of Agriculture, Human Nutrition Information Service, Home Economics Research Report No. 49, U. S. Department of Agriculture, Beltsville, MD, 1989, pp. 118–156.

Calloway, D. H., Zanni, E. Energy requirements and energy expenditure of elderly men. *Am. J. Clin. Nutr. 33*: 2088–2092 (1980).

Campbell, V. A., Dodds, M. L. Collecting dietary information from groups of older people. *J. Am. Diet. Assoc. 51*: 29–33 (1967).

Caspersen, C. J., Powell, K. E., Christenson, G. M. Physical activity, exercise, and physical fitness: Definitions and distinctions for health-related research. *Public Health Reports 100*: 126–131, 1985.

Committee on Diet and Health. *Diet and Health: Implications for Reducing Chronic Disease Risk.* National Research Council, National Academy Press, Washington, DC, 1989.

DeBoer, J. O., VanEs, A. J. H., Roovers, L. A., VanRaiij, J. M. A., Hautrast, J. G. V. A. Adaptation of energy metabolism of overweight women to low energy intake, studied with whole body calorimeters. *Am. J. Clin. Nutr. 44*: 585–595 (1986).

Dishman, R. K., Sallis, J. F., Orenstein, D. R. The determinants of physical activity and exercise. *Public Health Reports 100*: 158–171 (1985).

Donato, K., Hegsted, D. M. Efficiency of utilization of various sources of energy for growth. *Proc. Nat. Acad. Sci. USA 82*: 4866–4870 (1985).

Durnin, J. V. G. A. Is satisfactory energy balance possible in low energy intakes? *NFI Bulletin 11*(2):1–3 (1990).

Durnin, J. V. G. A., Passmere, R. *Energy, Work, and Leisure.* Heinemann Educational Books, London, 1967.

Edholm, O. G., Adam, J. M., Healy, M.J., Wolff, H. S. Goldsmith, R., Best, T. N. Food intake and energy expenditure of army recruits. *Br. J. Nutr. 24*: 1091–1107 (1970).

Elia, M., Laumert, O., Zed, C., Neale, G. Energy metabolism during exercise in normal subjects undergoing total starvation. *Human Nutrition, Clinical Nutrition 38C*: 355-362 (1985).

Eppright, E. S., Patten, M. B., Marlatt, A. L., Hathaway, M. L. Dietary study methods V. Some problems in collecting dietary information about groups of children. *J. Am. Diet. Assoc. 28*: 43–48 (1952).

Flores, M., Nelson, M. Methods for data collection at household or institutional level, In *Manual on Methodology for Food Consumption Studies* (M. E. Cameron and W. A. Von Staveren, eds.), Oxford University Press, Oxford, 1988, pp. 33–52.

Food and Nutrition Board, National Research Council. *Assessing Changing Food Consumption Patterns*, National Academy of Sciences Press, Washington, DC, 1981.

Food and Nutrition Board, National Research Council, *National Survey Data on Food Consumption: Uses and Recommendations*, National Academy Press, Washington, DC, 1984.

Food and Nutrition Board, National Research Council, *Nutrient Adequacy; Assessment Using Food Consumption Surveys*, National Academy Press, Washington, DC, 1986.

Forbes, G. B. *Human Body Composition: Growth, Aging, Nutrition, and Activity*. Springer-Verlag, New York, 1987a.

Forbes, G. B. Lean body mass—body fat interrelationships in humans *Nutr. Rev. 45*: 225-231 (1987b).

Fredriksson, M., Bengtsson, N. O., Hardell, L., Axelson, O. Colon Cancer, physical activity & occupational exposures: A case control study. *Cancer 63*: 1838-1842 (1989).

Frisch, R. E., Wyshak, G., Albright, N. L., Albright, T. E., Schiff, I., Jones, K. P., Witschi, J., Ishiang, E., Koff, E., Marguglio, M. Lower prevalence of breast cancer and cancers of the reproductive system among former college athletes, compared to nonathletes. *Br. J. Cancer 52*: 885-891 (1985).

Garabrant, D. H., Peters, J. M., Mack, T. M., Berstein, L. Job activity and colon cancer risk. *Am. J. Epidemiol. 119*: 1005-1014 (1984).

Garby, L., Laumert, O., Nielsen, E. Within subjects' between-weeks variation in 24-hour energy expenditure for fixed physical activity. *Human Nutrition: Clinical Nutrition 38*C: 391-394 (1984).

Garfinkel, L., Stillman, S. D. Mortality by relative weight and exercise. *Cancer 62*: 1844-1850 (1988).

Garrow, J. S. *Energy Balance and Obesity in Men*, 2d ed. Elsevier-Worth Holland, Amsterdam, 1978.

Gerhardsson, M., Norell, S. E., Kiviranth, H., Pedersen, N. L., Ahlbom, A. Sedentary jobs and colon cancer. *Am. J. Epidemiol 123*: 775-780 (1986).

Gibson, R. S. *Principles of Nutritional Assessment*. Oxford University Press, New York, 1990.

Gopalan, C. Low energy intakes. *W.F.I. Bulletin 11*(2):5 (1990).

Hackett, A. F., Rugg-Gunn, A. J., Appleton, D. R. Use of a dietary diary and interview to estimate the food intake of children. *Human Nutr., Applied Nutr. 37*A:293-300 (1983).

Haras, S. Macronutrients and cancer. *Clin. Nutr. 9*: 49-55 1990.

Hoffer, L. J. Starvation, In *Modern Nutrition in Health and Disease*, 7th ed. (M. E. Shils and V. R. Young, eds.) Lea & Febiger, Philadephia, PA, 1988.

Hofstetter, A., Schultz, Y., Jequier, E., Warren, J. Increased 24-hour energy expenditure in cigarette smokers. *N. Engl. J. Med. 314* (1986).

Holdstock, D. J., Misiewicz, J. J., Smith, T., et al. Propulsion (mass movement) in the human colon and its relationship to meals and somatic activity. *Gut 11*: 91-99 (1970).

Howe, G. R., Miller, A. B., Jain, M. Re: Total Energy Intake: Implications for Epidemiologic Analyses. *Am. J. Epidemiol 124*: 156-157 (1986).

Huenemann, R. L., Turner, D. Methods of dietary investigation *J. Am. Diet. Assoc. 18*: 562-568 (1942). Hultman, E., Thomson, J. A., Harris, R. C. Work and exercise, In *Modern Nutrition in Health and Disease*, 7th ed. (M. E. Shils and V. R. Young, eds.) Lea and Febiger, Philadelphia, PA,1988, pp. 1001-1022.

IARC Large Bowel Cancer Group. Second IARC International Collaborative Study on diet and large bowel cancer in Denmark and Finland. Nutrition and Cancer 4: 3-79 (1982).

Isaksson, B. Urinary nitrogen output as a validity test in dietary surveys. *Am. J. Clin. Nutr. 33*: 4–5 (1980).

Jain, M., Cook, G. M., Davis, F. G., Grace, M. G., Howe, G. R., Miller, A. B. A case control study of diet and colorectal cancer. *Int. J. Cancer 26*: 757–768 (1980).

Johnson, R. E. Calorie requirements under adverse environmental conditions. *Fed. Proc. 22*: 1439–1446 (1963).

Karvetti, R. L., Knuts, L. R. Validity of 24-hour recall *J. Am. Diet. Assoc. 85*: 1437–1442 (1985).

Kinney, J. M. Food as fuel: The development of concepts, In *Modern Nutrition in Health and Disease*, 7th ed. (M. E. Shils and V. R. Young, eds.), Lea and Febiger, Philadelphia, PA, 1988, pp. 516–532.

Kleiber, M. *The Fire of Life: An Introduction to Animal Energetics*. Robert E. Krieger, Huntington, NY, 1985.

Kromhaut, D. Changes in energy and maronutrients in 871 middle-aged men during 10 years of follow-up (the Zutphan Study). *Am. J. Clin. Nutr.37*: 287–294 (1983).

Kromhaut, D. Energy and Macronutrient intake in lean and obese middle-aged men (the Zutphan study). *Am. J. Clin. Nutr. 37*: 295–299 (1983).

LaPorte, R. E., Montoye, H. J., Casparsen, C.J. Assessment of physical activity in epidemiologic research: Problems and prospects. *Public Health Reports 100*: 131–146 (1985).

Life Sciences Research Office, Federation of American Societies for Experimental Biology, *Nutrition Monitoring in the United States, An Update on Nutrition Monitoring*, Prepared for the U.S. Department of Agriculture and the U.S. Department of Health and Human Services, DHHS Publication No. (PHS) 89–1255, Public Health Service, Washington, DC, U.S. Government Printing Office, September 1989, pp. 48–50.

Lyon, J. L., Mahoney, A. N. West, D. W. et al. Total food intake: A risk factor in colon cancer. *JNCI 78*: 853–861 (1987).

Manson, J. E., Stampfer, M. J., Hennekers, C. H., Willett, W. C. Body weight and longevity. *JAMA 257*: 353–358 (1987).

Marr, J. N. Individual dietary surveys, purposes, and methods. *World Review of Nutrition and Dietetics 13*: 106–164 (1971).

Marshall, J. R., Priore, R., Graham, S., Brasura. On the distortion of risk estimates in multiple exposure level case-control studies. *Am. J. Epidemiol 113*: 464–473 (1981).

Matthews, D. E., Bier, D. M. Stable isotope methods for nutritional investigation. *Am. Rev. Nutr. 3*: 309–339 (1983).

McArdle W.D., Katch, F.I. and Katch, V. L. *Exercise Physiology: Energy Nutrition and Human Performances*, 2nd Ed., Lea and Febiger, Philadelphia (1986).

McLean, J. A., Tobin, G. *Animal and Human Calorimetry*. Cambridge University Press, New York, 1988.

McMichael, A. J., Potter, J. D. Reproduction, endogenous, and exogenous sex hormones and colon cancer: A review and hypothesis. *JNCI 65*: 1201 (1980).

Merrill, A. L., Watt, B. K. *Energy Value of Foods, Basis and Derivation*. Agricultural Handbook No. 74, Human Nutrition Research Branch, Agricultural Research Service, U. S. Department of Agriculture, U.S. Government Printing Office, Washington, DC, 1955.

National Research Council. *Nutrient Adequacy: Assessment Using Food Consumption Surveys*. Report of the Subcommittee on Criteria for Dietary Evaluation, Food and Nutrition Board Commission on Life Sciences, National Academy Press, Washington, DC, 1986.

Nelson, M., Morris, J. A., Black, A. E., Cole, T. J. Between and within subject variation in nutrient intake from infancy to old age (in press).

Nettleton, P. A., Day, K. C., Nelson, M. Dietary Survey Methods 2. A comparison of nutrient intakes within families assessed by household measures and semi-weighed method *J. Human Nutrition 34*: 349-354 (1980).

Owen, O. E., Kavle, E., Owen, R. S., Polonsky, M., Caprio, S. Mozzoli, M. A., Bushman, M. C. and Boden, G. A reappraisal of colonic requirements in healthy women. *Am. J. Clin. Nutr. 44*:1-19 (1986).

Owen, O. E., Holup, J. L., D'Alession, D. A., Craig, E. S., Polansky, M., Smalley, K. S., Kavle, E. C., Bushman, M. C., Owen L. R., Mozzoli, M. A., Kendrick, Z. V., and Boden, G. H. A reappraisal of the colonic requiremenets of men. *Am J. Clin. Nutr. 46*:875-885, 1987.

Paffenbarger, R. S., Hyde, R. T., Wing, A. L., Hsieh, C. Physical activity, all-cause mortality, and longevity of college alumni. *N. Engl. J. Med. 314*: 605-613 (1986).

Paffenbarger, R. S., Hyde, R. T., Wing, A. L., Steinmetz, C.H. A natural history of athleticism and cardiovascular health. *JAMA 252*: 491-495 (1984).

Paffenbarger, R. S., Hyde, R. T., Wing, A. L. Physical activity and incidence of cancer in diverse populations: A preliminary report. *Am. J. Clin. Nutr. 45*: 312-317 (1987).

Pao, E., Cypel, Y. Estimation of dietary intake, In *Present Knowledge in Nutrition*, 6th ed. (M. L. Brown, ed.), International Life Sciences Institute, Nutrition Foundation, Washington, DC, 1990, pp. 399-406.

Pi-Sunyer, F. X. Obesity, In *Modern Nutrition in Health and Disease*, 7th ed. (M. E. Shils and V. R. Young, eds.), Lea and Febiger, Philadelphia, PA, 1988, pp. 795-816.

Poehlman, E. T., Horton, E. S. The impact of food intake and exercise on energy expenditure. *Nutr. Rev. 47*: 129-137 (1989).

Prentice, A. M., Black, A. E., Coward, W. A., et al. High levels of energy expenditure in healthy women *292*: 983-987 (1986).

Prentice, A. M., Coward, N. A., Davies, H.L., et al. Unexpectedly low levels of energy expenditure in healthy women. *Lancet ii*: 1419-1422 (1985).

Prentice, A. M., Coward, W. A. Measurement of energy expenditure in free living subjects using stable isotopes. *Proc. Assoc. Phys.* (in press).

Roberts, S. B., Young, V. R. Energy costs of fat and protein deposition in the human infant. *Am. J Clin. Nutr. 48*: 951-955 (1988).

Sallis, J. F., Haskell, W. L., Wood, P. D., Fortmann, S. P., Rogers, T., Blair, S. N., Paffenbarger, R. S. Physical activity assessment methodology in the Five City Project. *Am. J. Epidemiol. 121*: 91-106 (1985).

Schoeller, D. A. How accurate is self-reported dietary intake? *Nutr. Rev. 48*: 373-379 (1990).

Schoeller, D. A., Ravussin, E., Schutz, Y., Acheson, K. J., Baertschi, P., Jequier, E. Energy expenditure by doubly-labeled water: Validation in humans and proposed calculation. *Am. J. Physiol. 250*: R832-R830 (1986).

Schofield, W. N., Schofield, C., James, W. P. T. Basal metabolic rate. *Hum. Nutrition, Clinical Nutrition 39C* (Suppl 1):1–96 (1985).

Sempos, C., Johnson, N. E., Smith, E. L., Gilligan, C. Effects of intraindividuals and interindividual variation in repeated dietary records. *Am. J. Epidemiol. 121*: 120–130 (1985).

Severson, R. K., Normua, A. M. Y., Grove J. S., Stemmermann, G. N. A prospective analysis of physicial activity and Cancer. *Am. J. Epidemiol. 130*: 522–529 (1989).

Shils, M. E. Nutrition and diet in cancer, In *Modern Nutrition in Health and Disease*, (M. E. Shils and V. R. Young, eds.)., 7th ed. Lea and Febiger, Philadelphia, 1988.

Slattery, M. L., Schumacher, M. C., Smith, K. R., West, D. W., Abd-Elghany, N. Physical activity, deit and risk of colon cancer in Utah. *Am. J. Epidemiol. 128*: 989–999 (1988).

Sopko, G., Jacobs, D. R., Taylor, H. L. Dietary measures of physical activity. *Am. J. Epidemiol. 120*: 900–911 (1984).

Steen, B., Isaksson,B., Svanborg, A. Intake of energy and nutrients and meal habits in 70-year-old males and females in Gothenberg, Sweden: A population study. *Acta Med. Scand. Suppl. 611*: 39–86 (1977).

Stephens, T., Jacobs, D. R., White, C. C. The descriptive epidemiology of leisure time physical activity. *Public Health Report 100*: 147–158 (1985).

Subcommittee on the Tenth Edition of the RDA's Food and Nutrition Board, Commission on Life Sciences, National Research Council. *Recommended Dietary Allowances*, 10th ed. National Academy Press, Washington, DC, 1989.

Taylor, H. L., Jacobs, D. R., Schucker, B., et al. A questionnaire for the assessment of leisure time physical activities. *J. Chronic Disease 31*: 741–755 (1978).

Thompson, M. Logan, R. L. Sharmon, M., Lockerbie, L., Riemersma, R., Oliver, M. F. Dietary survey in 40-year-old Edinburgh men. *Human Nutrition, Applied Nutrition 36*A:272–281 (1982).

Todd, K. S., Hudes, M., Calloway, D. H. Food intake measurement: Problems and approaches. *Am. J. Clin. Nutr. 37*: 139–146 (1983).

Vera, J. E., Graham, S. Zielezny, M. Swanson, M. K., Barnes, R. E. Nolan, J. Lifetime occupational exercise and colon cancer. *Am. J. Epidemiol. 122*: 357–365 (1985).

Walker, M. A., Blettner, M. Comparing imperfect measures of exposure. *Am. J. Epidemiol. 121*: 783–790 (1985).

Warnold, I., Carlgren, G., Krofkiewski, M. Energy expenditure and body composition during weight reduction in hyperplastic obese women. *Am. J. Clin. Nutr. 31*: 750–763, (1978).

Widdowson, E. M., McCance, R. A. A study of English diets by the individual method, Part 1. Men. *J. Hygiene 36*: 269–292 (1936a).

Widdowson, E. M., McCance, R. A. A study of English diets by the individual method: Women. *J. Hygiene 36*: 293–309 (1936b).

Willett, W. Implications of Total Energy Intake for Epidemiologic Analyses, *Nutritional Epidemiology*, (W. Willett, ed.), Oxford University Press, New York, 1990, pp. 245–271.

Willett, W. C. Implications of total energy intake for epidemiologic studies of breast and large bowel cancer. *Am. J. Clin. Nutr. 45*: 5–60 (1987).

Willett, W. C., Sampson, L., Stampfer, M.J., et al. Reproducibility and validity of a semi-quantitative food frequency questionnaire. *Am. J. Epidemiol. 122*: 51–68 (1985).
Willett, W. C., Stampfer, M. J. Total energy intake: Implications for epidemiologic analyses. *Am. J. Epidemiol. 124*: 17–27 (1986).
Woo, R. R., Daniels-Kush, R., Horton, E. S. Regulation of energy balance. *Ann. Rev. Nutr. 5*: 411–433 (1985).
World Health Organization. *Energy and Protein Requirements*. Report of a Joint FAO/WHO/UNU Expert Consultation, Technical Report Series 724, World Health Organization, Geneva, 1985.
Wu, A. H., Paganini Hill, A., Poss, R. K., Henderson, B. E. Alcohol, physical activity, and other risk factors for colorectal cancer: A prospective study. *Br. J. Cancer 55*: 687–694 (1987).
Young, C. M., Chalmers, F. W., Church, H. N., Clayton, M. M., Murphy, G., Ticker, R. E. Subjects' Estimation of Food Intake and Calculated Nutritive Value of the Diet. *J. Am. Diet. Assoc. 29*: 1216–1220 (1953).
Young, C. M., Franklin, R. E., Foster, W. D., Steele, B. F. Weekly variation in nutrient intake of young adults. *J. Am. Diet. Assoc. 29*: 459–464 (1953).

6

Anthropometry and Dietary Assessment in Nutrition and Cancer Studies

Marc S. Micozzi
National Museum of Health and Medicine
Armed Forces Institute of Pathology
Washington, D.C.

INTRODUCTION

Anthropometry, literally "measuring man," is the technique of expressing quantitatively the form of the human body. Various dimensions of the human body may be measured and studied in relation to nutritional patterns. One potential of anthropometry in cancer research lies in its application as an indirect means of nutritional assessment, especially assessment of past nutritional experience. Anthropometry may add a useful dimension to investigation of the relations between diet and cancer, especially in light of the difficulties associated with other means of dietary assessment and validation (Block, 1982; Block and Hartman, 1989).

In this chapter, the developmental history and scope of anthropometry in cancer research is briefly reviewed and a rationale for the application of anthropometry to diet and cancer studies presented. Guidelines for future applications of anthropometric techniques to epidemiologic studies of diet and cancer are also proposed. A theoretical and methodologic framework is presented in which anthropometry may be considered in the design and interpretation of studies on diet and cancer. Detailed protocols for the use of anthropometric techniques have been adequately addressed elsewhere (Lohman et al., 1988).

LIMITATIONS OF NUTRITIONAL ASSESSMENT METHODS

Nutritional epidemiology relies upon nutritional assessment methods to determine dietary intake and nutritional status in individuals who currently have or may develop cancer. The methods available to nutritional epidemiology have been limited to collection of dietary intake information through survey research techniques or measurements of individual nutrients in biological fluids. However, the human diet is varied and complex and cannot be easily assessed or simply characterized. The precision and accuracy of information collected by dietary interview is limited by the human capacity for recall. Humans eat foods, not nutrients, and the ability to reconstruct nutrient intake from dietary information is limited due to inaccuracy and incompleteness of available food composition tables. Furthermore, much of the existing food composition data is not generalizable in terms of nutritional productivity due to variations in cultigen (varieties of a food), climate, harvesting, processing, storage, and preparation of foods as actually consumed by different human populations (Micozzi, 1989). Measurement of nutrients in biological fluids (biochemical epidemiology) has been another approach to nutritional assessment. However, adequate analytical techniques are not available for measuring many nutrients of interest. Further, for many nutrients, little or no data are available on the relation of a single measurement at one point in time to long-term nutritional status. If nutrient intake in early life is relevant to long-term cancer risk, measurements of nutrients in adults may not be sufficient to illustrate the definitive role of nutrition in cancer. Biological fluids or tissue materials may also be difficult or complicated to obtain for measurements of nutrient levels. A related consideration is that study participants may be less willing to provide biological materials then they are to participate in other aspects of a study.

The design of diet and cancer studies also presents limitations. Analytical research in cancer epidemiology is often conducted in large, multicenter studies. Many of these studies are collecting dietary intake data that can be only characterized as imprecise (Block and Hartman, 1989). Training, standardization, and quality control for dietary assessment are of particular concern in such studies. Case-control studies of diet and cancer have the added complication of considering the effects of the disease or treatment on reported or measured variables and other parameters of interest to the study.

Case-control studies may suffer from problems of recall bias. Controls may underestimate dietary intake compared to cases. The obese may underestimate diet compared to the lean. The elderly may underestimate compared to the young. Some of these biases may result in artifactual differences between cancer cases and controls. Biological measurement of nutrient levels on cancer patients may also be influenced by the effects of disease on the nutrient of interest.

There are also a number of other reasons why case-control studies on diet and cancer, which collect data on individuals within a population, may not adequately test diet-cancer hypothesis (Miller, 1977). For example, the variability in dietary patterns may be insufficient to detect an effect of diet on cancer within any one population analyzed. Furthermore, existence of "threshold" levels for dietary intake and cancer risk as observed in animal models may preclude observation of an effect in any one population if the dietary intake of all individuals studied is grouped above or below the threshold level. The time in life at which dietary exposures influence cancer risk may not be observable in analytic studies. For example, if nutrient intake in early life is important to the long-term risk of cancer, analytic studies on elderly cancer cases may not be the optimal manner in which to test diet-cancer hypotheses. In migrant studies on diet and cancer, the time of dietary acculturation may be strongly related to the age at migration and the year of migration, as well as the time since migration (Albanes et al., 1987). The influence of a nutritional factor on cancer appears to depend upon the timing, duration, and magnitude of dietary exposures. Studies that do not permit comparison along these lines may lead to incomplete conclusions.

ANTHROPOMETRIC DIMENSIONS OF CANCER RESEARCH

Human epidemiologic and animal experimental evidence has suggested that excess intake of macronutrients (fat, protein, total calories) may be associated with increased incidence and decreased survival for some site-specific cancers among different populations (Armstrong and Doll, 1975; Caroll and Khor, 1975; Hems, 1978,1980; Gaskill, et al., 1979; Gray et al. 1979; Kolonel et al., 1981; Ross et al., 1983). The epidemiologic evidence, including studies on migrant populations (Buell and Dunn, 1965; Buell, 1973; Dunn, 1977), has further suggested that dietary patterns in early life may be important to the long-term risk of cancer (Miller, 1977). Since cancer is currently thought to be a multistage process with a long latent period, early childhood growth and nutritional patterns which influence adult body size and composition may also influence the adult risk of cancer.

Enduring indicators of growth that can be measured in adults (e.g., stature, sitting height, frame size, and aspects of body composition) may be reflective of early growth and nutritional patterns that place individuals at an increased risk of certain cancers in later life (Micozzi, 1985). In addition, anthropometric variables which are associated with adult as well as childhood nutritional patterns (e.g., total body fat, percent body fat) have been related to the risk of certain cancers in defined groups (Choi et al., 1978; Miller et al., 1978; Lubin et al., 1985).

The anthropometric sites of measurement and techniques of measurement that are important to cancer research are those that permit accurate and precise description of body size and body composition in large numbers of individuals in the field situation, and may be related to childhood growth and/or adult nutritional patterns. Accordingly, elucidation of the specific relations between body size, body composition, and childhood and adult nutrition is essential to research on diet and cancer. Some specific anthropometric dimensions important to cancer research have been suggested by epidemiologic observations.

Stature

Stature is an index of growth and nutrition during childhood and adolescence, which may be important for the long-term risk of certain cancers. Adult stature is established through growth by age 18 years and does not change appreciably during normal adult life. Although adult decline in stature begins relatively early, the cumulative effects are not large until old age. Stature provides a biological marker of early nutritional experience. Stature is mediated by the growth process and time of maturity, is reliably measured in adults, and may be related to cancer risk as an enduring indicator of growth and nutritional status in children.

DeWaard (1975) first suggested that increased stature accounts for most breast cancer risk attributable to body size or body mass. Using body mass indices that are almost uncorrelated to stature in adults, he found no association of excess weight with breast cancer in premenopausal women. The cross-cultural correlations of average adult stature with age-adjusted breast cancer rates in women among different populations was high ($r = 0.8$) in a recent ecologic study (Micozzi,1987).

In a descriptive study of migrants, Buell (1973) noted increasing incidence of breast cancer in successive generations of Japanese women in the United States compared to Japan. These changing cancer rates were attributed to dietary acculturation during childhood and increased stature and weight. The result of increased cancer rates in Japanese-American women is reflected in the age-specific cancer rates of a large Asian-american population in Los Angeles, 1972–1977. (Waterhouse et al., 1982). The younger Japanese-American women have much higher breast cancer rates (like U.S. Caucasian women) than do older Japanese-American women, who reflect lower breast cancer rates (historically like women of that age-group in Japan).

There has also been a recent observation in Japan itself of a secular tend for both body size and certain cancer rates (Hirayama, 1978). This cohort effect is also seen in the growth patterns of Japanese-American children over successive generations. The mean adult stature of samples of Japanese-American women born in 1940 is 154 cm (Greulich, 1957), while that of Japanese-American women born one generation later is 158 cm (Kondon and Eto, 1975). Increased breast cancer rates in Japanese migrants may be a reflection of increased nutrition and growth in childhood, since stature increases are apparent in successive generations of Japanese women in the United States. Japanese women of various generations in California all appear to have similar growth patterns until the time of puberty (Greulich, 1976). However, later generations of Japanese women in California have greater growth at ages 15, 16, and 17 years, accounting for greater adult stature (Eveleth and Tanner, 1976). This period represents the time in life when age-specific anthropmetric variables become increasingly highly correlated to adult rates of breast, prostatic, pancreatic, and other cancers among human populations (Micozzi, 1986a).

Given that growth is partially a function of dietary intake (Johnston, 1981, 1983), cross-cultural among different population samples of cancer rates (age-adjusted for differences in average lifespan) with anthropometic measurements taken at different points during childhood provide additional information about the impact of diet, especially increased nutrition, on cancer. For example, correlations were found between breast cancer incidence and mortality rates and mean age-specific stature, weight, and biacromial diameter. The correlations between breast cancer and each of these anthropometric variables was highest for the oldest age group (Micozzi, 1987).

As observed in the divergence of growth curves, differences between populations are cumulatively reflected in size differences at later, rather than earlier, ages in children. The trend that anthropometric-cancer correlations are also stronger for older ages may lend further support to the relation beween diet and cancer. The nutrition, body size, and cancer correlations hold up independently when UNICEF (1981) measures of socioeconomic status (SES) are taken into account (Micozzi, 1987) and explain cancer rates in various populations around the world that cannot be explained by SES alone or are contradictory to SES hypothesis (e.g., Henderson, 1979).

In a prospective study of cancer recently conducted on a probability sample of U.S. men and women from the first National Health and Nutritional Examination Survey (NHANES I), greater stature and frame size (but not weight or body fatness) were associated with increased rates of breast cancer in women (Micozzi, 1986b), as well as total cancer rates and site-specific rates of lung and prostate cancer in men and colon and rectal cancer in men and women (Albanes et al., 1988). These observations do not suggest a primary role for adult nutrition, but maintain a role for childhood growth and nutrition in determining cancer risk.

Furthermore, there was a "threshold" effect for stature, such that the shortest quartile of individuals had significantly lower cancer rates. This effect is consistent with the observation that in a well-nourished population (like that of the United States) it may only be among the shortest individuals that there are those who are short primarily due to nutritional restriction during the growth period (Willett, 1987). In addition, males may be more sensitive to environmental and nutritional influences over growth than are females (Malina et al., 1985), and the association of adult stature and cancer was stronger in men than in women. There was also a stronger cancer association for the leg length component of stature, which may be more sensitive to nutritional and environmental differences than sitting height, especially during adolescence (Johnston et al., 1978).

In prospective studies such as those from NHAMES I (Micozzi, 1986b; Albanes et al., 1988), the effects of disease do not influence the anthropometric or other variables of interest to diet and cancer hypotheses because the anthropometric dimensions are taken prior to the development of cancer.

Weight

Conditions potentially related to overnutrition have been associated with increased cancer risk in adults. Relative weight has been directly associated with cancer death rates in men and women (Lew and Garfinkel, 1975). Among 750,000 individuals, increased relative weight was a risk factor for seveal site-specific cancers, including biliary, breast, cervical, colon, endometrial, ovarian, and renal cancer. Decreased relative weight in men (but not women) was also associated with overall cancer death rates, probably due to the association between smoking duration, body leanness, chronic illness, and lung and other cancers in men (Albanes et al., 1986).

Observations on body weight may be directly related to nutritional patterns. Hems (1980) assessed secular trends of dietary factors and cancer mortality for the United Kingdom for 60 years from 1911 to 1971. The trend for breast cancer mortality was seen to parallel that for dietary fat, animal protein, and sugar intake over time. The great increase in cancer rates beginning circa 1960 occurred 10–20 years after the increasing trend in dietary intake. The correlation between diet and breast cancer was greater when dietary intake 10 years earlier was used ($r = 0.6$) than when concurrent diet was used ($r = 0.4$) in the analysis. Studies by Choi et al. (1978), Miller et al. (1978), and Lubin et al. (1984) indicate that the effect of weight and body size on breast cancer risk increase with increasing age, following the effects of increased nutrient intake, in elderly postmenopausal women. Weight is elastic in response to nutritional patterns and exercise during adult life. Adult weight and weight indices may, therefore, provide an index or nutrition that correlates the cancer risk. Cancer risk is also associated with other aspects of body size, which are relatively inelastic during adulthood.

Other Anthropometric Dimensions

Different anthropometric dimensions either do or do not combine measures of linear growth, frame size, and lean body mass with measures of body fat. Childhood growth and nutritional patterns may be reflected by these indices in adults (Garn et al., 1982; Roche, 1984; Himes and Roche, 1985). Additional information may be obtained by comparing the correlations of different age-specific anthropometric measurements in childhood with adult cancer rates. For example, for prostatic and pancreatic cancer in male, cross-cultural correlations between age-specific weight, arm and chest circumferences in childhood (which measure frame size and lean body mass together with body fatness) are significantly greater than for triceps skinfold thickness (measuring fatness alone). The same relations hold true for pancreatic and ovarian cancer in women (Micozzi, 1986a).

The only early case-control study of breast cancer that collected additional information beyond stature and weight (and body mass indices derived therefrom) found that increased weight, sitting height, and biacromial and biiliac diameters were risk factors (Brinkley et al., 1971). In this study increased sitting height was a risk factor for cancer, while stature was not. It is well established that early age at menarche is a risk factor for breast cancer in women and early maturers generally have increased sitting height relative to stature, since the period during preadolescense when the lower body is growing relatively faster than the upper body is shorter in early maturers (Eveleth and Tanner, 1976). Increased sitting height may best discriminate an individual who had greater nutrient intake during childhood and earlier age at menarche within a population. In the cancer cases, it was demonstrated that cancer chemotherapy had no effect on indices of frame size, nor can nonmetastatic cancer be expected to affect these parameters. However, malignant disease and cancer therapy can be expected to affect body weight, body fat, and lean body mass, perhaps differentially (Cohn and Ellis, 1985).

In a recent study of prostate cancer in Japanese-American men in Hawaii, increased body mass index (weight/stature^2) and mid-upper arm circumference were associated with increased cancer rates, while triceps skinfold thickness was not (Severson et al., 1988). Both arm circumference and body mass index reflect lean body mass as well as body fat (Micozzi et al., 1986,1987), while triceps skinfold thickness reflects body fat alone. Therefore, the discrimination of cancer risk by various anthropometric dimensions as indicators of growth may vary with the specific dimensions measured.

The overall pattern of epidemiologic evidence suggests that early growth and nutrition may be important in determining adult cancer rates. These observations do not yet suggest strategies for clinical intervention. They do provide a framework for consideration of the influence of early growth and nutrition on cancer risk. They also suggest strategies for the application of anthropometry to epidemiologic research on diet and cancer. Measurement of anthropometric dimensions should be selectively incorporated into diet and cancer studies. The importance of anthropometry in such studies should not be underestimated, especially in light of the present limitations of nutritional epidemiology.

SELECTION OF ANTHROPOMETRIC METHODS IN DIET AND CANCER STUDIES

Measurement of nutrition-mediated variables which reflect growth (and can also be determined in adults) may be meaningful for the asssessment of past nutritional patterns and future cancer risk. Anthropometry provides a reliable means of assessing past, as well as current, nutritional patterns (Johnston, 1981). Increased intake of macronutrients during the growth period is associated with increased stature and lean body mass and accelerated rates of maturation. The former are reflected in increased stature and body size in adults, and the latter by early age at menarche in women.

Human Growth and Development

Increased nutrient intake during childhood is also related to increased childhood and adult fatness; and fatter children are taller, heavier and developmentally more advanced than the lean (Garn et al., 1982; Roche, 1984). These tendencies may begin early in life. Excessive macronutrient consumption during the postnatal period may lead to increased muscle growth, fat deposition, or, most probably, both. Thus, increased macronutrient intake during growth and development may eventually lead to an adult whose body size is close to the maximum for that genotype (Stini, 1978). Variations in stature and weight among different populations of children have been explained primarily by environmental factors, and not ethnic differences (Habicht et al., 1974). Environmental factors, such as nutrition, may have a greater influence on producing differences in body size during childhood than do genetic factors (Frisancho et al., 1980). Under conditions of restricted nutrition, the genetic control of growth may be further diminished (Frisancho et al., 1973).

However, variations in body size and body composition may be partially explained by genetic influences in some instances, e.g., heritability estimates of stature and fat patterning. Certainly, among populations in most industrialized nations, the majority of individuals may attain body size close to his or her genetic potential (Eveleth and Micozzi, 1988). In industrialized nations, diet may have less effect on population variation in stature and other anthropometric dimensions than it has in third world populations. For example, in the United States, it may be only among the shortest quantile of the population that there are individuals who are short due to nutritional restriction during the growth period (Willett, 1987; Albanes et al., 1988).

Thus, the capacity of particular anthropometric measurements to predict susceptibility to certain cancers may not always implicate nutritional factors to the exclusion of genetic ones. Since cancer is a cellular growth phenomenon, a genetic program for a particular pattern of growth and development may be associated with, and may contribute to, an increased susceptibility to specific neoplasms given certain nutritional intakes during childhood.

Furthermore, there are other factors, in addition to nutrition and genetics, which may influence growth and body size. These factors include terrestrial altitude, exposure to infectious diseases, industrial noise and pollution, environmental temperature, physical activity and exercise level, place of residence (urban vs. rural), and socioeconomic status (Eveleth and Tanner, 1976). Some of these variables, such as place of residence and socioeconomic status, may be highly intercorrelated with genetic and nutritional status. Therefore, in epidemiologic terms, growth has a high sensitivity to diet but may have a low specificity within a population.

Care should therefore be exercised in attributing growth outcomes to diet per se within a population. Comparisons between populations in ecologic studies do not provide definitive tests of hypotheses, but may be important in generating hypotheses about the relations of early diet to adult cancer. Cross-sectional anthropometric data in different populations are based upon physical measurements taken in children or adults that are partially related to nutrition during youth. As an alternate means of nutritional assessment, growth patterns may be used to observe possible relations between early diet and adult cancer. Whether anthropometry has as its greatest strength the ability to (a) substitute as a proxy dietary measure for the limited approaches undertaken by epidemiologists for human nutritional assessment, or (b) provide a greater understanding of existing relations between diet and cancer, the issue can only be resolved by collecting more anthropometic data in epidemiologic studies.

Choosing Measurements

Several factors enter into the appropriate selection of various anthropometric dimensions for cancer epidemiology studies in general, whether prospective or retrospective. Anthropometric techniques must be justified by both theoretical and methodologic considerations. Theoretically, they must be directly useful in assessing the hypothesized relation between nutrition, body size, and cancer with respect to the timing, duration, and magnitude of nutritional exposures. Data collected in a study that is designed to test a specific hypothesis about diet and cancer will be potentially more appropriate and useful than are anthropometric data collected in surveys.

Anthropometric measurements sites and techniques can be selected optimally to test specific hypotheses about the relations of, for example, fat and fat patterning to cancer, within the constraints of epidemiologic studies by giving proper consideration to the reliability of the measurements to be taken, the logistical accessibility of the measurement site, including subject participation, and the biologic meaning of the dimensions selected for study. Anthropometric techniques must generally be applied in a field or clinical situation taking into consideration (a) accessibility of the site, (b) correlation to other body dimensions and body composition, (c) comparability to dimensions and body composition measured in other studies, and (d) reliability, accuracy, and repeatability. Many of these factors are influenced by the necessity of conducting diet and cancer epidemiology studies on relatively large numbers of individuals.

Sample Size

Anthropometry has considerable advantages for application to epidemiologic research where sample size is large. Epidemiologic analyses must be obtained on a relatively large sample even in case-control studies in order to adequately test hypotheses about diet and cancer where relative risks are small (Micozzi, 1989). This concern was evident early in the development of diet and cancer studies (Wynder and Bross, 1961). There are also sigificant constraints on the degree of dietary variability observable wtihin human populations. In order to obtain large sample size, studies are often conducted in multiple centers. Thus, cancer epidemiologic studies often involve large numbers of study subjects in multiple locations, as well as large numbers of observers, and large numbers of (hopefully random) errors. Systematic error in individualized techniques may be randomized by having a large number of observers, as expected in large multicenter studies, although individualized techniques may be specific to a given study site.

Accessibility and Subject Participation

Large sample size also partially determines which anthropometric measurements may be realistically selected on the basis of accessibility and subject participation. The accessibility of a measurement site has both a logistic dimension and a technical dimension in the context of a large-scale study. The amount of undressing required in a large-scale ambulatory study may preclude practical selection of certain measurement sites. For example, in the U.S.-Finland Diet and Cancer Study conducted year-round in frigid areas, some north of the Arctic Circle (Helenius et al., 1986), the time taken to undress was greater than the time initially allocated for anthropometric measurements, and a more limited examination was eventually required. Large-scale studies also impose the requirement of measurement positioning for the comfort of the observer versus that of the subject. Time required for measurement and technical difficulty are important considerations, particularly since replicate measurements are required for reliability and quality control.

In case-control studies, the side of measurement should always be the one (right or left) that is not involved by cancer, if possible, due to the pathophysiologic effects of disease, surgery, and treatment. Martorell et al. (1988) have demonstrated that the side of measurement is probably not a critical variable in anthropometric studies of human populations in normal participants.

In addition to these technical and logistical considerations of accessibility for the observer, there are important issues regarding the willingness of subject participants to provide access to anthropometric sites of measurement. Complete undressing may be a subjective concern of the participants apart from the time restrictions imposed on the procedures. However, subjects may be more willing to permit anthropometric measurements to be taken than they are to undergo complicated and/or painful procedures for providing biologic samples for analysis.

For example, in the U.S.-Asian Women's Health Study, conducted on a census of all breast cancer cases among Chinese-, Japanese-, and Filipino-American women in Hawaii, Los Angeles, and San Francisco, only 30–50% of Asian-American women interviewed provided blood samples for nutrient analysis. However, nearly 90% of these women permitted a complete set of anthropometric measurements to be obtained. Reluctance to provide biologic samples may be an even greater problem in large populations in Asia, where diet and cancer studies appear otherwise to be very promising (Ershow et al., 1984).

Inadequate subject participation rates in a study may bias the results of that study. Thus far, subject participation for anthropometry in large cancer epidemiology studies appears promising in comparison to other methods for nutritional assessment.

Reliability

Stature and weight can generally be obtained fairly reliably in epidemiologic studies whether the dimensions are measured by the investigators or self-reported by the participants (Schlichting et al., 1981; Palta et al., 1982; Himes and Roche, 1982; McKenna et al., unpublished). There may be a systematic tendency for tall and heavy persons to underestimate their height and weight and, conversely, for small and thin persons to overestimate these measurements (Schlichting et al., 1981). In addition, elderly individuals may slightly overestimate stature, while young adults may slightly underestimate (Himes and Roche, 1982). It is tempting to conclude that the elderly, who have undergone some late adult contraction in stature, may accurately remember a somewhat taller adult stature, whereas young adults, who may still be growing slightly, accurately recall a somewhat shorter stature at the time of measurement. However, our current analysis of the NHANES I reveals correlations between self-reported and measured weight in the range of $r = 0.96–0.98$, including the elderly, ages 65–80 years (McKenna et al. unpublished), although high correlations do not rule out the possibility of systematic bias. Investigators may also choose to obtain stature and weight from subject drivers licenses; some have found such data to be sufficiently accurate for study purposes (LeMarchand et al., 1988), while others have not (Willey and Falsetti, 1987).

An important paradox for the application of anthropometric techniques to epidemiologic studies is that while stature and weight may generally be reported or measured reliably (Roche 1984; Abdel-Malek, et al., 1985) and permit computation of various body mass indices (Micozzi et al., 1986), stature, weight, and body mass indices may have less biologic meaning or utility for a given analysis than do more specific anthropometic measurements which are albeit measured less reliably. Body mass indices (BMIs), even when calculated to have maximum correlation to weight and independence from stature, do not provide pure measures of body fatness (Micozzi et al., 1986; Micozzi and Harris, 1989). These BMIs remain significantly correlated to lean body mass, frame size, and sitting height, in addition to body fat (Garn et al., 1982; Micozzi and Albanes, 1987,1988). Furthermore, there are significant age and sex variations in these correlations such that BMIs may be even more highly correlated to lean body mass than to body fat in some elderly men (Micozzi and Harris, 1989). Lee and Kolonel (1984) have demonstrated that various ratios of weight-for-height are not interchangeable in detecting associations between BMI and cancer. Therefore, limiting anthropometic measurements to stature and weight may be problematic in cancer studies.

On the other hand, more biologically specific or meaningful anthropometric dimensions, such as body circumferences and skinfolds, are measured less reliably than are stature and weight. Haas and Flegal (1981) have determined the magnitude of unreliability due to both undependability and imprecision (intraobserver and interobserver error) for each of seven skinfold sites in 99 individuals, ages 19–92 years. There was significant variability in the estimates of unreliability, ranging from less than 4% error for triceps skinfold to over 16% error (as percent of total variance) for suprailiac skinfold. Most of the imprecision was due to interobserver rather than intraobserver error. Skinfolds were also more prone to measurement error than was mid-upper arm circumference, for which only 2% of the variance was estimated as measurement error (Haas and Flegal, 1981).

Arm circumference was more highly correlated to BMIs than was triceps skinfold thickness in NHANES I, possibly due to greater technical errors of measurement for skinfolds, compared to arm circumference (Micozzi et al., 1986) or due to the correlation of BMIs with both fat and lean body mass (Micozzi and Albanes, 1988). Ashwell et al. (1982) have suggested that body fat and fat distribution may be better described by body circumferences, which are more reliable and generally simpler to measure than are skinfolds. Mueller and Malina (1987) also found that body circumferences are more reliable than skinfolds among adolescents in NHANES I. However, body circumferences incorporate aspects of frame size and lean body mass together with body fat. The calculation of arm muscle area, for example, as a pure measure of lean body mass requires both mid-upper arm circumference and triceps skinfold thickness, such that the reliability of the pure estimate of lean tissue is limited by the reliability of the skinfold.

Conversely, it has been suggested that arm fat area (also calculated from arm circumference and triceps skinfold) provides a better estimate of total body fat than does triceps skinfold thickness alone (Himes et al., 1980) and therefore results in less misclassification of obesity in children and adults (Frisancho, 1981). However, the reliability of any area estimate based upon skinfold thickness will still be limited in practice.

Overall Applicability

The overall applicability of a given anthropometric measurement in an epidemiologic study must therefore take into account large sample size, factors of accessibility and subject participation, technical reliability of measurements, comparability to other databases, and the biologic meaning of the measurement for the hypothesis under study. Attempts at standardization of anthropometric measurements (Micozzi, 1988; Lohman et al., 1988) will help ensure that data is collected in a replicable manner and that the types of data collected will be useful in comparison of different populations and study results. While more anthropometric dimensions are being collected, epidemiologists will continue to make use, appropriately or otherwise, of large data sets limited to relatively reliable information on stature and weight, as well as the health outcome(s) of interest. In the meantime, efforts should be made to employ appropriate ratios of weight-for-stature that are properly representative of the intended measure or estimate of body size or body composition and properly described for a specific population (Micozzi et al., 1986).

In selecting other dimensions that may be appropriate for measurement and analysis, skinfold(s), for example, various subjective and objective considerations must be taken into account such that appropriate weight is given to factors in addition to simple reliability. These factors are summarized in Table 1 for selected skinfold sites. Absolute reliability is just one factor that may be compared for the various skinfolds for appropriateness to a study. What cannot be reflected in Table 1 are the specific diet and cancer hypothesis to be tested and the biologic meaning of each measurement for a given hypothesis. For example, in the selection of a skinfold to estimate fatness of the upper trunk, subscapular and midaxillary sites both have the same correlation, and average accessability and reliability. However, subscapular skinfold is commonly used while the midaxillary site is rarely used in other studies for purposes of comparability of the database. Nonetheless, in a given study, if chest circumference is also measured, midaxillary skinfold taken at a site in the plane of the chest circumference measurement will permit correction of circumference for upper trunk fat as an estimate of frame size and lean body mass. If time does not permit obtaining both measures of upper trunk fat, a choice will have to be made that best suits the goals of the study.

Quality Control

Training, equipment, and quality control should be adequate to ensure maximum reliability and utility of the anthropometric measurements selected. It should be kept in mind that different standards of practice may be applied to the uses of anthropometry in cancer research, as opposed to, for example, human growth studies. In longitudinal growth studies, *changes* in anthropometricc dimensions

Table 1 Applied Considerations for Selection of Skinfold Measurements in Cancer Epidemiologic Studies

Skinfold site	Correlation	Accessibility and participation	Comparability	Reliability
Triceps	upper extremity	good	good	good
Subscapular	upper trunk	average	good	average
Midaxillary	upper trunk	average	poor	average
Suprailiac	lower trunk	poor	average	poor
Medial calf	lower extremity	poor	poor	good

(1) Accessibility and subject participation

good — minimal amount of undressing, brief time required for measurement, limited technical difficulty, little discomfort for observer or subject.

average — intermediate

poor — maximum amount of undressing, long time required for measurement, significant technical difficulty, great discomfort for observer or subject.

(2) Relative frequency of usage in epidemiologic studies

good — commonly used, popular

average — less commonly used

poor — rarely used, unusual

(3) Reliability

error as percent of total variance

good — < 5%

average — 5–10%

poor — >10%

are the unit of measurement, and it is important to maximize study conditions so that any variations in measurements are due, in fact, to growth and not to measurement errors. However, in cancer epidemiology studies cross-sectional data on large populations are collected in the field under conditions that result in relatively large numbers of random errors. Continuous anthropometric variables producing a normal or skewed distribution in the study population are utilized to categorize individuals into quantiles and to identify individuals at the extremes of the distribution.

Anthropometric data are combined with other data collected (or controlled for) and correlated to cancer outcome in an attempt to derive relative risks of cancer among individuals in the population. Individuals or groups at the extremes of the measurement distributions may be of particular interest for determining significant relative risks. Equipment, techniques, and equations (e.g., body mass indices) must be carefully selected and determined to be accurate at extremes of measurements, as well as within the nromal range of variation. Thus, as recommended in other contexts (Roche, 1984; Abdel-Malek et al., 1985), standardization of all indirect techniques against a more direct technique should be accomplished in a representative sample of the study population. In addition, the statistical characteristics of any body mass index used should be reported specifically for the population under study (Micozzi et al., 1986).

Given the multicenter, multipersonnel nature of many cancer epidemiology studies, replicate measurements on the total population, or on a representative sample, to determine inter- and intra-observer variability are also important components of quality control. Establishing reference standards between population centers is also important. Various intraclass correlation reliability coefficients may be determined that are more, or less, appropriate to analysis of variance (Bartko, 1976) for monitoring data collection and interpreting study results. Appropriate reliability statistics may be utilized for data sets with two observers, more than two observers, and varying numbers of observers with discontinuous or quantitative data (Bartko and Carpenter, 1976).

Anthropometry may provide a useful service to cancer research by facilitating implementation of appropriate quality control procedures and assessment of the quality of data that cannot be collected under controlled, "growth study" laboratory conditions. There is also a need to emply better and more specific anthropometric equipment, techniques, and dimensions than those currently used in many epidemiologic studies of cancer, as well as conducting appropriate analysis and interpretation of results. Epidemiologic studies often rely on stature, weight, and body mass indices derived therefrom as the only estimates of body size and composition in a study. Even here, body mass indices are not always employed in the most statistically suitable manner (Micozzi et al., 1986). Much of the current controversy over the use, improper or otherwise, of body mass indices in epidemiologic studies could answered by the addition of standard anthropometric measurements, as described above, which provide more complete and direct estimates of body size and composition.

However, the limitations of anthropometric measurements are also important criteria for their selection in epidemiologic studies and should be acknowledged in investigations of diet and cancer. Anthropometry is indirect, like most techniques of nutritional assessment used in cancer epidemiology. Obviously no single measurement can be taken as representative of total nutritional experience over a lifetime, the dimensions of the entire body, or overall cancer risk. Furthermore, several different anthropometric dimensions that may be relevant to cancer and chronic disease research may not be sensitive to isolated or acute nutritional events that may be of interest to other areas of clinical medicine. For example, anthropometric data are being increasing used, together with clinical and biochemical information, in nutritional monitoring of the elderly and the cancer patient (Mc Evoy and James, 1982, Heymsfield et al., 1982, Cohn and Ellis, 1985). Recognition of the effects of age, disease, and treatment on measurement of anthropometric dimensions is important to proper interpretation of study results. Selection of anthropometric measurements should not be random but suited to the hypothesis under study. Although the measurement of each dimension should be standarized (Lohman et al., 1988), the same set of measurements need not be used in every cancer study. For example, an anthropometric protocal suitable to estimating childhood nutritional intake in a breast cancer study would not be the most appropriate protocol for an endometrial cancer study in which fat and fat patterning in adult life is a major concern. Appropriate criteria should be applied for selection of a set of measurements that will best test a given hypothesis with respect to both biological and statistical considerations, as well as limitations.

CONCLUSIONS

Anthropometry is an important methodology for cancer research which can be used to help understand the relations between human diet and cancer and lead to identification of individuals and populations at increased cancer risk. It is not presently clear whether the greatest utility of anthropometry in cancer epidemiologic studies lies in its ability to substitute as a proxy dietary estimate or to provide a greater understanding of established relations between nutrition and cancer. These scientific issues can only be resolved by collecting more anthropometric data in epidemiologic studies. In this manner, anthropometry may possibly help answer questions about the adaptiveness of growth and body size in humans populations. As the relations between nutrition and anthropometric dimensions become better understood, there will be increasing applications for anthropometry in studying associations between nutrition and cancer.

SUMMARY

Epidemiologic research on cancer has recently expanded into new areas of investigation directly related to aspects of human biology, such as human diet and nutrition. The overall pattern of scientific evidence has suggested that dietary patterns in early life, as well as adulthood, may be related to the long-term risk of certain cancers. Anthropometry has considerable potential in cancer research as an indirect means of both childhood and adult nutritional assessment. Anthropometry has advantages in application to cancer studies where the sample size is large, as it must be to test most contemporary diet-cancer hypotheses. The anthropometric dimensions selected for measurement should be reliable, readily accessible in field or clinical situations with high rates of subject participation, have established correlations to other body dimensions, and be comparable to dimensions measured in other studies. Appropriate standards of practice and quality control procedures in cancer studies may differ somewhat from those employed in human growth studies. Anthropometry is an important biomedical research methodology, which may be used to study the relations between nutrition, body size, and cancer, leading to better identification of individuals and human populations at increased risk.

REFERENCES

Abdel-Malek, A. K., Mukherjee, D., Roche, A. F. A method of constructing an index of obesity. *Human Biology 57*: 415–430 (1985).

Albanes, D. A., Jones, D. Y., Micozzi, M. S., Mattson, M. Association between smoking and body weight in the U.S. population: Analysis of NHANES II. *American Journal of Public Health 77*: 439–444 (1986).

Albanes, D., Schatzkin, A. F., Micozzi, M. S. Survey of time-related factors in research on diet and cancer. *Journal Chronic Diseases 40* (Suppl. 2): 39S–44S (1987).

Albanes, D., Jones, D. Y., Schatzkin, A. G., Micozzi, M. S., Taylor, P. R. Adult stature and risk of cancer. *Cancer Res. 48*: 1658–1662 (1988).

Armstrong, B., Doll, R. Environmental factor and cancer incidence and mortality in different countries, with special reference to dietary practices. *Int. J. Cancer 15*: 617–631 (1975).

Ashwell, M., Chinn, S., et al. Female fat distribution. *Int. J. Obes. 6*: 143–152 (1982).

Bartko, J. J., Carpenter, W. T. On the methods and theory of reliability. *J. Nervous Mental Dis. 163*: 307–317 (1976).

Bartko, J. J. On various intraclass correlation reliability coefficients. *Psychological. Bull. 83*: 762–7650 (1976).

Block, G. A review of validations of dietary assessment methods. *Am. J. Epidemiol. 115*: 492–505 (1982).

Block, G., Hartman, A. In *Nutrition and Cancer Prevention: Investigating the Role of Micronutrients* (T. E. Moon and M. S. Micozzi, eds.), Marcel Dekker, New York, 1989, pp. 159–180.

Brinkley, D., Carpenter, R. G., Haybittle, J. L. An anthropometric study of women with cancer. *Br. J. Prev. Soc. Med. 25*: 65–75 (1971).

Buell, P., Dunn, J. Cancer mortality of Japanese Isei and Nisei of California. *Cancer 18*: 656–664 (1965).

Buell, P. Changing incidence of breast cancer in Japanese-American women. *JNCI 51*: 1479–1483 (1973).

Carroll, K. K., Khor, H. T. Dietary fat in relation to tumorigenesis. *Prog. Biochem. Pharmacol. 10*: 308–353 (1975).

Choi, N. W., Howe, G. R., Miller, A. B., Matthews, V., Morgan, R. W., Munan, L., Burgh, J. D., Feather, J., Jain, M., Kelly, A. An epidemiologic study of breast cancer. *Am. J. Epidemiol. 107*: 510–521 (1978).

Cohn, S. H., Ellis, K. J. *Body Composition by Means of In Vivo Neutron Activation Analysis*. USDA Conference for Federal Supported Human Nutrition Research Units and Centers, Chevy Chase, MD, 1985.

DeWaard, F. Breast cancer incidence and nutritional status with particular reference to body weight and height. *Cancer Rev. 35*: 3351–3356 (1975).

Doll, R., Peto, R. The causes of cancer: Quantitative estimates of avoidable risks of cancer in the United States today. *JNCI 66*:1191–1308 (1981).

Dunn, J. E. Breast cancer among American Japanese in the San Francisco Bay area. In *Epidemiology and Cancer Registries in the Pacific Basin—I. National Cancer Institute* Monograph 47, 1977, pp. 157–160.

Ershow, A. G., Zheng, S. F., Li, G. Y., Yang, C. S. Blot, W. J. Compliance and nutritional status during feasibility study for an intervention trial in China. *JNCI 73*(6): 1477–1481 (1984).

Eveleth, P. B., Tanner, J. B. *Worldwide Variations in Growth*. Cambridge University Press, Cambridge, 1976.

Eveleth, P. B., Micozzi, M. S. Growth variations in children and chronic disease in adults. In *Crecimiento y Desarrollo del Nino en las Americas* (M. Cusminsky and N. Saurez-Ojeda, eds.), Pan American Health Organization, Washington, DC, 1988.

Frisancho, A. R. New norms of upper limb fat and muscle areas for assessment of nutritional status. *Am. J. Clin. Nutr. 34*: 2540–2545 (1981).

Frisancho, A. R., Guire, K., Babler, W., Borkan, G., Way, A. Nutritional influence on childhood development and genetic control of adolescent growth of Quechuas and Mestizos from the Peruvian lowlands, *Am. J. Phys. Anthropol. 52*:367–375 (1980).

Frisancho, A. R., Sanchez, J., Pallardel, D., Yanez, L. Adaptive significance of small body size under poor socioeconomic conditions in southern Peru. *Am . J. Phys. Anthropol. 39*: 255–262 (1973).

Garn, S. M., Ryan, A. S., Higgins, M. W. Implications of fatness and leanness. *Am. J. Phys. Anthropol 57*: 191 (1982).

Gaskill, S. P., McGuire, W. L., Osborne, C. K., Stern, M. P. Breast cancer mortality and diet in the United States. *Cancer Res. 39*: 3628–3637 (1979).

Gray, G. E., Pike, M. C., Henderson, B. E. Breast cancer incidence and mortality rates in different countries in relation to known risk factors and dietary practices. *Br. J. Cancer 39*: 1–7 (1979).

Greulich, W. W. A comparison of the physical growth and development of native and American-born Japanese children. *Am. J. Phys. Anthropol. 15*: 489–515 (1957).

Greulich, W. W. Some secular changes in the growth of American-born and native Japanese children. *Am. J. Phys. Anthropol. 45*: 553–568 (1976).

Haas, J. D., Flegal, K. M. Anthropometric measurements, in *Nutrition and Cancer: Etiology and Treatment*. Raven Press, New York (G. R. Newell and N. M. Ellison, eds.), 1981, pp. 123–139.

Habicht, J. P., Martorell, R., Yarbrough, C., Malina, R. M., Klein, R. E. Height and weight standards for preschool children: How relevant are ethnic differences in growth potential? *Lancet 1*: 611–615 (1974).

Helenius, M. Y. T., Albanes, D. A., Micozzi, M. S., Heinonen, O. P. Studies of bioelectric resistance in overweight, middle-aged subjects. In *Symposium on Bioelectric Estimation of Body Composition*, (A. F. Roche, ed.), Human Biology, 59:271–279, 1986.

Hems, G. Contributions of diet and childbearing to breast cancer rates. *Br. J. Cancer 37*: 982 (1978).

Hems, G. Associations between breast cancer mortality rates, childbearing and diet in the United Kingdom. *Br. J. Cancer 41*:429–436 (1980).

Henderson, B. E. *Discussion of "The hormonal basis of breast cancer."* National Cancer Institute Monograph 53, 1979, pp. 192–193.

Heymsfield, S. B., Stevens, V., Noel, R., McManus, C., Smith, J. Nixon, D. Biochemical composition of muscle in normal and semi-starved human subjects: Relevance to anthropometric measurements. *Am. J. Clin. Nutr. 36*:131–142 (1982).

Himes, J. H., Roche, A. F. Reported versus measured adult statures. *Am. J. Phys. Anthropol. 58*: 335-341 (1982).

Himes, J. H., Roche, A. F. Subcutaneous fatness and stature: Relationships from infancy to adulthood. *Ann. Hum. Biol. 12* (Suppl. 1): 55 (1985).

Himes, J. H., Roche, A. F., Webb, P. Fat areas as estimates of total body fat. *Am. J. Clin. Nutr. 33*: 2093–2100 (1980).

Hirayama, T. Epidemiology of breast cancer with special reference to the role of diet. *Prev. Med. 7*: 173–195 (1978).

Johnston, F. E. Physical growth and development and nutritional status: Epidemiological considerations. *Fed. Proc. 40*: 2583–2587 (1981).

Johnston, F. E. The uses of anthropometry. *Acta. Med. Auxol. 15*: 69–74 (1983).

Johnston, F. E., Wainer, H., Thissen, D., MacVean, R. Hereditary and environmental determinants of growth in height in a longitudinal sample of children and youth of Guatamalen and European ancestry. *Am. J. Phys. Anthropol. 44*: 469–476 (1976).

Kolonel, L. N., Hankin, J. H., Lee, J., Chu, S. Y., Nomura, A. M. Y., Hinds, M. W. Nutrient intakes in relation to cancer incidence in Hawaii. *Br. J. Cancer 44*: 332–339 (1981).

Kondo, S., Eto, M. Physical growth studies on Japanese-American children in comparison with native Japanese. In *Proceedings of Meeting for Review and Seminar of the U. S. Japan Co-operative Research on Human Adaptabilities*, University Press, Tokyo, 1975, pp. 13–45.

Lee, J., Kolonel, L. N. Are body mass indices interchangeable in measuring obesity-disease associations? *Am. J. Public Health 74*: 376–377 (1984).

LeMarchand L. L., Yoshizawa, C. N., Normura, A. M. Y. Validation of body size information on drivers license. *Am. J. Epidemiol. 128*: 874–877 (1988).

Lew, E. A., Garfinkel, L. Variations in mortality by weight among 750,000 men and women. *J. Chronic Dis. 32*: 563–576 (1975).

Lohman, T. G., Roche, A. F. , Martorell, R. *Anthropometric Standardization Reference Manual*, Human Kinetics Publishers, Champaign, IL, 1988.

Lubin, F., Ruder, A. M., Wax, Y., Modan, B. Overweight and changes in weight throughout adult life in breast cancer etiology. *Am. J. Epidemiol. 122*: 579–588 (1984).

Malina, R. M., Little, B. B., Buschang, P. H., DeMoss, J., Selby, H. A. Socioeconomic variation in the growth status of children in a subsistence agricultural community. *Am. J. Phys. Anthropol. 68*: 385-391 (1985).

Martorell, R., Mendoza, F., Mueller, W., Pawson, I. G., Which side to measure: Right or left? *Anthropometric Standardization Reference Manual* (T. G. Lohman, A. F. Roche, and R. Martorell, eds.), Human Kinetics Press, Champaign, IL, 1988, pp. 87–92.

Mc Evoy, A. W., James, O. F. W. Anthropometric indices in normal elderly subjects. *Age and Ageing 11*: 97–100 (1982).

Micozzi, M. S. Nutrition, body size, and breast cancer. *Yearbook of Physical Anthropology, 28*: 175–206 (1985).

Micozzi, M. S. Cross-national correlations of food consumption, childhood growth, and cancer rates. *Am. J. Phys. Anthropol 69*: 240 (1986a) (abstract).

Micozzi, M. S. Childhood nutrition, growth, and development: Relation to the long term risk of breast cancer in human populations. Ph.D. dissertation, University of Pennsylvania, Ann Arbor, MI, University Microfilms International, 1986b.

Micozzi, M. S. Cross-cultural correlations of childhood growth and adult breast cancer. *Am. J. Phys. Anthropol. 73*: 525–537 (1987).

Micozzi, M. S. Cancer, In *Anthropometric Standardization Reference Manual* (T. G. Lohman, A. F. Roche, and R. Martorell, eds.), Human Kinetics Publishers, Champaign, IL, 1988, pp. 151–154.

Micozzi, M. S. Foods, micronutrients and reduction of human cancer, in *Nutrition and Cancer Prevention: Investigating the Role of Micronutrients* (T. E. Moon and M. S. Micozzi, eds.), Marcel Dekker, New York, 1989, pp. 213–241.

Micozzi, M. S., Albanes, D., Jones, D. Y., Chumlea, W. C. Correlations of body mass indices with weight, stature, and body composition in men and women NHANES I and II. *Am. J.Clin. Nutr. 44*: 725–731 (1986).

Micozzi, M. S. Albanes, D. Expanding on the three limitations of body mass indices. *Am. J. Clin. Nutr. 46*: 376–377 (1987).

Micozzi, M. S., Albanes, D. More on the three limitations of body mass indices, *Am. J. Clin. Nutr. 48*: 691–692 (1988).

Micozzi, M. S., Harris, T. M. Age variations in the relation of body mass indices to estimates of body fat and muscle mass. *Am. J. Phys. Anthropol 81*:375–379 (1990).

Miller, A. B. Role of nutrition in the etiology of breast cancer. *Cancer 39*: 2704–2708 (1977).

Miller, A. N., Kelly, A., Choi, N. W., Matthews, V., Morgan, T. W., Munan, L., Burch, J. D., Feather, J., Howe, G. R., Jain, M. A study of diet and breast cancer. *Am. J. Epidemiol. 10*: 499–509 (1978).

Mueller, W. H., Malina, R. M. Relative reliability of circumferences and skinfolds as measures of body fat distribution. *Am. J. Phys. Anthropol. 72*: 437–439 (1987).

Palta, M., Prineas, R. J., Berman, R., Hannan, P. Comparison of self-reported and-measured height and weight. *Am. J. Epidemiol. 115*: 223–230 (1982).

Roche, A. F. Anthropometric methods: New and old, what they tell us. *Int. J. Obesity 8*: 509–523.

Ross, M. H., Bras, G., Lustbader, E. D. *Diet, Body Weight and Tumor Susceptibility.* Twenty-eighth Scientific Report, Institute for Cancer Research, Fox Chase Cancer Center, Philadelphia, PA, 1983, pp.18–20.

Schlichting, P., Hoilund-Carlsen, P. F., Quaade, F. Comparison of self-reported height with controlled height and weight in women and men. *Int. J. Obesity 5*: 67–76 (1981).

Severson, R. K., Grove, J. S., Nomura, A. M. Y., Stemmermann, L. N. Body mass and prostatic cancer: A prospective study. *Br. Med. J. 297*: 713–715 (1988).
Stini, W. A. Early nutrition, growth, disease and human longevity. *Nutr. Cancer. 1*: 31–39 (1975).
UNICEF *The State of the World's Children*. Oxford University Press, London, 1981.
Waterhouse, J. C., Muir, K., Shanmugaratnam, S., Powell, J. *Cancer Incidence in Five Continents*, Vol. IV. International Agency for Research on Cancer, Lyons, France, 1982.
Willett, W. C. Implications of total energy intake for epidemiologic studies of breast and large-bowel cancer. *Am. J. Clin. Nutr. 45*: 354–360 (1987).
Willey, P., Falsetti, T. The inaccuracy of height and weight information on driver licenses. Abstracts. American Academy of Forensic Sciences, 39th Annual Meeting, San Diego, CA, 1987, p. 35.
Wynder, E. L., Bross, I. J. A study of etiological factors in cancer of the esophgus. *Cancer 14*: 389–413 (1961).

7

Biomarkers of Macronutrient Intake

Anna R. Giuliano and Thomas E. Moon
The University of Arizona Health Sciences Center
Tucson, Arizona

INTRODUCTION

At the present time, there are few firmly established and widely accepted scientific facts about the specific dietary causes or prevention of cancer in humans. Part of the current confusion may be attributed to methodologic limitations of quantifying dietary intake (Bazzarre and Myers, 1980; Staveren et al., 1988). The currently available methods to quantitate dietary intake have not been highly successful or consistent in identifying specific dietary patterns or specific nutrients that are related to cancer. The role of dietary fat in the etiology of breast cancer continues to be highly controversial, for example. Fats have been hypothesized to facilitate absorption of toxic fat-soluble chemicals, influence cell membrane composition, serve as precursors for the formation of prostaglandins and leukotriene, and impact the immune system (Berry et al., 1986). Each of the currently available dietary survey methods have weaknesses. Their limitations include the cost, the burden on the subject, responder bias and the availability of accurate and complete food composition tables. In some circumstances, dietary survey methods can be combined to improve the accuracy of quantifying dietary intake (Dweyer, 1988). However, even if the unobtainable goal of a precise and valid dietary intake method did exist and could be utilized in large-scale population-based studies, such a dietary intake method would not consider variation between individuals in digestion, absorption, and metabolism of nutrients. Such variation has likely contributed to the inconsistencies in evaluating the role of diet and cancer. Because of these limitations with dietary intake methods, biochemical markers are receiving more attention as independent composite quantitative measures of dietary intake, digestion, absorption, and metabolic breakdown. Additional research is required to fully evaluate the association between biomarkers of dietary intake and risk of cancer plus the evaluation of the relationship between biomarkers and dietary intake. Few studies using biomarkers of diet have been reported for studying the etiology of cancer.

To determine if diet is associated with cancer, epidemiologists have studied populations and subgroups, including entire nations and migrants to the United States, to evaluate the relationship between dietary patterns, changes in dietary patterns, and the risk of particular cancers. In general, variation in the pattern of dietary intake has tended to be associated with changes in cancer incidence (NRC, 1982). It has proven to be much more difficult to establish causal relationships and to determine which, if any, of the dietary components are involved in carcinogenesis and thus amenable to prevention strategies.

Even in experiments with laboratory animals, difficulties were encountered. Like humans, many animals have a significant incidence of cancer in older age, and the rates of these cancers often tend to be associated with changes in diet. Even with the advantages of laboratory experimentation that include more homogeneous inbred populations, tumor initiation using a known carcinogen, often at high dose, and controlled laboratory conditions there continues to be controversy as to whether the key dietary factors are total caloric intake or specific excess and deficiencies in macro- or other nutrients. The report by Freedman and et al. (1990) supports the role of dietary fat and total calories in enhancing the risk of mammary cancer in rats and mice.

Clinical pharmacology research using therapeutic drugs demonstrates that there is great variation between individuals in the bioavailability of a drug even when the same dose is consumed (Chabner, 1982). It has thus been generally accepted by clinical pharmacologists that it is not the dose of the drug administered but the actual tissue bioavailability that corresponds with therapeutic and toxic effects of a drug. It is widely recognized that the bioavailability of a drug may differ by as much as 10- to 100-fold between individuals receiving the same drug dose. It may also be anticipated that the bioavailability of nutrients substantially differs between individuals. A similar philosophy has not been widely embraced by epidemiologists in the study of diet and cancer. Research studies that not only quantify dietary intake but also use biomarkers of nutrients, thus accounting for between—individual differences in digestion, absorption, and metabolism, may provide a better understanding and more consistent association between foods, nutrients, and cancer incidence.

The goal of this chapter is to summarize the methods available to quantitate macronutrients in different biologic compartments including blood and other tissues as well as breath markers. Research on nutrient biomarkers may also provide better insights into the interaction between macronutrients, micronutrients, alcohol, and other toxicants such as cigarette smoke. Since nutrients exert their actions at specific tissue sites, adequate tissue concentrations of the nutrients and nutrient by carcinogen interactions may be critical in the prevention of cancer. This chapter will begin by briefly outlining the metabolic breakdown of dietary macronutrients, lipids, carbohydrates, and proteins. A discussion of the use of erythrocyte membrane fatty acid composition, adipose tissue fatty acid comparison, and breath gases as markers of macronutrient intake will follow. Studies utilizing these methods in the area of cancer etiology and prevention will be reviewed.

METABOLIC BREAKDOWN OF DIETARY LIPIDS, CARBOHYDRATES, AND PROTEINS

The liver is the regulatory site of macronutrient breakdown. The metabolic breakdown of each of the macronutrients is determined primarily by the energy requirements of the body. In the simplest of terms, when the host energy requirements are in excess of or equal to dietary intake, then dietary lipids and carbohydrates are metabolized for the production of the high energy compound adenosine triphosphate (ATP). If the dietary intake is in excess of energy requirements, then lipids, carbohydrates, and certain amino acids from proteins are metabolized to fat either in the form of triglycerides stored in adipose tissue or as part of phospholipids in cell membranes. Metabolism of excess dietary carbohydrates or protein results in the synthesis of fatty acids. The lipoproteins are the carriers in plasma of fatty acids bound for cell membranes or adipose tissue storage sites. An understanding of the interactions between lipids, carbohydrates, and proteins during their metabolism is essential in interpreting the results obtained from studies utilizing biomarkers of macronutrient intake and risk of cancer.

Dietary lipids consist primarily of triglycerides—a molecule of glycerol esterfied with three fatty acid molecules (Linscheer and Vergroesen, 1988). The fatty acids that are esterified to glycerol vary depending upon dietary intake. In general three classes of fatty acids are found in the diet: saturated fatty acids that have no double carbon bonds, monounsaturated fatty acids with one double carbon bond, and polyunsaturated fatty acids having two or more double bonds. Two systems are commonly used to identify the fatty acids. The first naming system uses English words (e.g., linoleic acid). The second naming system uses numbers to indicate the number of carbon atoms in the fatty acid chain and the number and position of any double bonds from the methyl and of the molecule. Linoleic acid would be C18:1 (n-6,9). Linoleic acid is therefore designated as a n-6 series fatty acid. The polyunsaturated fatty acids, linoleic acid (n-6) and linolenic acid (n-3), are essential fatty acids that humans are unable to synthesize, due to the location on the carbon chain of the first *cis* double bond (Devlin, 1982). Table 1 lists some commonly consumed lipids and their fatty acid composition.

Table 1 Fatty Acid Composition of Selected Lipids[a]

Fatty acids[b]	Coconut	Corn	Olive	Soy	Rapeseed	Menhaden[c] (fish oil)	Chicken	Beef	Pork
Saturated									
Total	86.5	12.7	13.5	14.4	6.8	32.5	29.8	49.8	39.2
12:0	44.6						0.1	0.9	0.2
14:0	16.8					7.0	0.9	1.3	1.3
16:0	8.2	10.9	11.0	10.3	4.8	22.3	21.6	24.9	23.8
18:0	2.8	1.8	2.2	3.8	1.6	3.2	6.0	18.9	13.5
Monounsaturated									
Total	5.8	24.2	73.7	23.3	55.5	29.1	44.7	41.8	45.1
16:1			0.8	0.2	0.5	14.2	5.7	4.2	2.7
18:1	5.8	24.2	72.5	22.8	53.8	15.0	37.3	36.0	41.2
20:1			0.3	0.2	1.0		1.1	0.3	1.0
22:1					0.1				
Polyunsaturated									
Total	1.8	58.7	8.4	57.9	33.3	30.3	20.9	4.0	11.2
18:2	1.8	58.0	7.9	51.0	22.1	1.5	19.5	3.1	10.2
18:3		0.7	0.6	6.8	11.1	2.1	1.0	0.6	1.0
18:4						2.0			
20:4						1.5	0.1		
20:5						14.7			
22:5						1.8			
22:6						7.0			
Other	5.9	4.4	4.4	4.4	4.4	8.1	4.6	4.6	4.5

[a]Amount in 100 g edible portion.
[b]From USDA, 1979.
[c]From Stansky, 1986.

Absorbed fatty acids are incorporated by intestinal epithelial cells into chylomicron lipoproteins as triglycerides, phospholipids, and cholesterol esters. Table 2 lists the various lipoprotein fractions found in plasma. Chylomicrons are secreted into the lymphatic circulation and subsequently into the bloodstream by way of the thoracic duct. Once in the bloodstream, fatty acids are released from chylomicrons by the action of lipoprotein lipase. Free fatty acids are taken up by muscle and other tissues for use as an energy source, use as structural components of cell membranes, and storage as adipose tissue, for later use as a source of stored energy. Fatty acids are rapidly reesterfied into triglycerides in extrahepatic tissue. Plasma fatty acids remaining from lipoprotein lipase action on chylomicrons are taken up by the liver and incorporated into very low density lipoproteins (VLDL). Fatty acids endogenously produced in the liver from the

Table 2 Characteristics of Plasma Lipoproteins

	Lipoprotein Type			
Average percentage composition	Chylomicrons	Very low density lipoproteins (VLDL)	Low density lipoproteins (LDL)	High density lipoproteins (HDL)
Triacylglycerols	86	55	8	5
Phospholipids	8	20	20	30
Cholesterol	2	10	10	5
Cholesterol esters	2	6	37	15
Protein	2	9	25	45

metabolism of carbohydrates and proteins are also incorporated by the liver into VLDL. Very low density lipoproteins are subsequently secreted into plasma and acted on by lipoprotein lipase to release fatty acids for tissue uptake. With sequential removal of fatty acids from VLDL, low density lipoproteins (LDL) are formed. High density lipoproteins (HDL) are synthesized and secreted into plasma by the liver primarily to transport tissue cholesterol to hepatocytes for metabolism and subsequent excretion. For a more thorough review of lipoproteins and lipid metabolism see Schaefer et al. (1978), and Grundy (1979, 1986), Goldstein et al. (1983), and Berns et al. (1989).

Fatty acids that are found in adipose tissue and cell membranes are from either dietary fatty acids or from endogenously synthesized fatty acids from carbohydrate and protein metabolism. In humans, the liver is the primary site for fatty acid synthesis, producing all but the essential fatty acids, linoleic (n-6), and linolenic (n-3) (Linscheer et al., 1988).

Since the body has no special storage form for amino acids to accomodate excess dietary protein intake (Broquist, 1984), amino acid catabolism is operating continually making the assessment of protein status very difficult (Young et al., 1990). Absorbed dietary amino acids pass to the liver via the portal vein. The main site of catabolism for 7 of the 10 essential amino acids is the liver, while the three branched-chain amino acids are degraded mainly in muscle and kidney (Munro and Crinn, 1988). The liver monitors the absorbed amino acids and adjusts the rate of their metabolism according to the body's needs (Devlin, 1982; Munro and Crinn, 1988). Amino acids have essentially three fates: (a) incorporation into tissue proteins, (b) synthesis of new nitrogen-containing compounds (e.g., purine bases, creatine, or epinephrine), and (c) catabolism to pyruvate and/or intermediates of the tricarboxylic acid cycle (TCA) (glycogenic amino acids) or acetyl CoA (ketogenic amino acids) for either ATP production or the subsequent synthesis of glucose and fatty acids (Devlin, 1982).

Throughout the world, 65% of food energy comes from carbohydrates. The population of some developing countries consume up to 90% of their food energy from carbohydrates, while the population of developed countries consume approximately 50% of food energy from carbohydrates (Dahlqvist, 1984). One storage form of excess dietary carbohydrate is glycogen, a polymer of glucose. The size of this store, however, is negligible (Dahlqvist, 1984). Although glycogen is produced in the most efficient, energy-inexpensive process, fat is the largest and most practical storage form of excess carbohydrate intake.

Fatty acid synthesis occurs in the cytosol of hepatocytes and is regulated by the availability of glucose such that a high carbohydrate, low fat diet increases the synthesis of fatty acids (Table 3). Fasting, high dietary fat intake, increased glucagon, high fish oil intake (eicosapentanoic acid C20:5, n-3) or insulin deficiency markedly depress fatty acid biosynthesis (Iritami et al., 1980; Harris et al., 1984). Palmitic acid (C16:0) produced during fatty acid synthesis is modified by elongation and desaturation to form longer, unsaturated fatty acids (Devlin, 1982). In the endoplasmic reticulum of hepatocytes, palmitate (C16:0) condenses with malonyl-CoA to form stearic acid (C18:0). Palmitic acid and stearic acid are both substrates for stearoyl-CoA desaturase in the endoplasmic reticulum. The enzyme catalyzes the oxidation of palmitic and stearic acid to introduce a *cis* double bond producing palmitoleic acid (C16:1, n-7) and oleic acid (C18:1, n-9), respectively. A double bond can only be introduced in the fatty acid carbon chain after the sixth carbon position. Further desaturation of C16:1 and C18:1 as well as of the essential fatty acids C18:2 (n-6) and C18:3 (n-3) occurs via the delta-6 desaturase enzyme (Linscheer et al., 1988). A common product of the desaturation of linoleic acid (C18:2, n-6) is arachidonic acid (C20:4, n-6). However, arachidonic acid is also obtained in the diet. The activity of the desaturase enzymes is under both dietary and hormonal control such that a diet high in polyunsaturated fats decreases desaturation while insulin increases

Table 3 Regulation of Fatty Acid Synthesis and Desaturation

Activity	Increases activity	Decreases activity
Fatty acid synthesis	High carbohydrate Low fat diet Increased citrate	Low carbohydrate High fat diet Increased glucagon Insulin deficiency n-3 fatty acid Increased palmitate
Fatty acid desaturation	Increased insulin Increased triiodothyroxine Increased hydrocortisone	High dietary polunsaturated fatty acid

desaturation (Devlin, 1982). Nonessential fatty acids are desaturated only in the relative absence of essential fatty acids. Thus, the presence of C20:3 (n-9), a desaturation product of C18:0, in phospholipids is strong evidence of essential fatty acid deficiency (Linscheer et al., 1988). Apparently a critical concentration of long-chain unsaturated fatty acids is required to maintain cell membrane integrity. If the dietary supply of these fatty acids is insufficient to meet this requirement, then elongation and desaturation of saturated fatty acids will proceed (Devlin, 1982).

FATTY ACID COMPOSITION OF ERYTHROCYTE MEMBRANES: A SHORT-TERM BIOMARKER OF RECENT MACRONUTRIENT INTAKE

As early as 1959 investigators demonstrated compositional changes in erythrocyte membrane fatty acids within weeks of feeding a new dietary regimen (Horwitt et al., 1959; Leibetseder and Ahrens, 1959). The use of erythrocyte membrane fatty acids as a biomarker of recent macronutrient intake was advocated (Farquhar and Ahrens, 1963). To better understand the changes one can expect in erythrocyte membranes with dietary changes, discussion of the lipid composition of the erythrocyte membrane is necessary (Angelico et al., 1983; Shanmugasunduram et al., 1986; Berlin et al., 1989).

Unlike adipose tissue, which is composed primarily of fatty acids esterified as triglycerides, erythrocyte membranes are generally composed of 61% phospholipid, 25% free cholesterol, 3% cholesterol esters and glycerides, and less than 3% free fatty acids. Of the phospholipids, approximately 36% are phosphatidylcholine, mainly found in the outer cell membrane, 29% are phosphatidylethanolamine, 10% are phosphatidylserine, and 21% are sphingomyelin. The fatty acid composition of phosphatidylcholine appears to undergo the largest changes resulting from dietary changes, followed by phosphatidylethanolamine (Farquhar and Ahrens, 1963; Popp-Snijders et al., 1984, 1986). Since approximately 50% of the erythrocyte membrane fatty acids are unsaturated, the extent to which dietary unsaturated fatty acids can alter the fatty acids in erythrocyte membranes is relatively small compared to other tissues (Farquhar and Ahrens, 1963).

The percent of linoleic acid (C18:2) present in erythrocyte membranes can be as high as 18–20% of total lipid, achieved by feeding 25 grams of linoleic acid per day, and as low as 9–11% of total lipid when dietary linoleic acid intake is low (Witting and Lee, 1975). Within this range of linoleic acid concentration in erythrocyte membranes, the percent of linoleic acid in phospholipids appears to be linearly related to the dietary intake of linoleic acid. The incorporation of linoleic acid into erythrocyte membranes occurs simultaneous with the disappearance of oleic acid (C18:1), reaching plateau levels within weeks of feeding a diet high in linoleic acid. These data suggest that mature circulating erythrocytes are capable of exchanging fatty acids with plasma lipoproteins (Farquhar and Ahrens, 1963). That the erythrocyte membrane fatty acids composition mirrors the relative proportion of linoleic acid in the diet is evident from the fact that the percent of linoleic acid in the erythrocyte membrane of Americans has increased from 8 to 14% between 1960 and 1975. This change reflects the increased use of margarines containing linoleic acid during this same time period (Witting and Lee, 1975).

The fatty acid composition of erythrocyte membranes has been shown in several studies to reflect not only the percent of linoleic acid in the diet but also the carbohydrate and fatty acid composition of the diet. A fat-free, carbohydrate-rich diet fed to adult subjects for 4–11 weeks resulted in a significant increase in C16:0, C16:1, C18:0, and C18:1, the fatty acid products of lipogenesis. Concomitantly, there was a 50% decrease in linoleic acid (C18:2) in these subjects (Farquhar and Ahrens, 1963). In a cross-cultural study, the erythrocyte membrane fatty acid profile was found to most accurately reflect the dietary macronutrient intake, whereas the plasma lipids were found to be poor indicators of long-term dietary intake due to their fast turnover and large day-to-day variation in diet (Dougherty et al., 1987). In a study of healthy adult males, a cod liver oil supplement providing 3 g/day of n-3 fatty acids (C18:4, C20:5, and C22:6) was found to significantly increase the percentage of these fatty acids in the phosphatidylcholine fraction while significantly reducing the percentage of the n-6 fatty acids (C18:2 and C20:3). The erythrocyte membrane changes were reversible within 2 weeks of removing the cod liver oil supplement from the diet (Popp-Snijders et al., 1984). When this same supplement was given for 8 weeks instead of 2 weeks, a similar magnitude of increase of the n-3 fatty acids in erythrocyte membranes was noted (Popp-Snijders et al., 1986). These data suggest that only 2 weeks on a new diet are needed to significantly alter the fatty acid composition of erythrocyte membranes. Also, there appears to be competition for phospholipid-binding sites between the two series of essential fatty acids (n-3, n-6), such that a diet high in n-3 fatty acids will cause a decrease in the level of n-6 fatty acids in erythrocyte membranes.

Recently a study compared the use of erythrocyte membrane fatty acid composition to that of serum triglyceride and cholesterol esters as indicators of dietary lipid intake (Glatz et al., 1989). Subjects were alternately fed a diet with a high polyunsaturated-to-saturated fat (P/S) ratio of 2.0 and a diet with a low P/S ratio of 0.2 for 3 weeks on each diet. Although the percent change in fatty acid composition of plasma cholesterol esters was significantly greater than that observed for erythrocyte membranes, the between-persons variability of the erythrocyte membrane marker was significantly lower. Methodologically the erythrocyte membrane analysis of fatty acids is simpler, however, the membrane analysis is more susceptible to oxidation and therefore requires that analysis be completed within 1 week of sample collection, whereas serum cholesterol esters can be stored without degradation over a longer period of time (Farquhar and Ahrens, 1963; Glatz et al., 1989). Given the smaller magnitude of change that can be demonstrated with extremes in dietary P/S ratios, Glatz and coworkers (1989) question the sensitivity of erythrocyte membrane fatty acid changes in distinguishing more moderate changes in dietary intake.

The relationship between disease and changes in fatty acid composition of erythrocyte membranes has been evaluated in a limited number of studies. A higher content of unsaturated fatty acids increases the fluidity of erythrocyte membranes and thus increases the metabolic rates of many cellular enzymes (Sandeman, 1979; Quinn, 1983). It has been reported that the desaturation of the C18 fatty acids in cellular membranes, especially the conversion of C18:0 (stearic acid) to C18:1 (oleic acid), was increased by several viruses including herpessimplex type 2, Newcastle disease virus, and a putative interferon antagonist (Apostolov and Barker, 1984). Desaturation was reported to have been decreased by interferon, diphtheria toxin, and Sindbis and Coxsackieviruses (Apostolov and Barker, 1982 1984; Nozawa and Apostolov, 1982). Apostolov and coworkers (1985) have also reported that erythrocyte membranes of chronic leukemia patients contained a relatively higher C18:1 content and lower C18:0 content compared to erythrocyte membranes from normal subjects. Comparing a group of 60 patients with various solid tumors to 40 normal controls and to 41 control subjects with various non-malignant conditions, Wood and coworkers (1985) reported that the ratio of C18:0 to C18:1 was statistically lower for cancer patients. Collectively, these reports suggest that increased desaturation of C18:0 may be a useful biomarker of proliferative disease (Wood et al., 1985). Neoptolemos and coworkers (1988) reported that C18:0 and C18:1 were increased; C20:4 (arachidonic acid) decreased, and the ratio of C18:0 to C18:1 not changed when comparing colorectal cancer patients to a group of patients receiving elective surgery for benign diseases. The use of elective surgery patients as control subjects in the Neoptolemos et al. study makes interpretation of their results difficult. The ratios of C18:0 to C18:1 were similar for both the Wood et al. (1985) and the Neoptolemos et al. (1988) reports.

FATTY ACID COMPOSITION OF BUCCAL MUCOSAL MEMBRANES: A NONINVASIVE BIOMARKER OF RECENT MACRONUTRIENT INTAKE

A potentially useful biomarker of macronutrient intake is the use of buccal mucosal cells. The use of erythrocytes as a biomarker for short-term dietary intake and adipose tissue as a longer-term marker of dietary intake is discussed in other sections of this chapter. However, both erythrocyte and adipose tissues require invasive techniques to obtain tissue. One advantage for the use of buccal mucosal cells is that a relatively noninvasive method can be used.

Recent reports have indicated that fatty acids from buccal mucosal cell membranes may serve as biomarkers for macronutrient intake (McMurchie et al.,

1984; Sampaugna et al., 1988). Higher correlations were reported between dietary lipid intake and buccal mucosal cell membrane fatty acids when ratios were used. Sampaugna et al. (1988) reported that diets with higher polyunsaturated-to-saturated fat ratios correlated with ratios of buccal cell fatty acids, C18:1/saturated fatty acid ratio was decreased, and C18:2/C18:0, C18:2/C18:1, and C18:2/20:4 were increased. They did not fully consider the role of carbohydrates in the diet and fatty acid composition in membranes.

The use of buccal mucosal cell membrane fatty acids require added evaluation for their use as biomarkers of dietary intake and the extent that disease modifies the composition of buccal cell fatty acids.

FATTY ACID COMPOSITION OF ADIPOSE TISSUE: A BIOMARKER OF DIETARY INTAKE OVER THE PREVIOUS 1–3 YEARS

The fatty acid composition of adipose tissue provides an index of the quality of dietary fat intake and possibly the quantity of dietary fat, protein, and carbohydrate intake over the previous 1–3 years (Insull, 1987). Since the fatty acid profile of adipose tissue reflects not only macronutrient intake, but its absorption and metabolism, adipose tissue analysis may be a good marker with which to test the relationship between macronutrient intake and disease.

In 1960, Hirsch and coworkers published a microtechnique using syringe aspiration for sampling subcutaneous adipose tissue from humans that gave results very similar to those attained from the classic method using a fat biopsy. Subcutaneous adipose tissue is generally thought to consist of two pools: a relatively small, readily exchangeable pool and a large inert pool (Hirsch et al., 1960). An adipose tissue sample will be predominantly composed of the large inert pool representing long-term dietary intake and storage (Beynen et al., 1980). Estimates of adipose tissue half-life range from 350 to 680 days (Hirsch et al., 1960; Dayton et al., 1966; Fleischman et al., 1967; Beynen et al., 1980). The tissue half-life and thus the life span of adipose tissue determines the time required for an alteration in the fatty acid composition resulting from dietary changes (0.1–0.2% of adipose cells are replaced per day). Whether adipose tissue behaves as a homogeneous entity such that individual fatty acids within adipose tissue have similar turnover and utilization kinetics remains a research question (Field and Clandinin, 1984). Approximately 99% of an adipose tissue aspirate consists of triglycerides with the predominant fatty acids (Table 4) being myristic (C14:0), palmitic (C16:0), palmitoleic (C16:1), stearic (C18:0), oleic (C18:1), linoleic (C18:2), and linolenic (C18:3) acids (Hirsch et al., 1960; Field and Clandinin, 1984; Malcolm et al., 1989). Other less common but relevant fatty acids include C20:0 (arachidic acid) and C20:4 (arachidonic acid).

The fatty acid composition of subcutaneous adipose tissue is predominantly determined by the fatty acid and carbohydrate composition of the diet (Field

Table 4 Predominant Fatty Acids Composing Adipose Tissue

Name	Code	Formula
Myristic acid	C14:0	$CH_3-(CH_2)_{12}-COOH$
Palmitic acid	C:16:0	$CH_3-(CH_2)_{14}-COOH$
Palmitoleic acid	C16:1, n-7	$CH_3-(CH_2)_5-CH=CH-(CH_2)_7-COOH$
Stearic acid	C18:0	$CH_3-(CH_2)_{16}-COOH$
Oleic acid	C18:1, n-9	$CH_3-(CH_2)_7-CH=CH-(CH_2)_7-COOH$
Linoleic acid	C18:2, n-6,9	$CH_3-(CH_2)_4-CH=CH-CH_2-CH=CH-(CH_2)_7-COOH$
Linolenic acid	C18:3, n-3,6,9	$CH_3-CH_2-CH=CH-CH_2-CH=CH-CH_2-CH=CH-(CH_2)_7-COOH$

and Clandinin, 1984). Several international studies have demonstrated that race and gender have little influence on the fatty acid composition of subcutaneous fat (Scott et al., 1964; Insull and Bartsch, 1967; Shortland et al., 1969; Field and Clandinin, 1984). Similarly, in an adult population (20–60 yr), age has little effect on adipose tissue fatty acid composition (Hirsch et al., 1960; Insull and Bartsch, 1967). Instead, the relative composition of fatty acids in adipose tissue reflects the relative type and amount of macronutrients in the diet (Beynen et al., 1980; Schaffer and Overvad, 1990).

Variables other than diet may have minimal influence on the fatty acid composition of subcutaneous adipose tissue. The relative proportion of saturated fatty acids has been shown to be higher in adipose samples from arms and abdomen than from buttock (Pittet et al., 1979; Malcolm et al., 1989). No difference in adipose fatty acid composition was detected when samples from breast and buttock were compared (Eid and Berry, 1989). The percent of linoleic acid in each of these subcutaneous adipose sites did not vary, suggesting that regardless of the subcutaneous site sampled, the content of linoleic acid can be used as a valid indicator of its dietary intake (Field and Clandinin, 1984; Malcolm et al., 1989).

The correlation between dietary intake of macronutrients and the composition of subcutaneous adipose tissue may be weakened in subjects who are experiencing significant weight changes (Dayton et al., 1966; Staveren et al., 1986, 1988). A significant increase in the P/S ratio and the percent of polyunsaturated fatty acids in adipose sampled from arm, thigh, and abdomen was observed in adult women placed on a weight reduction diet for 1 month (Pittet et al., 1979). The loss of more than 3 kg in body weight caused a decrease in the correlation coefficient between dietary and adipose tissue linoleic from 0.82 to 0.62 (Staveren et al., 1986).

Several studies have demonstrated a proportional increase in the percent of linoleic acid (C18:2) and a decrease in the percent of saturated fatty acids in adipose tissue with increases in dietary linoleic acid. A significant increase in the percent of polyunsaturated fatty acids in adipose tissue was observed when subjects were placed on a high polyunsaturated, 30–33% of calories as fat diet containing a 1:1:1 ratio of polyunsaturated:monounsaturated:saturated fatty acids. Western diets generally have had a 0.5:1:1 ratio during the past decade. Parallel to this increase was a decrease in the percent of monounsaturated and saturated fatty acids in adipose tissue (Christakis et al., 1965). In similar experiments a significant increase in the porportion of adipose linoleic acid (a two- to threefold increase) and a significant decrease in the other fatty acids was observed when subjects were fed diets high in linoleic acid for periods up to 5 years (Dayton et al., 1966, 1967; Fleischman et al., 1967). The relative increase in the proportion of adipose linoleic acid was negatively correlated ($r = -0.58$) with the initial body weight of subjects. The greater the adiposity of the subject, the smaller the relative increase in adipose linoleic acid observed (Dayton et al., 1967). Linear regression analysis of data from several studies gives the following equation (Beynen et al., 1980) for the relationship between dietary polyunsaturated fatty acids and adipose polyunsaturated fatty acids: Percentage of adipose polyunsaturated fatty acids = 3.43 + 0.54 (Percentage of dietary polyunsaturated fatty acids) (Beynen et al., 1980). The percentages of fatty acids in the equation were relative to total fatty acids in tissue and diet.

A correlation of 0.70 between diet and adipose tissue linoleic acid was reported by Staveren and coworkers (1986). However, the high correlation was observed only when dietary intake was quantitated (by 24-hour recall) 19 separate times over a 30-month time period. Even with such a large number of diet assessments over a long period, the correlation was 0.70 and thus represents approximately 50% of the variation in the dietary tissue–fatty acid relationship. Staveren and coworkers (1986) determined that the correlation between dietary intake as measured using a single 24-hour recall and tissue fatty acid had a correlation of approximately 0.28 or less than 8% of the variation between the diet and tissue fatty acid data.

Correlations of approximately 0.30 have been reported by several investigators when they related different dietary methods such as 24-hour recall with a semiquantitative food frequency method. Table 5 shows the correlation between specific tissue fatty acids and dietary lipids as measured using a food frequency questionnaire adapted from the method of Block (1982, 1989). The study subjects were randomly selected adult Anglo-Americans residing in southern Arizona and serving as normal free-living controls for an ongoing study. The majority of the correlations shown in Table 5 were less than 0.30. These data indicate the low correlation between dietary and tissue fatty acids and underscores the possibility for obtaining different conclusions from studies comparing dietary lipids with risk of cancer.

The proportion of carbohydrate and saturated/monounsaturated/polyunsaturated

Table 5 Correlation[a] Between Dietary Lipids and Adipose Tissue Fatty Acids

	Dietary Lipids				
Tissue fatty acid	Saturated fat (g)	Oleic acid (g)	Linoleic acid (g)	Saturated fat (%)	Linoleic acid (%)
14:0	0.19	0.09	−0.02**	0.29	−0.22**
16:0	0.15	0.17	0.20**	0.03	0.09
16:1	−0.03	−0.09	−0.15**	0.19*	−0.17*
18:0	0.28**	0.23**	0.31**	0.11	0.20**
18:1	−0.06	−0.02	−0.03	0.02	0.01
18:2	−0.15*	−0.14	−0.03	−0.15*	0.19*
18:3	0.07	0.05	−0.03	0.11	−0.07
20:4	−0.01	−0.04	−0.06	0.11	−0.10

[a]Pearson correlation coefficients were calculated using data from 182 normal free-living randomly selected subjects.
*p-value $\leq$ 0.05; **p-value $\leq$ 0.01.

fatty acids in the diet causes a distinct fatty acid profile in adipose tissue. Berry and coworkers (1986) proposed a model for predicting the macronutrient composition of the diet based on the fatty acid profile of adipose: (a) a diet high in animal fat increases adipose tissue palmitoleic (C16:1) and oleic (C18:1) acids (fatty acids found in animal products); (b) a diet high in carbohydrates increases palmitic (C16:0) and stearic (C18:0) acids (fatty acid products of lipogenesis) and decreases linoleic acid (C18:2); and (c) a diet high in vegetable oil increases linoleic acid and decreases palmitic and stearic acids. Support for this model comes from studies of adults on habitually low fat, high carbohydrate diets who have significantly reduced levels of adipose tissue, linoleic acid, and significantly increased levels of palmitic and palmitoleic acids (Hirsch et al., 1960; Farquhar and Ahrens, 1963). Similarly, reports indicate that neonates during their last trimester in utero synthesize and deposit fat from maternal carbohydrates and have approximately twice as much palmitic acid (C16:0) as adults (Hirsch et al., 1960; Farquhar and Ahrens, 1963; Field et al., 1985; Berry et al., 1986).

The study of adipose tissue fatty acid composition has provided insights into the changing dietary patterns of Americans in the past decades. Analysis of the linoleic acid content of adipose tissue in Americans shows a linear increase in adipose linoleic acid from 8% in the early 1960s to 16% in 1981–1982. This suggests that the general U.S. population has in recent years been consuming more unsaturated fatty acids (Witting and Lee, 1975; Berry et al., 1986). The increase in unsaturated fatty acids has been predominantly due to an increase in salad and cooking oils and margarine, which also contain *trans*-isomers of polyunsaturated fatty acids (Hunter et al., 1985). Approximately 2.0–5.8% of unsaturated fatty acids in adipose tissue are *trans*-fatty acid, reflecting a dietary consumption of 2.3–6.6 g of *trans*-fatty acids per day (Ohlrogge et al., 1981; Hunter et al., 1985).

Unfortunately, there have been few reports to date that have evaluated the correlation between tissue fatty acids and cancer. Hietanen and coworkers (1980) reported that patients with breast cancer had increased polyunsaturated fatty acids and decreased saturated fatty acids in the phospholipid content of cancerous cells. Hill and coworkers (1986) also reported that postmenpausal breast cancer patients had increased linoleic acid and increased stearic acid but decreased palmitic acid and decreased oleic acid. In contrast Caleffi and coworkers (1987) and Eid and Berry (1980) did not see a significant difference between tissue fatty acids evaluated in breast cancer cases and their control groups. These latter reports utilize control subjects that had some pathology that required either a biopsy or surgery, and thus the disease or the treatment may have altered tissue fatty acid levels. All of the above studied had very modest numbers of subjects and thus limit the evaluation of the role of the tissue fatty acids in the etiology of cancer.

Several studies relating tissue fatty acids and melanoma have been reported by Mackie and colleagues (1980, 1982, 1987). These authors analyzed subcutaneous adipose tissue samples from 100 melanoma patients and 100 matched controls and analyzed the fatty acids. Their studies indicated that mean percentages of tissue fatty acids were statistically significantly elevated for melanoma cases including polyunsaturates, and individually for linoleic acid and arachadonic acid. Also, their analysis of tissue fatty acids illustrated a lower statistically significant level of other tissue fatty acids, including palmitoleic acid and oleic acid as well as total monounsaturates.

BIOMARKERS OF CARBOHYDRATE AND FIBER INTAKE

The identification and evaluation of other biochemical markers of carbohydrate and fiber intake have been reported to be influenced by the completeness of digestion in the small intestine and fermentation in the large intestine. The most common dietary carbohydrates include starches, sugars, cellulose, hemicellulose, pectin, and gums (Williams, 1985) and can be classified by their resistance to digestion. The starches and sugars are digested primarily in the small intestine. Dietary fiber includes a heterogeneous group of carbohydrates, including cellulose, hemicellulose, pectin and gums, and lignin, a noncarbohydrate, that are not digested in the small intestine and subject to fermentation in the large intestine. Table 6 lists the carbohydrate and fiber composition of common cereals, fruits, vegetables, and nuts.

Current evidence indicates that the large intestine is the primary location for fermentation, an anaerobic bacterial conversion of digestion resistant carbohydrates

Table 6 Carbohydrate and Fiber Composition of Selected Foods[a]

	Cereals			Fruits		Vegetables		Legumes
	Bread, whole wheat	Bread, white	Corn flakes	Straw-berries	Bananas	Carrots, raw	Cabbage, raw	Peanuts, roasted
Total carbohydrate[b]	47.70	50.40	86.10	7.02	23.43	10.48	5.41	19.86
Total fiber[c]	8.50	2.72	11.00	2.12	1.75	3.70	2.83	9.30
Carbohydrate, fiber cellulose	1.31	0.71	2.42	0.33	0.37	1.48	0.69	1.69
Hemicellulose	5.95	2.01	7.26	0.98	1.12	2.22	1.76	6.40
Noncarbohydrate, fiber	1.24	tr	1.32	0.81	0.26	tr	0.38	1.21
Total water[d]	8.00	7.90	2.60	91.57	74.26	87.38	92.00	2.71

[a]Percentage composition in 100 g edible portion.
[b]USDA, 1979.
[c]Adapted from Southgate, 1986.
[d]Percent protein and fat not shown but can be calculated as the difference (100 − carbohydrate–lignin-water).

and fiber, that yields short-chain fatty acids, energy (ATP), and gases. The establishment of a quantitative measure of fermentation could provide a biomarker for dietary carbohydrate and fiber intake and provide more consistent assessment of the association of diet and cancer, especially colon cancer (McBurney and Thompson, 1990; Le Marchand, personal communication).

Large intestinal fermentation is controlled by the quantity of carbohydrate and fiber intake (Cummings and Englyst, 1987). On average 50% of cellulose is broken down during fermentation. However, different sources of fiber are fermented to different extents. Cellulose from fruits and vegetables is more completely fermented than wheat bran (Cummings, 1982). The noncellulose polysaccharide types of fiber are in general fermented to a greater extent than cellulose. Pectin and other water-soluble noncellulose polysaccharides are completely fermented. Lignin, a fiber from plant cell walls, is not broken down to any great extent in the intestine. As a general rule, the more lignified a plant structure, the less completely is it fermented in the large intestine (Cummings, 1982).

Although many of the effects of fiber relate to its fermentation in the large intestine, the starch in the diet currently appears to have primary control on fermentation. Cummings and Englyst (1987) have demonstrated that 10–20% of dietary starch is not digested in the small intestine and thus becomes available for fermentation in the large intestine. A typical Western diet supplies 8–18 g of fiber and 8–40 g of starch to the large intestine for fermentation (Cummings, 1990). Since virtually all starch that enters the large intestine is fermented and, as discussed above, only a portion of fiber is fermented, it is dietary starch that appears to provide the largest amount of substrate for fermentation in the large intestine.

A marker for the combined effect of dietary fiber plus starch on fermentation in the large intestine may provide a greater association with risk of several diseases including cancer (Vahouny and Kritchevsky, 1982). Fermentation of increased dietary fiber and starch in the large intestine results in (a) dilution of carcinogens by increased fecal bulk and decreased stool transit time (Stephen and Cummings, 1980; Shetty and Kurpad, 1986), (b) increased fecal excretion of lipids (Southgate, 1982), (c) a decrease in the degradation of primary to secondary bile acids as a result of lowering the pH of the large intestine by the fermentation of short-chain fatty acids (Midtvedt and Norman, 1968; Fleming et al., 1989), and (d) increased DNA repair, increased cellular differentiation, and growth inhibition of the large intestine through production of the short-chain fatty acid butyrate (Leder and Leder, 1975; Kim et al., 1980; Smith, 1986). However, the extent of these changes related to increased fiber and starch intake and the resulting increased fermentation are a function of both type of fiber and amount of fiber (Vahouny and Kritchevsky, 1982).

The quantitation of breath methane and hydrogen may provide useful and practical biomarkers of fermentation of total dietary fiber and starch intake (Solomons and Viteri, 1978; Vahouny and Kritchevsky, 1982; Eastwood et al., 1986;

Le Marchand, personal communication). Methane and hydrogen are two of the three gases produced during fermentation. These gases are absorbed into the portal bloodstream, transported to the lungs, and excreted unchanged by the lungs. The potential usefulness of breath methane and hydrogen is supported by the high correlation between breath levels and concentrations produced in the large intestine (Levitt and Ingelfinger, 1968; Levitt, 1969; Bond et al., 1971). These breath gases have been utilized to investigate carbohydrate malabsorption (Solomons and Viteri, 1978; Haderstorfer et al., 1989) in populations at different disease risks (Tadesse et al., 1980; Segal et al., 1988). The use of breath methane and hydrogen requires additional research to fully evaluate their prognostic role in cancer etiology and prevention.

REFERENCES

Angelico, F., Arca, M., Calvieri, A., et al. Plasma and erythrocyte fatty acids: A methodology for evaluation of hypocholesterolemic dietary interventions. *Prevent. Med. 12*: 124–127 (1983).

Apostolov, K., Barker, W. Reversible increase in the saturation of 18-carbon fatty acids induced by diphtheria toxin in tissue culture cells. *Infect. Immun. 38*: 843–847 (1982).

Apostolov, K., Barker, W. Cyclic effects of interferon and its antagonist on the saturation of 18-carbon fatty acids. *Ann. Virol. 135*: 245–256 (1984).

Apostolov, K., Barker, W., Catovsky, D., et al. Reduction in the stearic to oleic acid ratio in leukemic cells—a possible chemical marker of malignancy. *Blut 6*: 349–354 (1985).

Bazzarre, T. L., Myers, M. P. The collection of food intake data in cancer epidemiology studies. *Nutr. Cancer 1*: 22–45 (1980).

Berns, M. A. M., DeVries, J. H. M., et al. Increase in body fatness as a major determinant of changes in serum total cholesterol and high density lipoprotein cholesterol in young men over a 10-year period. *Amer. J. Epidemiol. 130*: 1109–1122 (1989).

Berry, E. M., Hirsch, J., Most, J., et al. The relationship of dietary fat to plasma lipid levels as studied by factor analysis of adipose tissue fatty acid composition in a free-living population of middle-aged American men. *Am. J. Clin. Nutr. 44*: 220–231 (1986).

Berry, E. M., Elliot, M., Zimmerman, M. D., et al. Dietary fat, adipose tissue composition, and the development of carcinoma of the colon. *JNCL 77*(1): 93–97 (1986a).

Berry, E. M., Elliot, M., Hirsch, J., et al. Does dietary linolenic acid influence blood pressure. *Am. J. Clin. Nutr. 44*: 336-340 (1986b).

Berlin, E., Bhathena, S. J., et al. Dietary fat and hormonal effects on erythrocyte membrane fluidity and lipid composition in adult women. *Metabolism 38*(8): 790–796 (1989).

Beynen, A. C., Hermus, R. J. J., et al. A mathematical relationship between the fatty acid composition of the diet and that of the adipose tissue in man. *Am. J. Clin. Nutr. 33*: 81–85 (1980).

Block, G. A review of validation of dietary assessment methods. *Am. J. Epidemiol. 115*: 492 (1982).

Block, G., Hartman, A. M. Dietary assessment methods, *Nutrition and Cancer Prevention: Investigating The Role of Micronutrients* (T. E. Moon and M. S. Micozzi, eds.), Marcel Dekker, New York, 1989, pp. 159–180.

Bond, J. H., Engel, R. R., Levitt, M. D. Factors influencing pulmonary methane excretion in man. *J. Exp. Med. 133*: 572–588 (1971).

Broquist, H. P. Amino acid metabolism, In *Present Knowledge in Nutrition*, 5th ed. The Nutrition Foundation, Washington, DC 1984.

Caleffi, M., Ashraf, J., et al. A comparison of the fatty acid profiles of subcutaneous fat from women with breast cancer, benign breast disease and normal controls. *Anticancer Research 7*: 1305–1308 (1987).

Chabner, B. A. *Pharmacologic Principles of Cancer Treatment*. W. B. Saunders, Philadelphia, 1982.

Christakis, G. J., Rinzler, S. H., et al. Effect of serum cholesterol-lowering diet on composition of depot fat in man. *Am. J. Clin. Nutr. 16*: 243–251 (1965).

Cummings, J. H. *Consequences of the Metabolism of Fiber in the Human Large Intestine in Dietary Fiber in Health and Disease* (G. U. Vahouny and D. Kriteheusky, eds.) Plenum Press, 1982.

Cummings, J. H., Englyst, H. N. Fermentation in the human large intestine and the available substrates. *Am. J. Clin. Nutr. 45*: 1243–1255 (1987).

Cummings, J. H. Microbial fermentation of starch in the large intestine: products and their effects. *Can. J. Physiol. Pharmaco.* (1990).

Dahlqvist, A. Carbohydrates, In *Present Knowledge in Nutrition*, 5th ed. The Nutrition Foundation, Washington, DC, 1984.

Dayton, S., Hashimoto, S., Dixon, W., et al. Composition of lipids in human serum and adipose tissue during prolonged feeding of a diet high in unsaturated fat. *J. Lipid Res. 7*: 103–111 (1966).

Dayton, S., Hashimoto, S., Pearce, M. L. Adipose tissue linoleic acid as a criteria of adherence to a modified diet. *J. Lipid Res. 8*: 508–510 (1967).

Devlin, T. M. *Textbook of Biochemistry with Chemical Correlations*. John Wiley and Sons, New York, 1982.

Dougherty, R., Galli, C., et al. Lipid and phospholipid fatty acid composition of plasma, red blood cells, and platelets and how they are affected by dietary lipids: A study of normal subjects from Italy, Finland, and the USA. *Am. J. Clin. Nutr. 45*: 443–455 (1987).

Dweyer, J. T. Assessment of dietary intake. In *Modern Nutrition in Health and Disease*, 7th ed. (M. E. Shils and V. R. Young, eds.), Lea & Febiger, Philadelphia, 1988, pp. 887–905.

Eastwood, M. A., et al. Methane production and excretion: A marker of cecal fermentation. In *Dietary Fiber: Basic and Clinical Aspects* (G. V. Vahouny and D. Kritchevsky, eds.), New York, 1986, pp. 151–166.

Eid, A., Berry, E. M. The relationship between dietary fat, adipose tissue composition and neoplasms of the breast. *Nutr. Cancer 11*: 173–177 (1988).

Farquhar, J. W., Ahrens, Jr., E. H. Effects of dietary fats on human erythrocyte fatty acid patterns. *J. Clin. Invest. 42*(5): 675–685 (1963).

Field, C. J., Clandinin, M. T. Modulation of adipose tissue fat composition by diet: A review. *Nutr. Research 4*: 743–755 (1984).

Field, C. J., Angel, A., et al. Relationship of diet to the fatty acid composition of human adipose tissue structural and stored lipids. *Am. J. Clin. Nutr. 42*: 1206–1220 (1985).

Fleischman, A., Hayton, T., et al. The effect of a polyunsaturated diet upon adipose-tissue fatty acids in young coronary males. A five-year cohort study. *Lipids 3*(2): 147–150 (1967).

Fleming, S. E., Fitch, M. D., Chansler, M. W. High-fiber diets: Influence on characteristics of cecal digesta including short-chain fatty acid concentrations and pH. *Am. J. Clin. Nutr. 50*: 93–99 (1989).

Freedman, L. S., Clifford, C., Messina, M. Analysis of dietary fat, calories, body weight, and the development of mammary tumors in rats and mice: A review. *Cancer Res. 50*: 5710–5719 (1990).

Glatz, J., Soffers, A. Katan, M. Fatty acid composition of serum cholesteryl esters and erythrocyte membranes as indicators of linoleic acid intake in man. *Am. J. Clin. Nutr. 49*: 269–276 (1989).

Goldstein, J., Kita, T., Brown, M. Defective lipoprotein receptors and atherosclerosis. *N. Engl. J. Med. 309*: 288–296 (1983).

Grundy, S. M. Dietary fats and sterols, In *Nutrition, Lipids and Coronary Heart Disease*, (R. Levy, B. Rifkins, B. Dennis, N. Ernst, eds.), Raven Press, New York, 1979.

Grundy, S. M. Effects of fatty acids on lipoprotein metabolism in man: perspectives for actions of fish oil fatty acids, In *Health Effects of Polyunsaturated Fatty Acis in Seafoods* (S. P. Simpoub, R. R. Kifer, R. E. Martin, eds.), Academic Press, New York, 1986.

Haderstorfer, B., Psycholgin, D., Whitehead, W. E., et al. Intestinal gas production from bacterial fermentation of undigested carbohydrate in irritable bowel syndrome. *Am. J. Gastroenterol. 84*: 375–378 (1989).

Hietanen, E., Punnonen, K., et al. Fatty acid composition of phospholipids and neutral lipids and lipid peroxidation in human breast cancer and lipoma tissue. *Carcinogenesis 7*(12): 1965–1969 (1986).

Hirsch, J., Farquhar, W., Ahrens, Jr., E. H., et al. Studies of adipose tissue in man. A microtechnic for sampling and analysis. *Am. J. Clin. Nutr. 8*: 499–511 (1960).

Horwitt, M. K., Harvey, C. C., Century, B. Effect of dietary fats on fatty acid composition of human erythrocytes and chick cerebella. *Science 130*: 917–918 (1959).

Hunter, J. E., Clement, I. P., Hollenbach, E. J. Isomeric fatty acids and tumorigenesis: A commentary on recent work. *Nutr. Cancer 7*: 199–209 (1985).

Insull, Jr., W., Bartsch, G. E. Fatty acid composition of human adipose tissue related to age, sex, and race. *Am. J. Clin. Nutr. 20*: 13–23 (1967).

Insull, Jr., W. Dietary fats and lipids of adipose tissue and cell membranes in carcinogenesis. *Prevent. Med. 16*: 481–484 (1987).

Kim, Y. S., Tsao, D., et al. Effects of sodium butyrate on three human colorectal adenocarcinoma cell lines in culture, In *Colonic Carcinogenesis* (R. A. Malt and R. C. N. Williamson, eds.), Falk Symposium 31, MTP Press Ltd., Lancaster, 1980, pp. 485–503.

Leder, A., Leder, P. Butyric acid, a potent inducer of erythroid differentiation in cultural erythroleukemic cells. *Cell 5*: 319–322 (1975).

Leibetseder, F., Ahrens, Jr., E. H. The fatty acid composition of red cells in paroxysural nocturnal haemoglobinuria. *Brit. J. Haemat. 5*: 356 (1959).

Levitt, M. D., Ingelfinger, F. J. Hydrogen and methane production in man. *Ann. NY Acad. Sci. 150*: 75–81 (1968).
Levitt, M. D. Production and excretion of hydrogen gas in man. *N. Engl. J. Med. 281*: 122¢127 (1969).
Linscheer, W. G., Vergroesen, A. J. Lipids, In *Modern Nutrition in Health and Disease*, (M. E. Shils and V. R. Young, eds.), Lea and Febiger, Philadelphia, 1988.
McBurney, M. I., Thompson, L. U. Fermentative characteristics of cereal brans and vegetable fibers. *Nutr. Cancer 13*: 271–280 (1990).
McMurchie, E. J., Margetts, B. M., et al. Dietary-induced changes in the fatty acid composition of human cheek cell phospholipids: Correlation with changes in the dietary polyunsaturated/saturated fat rio. *Am. J. Clin. Nutr. 39*: 975–980 (1984).
Mackie, B. S., Mackie, L. E., et al. Melanoma and dietary lipids. *Nutr. Cancer 9*(4): 219–226 (1987).
Malcolm, G. T., Bhattacharyya, A. K., et al. Fatty acid composition of adipose tissue in humans: Differences between subcutaneous sites. *Am. J. Clin. Nutr. 50*: 288–291 (1989).
Midtvedt, T., Norman, A. Parameters in 7-alpha-dehydroxylation of bile acids by anaerobic lactobacilli. *Act. Path. Microb. Scand. 72*: 313–329 (1968).
Munro, H. N. Crinn, M. C. The proteins and amino acids, In *Modern Nutrition in Health and Disease* (M. E. Shils and V. R. Young, eds.), Lea and Febiger, Philadelphia, 1988.
Neoptolemos, J. P., Clayton, H., Heagerty, A. M., et al. Dietary fat in relation to fatty acid composition of red cells and adipose tissue in colorectal cancer. *Br. J. Cancer 58*: 575–579 (1988).
Nozawa, C. M., Apostolov, K. Association of the cytopathic effects of Sindbis virus with increased fatty acid saturation. *F. Gen. Virol. 59*: 219–222 (1982).
Nozawa, C. M., Apostolov, K. Increase in the saturation of C18 fatty acids induced by coxsackie B6 virus in Vero cells. *Virology 120*: 247–250 (1982).
NRC (National Research Council). *Diet, Nutrition, and Cancer*. Report of the Committee on Diet, Nutrition, and Cancer. Assembly of Life Sciences. National Academy Press, Washington, DC., 1982.
Ohlrogge, J. B., Emken, E. A., Gulley, R. M. Human tissue lipids: Occurrence of fatty acid isomers from dietary hydrogenated oils. *J. Lipid Res. 22*: 955–960 (1981).
Pittet, G., Halliday, D., Bateman, P. E. Site differences in the fatty acid composition of subcutaneous adipose tissue of obese women. *Br. J. Nutr.* 57–61 (1979).
Popp-Snijders, C., Schouten, J., DeJong, A., et al. Effect of dietary cod-liver oil on the lipid composition of a human erythrocyte membranes. *Scand. J. Clin. Lab. Invest. 44*: 39–46 (1984).
Popp-Snijders, C., Schouten, J. A., Van Bliherswijk, W. J., et al. Changes in membrane lipid composition of human erythrocytes after dietary supplementation of (n-3) polyunsaturated fatty acids. Maintenance of membrane fluidity. *Biochem. Biophys. Acta 854*: 31–37 (1986).
Quinn, P. J. Models for adaptive changes in all membranes. *Biochem. Soc. Trans. 11*: 329–330 (1983).
Sampaugna, J., Light, L., Enig, M. G., et al. Cheek cell fatty acids as indicators of dietary lipids in humans. *Lipids 23*(1): 131–136 (1988).

Sandeman, Jr., H. Regulation of membrane enzymes by lipids. *Biochem. Biophys. Acta 515*: 209–237 (1979).

Schaefer, E., Eisenberg, S., Levy, R. Lipoprotein metabolism. *J. Lipid Res. 19*: 667–682 (1978).

Schaffer, L., Overvad, K. Subcutaneous adipose-tissue fatty acids and vitamin E in humans: Relation to diet and sampling site. *Am. J. Clin. Nutr. 52*: 486–490 (1990).

Scott, R. F., Lee, K. T., et al. Fatty acids of serum and adipose tissue in six groups eating natural diets containing 7 to 40 per cent fat. *Am. J. Clin. Nutr. 14*: 280–290 (1964).

Segal, I., Walker, L. S., et al. Breath methane and large bowel cancer risk in contrasting populations. *Gut 29*: 608–613 (1988).

Shanmugasundaram, K., Visvanathan, A., et al. Effect of high-fat diet on cholesterol distribution in plasma lipoproteins, cholesterol esterifying activity in leucocytes, and erythrocyte membrane components studied: Importance of body weight. *Am. J. Clin. Nutr. 44*: 805–815 (1986).

Shetty, P. S., Kurpad, A. V. Increasing starch intake in the human diet increases fecal bulking. *Am. J. Clin. Nutr. 43*: 210–212 (1986).

Shortland, F. B., Czochanska, Z., Prior, I. A. Studies on fatty acid composition of adipose tissue and blood lipids of polynesians. *Am. J. Clin. Nutr. 22*: 594–605 (1969).

Smith, P. J. N-butyrate alters chromatin accessibility to DNA repair enzymes. *Carcinogenesis 7*: 423–429 (1986).

Solomons, N. W., Viteri, F. Development of an interval sampling hydrogen (H_2) breath test for carbohydrate malabsorption in children: Evidence for a circadian pattern of breath H_2 concentration. *Pediatr. Res. 12*: 816–823 (1978).

Southgate, D. A. In *CRC Handbook of Dietary Fiber in Human Nutrition* (G. A. Spiller, ed.), CRC Press, Boca Raton, Florida, 1986.

Southgate, D. A. T. Digestion and absorption of nutrients, In *Dietary Fiber in Health and Disease* (G. U. Vahouny and D. Kritchevsky, eds.), Plenum Press, 1982.

Stansky, M. E. Fatty acids in fish. In *Health Effects of Polyunsaturated Acids in Seafood* (A. P. Simopoulos, R. R. Kifer, and R. E. Martin, eds.), Academic Press, New York, 1986.

Staveren, W. A., Van, Deurenberg, P., et al. Validity of the fatty acid composition of subcutaneous fat tissue microbiopsies as an estimate of the long-term average fatty acid composition of the diet of separate individuals. *Am. J. Epidemiol. 123*: 455–463 (1986).

Staveren, W. A., Van, Burema, J., Deurenberg, P., et al. Weak associations in nutritional epidemiology: the importance of replication of observations on individuals. *Int. J. Epidemiol. 17*(Suppl.): 964–969 (1988).

Stephen, A. M., Cummings, J. H. The microbial contribution to human feces mass. *J. Med. Microb. 13*: 45–56 (1980).

Tadesse, K., Smith, D., Eastwood, M. A. Breath hydrogen and methane excretion patterns in normal man and in clinical practice. *Am. J. Exp. Physiol. 65*: 85–97 (1980).

Vahouny, G. U., Kritchevsky, D. *Dietary Fiber in Health and Disease*. Plenum Press, 1982.

Williams, S. R. *Nutrition and Diet Therapy*. Times Mirror/Mosby College Publishing, 1985.

Witting, L. A., Lee, L. Recommended dietary allowance for vitamin E: relation to dietary, erythrocyte and adipose tissue linoleate. *Am. J. Clin. Nutr. 28*: 577–583 (1975).

Wood, C. B., Habib, N. A., Thompson, A., et al. Increase of oleic acid in erythrocytes associated with malignancies. *Br. Med. J. 291*: 163–165 (1985).
Young, V. R., Marchini, J. S., et al. Assessment of protein nutritional status. *Am. Inst. Nutr.* 1496–1501 (1990).

part three

EVIDENCE FOR SPECIFIC MACRONUTRIENTS AND RELATED FACTORS

8

Energy Intake and Cancer

Demetrius Albanes
National Cancer Institute
National Institutes of Health
Bethesda, Maryland

INTRODUCTION

The relationship between energy intake and cancer has been the subject of a considerable quantity of research over the past several decades. Early recorded allusions to the deleterious health effects of excess food consumption include those from Hippocrates (1), Rabagliati (2), Chittenden (3), and Hoffmann (4), for example. Such writings and early observations concerning the geographical distribution of cancer in the world from some of the early geographical pathologists led to the experimental manipulation of tumor incidence through the restriction of total food or caloric intake in rodents. These earlier experiments in turn influenced later epidemiologic studies and additional laboratory investigations. Results from this sequence of research events are the subject of this chapter.

ANIMAL STUDIES

A large number of laboratory studies have demonstrated that tumor incidence in rodents is highly dependent upon daily calorie intake and body weight. The earliest reports of the tumor inhibitory effect of underfeeding were those of Moreschi (5) and Rous (6,7). In the experiment of Moreschi, the growth of transplanted sarcomas increased directly with total daily food intake (5). Rous demonstrated a similar trend for the incidence of both transplanted and spontaneous tumors and their recurrence following excision (6,7). Subsequent experiments by Bischoff (8), McCay (9), Lavik and Baumann (10), Visscher (11), and others provided additional evidence for the substantial preventive role of food and calorie restriction in the development of neoplasia. During the 1940s, Tannenbaum and colleagues conducted a systematic series of investigations in this field (12–23). These experiments, along with the earlier studies and ones that followed (such as those by Boutwell and coworkers (24,25), which further extended our knowledge in the area), established an unequivocal body of evidence for the role of total energy intake in tumorigenesis. These experiments demonstrate that tumor incidence increases with increasing energy intake and resulting body weight over a range of dietary intake. Fewer tumors, delayed tumor onset, retarded tumor growth, and fewer metastases were also observed among calorie-restricted animals compared with control animals that were fed more calories ad libitum. In various species and strains, these effects have been established for a variety of both "spontaneous" and chemically induced neoplasms including carcinomas, sarcomas, adenomas, and papillomas of the skin, mammary gland, lung, liver, subcutaneous tissue, hematopoietic elements, or other sites, including, most recently, the prostate (26). The calorie-restricted animals in these experiments generally lived longer and were often reported as being as active and healthy as their ad libitum-fed controls; therefore, the benefit of reduced tumor incidence was not accomplished through the substitution with other pathology or by decreasing the animals' lifespans. (For comprehensive treatise dealing with the beneficial effects of dietary restriction on aging, see Ref. 27.)

A recent analysis combined data from a large number of published experiments and evaluated the quantitative relationship between total caloric intake and tumorigenesis in mice, as well as the independence of these effects from those of dietary fat intake (28). Data for approximately 5000 animals included total energy, fat, protein, and carbohydrate intake, body weight, and final tumor incidence. Each experiment compared a restricted, "experimental" group consuming fewer calories to an ad libitum "control" group (i.e., higher and usually ad libitum caloric intake). Dietary regimens were fixed for the duration of each experiment. The types of fat, protein, and essential vitamins were the same within each experiment. With the exception of the "underfeeding" experiments, which resulted in reduced vitamin intake among calorie-restricted animals (12), equivalent essential vitamin intake was generally maintained and reported.

The results from this analysis show that the experimental groups consumed on average 29% fewer calories, 50% less fat, 11% less protein, 27% less carbohydrate, and derived approximately 30% fewer calories from dietary fat daily, compared to the control groups. In contrast, the percentage of calories derived from carbohydrate was equivalent, and protein calories were 25% higher among experimental groups. Final tumor incidence was substantially lower among experimental groups (by 42%), as was body weight (by 25%). Each of the experimental group-control group differences was statistically highly significant ($p \leq 0.001$). Cumulative tumor incidence increased in the experimental groups with increasing caloric intake in a nearly dose-response manner (Fig. 1). This relationship was observed for both major tumor sites studied: chemically induced skin and "spontaneous" mammary tumors. A more striking linear relationship was evident for caloric restriction in mammary tumorigenesis, however, including lower incidence among the most restricted animals. Similar patterns were observed in this investigation for the relationship between tumor incidence and animal body weight (28). Lower tumor yield and delayed tumor onset were also observed among the calorie-restricted animals in most studies. These analyses indicate that the incidence of chemically induced and "spontaneous" tumors in mice is proportional to the level of caloric intake and resulting body weight over a wide range of caloric, as well as other macronutrient, intake in a variety of experimental settings. Furthermore, the results exclude confounding by dietary fat intake as an explanation for the influence of energy intake in these experiments. Although most abundantly demonstrated for skin and mammary tumors (with evidence for greater efficacy in the mammary models), this effect was also observed for other sites including all-sites incidence. That tumor incidence responds in a graded fashion to the level of energy restriction is also well-supported by findings from individual studies (17,18,20,21,29).

Several experiments have established the independence of the tumor inhibitory effect of restricted energy consumption from that of its specific component sources. Lavik and Baumann were among the first researchers to demonstrate that high total caloric intake leads to higher tumor incidence regardless of the level of total fat intake (10). Similar observations were made subsequently by Tannenbaum (14,15) and by Boutwell (24). These experiments introduced the term "net energy" to convey the importance of the total intake of energy from all macronutrient sources, including, especially, dietary fat. One recent experiment further developed this concept using the term "relative net energy" and demonstrating effects on both lean and fat body tissues (30). Other recent experiments by Kritchevsky and colleagues (31,32) corroborate the earlier studies, demonstrating that both dietary fat and total dietary calories independently promote tumor incidence when fed in higher quantities, with greater tumor reduction resulting from caloric—rather than fat—restriction. In the "meta-analysis" described above (28), the strong promotional role for high energy intake was independent of fat intake (Fig. 1) and was demonstrated at both low and high dietary fat levels. Tumor incidence was 34, 52, 23, and 54%, respectively, for the experiments classified as low calorie–low fat, high calorie–low fat, low calorie–high fat, and high calorie–high fat.

Another important observation made in these studies concerns the relationship between energy and body size. Mature body weight and daily caloric intake were highly correlated in these experiments (Fig. 2). The Spearman correlation

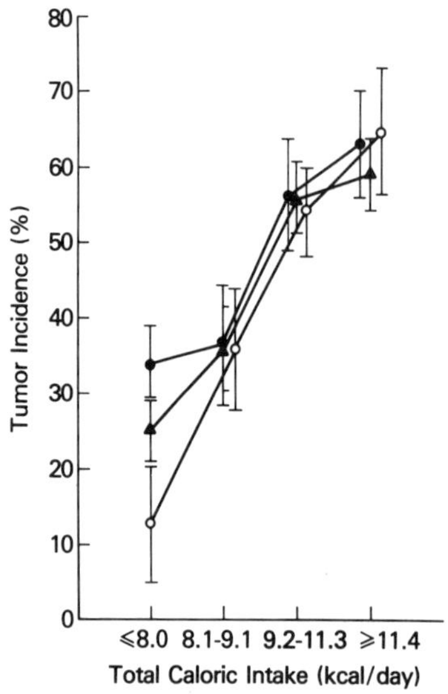

Figure 1 Relationship between cumulative tumor incidence and caloric intake in mice from 82 experiments: all tumor sites (▲); skin tumors (●); mammary tumors (○). Tumor incidence (percentage of animals developing one or more tumors by the end of the experiment) adjusted for incidence in control groups, site, and sex, and weighted by number of animals per experimental group. Caloric intake categorized by quartiles. Points, mean incidence; bars, SE.

coefficients corresponding to the two plots were 0.85 and 0.74 for males and females, respectively. This is in sharp contrast to results from human studies (see below). Of note was the reduced variability of body weight at lower levels (≤ 11 kilocalories) of caloric intake ($r = 0.90$ and 0.88 for male and female experimental groups, respectively), compared to that at higher energy intake ($r = 0.21$ and 0.39 for males and females, respectively). The correlations between body weight and fat or protein were much lower ($r = 0.07$ and 0.41, respectively) for all experiments combined, with little difference between sexes. The data confirm that under controlled, experimental conditions where basal metabolic and physical activity levels are relatively similar, body weight is directly proportional to caloric intake. Moreover, the close association between total intake, body weight, and tumor incidence in these experiments indicates that body weight is a sensitive indicator of energy balance as well as tumor risk. Experiments which have examined body composition demonstrate that calorie-restricted groups experience reductions in both lean and fat tissue mass, suggesting that the observed tumor

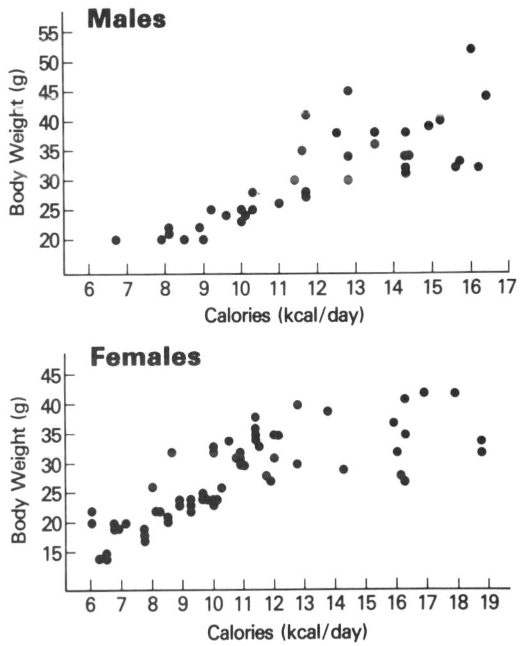

Figure 2 Relationship between adult body weight and daily caloric intake in mice from 82 experiments. Lifetime, fixed daily calorie diets were fed and body weight measured at the end of each experiment.

inhibition is mediated through the effects on both growth and overweight (30,33,34).

Animal experiments have been unique in their ability to elucidate other specific aspects of the relationships involved. For example, animals exposed to exogenous thyroxin or low environmental temperature, which result in lower body weight despite increased energy intake, experience reduced tumor incidence (35,36). Experimental data for rodents also demonstrate an antitumorigenic effect in the mammary gland and colon for regular physical activity (33,36–39). The combination of exercise and dietary caloric restriction led to even greater inhibition of mammary tumorigenesis than from exercise alone in one study (37). Efficiency of body weight gain throughout life is associated with increased tumor incidence (40). These studies, as well as others discussed earlier with respect to "net energy" (14,15,24,30), emphasize the importance of energy *balance*—that is, the net difference between energy intake and all expenditure combined—in experimental tumorigenesis. Finally, energy restriction inhibits tumorigenesis even when applied during presumably late stages of carcinogenesis, i.e, following exposure to a one-step or "complete" carcinogen (16), or among older animals fed ad libitum up to approximately "middle-age" but restricted thereafter (31,41). Still other experiments demonstrate that the inhibitory effect of restriction on tumorigenesis is greater when imposed later rather than earlier in life (42). Therefore, while reduced energy intake throughout life may be most efficacious, there is evidence that energy restriction instituted at older ages and after carcinogenic exposures is beneficial. This has important implications for anticarcinogenesis in humans, since the majority of cancers occur later in life and effects on promotion may be most relevant and useful for prevention through dietary restriction.

In summary, the wealth and consistency of results from rodent studies of energy intake and neoplasia is uncommon in nutrition-cancer research. Current experimental research is aimed at delineating the mechanisms responsible for the observed tumor inhibitory effects. Other seminal issues such as interactions with other specific nutrients and the effect of the timing of energy restriction on tumor prevention are also under investigation (see "Mechanisms" below).

HUMAN STUDIES

Whether total energy intake can affect the risk of developing cancer is a question that has received far less attention with respect to humans. Leading up to the 1982 National Research Council report entitled "Diet, Nutrition and Cancer" (43), a large number of epidemiologic investigations concerned with the relationship between food intake and cancer "risk" were conducted and published. Many of those studies had as their primary focus two food classes which were of great interest, namely, dietary fat intake, and fruits and vegetables known to be rich in a number of potentially cancer-preventive micronutrients. It is from some of the investigations of the role of dietary fat or other macronutrients, as well as other studies looking at diet in general, that evidence concerning cancer and total caloric intake is largely available.

ECOLOGICAL STUDIES

Five ecological investigations address the issue of whether caloric intake is related to the occurrence of cancer in humans. Four of these studies involve correlation analyses (two cross-nationally (44,45) and two intranationally (46,47)), and one other compares the diets and cancer rates between distinct socioeconomic classes (48). Ecological investigations usually employ per capita food "disappearance" data, such as those available for most nations from the Food and Agriculture Organization (49) or from other national data sources; alternatively, they are based on other estimates of group—rather than individual—food consumption. Analysis of such data assumes an average intake within each population. It also fails to take into account food wastage, which is particularly common in industrialized countries and may be group-specific in its magnitude within populations. Assuming that estimates of both individual foods and wastage are cumulative across food types, then error around the estimates for total calories are probably substantial. The cancer data from such studies also vary in their reliability between populations and may not necessarily be specific to the subpopulation from which food data were derived.

The international correlation study by Armstrong and Doll (44) demonstrated that total per capita caloric intake was correlated with cancer incidence and mortality. Site- and sex-specific correlation coefficients (r's) based upon concurrent food and cancer data for 33 countries were presented in the report, which demonstrated significant associations between total calories and cancer of the breast ($r = 0.57$), colon ($r = 0.66$), rectum ($r = 0.56$), uterus ($r = 0.65$), and kidney ($r = 0.64$) in women. Among men, total calories were correlated to cancer of the colon ($r = 0.60$), rectum ($r = 0.75$), kidney ($r = 0.55$), and nervous system ($r = 0.56$). A more recent but similar investigation by Kodama and Kodama (45) compared per capita food consumption to cancer mortality among 19 nations. The authors observed the following correlation coefficients for total calories and cancer: 0.77 (breast); 0.60 (prostate); 0.60 and .055 (male and female lung); −0.37 and −0.14 (male and female esophagus); −0.73 and −0.73 (male and female stomach); and 0.74 and 0.71 (male and female colon). In the cross-sectional study of colorectal cancer mortality in Hong Kong by Hill and colleagues (48), a greater than twofold rate increase was observed for persons in the highest of three family income categories compared to the lowest income group (in males, 26.7 vs. 11.7 per 100,000). This was related to increased consumption of all foods and estimated daily caloric intake among high-income individuals compared to the low-income population. Breast cancer mortality in the United States was also positively correlated with the regional demand for total food calories in the study of Gaskill and coworkers (46). Positive associations were also observed for protein, fat, milk, and beef, however, raising a problem pertinent to the previous study (44): namely, the collinearity of several dietary components across (or within) populations, and the resulting multiplicity of statistically significant factor-disease correlations. In contrast, Kato and others (47) failed to demonstrate any correlation between energy intake and breast or ovarian cancer mortality in Japan.

Although ecological investigations are often thought of as "hypothesis generating" rather than "hypothesis testing," those mentioned do provide some data in support of a positive total energy intake—cancer association. The inherent limitations of ecological analyses are well known and have been previously discussed in the context of diet-cancer relationships (44). They include such issues as validity and representativeness of risk factor and disease levels, appropriateness of the available measurement periods, and possible confounding. For example, these studies are generally not designed to exclude possible associations with other environmental factors. Furthermore, they lack data concerning physical activity, which varies greatly internationally. Differences in regional climates or even the heritable portion of basal metabolism may add to interpopulation differences in relative energy intake.

ANALYTICAL STUDIES

Most information concerning the relationship between cancer and energy intake in humans comes from analytical epidemiologic investigations. Many of these studies had other specific dietary components as their primary focus. A far greater number of case-control studies of diet and cancer have been unable to evaluate total caloric intake because of limitations inherent in the dietary methodology employed. With the exception of two cohort investigations, all of the reports concern hospital- or population-based case-control studies. Unless indicated otherwise, age-adjusted relative risk estimates are presented below.

Breast Cancer

Several studies from diverse populations shed light on the issue of whether energy intake is related to the occurrence of breast cancer in women. In the Canadian study by Miller and colleagues (50), which was the first case-control study of breast cancer to evaluate total energy intake, mean daily caloric intake of breast cancer cases was slightly (albeit significantly) higher than that of controls ($p = 0.01$). This association was stronger among postmenopausal women than among premenopausal women. No clear dose-response relation was demonstrated for caloric intake, however, with risk ratios of 1.3 and 1.1 for premenopausal women of moderate or high (>2500 kcal) daily intake compared to the ≤2000 kcal group, respectively. Among postmenopausal women, risk ratios of 1.0, 0.8 and 1.2 were obtained for three quartiles compared to the group ingesting less than 1500 calories daily. Similar modest case-control differences were observed by Rohan and coworkers in Australia (51). For their study group as a whole (including 451 cases), relative risk was only marginally increased in the highest quintile of energy intake (relative risk = 1.22 for >2371 kilocalories) compared to <1423 kilocalories. This association was only evident among postmenopausal women, however. In contrast, 120 cases reported nonsignificantly lower daily kilocalorie intake (1497 vs. 1556) compared to hospital controls in the investigation by Katsouyanni and colleagues in Athens, Greece (52). Quantile-related risk estimates were not presented for total calories.

Energy intake was substantially higher among 150 hospital-based, incident cases (mean, 2843 kilocalories) than for either neighborhood controls (2315 kilocalories) or hospital controls (2443 kilocalories) in the Argentine study by Iscovich and colleagues (53). Relative risk estimates for the increasing quartiles of energy intake were 1.00, 1.12, 3.13, and 8.65 using the neighborhood control series and quartile boundaries of <1969, −2425, −2890, and >2890 kilocalories. Somewhat lower estimates resulted from analysis of the hospital controls, although the elevated risk for the third and fourth quartiles were also highly statistically significant. Toniolo and coworkers observed similar differences in their population-based case-control study conducted in Italy (54). Cases reported higher mean calorie intake in their dietary histories than did controls subjects (2419 vs. 2294 kilocalories). Risk estimates increased from 1.0 to 1.5, 1.5, and 1.8 for quartiles one through four (lowest and highest quartile boundaries of <1900 and >2700 kilocalories). The most recent published data concerning energy intake and breast cancer risk are those of Knekt and colleagues, which are based on a cohort of Finnish women followed for up to 20 years (55). This investigation demonstrated somewhat lower mean daily energy intake among cases compared to noncases (2009 vs. 2141 kilocalories) and decreased relative risk for the second (1792–2334 kilocalories) and third (>2335 kilocalories) tertiles of energy intake (1.00 vs. 0.87 and 0.58; p-value for trend, 0.15). In this study, cases were taller and slightly leaner, on average, when compared with controls.

Of the six studies assessing the role of energy intake in breast cancer, four demonstrated a positive association between total caloric intake and cancer risk, one showed an inverse association, and one showed no clear relationship. These studies provide some evidence for a positive relationship between caloric intake and cancer of the breast. In the combined analysis of diet and breast cancer studies by Howe and colleagues (56), total calorie intake was positively related to breast cancer risk, increasing approximately 29% for every 2000 additional kilocalories of daily intake. The association was strong among postmenopausal women (40%, $p < 0.001$) and relatively weak premenopausally (8%; $p = 0.44$).

Colorectal Cancer

Large bowel cancer has also received much attention with respect to diet and macronutrients, including energy intake. Jain and colleagues observed a significant, positive dose-risk association for total calories among both men and women in their population-based study of cancer of the colon and rectum from Canada involving 400 cases (57). Relative risks of 1.5 and 1.8 were demonstrated among men for the middle (2485–3255 kilocalories) and high (>3255 kilocalories) intake groups compared to the low intake group (<2485 kilocalories). The corresponding risk ratios among the women were 1.6 and 2.2, using 1760 and 2360 kilocalories as tertile boundaries. An investigation of large bowel cancer by Bristol and coworkers in England showed substantially greater calorie intake for the 50 cases (mean = 2370 kilocalories) than for controls (2046 kilocalories), with relative risk increasing from 1.0 (<1936 kilocalories) to 2.2 and 23.0 (>2486 kilocalories) (58). Cases were also found to be taller and leaner in this study. Lyon and colleagues also found higher energy intake among colon cancer cases compared to controls in their population-based study in Utah (59). Relative risk ratios of 1.0, 2.0, and 3.6 for <1300 to >1800 kilocalories were observed in women, and 1.0, 2.5, and 2.5 for men (<1900 to >2600 kilocalories). Adjustment for differences in body mass index did not alter these findings for energy intake.

In contrast, two other studies of colorectal cancer demonstrated negligible case-control differences in caloric intake. Stemmermann and colleagues observed no material differences in mean calorie intake among colon or rectal cancer cases (combined n = 165) compared to controls in their cohort study of Japanese men in Hawaii (60). Small differences, inconsistent across sexes, were reported for energy intake for 715 cases compared to controls by Kune and coworkers in their population-based evaluation of dietary factors and large bowel cancer from Australia (61).

More recently, two studies demonstrated a positive association between energy intake and risk of colon cancer (62,63), and one did so for rectal cancer (64). The hospital-based study of 428 colon cancer cases in western New York by Graham and colleagues (62) demonstrated significant risk increases of from 1.00 to 1.45, 1.66, and 1.99 ($p = 0.01$ for trend) among men for the four quartiles of calories (boundaries not provided). Among women, risk increased from 1.00 to 1.09, 1.15, and 1.52 ($p = 0.13$). A population-based case-control study of 231 colon cancer cases was conducted in Utah by West and coworkers (63). In this study body mass index was strongly positively related to colon cancer risk: relative risk 2.1 and 2.3 for males and females, respectively, in the highest (compared to lowest) quintiles. Risk also increased with total caloric intake, from 1.0 to 1.5, 1.7, and 2.1 in men, and 1.0, 1.1, 1.8, and 1.5 in women (categories not given). A positive association between daily total calorie intake and cancer of the rectum has also been reported from western New York by Freudenheim and colleagues (64). In their hospital-based study of 422 cases, relative risk ratios of 1.00, 1.60, 1.85, and 2.57 were observed for the energy quartiles among men (categories not provided). For women relative risk increased from 1.00 to 1.71 and 1.40 for the increasing energy tertiles. Cases and controls did not differ with respect to height or body mass index.

In contrast to most of the above studies of large bowel cancer, Willett and colleagues showed energy intake to be unrelated to colon cancer (65). In their recently published study, over 88,000 female nurses in 11 states were followed for up to 6 years. Although other dietary factors such as fat and red meat were positively associated with colon cancer, relative risk estimates for the increasing quantiles of total calories were 1.00, 0.92, 1.07, 0.90, and 0.94 based on the following cuts: <1130, 1130–1389, 1390–1639, 1640–1959, and 1960+ kilocalories per day. Data concerning body size were not reported.

Of the nine analytic epidemiologic studies assessing the relationship between energy intake and risk of cancer of the large bowel, six demonstrated a positive association and three showed no association. These studies provide evidence for a positive relationship for all subsites of the colon, including the rectum. It is important to note that in none of the above investigations were data regarding physical activity energy expenditure and, therefore, true energy balance, presented. In some studies, however, adjustment for differences in body mass index had no effect on the calorie results (59,63,64). These investigations suggest that energy intake and body fatness are independently related to colorectal cancer. By contrast, the two studies in which body size was also analyzed separately demonstrated somewhat stronger positive associations between colon cancer and body mass index than they did for energy intake (62,63).

Other Sites

Four recent investigations provide data concerning energy intake and cancer at sites other than breast and large bowel (66–69). Shu and colleagues observed a positive association between total calories and risk of ovarian cancer in their population-based study of 172 cases from the People's Republic of China (66). Relative risks of 1.0, 1.0, 1.6 and 1.3 were demonstrated for the four increasing quartiles of energy intake (boundaries were not presented). A recent study of the nutritional epidemiology of gastric cancer conducted in western New York by Graham and coworkers showed that men and women reporting high calorie intake had significantly elevated risk of disease (67). Among men, risk increased significantly from 1.0 to 1.7, 4.1, and 2.4 for the four increasing calorie quartiles ($\leq$1567 to $\geq$2657 kcal/day). In women, the risk ratios were 1.0, 3.1, and 2.6 for three intake levels of $\leq$1440 to $\geq$1883 kcal/day. Two other studies have looked at pancreatic cancer (68, 69). Howe and colleagues found higher energy intake among 249 pancreas cancer cases compared to controls in their population-based study in Canada (68). The authors demonstrated somewhat greater total caloric intake among cases (means of 3495 and 2155 kilocalories for the male and female nonproxy cases, respectively) than for nonproxy controls (3087 and 2031 kilocalories for males and females). Relative risk ratios of 1.00, 1.65, 1.87, and 2.39 (p-value for trend 0.0004) were observed for women and men combined, using the energy intake cuts of $<$1735, −2295, −3009, and $>$3009 kilocalories. There were no case-control differences in body mass index. The investigation by Farrow and coworkers in New Mexico showed reduced energy intake for the 168 population-based male cases compared to controls (69). Although relative risk was not estimated for quantiles of daily calories, more cases (27%) compared to controls (23%) reported intakes of $<$ 1718 kilocalories, while fewer did so for $>$2705 kilocalories (22% vs. 27%). These studies provide additional evidence for three diverse sites that total energy intake may be associated positively with cancer risk.

Summary

These analytic epidemiologic studies from somewhat diverse populations provide evidence for a positive relationship between energy intake and risk of cancer. This is particularly true for cancer of the large bowel, for which the majority of studies are positive. Data concerning breast and pancreatic cancer are more equivocal, while the two positive investigations of ovary and gastric cancer can only be considered suggestive, pending additional studies. The pattern of sites associated with energy intake is probably more a reflection of the intensity of macronutrient-cancer research efforts for a few sites, breast and large bowel being among them. In general, for sites in which both women and men were included, the reported associations were of relatively similar magnitudes.

COMPARISON OF ANIMAL AND HUMAN STUDIES

The aforementioned animal studies were for the most part true experiments in that measured quantities of diets of known composition were fed for predetermined periods to nearly identical, randomized "subjects" preselected according to their well-delineated hereditary characteristics. These "subjects" were then scrupulously observed for neoplastic events. Such studies are relatively fast and uncomplicated, especially when compared to epidemiologic investigations. Although it can be argued whether the experimental design has distinct advantages over nonexperimental methods in research (70), a general comparison of epidemiologic studies of energy intake to the animal experiments described earlier is useful in highlighting the difficulties involved in human investigations in this area. Issues of relevance include: (a) the relationship between daily energy intake, body weight, and energy balance; (b) the range of dietary exposure (i.e., total calories); (c) the duration and timing of exposure; (d) the validity of measurement of dietary intake; (e) the high collinearity of total energy intake and its component macronutrients; (f) the degree of control over other cancer-causing exposures; and (g) the genetic composition of the study population.

Energy Intake, Body Weight, and Energy Balance

The relative homogeneity of animal characteristics and living conditions within specific experiments contributes to the close relationship between energy intake, body size, and "net energy balance" in animal studies. These factors include animal housing, physical activity, and the heritable components of physical attributes and metabolism, for example. In such settings, body weight serves as one reliable and readily available marker of daily caloric intake (28). This has also been shown in well-controlled feeding studies of humans (71–73). In contrast, epidemiologic studies fail to demonstrate a close and consistent relationship between energy intake and body size. Many have, for example, shown that obese individuals have somewhat lower caloric intake than the nonobese, with energy intake and body "fatness" being inversely associated (74–76). This has been attributed both to reduced activity levels and the underreporting of intake among overweight persons. Other studies demonstrate that energy intake is positively associated with height and, to a lesser degree, with absolute body weight (77). The explanation for this is probably manifold. To begin with, epidemiologic studies are not well-controlled feeding experiments, and they do not usually include large numbers of individuals on restricted diets. In free-living populations, total energy intake is a function of total energy expenditure (and to some degree, food availability). Expenditure, in turn, is determined primarily by basal metabolic requirements, and the thermic effects of muscular activity and food, with physical activity being the largest modifiable component among these factors. Another possible reason is suggested by the rodent experiments. The observation has been made that calories and body weight are related in a linear fashion at lower, more restricted intake levels, while body weight varies more at any given intake over the higher and ad libitum intake range (28). Marked variation in human body size and composition, physical activity, and resting metabolic rate greatly disengages the correspondence between energy intake, body size, and energy balance in observational studies. In such circumstances, the measurement of intake alone offers only one point of reference for the interpretation of any causal relationship.

Investigations with information regarding other energy-related parameters (e.g., body weight and physical activity) therefore would offer a more complete assessment of the relationship between energy and cancer. Ecological studies which have observed positive cancer–body size correlations are indirectly supportive of the findings for total calories (78–80). Although such data were not available from most of the human analytic investigations described above, they were from a few. In these studies, adjustment for differences in body mass index had no effect on the calorie results (54,55,59,63,64). This suggests that energy intake and body fatness may be independently related to cancer. By contrast, the three studies in which body size was also analyzed separately demonstrated somewhat stronger positive associations between cancer and body mass index than they did for energy intake (50,62,63). Further research is needed to determine the independence of the effects of increased energy consumption from those of greater body mass or fatness.

Regarding physical activity, there are several reported investigations of physical activity and cancer, most of these having examined either occupational activity (81–87) or involvement in athletics (88–92). For example, several studies demonstrate an inverse relationship between occupational physical activity, based on job classification, and the development of cancer, particularly colon cancer (81–87). Other studies have focused on whether the risk of cancer of current or former athletes differs from that of nonathletes (88–92). A number of these investigations support the notion that higher levels of physical activity may be protective against the development of cancer. Data are most available for colon, lung, and total cancer in men, and there is some evidence for a protective role in breast and endometrial carcinoma as well. Although such studies have not yet been directly related to those concerning calorie intake, future research should attempt to clarify whether the two sets of observations are related. As mentioned earlier, animal experiments would suggest they are. Few of these studies provide information concerning energy intake for even a crude assessment of energy balance, however.

Range of Intake

Rodent studies have been able to test the efficacy of long-term caloric restriction in preventing tumor incidence over a very wide range of intakes (20,28,31). Taking ad libitum as the maximum food and energy intake and assigning to it the value of 100%, long-term calorie reduction as great as 58% (i.e., a restriction to 42% of ad libitum control animals) has been achieved (12,28). Energy reduction in the range of 20–40% has been more commonly tested and found to be very effective in inhibiting the occurrence of tumors. As described above, body weight has been a highly sensitive marker of the level of energy intake in these experiments, and substantially diminished weight gain was achieved in entire experimental groups in large numbers of studies. In contrast, most epidemiologic investigations are conducted in affluent countries, and relatively few participants in these studies report very low caloric intake or have chronically low (but healthy) body weight. Leanness has in fact been associated with increased mortality in some studies (93), due in part to the association between chronic cigarette smoking, leanness, and lifetime weight loss (94). The power to reliably estimate true differences in the risk of developing cancer between high-calorie and low-calorie groups or individuals is greatly reduced if, for example, only 5% of the population consumes food at the lower intake levels.

Timing and Duration of Intake

Related to this issue is the timing and duration of energy restriction, with most experiments employing chronic feeding protocols beginning at the time of animal maturation and ending with the death of the animals or some earlier (and fixed) study termination. In most instances, the diets were fed daily and dietary composition remained unchanged for the duration of the experiments. Participants in human studies rarely experience such chronicity and uniformity in dietary habits, either with respect to the intake of total energy or other specific nutrients, and the true lifetime dietary experience is rarely (if ever) known. Dietary data used in human studies typically are obtained at one point in time, usually later in life, around the time (or age) of a cancer diagnosis and entry into an epidemiologic study. The analysis of such observational data presumes a correspondence between the more recent self-reported diets and food consumed several decades earlier, but this has not been substantiated (95). Quantities and patterns of food intake are often assumed to have been relatively constant throughout a lifetime, which is unlikely given reports of intraindividual variation in intake (96–98) and secular trends in food availability and consumption (99). In fact, changes in energy intake can have differential effects on body size depending on the period of exposure, with early caloric "exposure" affecting growth, maturation, and height and adult consumption modulating primarily adiposity.

Validity of Dietary Information

Experiments administer measured quantities of specific diets to the animals, in contrast to human analytic studies where usually one dietary instrument (e.g., a food frequency questionnaire or a dietary history) is given to subjects for the self-reporting of their dietary habits, present or past. The validity of such questionnaire methods has been the subject of tremendous study in recent years (96–98,100–103). Reported total energy intake has been shown to be only modestly correlated with actual dietary diaries in these studies, with correlation coefficients being in the range of 0.2–0.6. Since no better "markers" exist for energy intake as they do, for example, for micronutrients, human research in this field must for the most part rely upon the use of reported diets with their inherent limitations.

Calorie-Macronutrient Collinearity

Collinearity between macronutrient and energy intake is another potential problem in this area of study. Experiments can selectively manipulate and test one source of energy at a time (e.g., carbohydrates) at the same time that the amounts and proportions of all macronutrients are known and analyzable. In both cross-sectional studies, such as the international correlation analyses, and case-control studies, high and low energy "intake" are, for example, strongly associated with high and low dietary fat "intake," respectively. This is true both cross-nationally (44) and interindividually (104), making data analysis and the interpretation of results concerning similar cancer relative risk estimates for both total calories and fat difficult. This problem has been addressed in great detail recently (104), although it has yet to be completely resolved. In a similar vein, the association between caloric and micronutrient intake adds complexity because of the potential reduction in cancer risk afforded by the ingestion of some vitamins, for example. While animal experiments are able to control this directly, epidemiologic studies can only attempt to quantitate these intakes and adjust for them as necessary.

Positive associations between cancer risk and specific macronutrients were observed in several of the above investigations. In many studies, for example, dietary fat was more strongly related to breast or colorectal cancer than was energy intake (44,50,54,55,60,65). As previously mentioned, the very high correlation between fat and total calories ($r = 0.90$) (59,62,64,104) for example, creates methodological and interpretative difficulties for the cancer epidemiologist. Researchers have gone to great lengths to disentangle and clarify the resulting observed interrelationships with cancer (59,104). Animal studies demonstrate independent associations for calorie and fat intake, for example, with a stronger overall effect for total calories. Whether this tissue can be sufficiently resolved through human observational studies remains to be seen.

Other Carcinogenic Exposures

Carcinogenic exposures in tumor studies are limited to the one or two inducing agents (if any, as in the case of spontaneous tumor models) and the dietary exposures. By comparison, free-living humans are exposed to a great number of potentially carcinogenic substances (105,106), only some of which will be known to those exposed. In addition, few are reliably quantifiable in epidemiologic investigations. The more common factors include cigarette smoking, radiation, and several occupational exposures (105,106). Cigarette smoking is known, for example, to both affect energy balance (94,107) and promote cancer (108). Such factors can add substantial variability to the estimates of cancer "risk" found in epidemiologic studies.

Genetic Composition of Study Population

Rodent experiments will typically employ one strain of animal from a limited number of litters, thereby reducing the genetic variation between animals and experimental groups. Although epidemiologic studies are sometimes limited to one race or ethnic background, for example, or stratify according to such characteristics, substantial genetic heterogeneity exists within populations and studies which can potentially impinge on cancer risk directly (60), interact with energy intake or energy utilization, such as resting metabolic rate (109), or both.

It is useful to keep these differences in mind when interpreting data concerning energy intake and cancer in humans. They suggest that the assessment of cancer relative risks by categories of self-reported energy consumption reveals only one piece of the puzzle. Their combined effect would tend to diminish the observable relationship between energy intake and subsequent cancer risk. Some of the above problems are inherent in human studies of nutrition and cancer. The true range of total calorie intake and the period of "exposure" to those intakes are relatively fixed in observational studies (in contrast to intervention trials—see Part Four). That high energy consumption is strongly related to high fat intake is a characteristic of most affluent societies that may in the future change in several ways, but today poses great challenges to the nutritional epidemiologist. At present also, the genetic diversity of general populations and study participants is a fait accompli. In contrast, other of these issues can be addressed through changes in the design of individual epidemiologic studies. Unique populations can be chosen based on their dietary energy characteristics (110). The validity of measurement of energy intake can be improved with the use of high quality, well-studied questionnaires. Within limits, dietary patterns during remote periods of life can be queried (95). Relevant nondietary cancer risk factors, such as tobacco use or reproductive histories, should be ascertained and used for statistical adjustment during analysis. Future studies should attempt to collect as much energy-related information as possible, including energy intake and expenditure (physical activity and, where possible, resting metabolism) and anthropometry (height, weight, and measures of fatness such as skinfold thickness), in order to provide a more complete evaluation of the complex relationships involved.

MECHANISMS

While no single mechanism has been recognized as the mediator for the relationship between energy intake and cancer, several have been, and continue to be, investigated. Energy balance is known to influence a large number of physiologic functions including body temperature, basal metabolic rate, protein synthesis, the activity of several enzymes, cell-mediated immunity, and endocrine status (i.e., levels of pituitary hormones, insulin, T_3 and T_4, and estrogens) (72,73,111–115). In addition, DNA synthesis and cell division are positively related to energy balance (116–118). A role in human malignancy has been suggested for some of these factors (115,116,118), which represent mechanisms generalizable to multiple sites (i.e., immunity (115), free radical production (119), or cell number and the rate of cell division (118)). Others are site-specific. For example, hormonal mechanisms have received the greatest attention with respect to adenocarcinoma of the breast. It has long been hypothesized that enhanced estrogen production in overweight and obese women accounts for increased risk of developing breast cancer after the menopause (120). Mechanisms suggested to explain the observations concerning colon cancer, which has been linked to greater energy intake and body size, and to lower levels of physical activity include local effects from greater food intake (e.g., greater exposure of colonic mucosa to exogenous carcinogens or bile acids (121), greater rates of mucosal epithelium proliferation (122), and the possibility of longer intestinal transit time due to dietary differences (123) or physical inactivity (83)). Further research is needed to test these and other hypotheses of general or site-specific mechanisms.

CONCLUSIONS

Animal experiments in this field can be considered a more or less ideal situation for evaluating the efficacy of restricting energy intake in cancer prevention, and therefore probably portray a maximum achievable effect. These studies suffer primarily (and possibly solely) from the question of their generalizability to the human condition. Human observational studies, on the other hand, provide no similar test of the energy-cancer hypothesis and are fraught with a number of methodological limitations. Even so, they provide evidence for a positive energy intake-cancer association, particularly for colorectal and breast cancer. Dietary intervention trials may overcome some of these shortcomings. Although cancer prevention trials of energy restriction have not yet been undertaken, other randomized intervention trials investigating the effects of low dietary fat intake on breast cancer and adenomatous polyps of the colon have been started (124,125). (These prevention trials are described in greater detail in Chapter 17.) Although not designed to evaluate cancer prevention effects related to total caloric intake specifically, these trials may in any case shed light on the issue since energy intake is being quantified as part of the dietary evaluation, and weight loss has been associated with the intervention in one of these studies (124). It should be an important objective of future investigations to incorporate information regarding several energy-related parameters (e.g., body size and physical activity) in order to offer a more complete assessment of the relationship between energy and cancer.

REFERENCES

1. Hippocrates. On airs, waters, and places, *Medical Classics, 3*, 19 (1938).
2. A. Rabagliati, *Air, Food and Exercises. An Essay on the Predisposing Causes of Disease*, 3rd ed. Bailliere, Tindall and Cox, London, 1904.
3. R. H. Chittenden, *Physiological Economy in Nutrition, with Special Reference to the Minimal Protein Requirement of the Healthy Man; an Experimental Study*. A Stokes Co., New York, 1904.
4. F. L. Hoffmann, *The Mortality from Cancer Throughout the World*. Prudential, Newark, NJ, 1915.
5. C. Moreschi, Beziehungen zwischen ernährung und tumor-wachstum, *Z. Immunitatsforsch.*, *2*, 651 (1909).
6. P. Rous, The influence of diet on transplanted and spontaneous mouse tumors, *J. Exp. Med.*, *20*, 433 (1914).
7. P. Rous, The influence of dieting upon the course of cancer, *Johns Hopkins Hosp. Bull.*, *26*, 146 (1915).
8. F. Bischoff, M. L. Long, and L. C. Maxwell, Influence of caloric intake upon the growth of sarcoma 180, *Am. J. Cancer, 24*, 549 (1935).
9. C. M. McCay, M. D. Crowell, and L. A. Maynard, The effect of retared growth upon the length of life span and upon the ultimate body size, *J. Nutr.*, *10*, 63 (1935).

10. P. S. Lavik, and C. A. Baumann, Further studies on tumor promoting action of fat, *Cancer Res.*, *3*, 749 (1943).
11. M. B. Visscher, Z. B. Ball, R. H. Barnes, and I. Sivertsen, I. The influence of caloric restriction upon the incidence of spontaneous mammary carcinoma in mice, *Surgery*, *11*, 48 (1942).
12. A. Tannenbaum, The initiation and growth of tumors: Introduction: I, effects of underfeeding, *Am. J. Cancer*, *38*, 335 (1940).
13. A. Tannenbaum, The genesis and growth of tumors: II. Effects of caloric restriction per se, *Cancer Res.*, *2*, 460 (1942).
14. A. Tannenbaum, The genesis and growth of tumors: III. Effects of a high fat diet, *Cancer Res.*, *2*, 468 (1942).
15. A. Tannenbaum, The dependence of the genesis of induced skin tumors on the fat content of the diet during different stages of carcinogenesis, *Cancer Res.*, *4*, 683 (1944).
16. A. Tannenbaum, The dependence of the genesis of induced skin tumors on the caloric intake during different stages of carcinogenesis, *Cancer Res.*, *4*, 673 (1944).
17. A. Tannenbaum, The dependence of tumor formation on the degree of caloric restriction, *Cancer Res.*, *5*, 609 (1945).
18. A. Tannenbaum, The dependence of tumor formation on the composition of the calorie-restricted diet as well as on the degree of restriction, *Cancer Res.*, *5*, 616 (1945).
19. A. Tannenbaum, A., and H. Silverstone, Dosage of carcinogen as a modifying factor in evaluating experimental procedures expected to influence formation of skin tumors, *Cancer Res.*, *7*, 567 (1947).
20. A. Tannenbaum, Effects of varying caloric intake upon tumor incidence and tumor growth, *Ann. NY Acad. Sci.*, *49*, 5 (1947).
21. A. Tannenbaum and H. Silverstone, The influence of the degree of caloric restriction on the formation of skin tumors and hepatomas in mice, *Cancer Res.*, *9*, 724 (1949).
22. H. Silverstone and A. Tannenbaum, The effect of the proportion of dietary fat on the rate of formation of mammary carcinoma in mice, *Cancer Res.*, *10*, 448 (1950).
23. A. Tannenbaum and H. Silverstone, Effect of limited food intake on survival of mice bearing spontaneous mammary carcinoma and on the incidence of lung metastases, *Cancer Res.*, *13*, 532 (1953).
24. R. K. Boutwell, M. K. Brush, and H. P. Rusch, The stimulating effect of dietary fat on carcinogenesis, *Cancer Res.*, *9*, 741 (1949).
25. R. K. Boutwell, M. K. Brush, and H. P. Rusch, Some physiological effects associated with chronic caloric restriction, *Am. J. Physiol.*, *154*, 517 (1948).
26. M. Pollard, P. H. Luckert, and D. Snyder, Prevention of prostate cancer and liver tumors in L-W rats by moderate dietary restriction, *Cancer*, *64*, 686 (1989).
27. R. Weindruch and R. L. Walford, *The Retardation of Aging and Disease by Dietary Restriction*. Charles C. Thomas, Springfield, Illinois, 1988.
28. D. Albanes, Total calories, body weight, and tumor incidence in mice, *Cancer Res.*, *47*, 1987 (1987).
29. D. M. Klurfeld, C. B. Welch, M. J. Davis, and D. Kritchevsky, Determination of degree of energy restriction necessary to reduce DMBA-induced mammary tumorigenesis in rats during the promotion phase, *J. Nutr.*, *119*, 286 (1989).

30. G. A. Boissonneault, C. E. Elson, and M. W. Pariza, Net energy effects of dietary fat on chemically induced mammary carcinogenesis in F344 rats, *JNCI, 76*, 355 (1986).
31. D. Kritchevsky, M. M. Weber, and D. M. Klurfeld, Dietary fat versus caloric content in initiation and promotion of 7, 12-dimethylbenz(a)anthracene-induced mammary tumorigenesis in rats, *Cancer Res., 44*, 3174 (1984).
32. D. M. Klurfeld, C. B. Welch, L. M. Lloyd, and D. Kritchevsky, Inhibition of DMBA-induced mammary tumorigenesis by caloric restriction in rats fed high fat diets, *Int. J. Cancer, 42*, 922 (1989).
33. C. Moore and P. W. Tittle, Muscle activity, body fat, and induced rat mammary tumors, *Surgery, 73*, 329 (1973).
34. D. M. Klurfeld, L. M. Lloyd, C. L. Buck, M. J. Davis, O. L. Tulp, and D. Kritchevsky, Inhibition of mammary tumorigenesis by caloric restriction in LA/N-cp (corpulent rats), *Fed. Proc., 46*, 436 (1987).
35. H. Silverstone and A. Tannenbaum, Influence of thyroid hormone on the formation of induced skin tumors in mice, *Cancer Res., 9*, 684 (1949).
36. A. Tannenbaum and H. Silverstone, Effect of low environmental temperature, dinitrophenol, or sodium fluoride on the formation of tumors in mice, *Cancer Res., 9*, 403 (1949).
37. H. P. Rusch and B. E. Kline, The effect of exercise on the growth of a mouse tumor, *Cancer Res., 4*, 116 (1944).
38. G. D. Andrianopoulos, R. L. Nelson, A. Misumi, et al., Effect of activity-stress on experimental rat colon carcinogenesis: Early histopathologic changes and colon tumor induction, *Cancer Detection and Prevention, 13*, 31 (1988).
39. D. M. Klurfeld, C. B. Welch, E. Einhorn, and D. Kritchevsky, Inhibition of colon tumor promotion by caloric restriction or exercise in rats, *FASEB J., 2*, A433 (1988).
40. M. H. Ross, E. D. Lustbader, and G. Bras, Dietary practices of early life and spontaneous tumors of the rat, *Nutr. Cancer, 3*, 150 (1982).
41. R. Weindruch, and R. L. Walford, Dietary restriction in mice beginning at 1 year of age: Effect on life-span and spontaneous cancer incidence, *Science, 215*, 1415 (1982).
42. D. Kritchevsky, C. B. Welch, and D. M. Klurfeld, Response of mammary tumors to caloric restriction for different time periods during the promotion phase, *Nutr. Cancer, 12*, 259 (1989).
43. Committee on Diet, Nutrition and Cancer, Assembly of Life Sciences, National Research Council, *Diet, Nutrition, and Cancer*, National Academy Press, Washington, DC, 1982.
44. B. Armstrong and R. Doll, Environmental factors and cancer incidence and mortality in different countries with special reference in dietary practices, *Int. J. Cancer, 15*, 617 (1975).
45. M. Kodama and T. Kodama, Interelation between Western type cancers and non-Western type cancers as regards their risk variations in time and space. II. Nutrition and cancer risk, *Anticancer Res., 10*, 1043 (1990).
46. S. P. Gaskill, W. L. McGuire, C. K. Osborne, and M. P. Stern, Breast cancer mortality and diet in the United States. *Cancer Res., 39*, 3628 (1979).

47. I. Kato, S. Tomnaga, and T. Kuroishi, Relationship between westernization of dietary habits and mortality from breast and ovarian cancer in Japan, *Jpn. J. Cancer res.*, (Gann), *78*, 349 (1987).
48. M. Hill, R. Maclennan, and K. Newcombe, Letter to the editor: Dict and large bowel cancer in three socioeconomic groups in Hong Kong, *Lancet, 1*, 436 (1979).
49. Food and Agriculture Organization, *Food Balance Sheets and Per Capita Food Supplies*, 1961–1977, United Nations, Rome, 1980.
50. A. B. Miller, A. Kelly, N. W. Choi, et al., A study of diet and breast cancer, *Am. J. Epidemiol., 107*, 499 (1978).
51. T. E. Rohan, A. J. McMichael, and P. A. Baghurst, A population-based case-control study of diet and breast cancer in Australia, *Am. J. Epidemiol., 128*, 478 (1988).
52. K. Katsouyanni, W. Willett, D. Trichopoulos, P. Boyle, A. Trichopoulou, S. Vasilaros, J. Papadiamantis, and B. MacMahon, Risk of breast cancer among Greek women in relation to nutrient intake, *Cancer, 61*, 181 (1988).
53. J. M. Iscovich, R. B. Iscovich, G. Howe, S. Shiboski, and J. M. Kaldor, A case-control study of diet and breast cancer in Argentina, *Int. J. Cancer, 44*, 770 (1989).
54. P. Toniolo, E. Riboli, F. Protta, M. Charrel, and A. P. M. Cappa, Calorie-providing nutrients and risk of breast cancer, *JNCI, 81*, 278 (1989).
55. P. Knekt, D. Albanes, R. Seppanen, A. Aromaa, R. Jarvinen, L. Hyvonen, L. Teppo, and E. Pukkala, Dietary fat and risk of breast cancer, *Am. J. Clin. Nutr., 52*, 903 (1990).
56. G. R. Howe, T. Hirohata, T. G. Hislop, J. M. Iscovich, J. M. Yuan, K. Katsouyanni, F. Lubin, E. Marubini, B. Modan, T. Rohan, P. Toniolo, and Y. Shunzhang, Dietary factors and risk of breast cancer: Combined analysis of 12 case-control studies, *JNCI, 82*, 561 (1990).
57. M. Jain, G. M. Cook, F. G. Davis, et al., A case-control study of diet and colorectal cancer, *Int. J. Cancer, 26*, 757 (1980).
58. J. B. Bristol, P. M. Emmett, K. W. Heaton, and R. C. N. Williamson, Sugar, fat, and the risk of colorectal cancer, *Br. Med. J., 291*, 1467 (1985).
59. J. L. Lyon, A. W. Mahoney, D. W. West, et al., Energy intake: Its relationship to colon cancer risk, *JNCI, 78*, 853 (1987).
60. G. N. Stemmermann, A. M. Y. Nomura, and L. K. Heilbrun, Dietary fat and the risk of colorectal cancer, *Cancer Res., 44*, 4633 (1984).
61. S. Kune, G. A. Kune, and L. F. Watson, Case-control study of dietary etiological factors: The Melbourne colorectal cancer study, *Nutr. Cancer, 9*, 21 (1987).
62. S. Graham, J. Marshall, B. Haughey, A. Mittelman, M. Swanson, M. Zielezny, T. Byers, G. Wilkinson, and D. West, Dietary epidemiology of cancer of the colon in Western New York, *Am. J. Epidemiol., 128*, 490 (1988).
63. D. W. West, M. L. Slattery, L. M. Robison, K. L. Schuman, M. H. Ford, A. W. Mahoney, J. L. Lyon, and A. W. Sorensen, Dietary intake and colon cancer: Sex- and anatomic site-specific associations, *Am. J. Epidemiol., 130*, 883 (1989).
64. J. L. Freudenheim, S. Graham, J. R. Marshall, B. P. Haughey, and G. Wilkinson, A case-control study of diet and rectal cancer in western New York, *Am. J. Epidemiol., 131*, 612 (1990).
65. W. C. Willett, M. J. Stampfer, G. A. Colditz, B. A. Rosner, and F. E. Speizer,

Relation of meat, fat, and fiber intake to the risk of colon cancer in a prospective study among women, *N. Engl. J. Med.*, *323*, 1664 (1990).
66. X. O. Shu, Y. T. Gao, J. M. Yuan, R. G. Ziegler, and L. A. Brinton, Dietary factors and epithelial ovarian cancer, *Br. J. Cancer, 59*, 92 (1988).
67. S. Graham, B. Haughey, J. Marshall, J. Brazure, M. Zielezny, J. Freudenheim, D. West, J. Nolan, and G. Wilkinson, Diet in the epidemiology of gastric cancer, *Nutr. Cancer, 13*, 19 (1990).
68. G. R. Howe, M. Jain, and A. B. Miller, Dietary factors and risk of pancreatic cancer: Results of a Canadian population-based case-control study, *Int. J. Cancer, 45*, 604 (1990).
69. D. C. Farrow and S. Davis, Risk of pancreatic cancer in relation to medical history and the use of tobacco, alcohol and coffee, *Int. J. Cancer, 45*, 816 (1990).
70. A. R. Feinstein, Scientific standards and epidemiologic methods, *Am. J. Clin. Nutr.*, *45*, 1080 (1987).
71. G. B. Forbes, Energy intake and body weight: A reeamination of two 'classic' studies, *Am. J. Clin. Nutr.*, *39*, 349 (1984).
72. A. Keys, J. Brozek, A. Henschel, et al., *The Biology of Human Starvation*, University of Minnesota Press, Minneapolis, 1950.
73. H. L. Taylor and A. Keys, Adaptation to caloric restriction, *Science, 112*, 215 (1950).
74. L. E. Braitman, E. V. Adlin, and J. L. Stanton, Obesity and caloric intake: The national health and nutrition examination survey of 1971–1975 (HANES I), *J. Chronic Dis.*, *38*, 727 (1985).
75. D. Kromhout, W. H. M. Saris, and C. H. Horst, Energy intake, energy expenditure, and smoking in relation to body fatness: The Zutphen study, *Am. J. Clin. Nutr.*, *47*, 668 (1988).
76. I. Romieu, W. C. Willett, M. J. Stampfer, G. A., Colditz, L. Sampson, B. Rosner, C. H. Hennekens, F. E. Speizer, Energy intake and other determinants of relative weight, *Am. J. Clin. Nutr.*, *47*, 406 (1988).
77. A. M. Thompson and W. Z. Billewicz, Height, weight and food intake in man, *Br. J. Nutr.*, *15*, 241 (1961).
78. G. E. Gray, M. C. Pike, and B. E. Henderson, Breast cancer incidence and mortality rates in different countries in relation to known factors and dietary practices, *Br. J. Cancer, 39*, 1 (1979).
79. M. S. Micozzi, Cross-cultural correlations of childhood growth and adult breast cancer, *Am. J. Phys. Anthropol.*, *73*, 525 (1987).
80. D. Albanes and P. R. Taylor, International differences in body height and weight and their relationship to cancer incidence, *Nutr. Cancer, 14*, 69 (1990).
81. I. Sivertsen and A. W. Dahlstrom, Relation of muscular activity to carcinoma, *J. Cancer Res.*, *6*, 365 (1922).
82. H. Taylor, E. Klepetar, A. Keys, et al., Death rates among physically active employees of the railroad industry, *Am. J. Public Health, 52*, 1697 (1962).
83. D. H. Garabrant, J. M. Peters, T. M. Mack, et al., Job activity and colon cancer risk, *Am. J. Epidemiol.*, *119*, 1005 (1984).
84. J. E. Vena, S. Graham, M. Zielezny, et al., Lifetime occupational exercise and colon cancer, *Am. J. Epidemiol.*, *122*, 357 (1985).

85. M. Gerhardsson, S. E. Norell, H. Kiviranta, et al., Sedentary jobs and colon cancer, *Am. J. Epidemiol.*, *123*, 775 (1986).
86. R. S. Paffenbarger, R. T. Hyde, and A. L. Wing, Physical activity and incidence of cancer in diverse populations: A preliminary report, *Am. J. Clin. Nutr.*, *45*, 312 (1987).
87. D. Albanes, A. Blair, and P. R. Taylor, Physical activity and risk of cancer in the NHANES I population, *Am. J. Public Health, 79*, 744 (1989).
88. L. Schmid, Malignant tumors as causes of death of former athletes. In *Metabolic Adaptation to Prolonged Exercise* (H. Howald and J. R. Poortsmans, eds.), Birkhauser Verlag, Basel, 1975.
89. J. Burian, Contribution to the problem of timely diagnosis and mass investigation of stomach and cardiac cancer, *Rozhledy Chirurgia, 33*, 437 (1954).
90. A. P. Polednak, College athletics, body size, and cancer mortality, *Cancer, 38*, 382 (1976).
91. R. E. Frisch, G. Wyshak, N. L. Albright, et al., Lower prevalence of breast cancer and cancer of the reproductive system among former college athletes compared to non-athletes, *Br. J. Cancer, 52*, 885 (1985).
92. R. E. Frisch, G. Wyshak, N. L. Albright, et al., Lower lifetime occurrence of breast cancer and cancers of the reproductive system among former athletes, *Am. J. Clin. Nutr.*, *45*, 328 (1987).
93. J. E. Manson, M. J. Stampfer, C. H. Hennekens, and W. C. Willett, Body weight and longevity, *JAMA, 257*, 353 (1987).
94. D. Albanes, Y. Jones, M. S. Micozzi, and M. E. Mattson, Associations between smoking and body weight in the U.S. population: Analysis of NHANES II. *Am. J. Public Health, 77*, 439 (1987).
95. T. Byers, R. Rosenthal, J. Marshall, et al., Dietary history from the distant past: A methodological study, *Nutr. Cancer, 5*, 69 (1983).
96. G. H. Beaton, J. Milner, P. Corey, et al., Sources of variance in 24-hour dietary recall data: Implications for nutrition study design and interpretation, *Am. J. Clin. Nutr.*, *32*, 2446 (1979).
97. W. C. Willett, L. Sampson, M. J. Stampfer, et al., Reproducibility and validity of a semiquantitative food frequency questionnaire, *Am. J. Epidemiol.*, *122*, 5 (1985).
98. P. Pietinen, A. M. Hartman, E. Haapa, et al., Reproducibility and validity of dietary assessment instruments I: A self-administered food use questionnaire with a portion size picture booklet, *Am. J. Epidemiol.*, *128*, 655 (1988).
99. W. A. Gortner, Nutrition in the United States, 1900 to 1974, *Cancer Res.*, *35*, 3246 (1975).
100. B. S. Burke, The dietary history as a tool in research, *J. Am. Diet. Assoc.*, *23*, 1041 (1947).
101. G. Block, A review of validations of dietary assessment methods, *Am. J. Epidemiol.*, *125*, 164 (1985).
102. G. Block, A. M. Hartman, C. M. Dresser, et al., A data-based approach to diet questionnaire design and testing, *Am. J. Epidemiol.*, *124*, 453 (1986).
103. K. M. Flegal, F. A. Larkin, H. L. Metzner, et al., Counting calories: Partitioning

energy intake estimates from a food frequency questionnaire, *Am. J. Epidemiol.*, *128*, 749 (1988).
104. W. Willett and M. J. Stampfer, Total energy intake: Implications for epidemiologic analyses, *Am. J. Epidemiol.*, *124*, 17 (1986).
105. R. Doll and R. Peto, *The Causes of Cancer*, Oxford University Press, Oxford, 1981.
106. D. Schottenfeld and J. F. Fraumeni, *Cancer Epidemiology and Prevention*, W. B. Saunders, Philadelphia, 1982.
107. R. C. Klesges, L. H. Eck, T. R. Isbell, W. Fulliton, and C. L. Hanson, Smoking status: Effects on the dietary intake, physical activity, and body fat of adult men, *Am. J. Clin. Nutr.*, *51*, 784 (1990).
108. United States Department of Health and Human Services, *The Health Consequences of Smoking. A Report of the Surgeon General*. DHHS Pub. No. 0-377-301, Govt. Printing Office, Washington, DC, 1982.
109. E. Ravussin, S. Lillioja, W. C. Knowler, L. Christin, D. Freymond, W. G. H. Abbott, V. Boyce, B. V. Howard, and C. Bogardus, Reduced rate of energy expenditure as a risk factor for body-weight gain, *N. Engl. J. Med.*, *318*, 467 (1988).
110. Y. Kagawa, Impact of westernization of the nutrition of Japanese: Changes in physique, cancer, longevity and centenarians, *Prev. Med.*, *7*, 205 (1978).
111. E. Forsum, P. E. Hillman, and M. C. Nesheim, Effect of energy restriction on total heat production, basal metabolic rate and specific dynamic action of food in rats, *J. Nutr.*, *111*, 1691 (1981).
112. J. C. Waterlow, Metabolic adaptation to low intakes of energy and protein, *Annu. Rev. Nutr.*, *6*, 495 (1986).
113. F. Grande, Man under caloric deficiency, In *Handbook of Physiology* (D. B. Dill, ed.), Section 4 American Physiological Society, Washington, D.C. 1964.
114. R. A. Chandra, Immune response in overnutrition, *Cancer Res.*, *41*, 3795 (1981).
115. R. Weindruch, S. R. S. Gottesman, and R. L. Walford, Modification of age-related immune decline in mice dietarily restricted from and after midadulthood. *Proc. Natl. Acad. Sci. USA*, *79*, 899 (1982).
116. W. S. Bullough, Mitotic activity and carcinogenesis, *Br. J. Cancer*, *4*, 329 (1950).
117. M. Winick and A. Nobel, Cellular response in rats during malnutrition at various ages, *J. Nutr.*, *89*, 300 (1966).
118. D. Albanes and M. Winick, Are cell number and cell proliferation risk factors for cancer? *JNCI*, *80*, 772 (1988).
119. D. Harman, Nutritional implications of the free-radical theory of aging, *J. Am. Coll. Nutr.*, *1*, 27 (1982).
120. F. De Waard and D. Trichopoulos, A unifying concept of the aetiology of breast cancer, *Int. J. Cancer*, *41*, 666 (1988).
121. L. R. Jacobs, Role of dietary factors in cell replication and colon cancer, *Am. J. Clin. Nutr.*, *48*, 775 (1988).
122. M. Lipkin, Biomarkers of increased susceptibility to gastrointestinal cancer: Their development and application to studies of cancer prevention, *Gastroenterology*, *82*, 1083 (1987).
123. O. M. Jensen, R. MacLennan, and J. Wahrendorf, Diet, bowel function, fecal

characteristics, and large bowel cancer in Denmark and Finland, *Nutr. Cancer, 4*, 5 (1982).
124. W. Insull, M. M. Henderson, R. L. Prentice, D. J. Thompson, C. Clifford, S. Goldman, S. Gobrach, M. Moskowitz, R. Thompson, and M. Woods, Results of a randomized feasibility study of a low-fat diet, *Arch. Intern. Med.*, *150*, 421 (1990).
125. A. Schatzkin, E. Lanza, and R. Ballard-Barbash, The case for a dietary intervention study of large bowel polyps, *Cancer Prev.*, *1*, 106 (1990).

9

Dietary Fat

Anthony B. Miller
University of Toronto
Toronto, Canada

INTRODUCTION

Of the known causes of cancer, dietary factors collectively contribute to a large proportion of potentially preventable cancers. Estimates have varied but tend to be around 30–35%, though the evidence is not precise, and several years ago Doll and Peto suggested a range of 10–70% (1). Dietary fat intake contributes substantially to such estimates (2). The importance of dietary fat is potentially almost as great in developing countries as it is for the technically advanced countries, because of the tendency for developing countries to acquire Western-type dietary patterns as they increase in affluence, though most but not all of the data have been derived from technically advanced countries. The stage has now been reached where appropriate and acceptable recommendations can be made on optimal dietary patterns. These will be reviewed at the end of this chapter, which shall mainly review the scientific basis for the recommendations, concentrating on that derived from epidemiology.

THE EVIDENCE RELATING TO DIETARY FAT

Of all dietary factors believed to affect cancer incidence, dietary fat has perhaps attracted the most interest. This is in part due to the strong correlations noted in international data between the incidence of or mortality from certain cancer sites and estimated population intake of dietary fat (3), and in part because of observations from animal experimental models. The international correlation studies (ecologic studies) cannot be used to infer causality, but they are useful in raising hypotheses. They may also provide some indication of the range of the effect, which may be difficult to determine within a country if dietary patterns are relatively homogeneous. In practice, the most attention has been paid to correlations of dietary fat disappearance data with incidence or mortality from breast and colorectal cancer, but equally strong associations have been noted with endometrial cancer, as well as associations with prostate, ovarian, renal, and pancreatic cancer. One study of this type has based the associations on dietary data from personal interviews of samples of individuals in Hawaii (4). Significant associations were found for ethnic patterns of incidence of breast, prostate, and corpus uteri cancer incidence but not of colon cancer with estimated total fat, animal fat, and saturated and unsaturated fat consumption. Although for both mammary cancer and colon cancer in rodents strong associations have been noted with high fat in the diet, particularly with regard to colorectal cancer, the animal models have been developed specifically to explore mechanisms potentially relevant to the fat hypothesis and therefore cannot be used to confirm the validity of that hypothesis (5).

In the absence of human intervention studies, emphasis has to be placed on the results of analytic epidemiology, namely, case-control and cohort studies. In case-control studies dietary histories of newly diagnosed cases are compared with those from comparable controls, preferably drawn from the same population as the cases. In cohort studies, dietary data are collected from an identified group or cohort, usually with a self-administered questionnaire, and the cohort is followed to determine the subsequent incidence of (or mortality from) cancer. Unfortunately, many of the reported studies were based on inadequate dietary methodology, often with a very indirect assessment of dietary fat intake, so that misclassification of intake, even into tertiles, is very likely. This would tend to bias the reported associations towards the null. Further, all the case-control studies provide estimates of fat intake which relate to current or recent diet, and which therefore only imperfectly, if at all, reflect diet at the relevant time period for cancer induction. For both these reasons, negative studies or weak associations may be expected. Indeed, in the absence of any indication of a systematic bias, reported positive associations, especially if there is a dose-response relationship, provide strong evidence for a causal association.

Breast Cancer

For breast cancer, the ecologic studies have shown strong associations with dietary fat (3). One recent study of international data has shown that the effect is largely restricted to fat calories, calories from protein, carbohydrate, and alcohol having no significant effect (6). Much of the other positive evidence associating dietary fat with increased risk comes from case-control studies, though in many the associations have been weak. Some of these studies collected data only on fat-containing foods, such as a study in Seventh-day Adventists in California in which there were positive associations with fat-containing foods (7), a study in Canada in which increasing risk with increasing consumption of whole milk, beef, and a protective effect from fish consumption was found (8), and a study in France where increased risk from consumption of full-cream milk and cream was found (9). In other studies it was possible to characterize respondents in terms of dietary fat intake. Two such studies have been performed in Canada. In the first, suggestive associations were found with total fat intake in both pre- and postmenopausal women with a relative risk of 1.5 with dichtomized exposure to total fat intake (only the association in postmenopausal women was significant), though without a dose-response relationship (10). In a subsequent reanalysis of this study using the data from a 24-hour recall and a quantitative dietary history, the strongest association (with a dose-reponse relationship) was found in premenopausal women (11). In the second, increasing risk with increasing consumption levels of beef, pork, animal fat, and animal protein were found, with suggestive dose-response relationships (12). Although this study can be criticized on methodological grounds, because the control group was interviewed by a completely different team at a different time period, it is not clear why this should have been a source of systematic bias. A large study in Israel pointed to the importance of dietary pattern (13). Risk was increased in those with a high consumption of fat and protein and a low consumption of fiber, whereas risk was lowest in those with a low consumption of fat and protein, and a high consumption of fiber. Further evidence in support of the hypothesis that dietary fat is a risk factor for breast cancer was derived by a study of benign breast disease by the same investigators, in which the cases were classified by the degree of ductal atypia (14). Women with atypic lesions reported a higher intake of foods containing 10% or more of fat compared to both surgical and neighborhood controls. Odds ratios associated with the highest fat consumption quartile were close to 3.0. A study of diet and breast cancer in Italy showed a significant increased risk with increasing total and saturated fat consumption (15). Positive associations were also found with consumption of dairy products, particularly those rich in fat, such as high-fat cheese and whole milk. These associations were characterized by significant dose-response trends and were not modified by adjustment for total calorie intake or for other risk factors for breast cancer. In The Netherlands a case-control study also found elevated risk for high fat consumption, with a positive trend with increasing fat intake (16). The association could not be attributed to energy intake, nor to the degree of saturation of the fat, nor to any specific dietary source of fat. Preliminary results have also been reported from a large case-control study in Denmark involving 1457 cases and 1304 controls

(17). A significant trend of increasing breast cancer risk with increasing fat intake was found ($p < 0.001$). Compared to the lowest quartile, the top quartile was associated with a 50% increase in risk.

In general the level of increased risk found in these studies was of the order of 1.5–2.0, though risks >3.0 in the highest quartile or quintile relative to the lowest were found in the studies in Italy (15) and The Netherlands (16).

Some other case-control studies, however, have been negative, including studies in New York state (18) where a limited dietary instrument was used, Greece (19) where fat consumption is low and all subjects may have been at low risk of breast cancer, Hawaii (20) where only a limited dietary instrument was used and where there was a suggestion that cases consumed more saturated fat and oleic acid that did controls, and Australia (21) where a self-administered dietary questionnaire was used.

The findings from 12 of the case control studies, including several of the "negative" studies, have been reanalyzed in combination, using the original data rather than the data in published reports (22). This analysis shows a statistically significant increase in risk with increasing fat intake, especially in postmenopausal women. The findings in premenopausal women were not significant, though there was a suggestion of an increase in risk with increasing fat consumption. The degree of increase in risk, even in postmenopausal women, was not large (a relative risk of 1.48 for an increase in consumption of 100 g/day total fat), but this could have been due to the attenuation in risk because of relative poor dietary methodology in some of the studies.

One of the potential problems with case-control studies is the possibility of recall bias, namely that cases may associate their illness with suspect causal factors and may be more likely to report elevated exposure to factors such as dietary fat than controls. In practical recall bias for dietary enquiries has never been demonstrated, yet many prefer cohort studies where this bias is eliminated. There have been fewer dietary cohort studies than case-control studies, but a large cohort study of American nurses was negative (23), as was a smaller study based on the NHANES I survey (24). Nevertheless, the difference in intake between the upper and the lower quintiles of fat intake in the nurses study could not be expected to demonstrate more than a relative risk of 1.4 if the international correlation studies are a guide, while the NHANES cohort data, which showed an inverse association with dietary fat intake, no longer significant when adjusted for total energy intake, were based on a 24-hour recall of intake, recognized as poor in providing estimates of individual intake. Further, with a weak risk anticipated, and the possibility of greater measurement error from a self-administered questionnaire than from an interviewer-administered detailed quantitative dietary history, it is perhaps not surprising that such studies should be negative. A third cohort recently reported comprises 20,342 California Seventh-day Adventist and largely postmenopausal women who completed a detailed lifestyle questionnaire in 1976 and who were followed for 6 years, among whom 215 breast cancers were diagnosed (25). Increasing consumption of high animal fat-containing foods was not associated with increased risk of breast cancer in a consistent fashion, though there was a significant trend of increasing risk with increasing consumption of cheese. Results from a fourth cohort based on the National Breast Screening Study in Canada have also been evaluated (26). In this study, 56,837 participants age 40–59 completed a self-administered dietary questionnaire. Follow-up has so far revealed 519 women who developed breast cancer within 6 years after the questionnaire was completed. Their fat intake has been assessed in comparison to that from an equal number of matched controls. A small but significant increase in risk for dietary fat calories was found (a relative risk of 1.35 for the highest quartile relative to the lowest, 95% confidence intervals (CI 1.0–1.82) in a model incorporating other sources of calories, the effect of carbohydrate calories being protective (RR 0.72, 95% CI 0.52–0.99).

The problem of misclassification of fat intake, especially in self-administered questionnaires, is likely to be particularly severe for breast cancer, and may explain some of the inconsistency in results. This is because it seems likely that all dietary studies of breast cancer, both case-control and cohort, have been timed inappropriately in terms of the dietary data, as the period in life when effects may be most relevant may be in adolescence or early adult life, in the time from menarche to first birth. This is supported by a study of two groups of nuns who adopted low-fat diets in early adult life, in whom no reduction in risk for breast cancer was found in comparison with that expected from the general population after correcting for nulliparity (27).

In summary, the overall evidence associating dietary fat intake with breast cancer is inconsistent, though several recent case-control studies have been positive, as was a combined analysis of 12 case-control studies and a cohort study in Canada. There are several reasons why the analytic epidemiology studies should produce such weak evidence, compared to the strong associations noted in the ecologic and animal studies. Among the most important of these are misclassification of dietary exposure, and dietary enquiries that are poorly timed in relation to the natural history of breast cancer. Although one possible approach that may resolve the issue is a trial of dietary fat reduction, this may not overcome the problem of the timing of the intervention in relation to the natural history of breast cancer, unless very young women are recruited and the follow-up period is very prolonged.

Colorectal Cancer

For colorectal cancer, although there have been negative studies, the evidence is becoming more consistent. A case-control study of Seventh-day Adventists showed that meat of any type, beef products, beef hamburger, and lamb increased risk (7). In a study of San Francisco Bay area blacks, the highest risk was found in those with a high consumption of saturated fat-containing foods and a low consumption of fiber-containing foods, while conversely the lowest risks were in those with a high consumption of fiber-containing foods and a low consumption of fat-containing foods (28). A study in Canada of 348 cases of colon cancer and 194 cases of rectal cancer, 542 neighborhood controls, and 535 hospital controls who had undergone an abdominal operation showed a dose-response relationship for fat intake which was strongest for saturated fat. For colon and rectal cancer in both sexes combined, the risk in the highest saturated fat intake category relative to the lowest was of the order of 2.5 (29). In a further analysis of this study, the risk for a number of food groups was evaluated taking account of the effect of saturated fat intake (30). For most food groups, there did not appear to be an effect of the food independent of the saturated fat effect. In females the saturated fat effect consistently increased risk for colon cancer and also had an important effect over and above an apparent effect of some meats in increasing the risk of rectal cancer. In males, different meat products appeared to increase risk of rectal but not colon cancer, and only for rectal cancer did intake of saturated fat not appear to have an independent effect. There has been some controversy over whether the effect of total energy intake was appropriately considered in this study, and whether the effect of saturated fat persists with a nutrient density approach to analysis (31). This led to a reanalysis of the findings, with logistic regression models that included variables representing the effect of saturated fat and calories from sources other than saturated fats (32). In this analysis, the risk for the highest relative to low consumption levels of saturated fat was found to be 2.0 for males and 2.3 for females. No independent effect was found for other sources of calories or for fiber. Similar findings were seen in a study in western New York of 428 cases of colon cancer and neighborhood controls (33). In both sexes and for all sites of the colon, risk increased with the frequency and amount of ingestion of total fats and total calories. The risk for the highest ingestion quartile relative to the lowest approximated to 4 in males and approached 3 in females, with risks slightly higher for calories than total fats. However, the authors noted that the consumption of total fats and calories was highly correlated, and they did not attempt to separate the effect using the analytic methods in the reanalysis of the Canadian study, and now preferred for this problem (34).

A similar problem may have affected the results reported for a study in Utah, where fat, protein, and carbohydrate intake had elevated risks but "could not be assessed as risk factors independent of energy intake because of their strong correlations with total calories" (35). In a further analysis of the findings from this study, total dietary fat (OR = 1.9) and energy intake (OR = 1.5) were associated with increased colon cancer risk after adjusting for age, body mass index (associated with increased risk in both sexes), and crude fiber intake in females (36). In males adjusted risk estimates were 2.0 for total dietary fat, 3.8 for polyunsaturated fat, fat 2.1 for monounsaturated fat, and 2.1 for energy intake. In a study of rectal cancer in western New York increased risk with increasing intake of kilocalories and fat (37) with significant trends for males, but not females, was found. In this analysis, the association with fat intake was adjusted for total kilocalorie intake by the method of Willett and Stampfer (31). Thesc findings for dietary fat are therefore consistent for both colon and rectal cancer, as they were for a study of diet related to proximal and distal colon cancer in Wisconsin, where for both sites high fat-containing foods, such as processed lunchmeat and pan-fried foods, showed increased risks with high consumption levels for both subsites (38).

That the findings from case-control studies may be sensitive not only to the approach used in the analysis but also to the nature of the questionnaire and the main sources of fat used by the population is indicated by two studies from Europe and one in Singapore. In a study in the Marseilles region of France, where the main source of dietary fat is olive oil, there was no evidence of increased risk from total consumption of dietary fat (39). However, a reduced risk was associated with increasing consumption of oil, with a risk of 0.54 for the highest consumption quartile relative to the lowest ($p = 0.002$ for trend). Very similar results were found by the same group of investigators in a study of colorectal polyps and diet in Marseilles (40), though there was a nonsignificantly slightly higher intake of saturated fat in the cases compared to the controls. In a study in Belgium, using a similar questionnaire as in the studies in Marseilles, no effect was found for dietary fat in increasing risk, though there was a clear dose-response effect for intake of mono- and disaccharides (not so far replicated in any other study of colorectal cancer) and a suggestion of a protective effect for linoleic acid, a constitutent of vegetable oils (41). In a study in Singapore there were no consistent trends for fat or fiber intakes, though cruciferous vegetable intake was protective, while a high ratio of meat to vegetable intake (80–100%) showed increased risk (OR 1.97, 95% CI 1.32–2.93 for cancers of the colon and rectum combined) (41).

In two studies in Australia (43,44), there were similar findings to the North American studies, in that both dietary fat and sources of animal protein appeared to increase risk. In one, conducted in Adelaide (43), there was evidence of increasing risk with increasing consumption of a number of nutrients, and a pattern of food intake involving high dietary fat and protein and possibly saturated fats. It was the impression of the authors, however, that the major contribution to increased risk came from protein. In the other, conducted in Melbourne (44), fat intake was found to be a risk factor for both males and females. The relative risk associated with high fat intake was 1.4 after adjustment for meat and vegetable intake. The effect seemed to be similar for colon and rectal cancer.

A particularly informative case-control study of diet and colorectal cancer among Chinese living in North America and Chinese living in China has recently been reported (45). This population-based study, conducted simultaneously in people of similar genetic origin but with one (the North American) group known to have shown an increase in incidence in colorectal cancer since migration, showed increasing risk with increasing consumption of saturated fat. The odds ratios were much higher and statistically significant for the North American group, being 2.1 (95% CI 1.6–2.7) for colorectal cancer in males per 100 calories contributed by saturated fat and 2.2 (95% CI 1.5–3.5) in females. The corresponding odds ratios for the group from the People's Republic of China were 1.2 (0.84–1.7) in males and 1.4 (0.87–2.3) in females. No excess risk was found for other sources of calories. The risks were particularly elevated for those with sedentary lifestyle or jobs and for those who had lived 20 or more years in North America. These findings are precisely in line with those predicted from the dietary fat hypothesis, and suggest that the major reason for the increase in incidence of colorectal cancer after migration to North America is a change to a diet involving greater consumption of dietary fat. Indeed the authors calculated that saturated fat intakes exceeding 10 g/day, in combination with physical inactivity, could account for 60% of colorectal cancer incidence among Chinese-American men and 40% among Chinese-American women, proportions very similar to those computed for the Canadian case-control study conducted a decade earlier (29).

Three cohort studies with negative data relevant to the dietary fat hypothesis and one positive study have so far been reported. In a cohort study of 8006 Japanese men in Hawaii, the dietary information was collected by 24-hour recall at baseline (46). Over a 14–17-year follow-up there were 99 cases of colorectal cancer, with an estimated mean intake of fat of 69 g/day. This was assessed in comparison to a mean intake of 77 g/day for 378 controls. Thus the fat intake in both groups was low, but the findings were not in accord with the dietary fat hypothesis. Similarly, in a follow-up of 1954 men in the Western Electric cohort, no differences were found between men who developed colorectal cancer and those who did not in the percent of calories from fat or animal protein, or in mean caloric intake (47). Further, in a 21-year follow-up of colorectal cancer mortality among over 25,000 Seventh-day Adventists, there was no clear association between consumption of high fat foods and colon cancer risk (48). Nevertheless, all of these studies used dietary instruments that were not fully able to characterize dietary fat intake, and two were specifically designed to study cardiovascular disease. However, in the large cohort study of 88,751 American nurses, 150 incidence cases of colon cancer were documented in a 6-year follow-up (49). After adjustment for total energy intake, animal fat was positively associated with risk of colon cancer, the relative risk for the highest versus lowest quintile being 1.89 (95% CI 1.13–3.15). No association was found for vegetable fat or cholesterol intake. It is of interest that no association was found between dietary fat intake and breast cancer risk in this cohort (23); it is possible that the effect of dietary fat on risk of colon cancer is more immediate, as might be expected by the more rapid change of colon cancer risk on migration than that of breast cancer.

In summary, the weight of the evidence points to a causal association between colorectal cancer and a pattern of food intake involving high dietary fat, perhaps particularly saturated fat. To fully clarify the effect of fat in relation to total energy intake, it would be appropriate to reanalyze the reported studies in the same way as has been possible for breast cancer (22). Such a reanalysis is now planned.

Prostate Cancer

Several studies have evaluated the role of dietary fat in prostate cancer (50). One of the largest case-control studies, conducted in Hawaii, found a dose-response gradient in risk of prostate cancer associated with saturated fat intake in men age 70 years and older (51). The risk for the highest relative to the lowest quartile of saturated fat intake was 1.7. In contrast, a much smaller study conducted in American blacks (who have a higher incidence of prostate cancer than whites) found increased risk associated with fat intake only for those under the age of 50 (52). A further American study of whites found elevated risk associated with increasing consumption of animal fats, with no apparent differential effect by age (53). A risk of the order of 2.0 was found for fat consumption greater than 2100 g/month relative to fat consumption of less than 1200 g/month. There have been two relevant cohort studies reported, both in Seventh-day Adventist men. The first was a study of 6763 white males who were followed from 1960 to 1980 in terms of mortality (54). Suggestive positive associations were found for fatal prostate cancer and the consumption of milk, cheeses, eggs, and meat, together with a dose-response relationship. The relative risk for heavy consumption of all four animal products was 3.6. Although the dietary instrument used in 1960 could not provide an estimate of fat intake, it seems likely that dietary fat contributed to the associations seen. The second was a cohort of approximately 14,000 men who completed a lifestyle questionnaire in 1976 and were monitored for cancer incidence in 1982 with 180 prostate cancers detected (55). There were suggestive relationships between increasing animal product consumption and increased risk of prostate cancer, the relative risk for daily use of meat, poultry, or fish being 1.41 (95% CI 0.79–2.51) in a multivariate analysis. In the same analysis some indices of fruit and vegetable consumption were protective. It was apparently not possible, however, to determine fat consumption.

Other Cancers

For other cancers, there is less evidence. Some studies suggest increased risk from fat intake for ovarian cancer, while a few suggest similar effects for pancreas, kidney, and even lung cancer (50).

For ovarian cancer there have been three positive (56–58) and two negative (59,60) studies. In one of the positive studies conducted in the United States it was found that the 215 white women with ovarian cancer favored and consumed greater amounts of foods high in animal fats and less vegetable fat than the 215 control women (56). The second study was conducted in Italy (57). In this study significantly elevated risks were found for women who reported frequent consumption of meat, ham, and fats, especially butter. The most recent study was conducted in China with 172 case-control pairs (58). A significant ($p < 0.01$) dose-response relationship was found between intake of fat from animal sources and risk of ovarian cancer, but plant fat was not associated with increased risk.

For pancreatic cancer, a case-control study conducted in Toronto showed little effect of dietary fat, but a significant effect of kilocalories in increasing risk, the RR for the highest compared to the lowest quartile being 2.39 (95% CI 1.18–4.83) (61). Positive correlations between international rates of pancreas cancer and egg consumption have been reported (3,62), and a positive association between egg intake and fatal pancreas cancer in a cohort study of Seventh-day Adventists (63). Dietary cholesterol has been found to be associated with increase in risk in a study of bladder cancer (64) and in several studies of lung cancer (65–68). In one of these, a study in Toronto (68), although there was a statistically significant association with saturated fat intake, this effect was weaker than the cholesterol effect, and in models in which both were included simultaneously the saturated fat effect disappeared entirely. The odds ratio for each 400-mg dietary cholesterol consumption was 1.5, though the effect seemed largely limited to those in the upper quartile of consumption. In international correlations, fat intake is associated with increased risk of lung cancer, and a positive, but nonsignificant, association was also found in one case control study (66).

CONCLUSION AND IMPLICATIONS

Increasingly, data from several types of epidemiologic studies, conducted in several different countries, show that dietary fat intake is associated with increased risk for several types of cancers, most consistently with colon cancer, but also with breast, prostate, and ovarian cancer. In addition, dietary cholesterol is associated with increased risk of lung and bladder cancer. It is notable that the strongest evidence has come from studies in which a detailed quantitative dietary questionnaire has been administered. The few epidemiologic studies that have been able to adequately characterize saturated fat intake in contradistinction to other types of fat have in general found that risk is more associated with saturated fat intake than with other types of fat.

The Committee on Diet and Health of the National Research Council (2), having carefully reviewed the evidence associating dietary factors with the risk of chronic diseases, including cancer, concluded that a number of recommendations were appropriate for the general population. Although the evidence for these was greater for heart disease than cancer, the committee concluded that they can be expected to reduce cancer incidence, some being largely adopted on the basis of data on cancer. The strongest recommendation concerned dietary fat and can be summarized: Reduce fat intake to between 25 and 30% of total calories with no more than 10% of total calories from saturated fats, 6–8% as polyunsaturated fats, and the remainder as monounsaturated fats.

The remaining recommendations related to a dietary pattern compatible with reduced fat consumption, including consumption of a variety of green and yellow vegetables, and increased consumption of carbohydrates.

The implementation of such recommendations is likely to require concerted action on several fronts. These include increasing the knowledge of the public through public education, obtaining the cooperation of the food producing, manufacturing, and distributing industries to ensure that the public has the necessary choices available, and some actions from governments. Government support of the food industry can have adverse consequences. Government grants or subsidies have sometimes been made to promote the development of animal husbandry, encourage high fat content of meat, and encourage the provision of high fat milk and cream, even to schools. For example, the agricultural policies of the European Economic Community have for some time encouraged the production of fat and alcohol. An increase in fat intake and particularly in saturated fat resulting from such policies may specifically effect areas of southern Europe where some dietary associated cancers are much lower in incidence than in northern or western Europe. Similarly, in developing countries, it is often believed that an advantage of increasing affluence is the ability to consume increasing amounts of animal products, rich in fat. There is, therefore, a risk of a major increase in incidence of dietary associated cancers in many parts of the world. National government policies should be directed to reducing dietary fat and alcohol consumption and supporting prudent dietary recommendations (69).

SUMMARY

Diet is one of the major causes of cancer. The epidemiologic data on which this conclusion is based has been derived from analytic epidemiologic studies, buttressed by descriptive (ecologic) epidemiology and studies in experimental animals. Although the evidence is not entirely consistent, high dietary fat intake appears to be a major cause of breast cancer and, more consistently, of colorectal cancer and probably prostate cancer as well. High fat intake is also associated with increased risk of ovarian cancer, while fat-associated nutrients (especially dietary cholesterol) may increase the risk of lung and bladder cancer. These data are of sufficient importance that they justify including modification of dietary fat intake into general food policy in Western populations, and taking measures to avoid an increase in dietary fat intake in developing countries.

REFERENCES

1. R. Doll and R. Peto, *JNCI, 66*, 1191 (1981).
2. Committee on Diet and Health, National Academy Press, Washington, DC, 1989.
3. B. Armstrong and R. Doll, *Int. J. Cancer, 15*, 617 (1975).
4. L. N. Kolonel, J. N. Hankin, J. Lee et al., *Br. J. Cancer, 44*, 332 (1981).
5. M. J. Hill, in *Diet and the Aetiology of Cancer*. (A. B. Miller, ed.) Springer-Verlag, Berlin, 1989, p. 31.
6. R. L. Prentice F. Kakar, S. Hursting, et al., *JNCI, 80*, 802 (1988).
7. R. L. Phillips, *Cancer Res., 35*, 3513 (1975).
8. T. G. Hislop, A. J. Coldman, J. M. Elwood, et al., *Cancer Detect. Prev., 9*, 47 (1986).
9. M. G. Le, L. H. Moulton, C. Hill, and A. Kramer, *JNCI, 77*, 633 (1986).
10. A. B. Miller, A. Kelly, N. W. Choi, et al., *Am. J. Epidemiol., 107*, 499 (1978).
11. G. R. Howe, *J. Chron. Dis., 38*, 663 (1985).
12. J. H. Lubin, P. E. Burns, W. J. Blot, et al., *Int. J. Cancer, 28*, 685 (1981).
13. F. Lubin, Y. Wax, and B. Modan, *JNCI, 77*, 605 (1986).
14. F. Lubin, Y. Wax, E. Ron, et al., *Am. J. Clin. Nutr., 50*, 551 (1989).
15. P. Toniolo, E. Riboli, F. Protta, et al., *JNCI, 81*, 278 (1989).
16. P. van't Veer, F. J. Kok, H. A. M. Brants, et al., *Int. J. Epidemiol., 19*, 12 (1990).
17. O. M. Jensen, M. Ewertz, H. Møller, and A. Tjønneland, in *Recent Progress in Research on Nutrition and Cancer* (C. J. Mettlin and K. Aoki, eds.), Wily-Liss, New York, 1990, pp. 67–82.
18. S. Graham, J. Marshall, C. Mettlin, et al., *Am. J. Epidemiol., 116*, 68 (1982).
19. K. Katsouyanni, D. Trichopoulos, P. Boyle, et al., *Int. J. Cancer, 38*, 815 (1986).
20. T. Hirohata, A. G. Nomura, J. H. Hankin, et al., *JNCI, 78*, 595 (1987).
21. T. Rohan, A. J. McMichael, and P. A. Baghurst, *Am. J. Epidemiol., 128*, 478 (1988).
22. G. R. Howe, T. Hirohata, T. G. Hislop, et al., *JNCI, 82*, 561 (1990).
23. W. C. Willett, M. J. Stampfer, G. A. Colditz, et al., *N. Engl. J. Med., 316*, 22 (1987).
24. D. Y. Jones, A. Schatzkin, S. B. Green, et al., *JNCI, 79*, 465 (1987).
25. P. K. Mills, L. Beeson, R. L. Phillips, et al., *Cancer, 64*, 582 (1989).
26. G. R. Howe, C. M. Friedenreich, M. Jain, and A. B. Miller, *JNCI, 83*, 336 (1990).
27. L. J. Kinlen, *Lancet, i*, 946 (1982).
28. L. G. Dales, G. D. Freidman, H. K. Ury, et al., *Am. J. Epidemiol., 109*, 132 (1979).
29. M. Jain, J. M. Cook, F. G. Davis, et al., *Int. J. Cancer, 26*, 757 (1980).
30. A. B. Miller, G. R. Howe, M. J. Jain, et al., *Int. J. Cancer, 32*, 155 (1983).
31. W. Willett and M. J. Stampfer, *Am. J. Epidemiol., 124*, 17 (1986).
32. G. R. Howe, A. B. Miller, and M. Jain, *Am. J. Epidemiol., 124*, 157 (1986).
33. S. Graham, J. Marshall, B. Haughey, et al., *Am. J. Epidemiol., 128*, 490 (1988).
34. G. R. Howe, *Am. J. Epidemiol., 129*, 1314 (1989).
35. J. L. Lyon, A. W. Mahoney, D. W. West, et al., *JNCI, 78*, 853 (1987).
36. D. W. West, M. A. Slattery, L. A. Robison, et al., *Am. J. Epidemiol., 130*, 883 (1989).
37. J. L. Freudenheim, S. Graham, J. R. Marshall, et al., *Am. J. Epidemiol., 131*, 612 (1990).
38. T. B. Young and D. A. Wolf, *Int. J. Cancer, 42*, 167 (1988).

39. G. Macquart-Moulin, E. Riboli, J. Cornee, et al., *Int. J. Cancer, 38*, 183 (1986).
40. G. Macquart-Moulin, E. Riboli, J. Cornee, et al., *Int. J. Cancer, 40*, 179 (1987).
41. A. J. Tuyns, M. Haelterman, and R. Kaaks, *Nutr. Cancer, 10*, 181 (1987).
42. H. P. Lee, L. Gourley, S. W. Duffy, et al., *Int. J. Cancer, 43*, 1007 (1989).
43. J. D. Potter and A. J. McMichael, *JNCI, 76*, 557 (1986).
44. S. Kune, G. A. Kune, and L. F. Watson, *Nutr. Cancer, 9*, 21 (1987).
45. A. S. Whittemore, A. H. Wu-Williams, M. Lee, et al., *JNCI, 82*, 915 (1990).
46. G. N. Stemmermann, A. M. Y. Nomura, and L. K. Heilbrun, *Cancer Res., 44*, 4633 (1984).
47. C. Garland, R. B. Shekelle, E. Barrett-Connor, et al., *Lancet, i*, 307 (1985).
48. R. L. Phillips and D. A. Snowdown, *J. Natl. Cancer Inst., 74*, 307 (1985).
49. W. C. Willett, M. J. Stampfer, G. A. Colditz, et al. *N. Eng. J.Med., 323*, 1664 (1990).
50. J. Wahrendorf, in *Diet and the Aetiology of Cancer* (A. B. Miller, ed.), Springer-Verlag, Berlin, 1989, p. 13.
51. L. N. Kolonel, C. N. Yoshizawa, and J. H. Hankin, *Am. J. Epidemiol., 127*, 999 (1988).
52. M. Y. Heshmat, L. Kaul, J. Kovi, et al., *Prostate 1, 6*, 7 (1985).
53. S. Graham, B. Haughey, J. Marshall, et al., *JNCI, 70*, 687 (1983).
54. D. A. Snowdon, R. L. Phillips, and W. Choi, *Am. J. Epidemiol., 120*, 244 (1984).
55. P. K. Mills, W. L. Beeson, R. L. Phillips, and G. E. Fraser, *Cancer, 64*, 598 (1989).
56. D. W. Cramer, W. R. Welch, G. B. Hutchinson, et al., *Obstet. Gynecol., 63*, 833 (1984).
57. C. La Vecchia, A. Decarli, E. Negri, et al., *JNCI, 79*, 663 (1987).
58. X. O. Shu, Y. T. Gao, J. M. Yuan, et al., *Br. J. Cancer, 59*, 92 (1989).
59. T. Byers, J. Marshall, S. Graham, et al., *JNCI, 71*, 681 (1983).
60. M. L. Slattery, K. L. Schuman, D. W. West, et al., *Am. J. Epidemiol., 130*, 497 (1989).
61. G. R. Howe, M. Jain and A. B. Miller, *Int.J. Cancer 45*, 604 (1990).
62. A. J. Lea, *Ann. Roy. Coll. Phys., 41*, 432 (1967).
63. P. K. Mills, L. Beeson, D. E. Abby, et al., *Cancer, 61*, 2578 (1988).
64. H. A. Risch, J. D. Burch, A. B. Miller, et al., *Am. J. Epidemiol., 127*, 1179 (1988).
65. M. W. Hinds, L. N. Kolonel, J. Lee, and J. H. Hankin, *Am. J. Clin. Nutr., 37*, 192 (1983).
66. T. E. Byers, S. Graham, B. P. Haughey, et al., *Am. J. Epidemiol., 125*, 351 (1987).
67. M. T. Goodman, L. N. Kolonel, C. N. Yoshizawa, and J. H. Hankin, *Am. J. Epidemiol., 128*, 1241 (1988).
68. M. Jain, J. D. Burch, G. R. Howe, et al., *Int. J. Cancer, 45*, 287 (1990).
69. WHO Technical Report Series 797 (1990).

10

Alcohol

Robert A. Hiatt
Kaiser Permanente Medical Care Program
Oakland, California

INTRODUCTION

> Wine has been with us since the beginning of civilization. It is the temperate, civilized, sacred, romantic mealtime beverage recommended by the Bible. Wine has been praised for centuries by statesmen, philosophers, poets and scholars. Wine in moderation is an integral part of our culture, heritage and the gracious way of life.
>
> GOVERNMENT WARNING: (1) According to the Surgeon General, women should not drink alcoholic beverages during pregnancy because of the risk of birth defects. (2) Consumption of alcoholic beverages impairs your ability to drive a car or operate machinery and may cause health problems.
>
> Robert Mondavi wine label, 1990

Human beings have consumed ethyl alcohol as part of their diet since recorded time (204). With the exception of Muslims and a few other cultures, alcoholic beverages have been a common feature of all human societies (204) and will continue to be consumed in the foreseeable future. Whereas the excess consumption of alcohol is generally perceived as a detriment to personal and social well-being, and its addictive potential and drug effects are well recognized, the moderate consumption of alcohol is frequently viewed as a source of personal pleasure, social cohesiveness, and celebration. It is because of the latter deeply established values that alcohol consumption has continued to be so prevalent in human populations.

The contrast between the pleasurable aspects of alcohol and its negative health effects presents a dilemma for the consumer and the scientist because the relationship of alcohol to disease is complex. Whereas heavier consumption of alcohol is clearly associated with increased mortality (91,121,204), principally from cirrhosis, accidents, hypertension, and certain cardiovascular disease, there is also good epidemiologic evidence that abstainers are at higher risk of cardiovascular mortality than persons who consume moderate amounts (91,121). However, persons who consume moderate levels of alcohol may also be at increased risk of cancers of the breast (225), colon, and rectum (10,203). This interaction of level of alcohol consumption, cancer, and cardiovascular risk presents a challenge to epidemiologists and other investigators that is currently unresolved.

Most of the evidence presented in this chapter will come from human epidemiologic studies, although there will be reference to some animal studies in the discussion of possible biologic mechanisms. For further reference, several reviews of this topic are available (56,63,189,200,204), and there is a recent comprehensive monograph on alcohol and cancer from the International Agency for Research and Cancer (IARC) (235).

The association of alcohol with human cancer was probably first reported by a Boston surgeon in 1837, when he attributed a case of cancer of the tongue to the "long use of ardent spirits" (125) by a seaman from Maine who also chewed tobacco. Perhaps the earliest recognition that excess consumption of alcohol was common to a series of cases was made by Lamy in 1910 in France (210) in a study where he noted that 80% of a group of esophageal cancer cases were men who were heavy alcohol drinkers, particularly of absinthe. Other early studies have also shown a relationship between alcohol and cancers of the upper airways and digestive tract (206). Late in the 1950s, large-scale retrospective epidemiologic studies of tobacco users were conducted by Wynder and his colleagues (96,111,124,177) and by Schwartz et al. (169), among others (172,218). These studies implicated both tobacco and alcohol in the etiology of cancers of the tongue, buccal activity, oropharynx, hypopharynx, larynx, and esophagus.

The independent role of alcohol consumption in the carcinogenesis of cancers of the upper respiratory and alimentary tract was difficult to isolate from tobacco use because they are so highly correlated (105,233). Because ethanol alone has not been shown to be carcinogenic (26,204), it was generally believed that heavy use of alcohol acted through direct contact with mucosal tissues to augment the carcinogenic effects of tobacco (248). There has also been a substantial amount of research into the possibility that alcoholic beverages contain substances that may be carcinogenic (200). In the last decade, however, evidence has accumulated that alcohol consumption may be linked to aerodigestive cancers and cancer of the liver independent of tobacco and the nonalcoholic contents of alcoholic beverages (45,95,235). Furthermore, new studies have implicated even light and moderate use of alcohol in cancers of the breast (81,119,120) and colorectum

(76,190,203). In studies of melanoma and cancers of the pancreas, bladder, lung, ovary, and prostate the effects of alcohol are either absent or much less consistent. Clearly alcohol must work through mechanisms other than or in addition to direct concentrated contact with tissues. Current hypotheses include a number of possible pathogenetic mechanisms that could explain alcohol's role in the development of cancer at sites distant from the upper aerodigestive tract (189).

As more cancers are etiologically linked to alcohol consumption, the public health implications potentially grow. A decade ago Doll and Peto (233) and Rothman (123) attributed 3% of cancer mortality to alcohol use. This estimate needs to be reexamined in light of new findings.

Before reviewing the epidemiologic studies that have relevance to the question of alcohol's role at each specific cancer site, several general issues about the measurement of alcohol intake will be presented. The interaction of alcohol with other putative agents, such as tobacco, and some proposed biologic mechanisms will also be presented.

GENERAL ISSUES

Validity of Reported Alcohol Intake

In the conduct and evaluation of studies of alcohol and disease, the validity of self-reported intake is frequently questioned. There is widespread concern that alcohol intake is underreported, and some investigators have gone so far as to call for a moratorium on alcohol-related research until a better means of assessing intake can be developed (240). Virtually all epidemiologic studies have relied on self-reported information on intake or that provided by collaterals (e.g., spouse, relative, friend, or employer). It is worthwhile, therefore, to review the nature and magnitude of this problem.

One should recognize that all efforts at evaluating the validity of alcohol intake are limited because they are simply comparisons of two or more imprecise estimates of true intake. In one commonly used method the reports by collaterals of the amounts of alcohol consumed are compared to that reported by the subject. Correlations by this method in studies of alcoholics have varied between studies with some providing no confidence in self-report and others indicating that they are extremely accurate (122). The use of diaries is another method that has been used to assess intake. However, the validity of this method is compromised because filling out the diary may influence the behavior being measured. Investigators have found that intake reported while keeping a diary is usually higher than that from self-administered questionnaire (122), although there are exceptions (268). Willet et al. (120) found very high correlations between data obtained from self-administered questionnaires given to nurses one year apart and with that from four one-week diaries kept during the intervening year.

In one study of clients at an alcohol clinic, results were highly correlated when intake that was self-reported into an interactive computer was compared to that received in face-to-face interviews or to that reported on a self-administered form (276). However, in a general population study in Edinburgh (238), the computer recorded amount was 33% higher than that reported in face-to-face interviews. So-called "bogus pipeline" techniques, in which the respondents are led to believe that the truthfulness of their answers will be checked by some physiologic test, have yielded conflicting results. In high school students the bogus pipeline technique produced no difference in the responses (237), but in pregnant women almost twice as many subjects reported alcohol use during pregnancy (27%) compared to controls (14%) (239).

It thus appears that the accuracy of an individual report of alcohol consumption depends on the interview situation, the respondent, how the specific information is elicited, and the context of the interview (122). Also, many validity studies have been performed among alcoholics or heavy users of alcohol, and the applicability of results from such studies to the behavior of the general population is not known.

Dose of Ethyl Alcohol

The use of widely different methods of defining alcohol intake has made the comparison of epidemiologic studies of alcohol and cancer difficult and introduced inaccuracies (271). Some investigators have used "drinks per day" or "per week," others have used "days per week," "units per day," or "current, past or never." Most recent studies attempt to translate reported consumption of specific types and amounts of alcoholic beverages into grams per day of alcohol. Although this summary measure has proven useful for comparisons across epidemiologic studies, any measure of total alcohol intake obscures patterns of alcohol intake, such as binge drinking (269).

Unfortunately the grams of ethanol assigned to a standard drink differ among studies reported in the literature. These variations depend upon the country (11,121) and changes over time in the standard size of containers and drinks (132). Among recent studies in the United States some investigators have used information from the Department of Agriculture to estimate that there is 13.2 g ethanol in a 12-oz beer, 10.8 g in a 4-oz glass of wine (or 13.5 g in 5 oz), and 15.1 g for a drink of liquor (120). Other investigators have considered 1 oz of ethanol approximately equal to 25 g and assigned 12.5 g to a standard 12-oz beer, 5-oz glass of wine, and a shot of liquor (119). Finally, the United States Surgeon General's Report on Nutrition and Health has used 15 g of ethanol as the approximate content of these same standard-sized drinks and specified a drink of spirits as 1.5 oz of 80 proof liquor (264,265). The lack of consistency in translating reported intake into grams per day of ethanol may account for as much as a 15% difference between studies in reported exposures.

When one is concerned about the possible carcinogenic effects of substances in alcoholic beverages, rather than ethanol itself, there is also the problem of how to determine risk associated with a beverage type when more than one type is consumed (e.g., the risk associated with beer consumption in someone who also drinks wine). Usually the problem is ignored and risk is simply reported for persons who consume a single type of beverage compared to persons who don't (e.g., beer drinkers versus nonbeer drinkers). Obviously, this simple approach does not account for the likely influence of other types of alcohol consumed by the same individual. Klatsky et al. (205) have tried to solve this problem by associating risk with the "beverage most frequently chosen" by "preferrers," those who drank a particular type of beverage more than one day per week and who drank other beverages less. Willet et al. (120) have used a multiple logistic model, simultaneously entering data on consumers of less than 5 g and 5 g or more of alcohol a day of a particular beverage, to estimate the independent effects of each beverage.

Within any particular study one can reasonably rely on the accuracy of relative levels of intake despite the problems mentioned above. This assumption is supported by evidence that underestimation of intake is proportional to level of consumption so that the ordinal relationship between heavy, moderate, and light drinkers is maintained (247). However, there is also some indication that heavy drinkers are most likely to underreport consumption and may even deny any alcohol use (269).

One frequently wishes to make comparisons between epidemiologic studies to assess the consistency of risks of disease for given levels of exposure. When making such comparisons, there is unfortunately less confidence that similarly reported exposure levels reflect similar exposures. This is particularly difficult when studies have used widely different dose ranges and when comparisons are made at low dose levels (5). Furthermore, current abstainers are often former heavy drinkers (270), and it is important to separate out former drinkers from lifelong abstainers. At the highest dose level offered to respondents in any survey, one would expect to find the heaviest drinkers despite any relative differences in underreporting of intake. Thus for the highest level of consumption more valid comparisons may be possible (225). The problem of clearly defining the lowest putative level of alcohol use is an unresolved, but important one.

Although the contribution of heavy alcohol intake to the cancers of the upper aerodigestive system has been well defined and consistently confirmed, the importance of light or moderate alcohol intake is less clear. Since so many of the early studies were performed among alcoholics, the risks associated with lower levels of alcohol use were not studied. In 1984 Broitman concluded that moderate drinking had not been associated with an increased risk of cancer at any site (191). Since that time evidence has been presented that moderate and even light levels of alcohol drinking may be associated with cancers of the breast

(81,119,120,128) and of the colorectum (76,190). A reassessment of the importance of moderate alcohol intake on upper aerodigestive cancer is needed.

Interaction Effects

In evaluating the effects of alcohol consumption on cancer, it is also important to understand its interaction with other agents such as tobacco. An interaction occurs when two variables have an effect on an outcome that is greater than what one would predict from the addition of their independent effects (95). Such interaction effects, sometimes referred to as synergistic effects, have been recognized for alcohol and tobacco for almost 25 years. First discussed by Flamant et al. (248), the interaction of these two agents was especially marked among heavy consumers of both substances. For some sites, such as the hypopharynx, heavy use of both substances can result in extremely high relative risks (45). The importance of these interactions, beyond their usefulness in defining individual risk, is that they suggest that alcohol augments the carcinogenic effect of tobacco use, thereby providing some clues about the biologic mechanisms of alcohol's role in carcinogenesis. Interaction effects have been observed between alcohol and dietary factors in some studies (43), but not in others (194).

Biological Mechanisms

The mechanism by which alcoholic beverages are carcinogenic is not clearly understood. Numerous studies have shown that ethanol itself is not carcinogenic, but mechanisms by which it might act as a cocarcinogen or promoter have not been firmly established. Several current reviews on this subject are available (26,34,44,56,189), and salient points of some of these theories will be summarized here.

The possibility that certain alcoholic beverages contain carcinogens, promoters, enzyme inducers, or inhibitors has been a subject of interest for some time (3,200,236). Early reports linking alcohol use to cancer tended to refer to specific types of beverages popular in the culture or to special populations under observation. For example, esophageal cancer among African populations was ascribed to a fermented drink derived from maize (100), among the French to absinthe (210), and to pai-kan in China (249,250).

While the presence of carcinogens in alcoholic beverages is clearly not the whole story, they may play a role in certain areas of the world (26) and with certain beverages, particularly dark liquors (62). Tuyns has studied esophageal cancer in Normandy, where rates are unusually high, and found that the risk associated with calvados (apple brandy) is higher than for similar amounts of alcohol consumed in other beverages (43). Studies of esophageal cancer in Puerto Rico (98) and localized areas of the southern United States (234) also indicate that the substances in certain alcoholic beverages may have a causative role. Rothman et al. (62) studied hypopharyngeal and laryngeal cancers and found independent effects for the consumption of dark liquors and for total lifetime alcohol consumed (thus the effect of alcohol itself).

Beer drinking has been inconsistently linked to rectal cancers in studies of brewery workers in different parts of the world (51,86,88). The relationship has now been confirmed in ethnically diverse populations (18,76,176). This raises the possibility of a substance in beer other than ethanol that acts in a specific way on the rectal mucosa.

Despite these examples, it is clear from numerous studies that all types of alcohol, whether beer, wine, or liquor, have been associated with increased risk of cancer (204). Mechanisms through which alcohol contributes to carcinogenesis, other that through nonalcoholic substances in alcoholic beverages, must be considered. There are several postulated mechanisms explaining how ethanol may act as a cocarcinogen, which include: (1) local action directly on tissues through a solvent or cytotoxic effect; (2) through the induction of microsomal enzymes that convert carcinogens into more active forms; (3) through metabolism of retinol and retinoic acid; (4) through the inhibition of DNA repair mechanisms; and (5) through immunosuppression (26,44,63). These mechanisms are not mutually exclusive.

The first of these is the intuitively attractive hypothesis that alcohol has some sort of direct solvent or cytotoxic activity that facilitates the penetration of tissues by carcinogens (126). This theory is still credible for cancers of the upper digestive and upper respiratory tract that come in direct contact with alcohol in an undiluted form. Williams and Horm (78) noted that the risk of cancer was highest where the direct contact of tissue with alcohol occurred in the upper aerodigestive tract and diminished further down the alimentary tract. However, there is little evidence that ethanol can facilitate the penetration of carcinogens across mucosal barriers (194), and the association of upper aerodigestive cancers with beer, a weak alcoholic drink, also argues against such an effect (26). For sites with no direct contact with high concentrations of alcohol, such as liver, breast, colon, and rectum, other mechanisms must be sought.

The second possible mechanism suggested is that of a systemic effect through the induction of microsomal enzymes (26,207). Ethanol can induce activity of the cytochrome P-450–dependent biotransformation system in the liver, intestines, and lung (273,242). This system is capable of the conversion of many different chemical substances into electrophilic metabolites that are carcinogenic (26,274). Alcohol also acts by directly stimulating the liver to release its stores of vitamin A (243) and by inducing the cytochrome P-450 system to metabolize retinol and retinoic acid (244). Since vitamin A may play a critical anticarcinogenic role (241), susceptibility to carcinogens may increase through this mechanism.

A fourth possible mechanism suggests that chronic alcohol consumption inhibits enzymes in the DNA-repair system that protect cells from chemical carcinogens that affect the integrity of DNA structures and sequences (245). Without an intact DNA-repair system the risk of somatic mutations and the expression of oncogenes is increased (26). Finally, it has also been proposed that alcohol or its metabolites can suppress aspects of the immune system (44). Garro and Lieber point out that most of the studies have been performed in persons who already have alcoholic liver disease and that associated nutritional deficiencies could affect the immune response (26). Nevertheless, animal studies have shown that exposure to ethanol or its metabolites can impair the immune system in the absence of any liver disease (26). The importance of this interference with the immune system is, however, questionable since the cancers one sees in immunosuppressed persons are lymphomas and leukemias and these tumors have not been associated with alcohol consumption (26).

One other effect of alcohol that requires mention is the possible role of dietary deficiencies that may contribute to increased cancer risk, particularly of the esophagus (116,124,194). Alcoholics, who may consume 30–50% of their calories from alcohol, easily become malnourished (63). Poor diets may lead to the reduced consumption of the potential dietary preventives contained in fruits and vegetables (241). Dietary deficiencies include those of iron, zinc, riboflavin, pyridoxine, vitamin E, and lipotropes (26). However, other than among alcoholics and other heavy users who do not maintain a balanced diet, the role of dietary deficiencies is probably minimal and holds little promise in explaining malignancy associated with moderate levels of intake.

EPIDEMIOLOGIC STUDIES

Epidemiologic studies of alcohol consumption and cancer have included cohort studies of alcoholics and special subpopulations that abstain from alcohol for religious reasons, as well as correlation studies, case-control and cohort studies in general populations. Most studies of alcohol and cancer have been retrospective case-control investigations. For the understandable reasons of cost and time, relatively few prospective studies with data on individual consumption patterns have been performed.

The interpretation of evidence from these studies needs to be tempered by an appreciation of their limitations. Correlation studies of grouped data on alcohol sales or other indices of presumed use and of cancer rates, so-called ecologic correlations, are flawed because they can produce results contrary to those obtained on the individual level within populations (76). Case-control studies potentially suffer from the problem of recall and interview bias and the difficulties of selecting an appropriate control group (76,195). Prospective studies can be limited in their generalizability if their subjects are a selected population unrepresentative of the general public.

This section will review studies of each type, but will focus primarily on the case-control and the population-based cohort studies that provide the strongest evidence for or against the role of alcohol consumption in the etiology of cancer. Because the quality of the data and indeed the mechanism of action may vary by cancer site, the evidence will be presented for each site separately. Only the data on the association of alcohol with breast cancer has been examined by meta-analysis (128), so studies for most sites are summarized without benefit of any systematic weighting according to their size or study design.

Mouth and Pharynx

Cancers of the mouth and pharynx, also referred to as cancer of the oral or buccal cavity, oropharynx, hypopharynx or as cancers of the head and neck, share much the same histologic and epidemiologic features and are discussed together. The key feature in the epidemiology of these cancers is a strong synergism or interaction between tobacco use and heavy consumption of alcohol (95). Recent studies have also shown an independent effect of alcohol in nonsmokers (3). Studies of dietary influences (47,49,145) have suggested that consumption of fruits and foods containing vitamin C has a protective effect after adjustment for alcohol and tobacco use. Few other risk factors have been identified for these cancers.

Cancers of the mouth and pharynx were the first to be recognized as related to alcohol consumption, primarily because the use of alcohol and tobacco were so common in the cases studied (107,206,210). Early quantitative studies of consumption in alcoholics (57,77,84,90) and in brewery workers given generous access to their product (88) all showed an increased risk of these cancers. However, the dose of alcohol was not recorded, and there was no control for tobacco consumption. On the other hand, among populations such as the Seventh-day Adventists (89,178,181) and Mormons (35,182,183,185), who presumably do not consume alcohol or tobacco in any form, the rates of these cancers were extremely low. A temporal relationship between increased oral and pharyngeal cancer rates with increased per capita consumption of alcohol has been observed in Denmark (36,42) and Australia (58).

Case-control studies have confirmed the association of cancers of the mouth and oropharynx with heavy consumption of alcohol in the United States (3,96,98,101,111,193) and other countries (42,47,48,106,109,169), adjusting for the effect of tobacco. The interaction between tobacco and alcohol was probably first examined by Wynder and Bross (111). Rothman and Keller (95) showed that risk increased for increasing levels of alcohol for each level of tobacco use and, likewise, risk increased for increasing levels of tobacco use at each level of alcohol consumption. Synergistic effects were also documented in that the risk for persons who used both alcohol and tobacco in large amounts was several times greater than one would expect on the basis of adding the two factors together (95). This same phenomenon has since been confirmed by others (3,106,208,236).

Few cohort studies have included enough cases of these relatively uncommon cancers to define the risk more clearly by amount and duration of alcohol use. Pollack et al. (76) and Kono et al. (19,93,94) did not separate out lesions of the oral cavity and pharynx in their studies of upper aerodigestive cancers. However, large case-control studies by Rothman and Keller (95) and others (3,106,208) have shown excess risk in persons who drink but do not smoke. Blot et al. (3), in the largest case-control study yet conducted, found a dose-response relationship of alcohol to oral and pharyngeal cancer among nonsmokers, with almost a sixfold increased risk among consumers of more than 30 drinks per week. Several studies have demonstrated that the risk associated with tobacco use returns to normal after about 10 years of abstinence (3,47), but the effect of stopping drinking has not been evaluated.

All types of alcoholic beverages have been implicated in the etiology of oral and pharyngeal cancers. Blot et al. (3) found consumption of over four drinks a day of either hard liquor, beer, or wine increased risk, although the relationship with wine was the weakest.

Oral cancers were estimated to account for 4% of male and 2% of female cancers in 1991 (209). For these cancers risk attributable to alcohol is difficult to separate from that of tobacco (3). Where it has been examined jointly (3,95), approximately 75% has been attributed to the effects of alcohol and tobacco together. Rothman estimated that if each factor is assumed to have independent effects, then perhaps 50% of oral cancer in men and 40% in women could be attributed to alcohol alone (123). Based on this assumption and the predicted number of these cancers expected in the United States in 1991 (209), approximately 14,380 oropharyngeal cancers could be attributed to alcohol use.

Larynx

The epidemiologic relationship of alcohol to laryngeal cancer is very similar to that of oral and pharyngeal cancers. Alcohol consumption and smoking are the two most important risk factors, and a multiplicative interaction between them has been reported (45). Laryngeal cancer is more dependent on smoking history than alcohol intake (108), and an increased risk independent of smoking may require an average alcohol intake of over 80 g per day (45). Even though most studies report higher risks for smoking than alcohol use, international differences in rates correlate more closely with alcohol consumption patterns than tobacco use patterns (45). Laryngeal cancer is about five times more common in men than women, in contrast to cancers of the mouth and pharynx, which are only twice as common (209). Various occupational exposures (31), including those of machinists (68), have been suspected of conferring additional risk, although residual confounding by the powerful effects of tobacco and alcohol may still be partially responsible (45).

Laryngeal cancer has been observed to occur more frequently than expected in brewery workers (51,86,88) and among alcoholics (57,77,82–84,90) and less than expected among subpopulations who abstain from alcohol (35). Numerous case-control studies have confirmed the increased risk among heavy drinkers in the United States (27,31,104,106,113,177), other Western societies (45,58,102), and Asian countries (53).

Although most studies have not distinguished subsites within the larynx (108), there does appear to be a noteworthy difference between cancers of the endolarynx, which is mainly exposed to inhaled substances and where the effects of smoking predominate, and the epilarynx and hypopharynx, which are exposed to ingested substances and where the effects of alcohol predominate (45). The strong interaction between alcohol and tobacco consumption in the etiology of laryngeal cancers leads to multiplicative risks among persons who both drink and smoke heavily (27,31,45,96,102,108,110,112).

The effects of smoking are more clear and demonstrate a linear increased risk with increased use, with the heaviest smokers having approximately 30 times the risk of nonsmokers (108). Whereas the independent role of alcohol has been called into question (104), more recent studies have shown that alcohol increases risk in nonsmokers (45,106,113). Tuyns et al. (45) have demonstrated that for the heaviest drinkers at the lowest level of tobacco use (0–7 cigarettes per day) alcohol can increase the risk of endolaryngeal cancer almost fourfold and almost 15-fold for epilaryngeal and hypopharyngeal cancers. Effects of dark liquors that are independent of smoking and level of alcohol consumption have been reported (62).

The risk attributed to drinking more than 40 g per day has been estimated at 28% for laryngeal cancer and 68% for epilaryngeal/hypopharyngeal cancer (45). Another estimate attributes 50% of all laryngeal cancer in men and 40% in women to alcohol (123). Based on this later estimate, approximately 6000 cancers of the estimated 12,500 laryngeal cancers in the United States in 1991 (209) could be attributed to alcohol.

Esophagus

There are several features that distinguish alcohol's relationship to esophageal cancer from that of the head and neck cancers discussed above. Although both tobacco and alcohol are again the most important risk factors, and independently confer increased risk, the role of alcohol in esophageal cancer is clearly more predominant (97). Also particular ingredients in alcoholic beverages probably have a carcinogenic effect in addition to the effect of ethanol itself (261). The other feature of interest for esophageal cancer is that there are markedly higher rates for some geographic locales and dietary deficiencies may influence the risk (200). The food groups most consistently implicated have been a lack of fresh fruits and vegetables (28,43,97,116,198).

Like head and neck cancer, excess numbers of esophageal cancer were recognized as occurring more frequently among alcoholics (57,77,79,84,85,90) and brewery workers (51,88). Also, like head and neck cancer, Seventh-day Adventists (226) and Mormons (35,185), who presumably abstain from use of alcohol, are known to have lower than expected rates of esophageal cancer. Tuyns has found that there is a geographic correlation of mortality from alcoholism and esophageal cancer by *departement* in France (99), and La Rosa et al. have shown that an increased consumption of hard liquor in Italy shows a temporal relationship with an increased standardized cohort mortality ratio for esophageal cancer (23).

Case-control studies from the United States (28,97,116), France (169,199), Puerto Rico (98), South America (117,118), Singapore (114), and India (41) have confirmed the association of alcohol consumption and esophageal cancer. A clear dose-response relationship has also been documented (28,199), and the nature of the interaction of smoking and alcohol has been studied by Tuyns et al. (216) and others (9) and shown to be multiplicative. Thus, like head and neck cancers, both alcohol and tobacco have demonstrable independent risks, but together act synergistically. In many studies, particular types of alcoholic beverages seem to confer an additional excess risk (199). In a cohort study of 5130 Japanese physicians, Kono et al. (19) found a significantly increased relative risk of 14.5 (95% CI 3.0–69.7) for drinkers of two or more *go* of sake per day (1 *go* = 27 ml alcohol) after adjustment for age and smoking.

The significance of the association with certain types of beverages is that substances in the beverage besides the alcohol may be partially responsible for the increased risk (199). In the early work of Wynder et al. (97), there was some suggestion that whiskey drinkers were at higher risk than beer or wine drinkers. Since that time, certain types of liquors, usually dark liquors, have been implicated (62). For example, Tuyns has shown that in Normandy, for those who drink calvados, an apple brandy popular in the region, the risk is greater than for other persons in the same population who consume the same amount of alcohol in wine and other beverages (199). Similar evidence for other beverages has been reported among black men in Washington, D.C., where risk was substantially higher among hard liquor consumers than among beer drinkers (116). In Los Angeles the risk from liquor was more than two times that from beer, while wine was intermediate (28).

As opposed to head and neck cancers, where roughly 50% could be attributed to alcohol, approximately 75% of esophageal cancer may be due to alcohol consumption (123). In 1991 an estimated 8175 esophageal cancers of those 10,900 predicted in the United States (209) could be attributed to alcohol use.

Stomach

Alcohol is probably not a risk factor for stomach cancer, except perhaps for the cardia, that portion of the stomach closest to the esophagus. Most of the studies that have looked at cancer mortality in alcoholics (77,84,90) or heavy consumers (51,86,88) have found no increased risk. In the United States as in other industrialized countries, where alcohol consumption has increased since the middle of the century, there has been a dramatic drop in stomach cancer incidence (209).

Case-control studies that have examined this question have usually found no difference in the alcohol consumption histories between cases and controls (147,157,174,211–213). Among the few positive studies the estimates of relative risk have usually been below 2.0, and no dose response has been observed (46,162,217). Correa et al. found an estimated relative risk of 2.0 (95% CI 1.2–3.2) for current drinkers of liquor among whites but not blacks in southern Louisiana (217). In France, the heavy intake of red wine was associated with a relative risk of 6.9 (95% CI 3.3–14.3) and dose-response was documented, with 800+ g per week being the highest level evaluated (160). A migrant study of Japanese-American immigrants (Issei) found a small increased risk for beer consumption without a dose response, but not for their offspring (Nisei) (148). Some studies have suggested that only persons who consume alcohol on an empty stomach are at excess risk (46,162).

One possible explanation for the discrepancy in studies to date may be that the site within the stomach is usually not considered. A recent case-control study by Wu-Williams et al. (33) separated cancers of the cardia, which is more proximal to the esophagus, from those of the fundus and those of the antrum and pylorus. Subsite was determined from hospital records. They found significantly increased risk for cancers of the cardia for consumers of all types of alcoholic beverages, with independent risks for both alcohol and smoking. For all ethanol combined, a relative risk of 3.0 (95% CI 1.1–8.77) was observed for consumers of over 80 g/day. No mention was made of the possible misclassification of lower esophageal adenocarcinomas as gastric cardia cancers in this study.

In a cohort study of 7990 Japanese-American men in Hawaii, Nomura et al. (2) found that alcohol drinkers had a nonsignificant increased risk of 1.2 that dropped to 1.1 after adjustment for cigarette smoking status. Three other cohort studies have been consistent in finding no increased risk (19,76,214), although none of them has controlled for subsite within the stomach.

Stomach cancer accounted for an estimated 23,800 new cancers in the United States in 1991 (209). Based on the weight of the epidemiologic data available, it seems unjustified to attribute any of these cancers to alcohol intake. If further studies confirm the relationship of alcohol consumption to cancer of the gastric cardia (33), this assessment should be reconsidered.

Colon and Rectum

The epidemiologic characteristics of colonic and rectal cancers are rather different, especially with regard to the much-reported association of beer drinking with cancer of the rectum (146). They are discussed together because studies frequently make no distinction between them. Dietary factors, in particular fat and fiber, have been identified as potential risk factors key to the etiology of these cancers (262), while alcohol may play a minor, but significant role.

The high risk among alcoholics for upper aerodigestive cancers does not hold for cancers of the colon and rectum (57,77,84). Among three follow-up studies of brewery workers, the increased risk of rectal cancer has been documented in two (51,88), but not the third (159). As with other alcohol-associated sites, Mormons (35,183,185) and Seventh-day Adventists (178) have significantly lower numbers than expected, although dietary practices in these groups probably also play some protective role (178).

The association of alcohol drinking with colorectal cancer was perhaps first suggested by Wynder and Shigematsu (176). Subsequent case-control studies that have considered the relationship of alcohol with large bowel cancer have been inconsistent, with slightly more studies supporting the association (18,20,21,144,163,190,202) than not (32,112,159,167,201,218). The most consistent finding is the relationship between beer and rectal cancer (18,20, 21,163,190). Beer consumption per capita has been correlated with colon and rectal cancers in the United States and 24 other countries (146,187,188,274), but in all cases the correlations have been stronger for rectal cancer. The disparity in results of these case-control studies may be partially due to the use of hospital controls in all but a few of them (144) and the possibility that alcohol-related diseases were more common among the controls than would be found in the general population (10).

To date, in the seven prospective studies that examined the relationship of alcohol and colon and rectal cancer (10,76,87,203,223,224), alcohol consumption has been implicated to some degree in all but one (224). Pollack et al. (76), in their prospective study of 7837 Japanese men in Hawaii, found a significant trend showing an increased risk of rectal cancer with increased reported levels of alcohol consumption (76). No such relationship was found for colon cancer. When men who consumed a particular type of beverage were compared to those who consumed none of that beverage, only beer showed a significant trend, with increasing dose. At $\geq$15 liters of beer per month, the relative risk was significantly elevated at 3.1 ($p < 0.01$). Klatsky et al. (203), in a study of 106,203 men and women in California, found an increased risk of rectal cancer with alcohol consumption (trend $p < 0.03$), but not for colon cancer (trend $p < 0.11$). At levels of three or more drinks a day, where the relative risk for rectal cancer was 3.2 (95% CI 1.1–9.6), colon cancer overall was of borderline significance

(RR 1.7,95% CI 0.9–3.2). For women alone the relative risk reached 2.6 (95% CI 1.0–6.4). No single type of beverage could be clearly implicated, although the relationship for beer with rectal cancer was the most suggestive.

In a third prospective study in a Los Angeles retirement community of 11,888 residents in whom 126 colorectal cancers developed, daily alcohol drinkers experienced a relative risk of 2.2 (95% CI 1.21–3.8) after adjustment for physical activity, body mass, and smoking (10). Age-adjusted relative risks showed a positive trend in both sexes, but the effect was stronger in men, where drinkers of from 1 to 30 ml a day had a risk of 2.2 (95% CI 1.1–4.4) and those who drank more than 30 ml had a risk of 2.4 (95% CI 1.3–4.5) compared to nondaily drinkers. Hirayama reported that daily beer drinkers among a large cohort of Japanese men were 1.7 times more likely to develop cancer of the colon than other groups (87). Thus, most prospective studies have supported some degree of association with cancer of the colon or rectum. Unfortunately none of these studies has included dietary factors in their analysis, so possible confounding by diet cannot be ruled out.

Proposed mechanisms for carcinogenesis of the large bowel are complex and include hypotheses related to dietary fiber, fat, animal protein, and total calories, in addition to the potential deleterious role of bile salts on gut bacteria (221,222,262). The modest risk posed by alcohol, if it is real, is not likely to explain as much of colorectal cancer incidence as these dietary factors. The repeatedly confirmed relationship between rectal cancers and beer, however, may suggest a unique role for the constituents in beer (163), although it is also possible that some unknown confounding factor associated with beer consumption is responsible. Known carcinogens including nitrosamines (189) are found in alcoholic beverages, and, as mentioned above, substances other than ethanol may play a role in the excess risk noted for head and neck (62) and esophageal cancers (115).

Although the strength of the relationship of alcohol with colon and rectal cancers is a weak one, if the relationship is real, the high incidence of these cancers would lead to a substantial proportion of colorectal cancers attributable to alcohol. It is especially difficult to estimate the population-attributable fraction due to alcohol for these cancers because of the variability of results and because these results have not always distinguished between men and women and between colon and rectum. In addition many studies have reported elevated risks for beer consumption and rectal cancer only. Nevertheless, if the relative risks reported from the prospective studies mentioned above are confirmed, one could estimate that 25% of rectal cancers and 15% of colon cancers are attributable to alcohol. In 1991 there will be an estimated 112,000 new colon and 45,000 new rectal cancers in the United States (209), and thus 16,800 and 11,375 could be attributable to alcohol, respectively.

Liver

The liver is another site where cancer has been associated with alcohol consumption, even though undiluted alcohol does not come in direct contact with hepatic tissues. Of all the nongastrointestinal cancer sites with reported associations with alcohol, such as breast, pancreas, and bladder, the evidence in support of some etiologic relationship with cancer of the liver is perhaps the strongest. However, among the established risk factors for hepatocellular carcinoma, alcohol is substantially less important than hepatitis B viral (HBV) infection (26).

In countries of Asia and Africa where primary liver cancer is most prevalent, the role of HBV in its etiology is most clearly prominent (60). Other risk factors include cigarette smoking (165,255), blood transfusions (25,50), and perhaps aflatoxins (60,253). The potential importance of alcohol, smoking, and perhaps other factors is suggested by the observation in Japan that the incidence of primary liver cancer has been increasing while the prevalence of hepatitis B surface antigen (HBsAg) positive among persons with this cancer has dropped substantially (50). However, some studies indicate no more than a weak contribution by both alcohol and cigarettes to primary liver cancer in the United States (7).

The role of alcoholic cirrhosis in hepatocellular carcinoma is controversial. Although the association has been shown in North America and western Europe, where alcoholic cirrhosis is common (200), there is some evidence that liver cancer occurs in alcoholics even without cirrhosis (207). Furthermore, evidence has been accumulating that infection with HBV is more prevalent in alcoholics than in the general population (259), and among cirrhotics those who are HBsAg positive are at substantially higher risk that those who are HBsAg negative (175).

In studies of brewery workers, alcoholics, and other heavy consumers of alcohol, evidence of an increased incidence of liver cancer has been found in Finland (82), Denmark (88), and Ireland (86), but not in Canada (84) or the United States (77). Among Mormons, a significantly lower incidence ratio was observed (35,184).

For case-control studies that have evaluated the relationship of alcohol consumption to liver cancer, there are again disparities between those conducted in different countries. In the United States (17,158,171,180), Europe (175,256), and Japan (25), the relationship is supported by most, although not all studies (175). In studies conducted in other parts of Asia (165,258) and Africa (257), where the prevalence of liver cancer is much higher, the connection with alcohol consumption is generally absent.

Case-control studies that have examined the role of alcohol, HBV, and cirrhosis together are few (175). Yu et al. found a dose-response relationship with alcohol, which was significant for women over 50 years at diagnosis (7). The estimated relative risk for women who consumed >1 drink per day versus <1 drink per day was 2.1 (95% CI 1.0–4.5). This analysis, which was controlled for smoking and other risk factors, did not include any measure of HBV infection.

A similar study by Austin et al. (17), which did control for HBsAg status, found no relation with cigarette smoking but an almost threefold increased risk associated with moderate alcohol consumption (one or more drinks per day). The study also showed a significant dose-response relationship with both the highest levels of lifetime consumption of alcohol and with cumulative alcohol consumption (17).

The putative dose of alcohol capable of increasing the risk of primary liver cancer is inconsistent among published studies. The threefold increase for persons who consumed one or more drinks per day reported by Austin et al. (17) contrasts with a similar level of risk only for heavy drinkers in other studies. In two recent case-control studies in Japan, which examined alcohol, HBV status, smoking status, and history of blood transfusions (25,50), both found an increased risk for all these factors with and an increased relative risks for heavy drinking of 2.5 (25) and approximately three (50).

Cohort studies, primarily performed in Japan (19,168,170), support the causal role of alcohol suggested by the case-control studies in Western countries. Strong positive associations between alcohol and liver cancer have been noted in studies among Japanese men who were HBsAg positive after control for smoking (168). Dose-response relationships with a relative risk of 8.0 for heavy (>80 ml alcohol per day) were found. Similarly, a long-term cohort study of 639 Japanese fishermen found a dose-response relationship with liver cancer for consumption of shoche, a distilled beverage containing approximately 25% alcohol, and a relative risk of 14.3 (95% CI 3.6–56.6) for the highest category (>360 ml per day) (170). In Germany a prospective study of cirrhotics with excess alcohol consumption found that those who also had HBV infection had a higher incidence of hepatocellular carcinoma than those without it (252). Likewise, Nakanuma and Ohta in Japan (254) found that the incidence of liver cancer among HBsAg-positive alcoholics was almost three times as high as in HBsAg negative alcoholics.

An attributable risk of 24% for heavy drinking has been calculated in Japan (50). Rothman estimated that in the United States the attributable risk was on the same order of magnitude at 30% (123). Thus, approximately 4500 of the 15,000 primary liver cancers estimated for 1991 in the United States (209) could have been due to alcohol.

Pancreas

An epidemiologic search for a direct link between pancreatic cancer and alcohol consumption has been pursued because this cancer is often observed in persons with chronic pancreatitis (16), which commonly results from habitual alcohol abuse (90). Recent reviews on this subject have concluded that the evidence for this association is weak (16,38). Several more recent studies have confirmed this conclusion (6,8,30,52,67).

Until recently, none of the prospective studies of alcoholics (77,82,84,85,90,92) or brewery workers (86,88) showed any increased risk. In one study of Swedish brewery workers, the relative risk was 1.7 (95% CI 1.2–2.3), but cigarette smoking, a known risk factor (6), was uncontrolled and could have been responsible for the association (51). Correlation studies of pancreatic cancer rates with per capita consumption of alcohol derived from tax figures (275,219) found positive associations, while other similar studies done with alcohol and tobacco consumption data collected from interviews in Hawaii have been negative (112). As mentioned above, the reliability of either positive or negative correlations from studies of this nature are limited (16).

Fourteen case-control studies, primarily motivated by an interest in a possible link between coffee and pancreatic cancer, have also examined alcohol intake. Eleven of these have been negative (8,30,52,67,149,151–154,164,166), while only three have suggested that alcohol might play some role (13,156,161). In England, Durbec et al. (156) found an estimated relative risk of 2.7 (95% CI 1.2–4.3) among persons who consumed more than 40 g of alcohol a day, and Cuzick and Babiker (13) found a relative risk of 3.2 ($p < 0.05$) for beer drinkers of >7 pints per week with a significant linear trend. Most recently, in a study of 212 pancreatic cancer cases in Minnesota, Olsen et al. (263) reported an odds ratio of 2.7 (95% CI 1.0–7.3) for heavy drinkers of four or more drinks per day.

At least four cohort studies have examined the association of alcohol and pancreatic cancer (6,91,150,220). Hirayama's most recent report from a large cohort study in Japan found no excess risk in 12 years of follow-up (220). Klatsky et al. originally reported on a cohort study of health plan members, where they found a nonsignificant elevated risk of 3.0 for heavy consumers (six or more drinks a day) compared to nondrinkers, based on only six cases. In a later cohort study in the same health plan population with more detailed information available on alcohol consumption and 48 incident cases, Hiatt et al. found no elevated risk (6). The only positive prospective study was that of Heuch et al. in Norway (150). A cohort of 16,713 men who reported frequent use of alcoholic beverages (>14 times a month) showed an elevated risk of 2.7 compared to nondrinkers and a "limited use" category. When men without histologically confirmed cancers and information on cigarette consumption were excluded, 13 of their 16 cases were eliminated and the relative risk increased to 8.0 with wide confidence intervals (91).

According to the current state of knowledge, it seems unlikely that alcohol consumption is linked to pancreatic cancer. Therefore, none of the estimated 28,200 incident cases anticipated in the United States in 1991 can be attributed to alcohol consumption (209).

Breast

Perhaps more has been written about alcohol and breast cancer in the last 5 years than any of the other cancers discussed thus far. Although part of this activity stems from the fact that the relationship between the two represents a new hypothesis, a motivating force for many has been the high prevalence of breast cancer and the relatively large impact even a small attributable risk could make on disease outcomes and the public health. Thus far, much of the evidence accumulated supports a causal relationship, but the data are not entirely consistent. Several comprehensive reviews have recently been published that highlight the results and controversial issues (129–131,225,277).

There is little literature to support the relationship between heavy consumption of alcohol and breast cancer, because most of the studies of heavy alcohol consumers are based on men only. Adelstein and White reported a twofold increase in breast cancer among women admitted to hospitals with a diagnosis of alcoholism in England (79), whereas Monson and Lyon found none in Massachusetts (77). Among Mormons in Utah the standardized incidence was significantly less than expected (35), and in Seventh-day Adventists in California breast cancer mortality was approximately 15% lower than for matched non–Seventh-day Adventists (226). Correlation studies of alcohol consumption and breast cancer mortality have been positive in the United States (275), although not internationally (61).

The hypothesis that alcohol might increase the risk of breast cancer was generated by the case-control study of Williams and Horm in 1977 (78), based on data from the Third National Cancer Survey in the United States. They estimated that women who drank over 51 ounces of alcohol a year were 60% more likely to develop breast cancer than nondrinkers. Rosenberg reported that hospitalized women with breast cancer were 90% more likely to drink alcohol than hospitalized women without cancer (80). Subsequently, at least 21 case-control and six cohort studies in the English language literature have examined this question. Among the studies that followed the study of Williams and Horm that generated the hypothesis (78), 13 have supported it (11,12,15,37,39,74,80, 134–138,140) and seven have not (14,22,64,133,141–143), including the Cancer and Steroid Hormone Study (64), with 3498 cases. Among studies where alcohol has been implicated, all types of alcoholic beverages have conferred increased risks and no particular type seems to be favored (225).

The first cohort study to focus on alcohol and breast cancer was published in 1984 and was based on 95,000 women who were members of a large health plan in California (81). Women who reported consuming three or more drinks a day had a 40% increased risk. Four more cohort studies have followed (29,119,120), plus a reanalysis of the data in a large American Cancer Society cohort study in which the association of alcohol and breast cancer was not fully examined (139). To date, five of six cohort studies have reported an association (29,81,119, 120,139), while a smaller report from the Framingham Heart Study was negative (132).

In almost all positive studies of alcohol and breast cancer, the magnitude of risk for moderate use has varied between 1.4 and 3.0, and is seldom higher. These have been referred to as "weak" associations (133). Although there is concern that the weaker the association, the more likely it is to be explained by bias, confounding factors, or by inappropriate analysis, this concern is diminished by the many studies consistently demonstrating the same rather low level of increased risk.

Simply summarizing studies as positive or negative inadequately represents their quality in terms of the influence of chance, confounding factors, and bias. Unlike studies of other sites, studies of breast cancer and alcohol have benefited from a meta-analysis in which all studies are placed in a hierarchy according to preset criteria of quality and the results of each study are expressed in a common form (128). Longnecker and his colleagues found a clearly elevated, although modest, risk of 1.4 (95% CI 1.0–1.8) in case-control studies and 1.7 (95% CI 1.4–2.2) in follow-up studies. Trends of increased risk with increasing levels of reported consumption were noted with both groups of studies (128).

In the studies that have been able to evaluate it, the effects of diet, a potential confounding factor, have not influenced the results in any important way (15,22,54,119,120,139). Most recognized breast cancer risk factors are weakly associated with the disease, and in order for some as yet confounding factor to explain away the alcohol association, it would have to be much more strongly related to breast cancer than those currently identified. In addition, since some studies have suggested that the relative risks of heavy drinking are above 2.5 (11,54,81,119), the possibility of an unrecognized confounder seems unlikely.

There is, as yet, no known biologic mechanism by which alcohol consumption leads to carcinogenesis in the breast, although research in this area is being actively pursued. A direct effect on breast tissue is possible since alcohol appears in human milk after alcohol is consumed (227). There could also be indirect effects through the influence of alcohol on liver enzymes, which are important in the metabolism of carcinogens (228). Alcohol also inhibits the hepatic metabolism of estrogens, which have long been of primary concern in the etiology of breast cancer (4). Alcohol has a direct stimulatory effect on prolactin secretion from the pituitary, and elevated prolactin has also been hypothesized to have a role (127). Finally, it has been suggested that reduced pineal melatonin production might increase the risk of breast cancer in humans (229), and alcohol has been shown to suppress melatonin production in rats (230). A possible biologic pathway is further suggested by the observation that melatonin suppresses prolactin production by the pituitary and estrogen by the ovary (231). With low levels of melatonin, increased prolactin and estrogen effects may act to promote carcinogenesis in the breast.

Stampfer and his colleagues summarized the data they reviewed and concluded that there is a 50–100% increased risk of breast cancer associated with one to two drinks per day (1). Two other investigators produced estimates of 13 and 14% (81,128) attributable risk for the general population. Since breast cancer is a common disease, these percentages would translate into 19,617–21,126 new breast cancer cases that could be attributed to alcohol consumption in 1991 in the United States alone (209). Since little is available in the way of primary prevention of breast cancer and only 25% breast cancer can be accounted for by known risk factors (232), the potential public health significance of alcohol is substantial.

Other Sites

Several other cancer sites have been the focus of studies of alcohol consumption including lung, bladder, ovary, prostate and cervix. For none of these sites is there strong support for a putative role of alcohol consumption.

Lung cancer mortality was elevated among cohorts of heavy alcohol consumers in Finland (82) and Canada (92), but these investigators concluded the association was confounded by smoking, which they could not control. Later Pollack et al. (76) found a significantly increased risk of 2.2 ($p = 0.03$) for Japanese men in Hawaii consuming 50 or more ounces of wine per month even after controlling for smoking. There was also a significant dose-response relationship.

One study from Germany has suggested that the risk of bladder cancer in men was 2.8 for drinkers of one liter of beer or more a day and 2.7 for more than 0.5 liters a week of spirits after control for smoking (40,66). However, at least six other case-control studies, both before and after publication of the German study, have not confirmed this finding (59,70,72,73,173,251).

Prostate cancer has been evaluated in an early case-control study by Wynder et al. (179), and in the Williams and Horm (78) study based on the Third National Cancer Survey, without any apparent positive associations. Other studies since that time, including a case-control study that used patients with benign prostatic hyperplasia as controls (55) and a large prospective study of 79,000 men taking a multiphasic health checkup (260), have confirmed the absence of any relationship of alcohol consumption with prostatic cancer.

Case-control studies of ovarian (65,69) and cervical cancer (278) that have examined alcohol intake have been negative. However, in the Cancer and Steroid Hormone study, nondrinking women actually had an increased risk of 1.83 (95% CI 1.11–3.01) for endometrial cancer relative to women who consumed an average of 150 g or more of alcohol per week (75). The authors offered the explanation that this elevated risk among abstainers, which was especially strong among overweight women, may be due to an attenuating effect of alcohol on the conversion of estrogen in adipose tissue. However, other studies that have examined alcohol consumption and endometrial cancer have found no such protective relationship (78,246).

Finally, a weak association of alcohol consumption with melanoma has been reported (71,267). Beer drinkers were more likely to develop nodular melanoma in a study by Holman et al. (267), and persons consuming more than 10 g per day (or less than a drink a day) had an odds ratio of 2.0. In another case-control study that included 204 cases of melanoma, a significant dose-response ($p < 0.03$) was observed with odds of 1.8 (95% CI 1.0–3.3) for persons who consumed over 10 g per day (71). Other investigations are compatible with no greater than a modest association (78).

CONCLUSIONS

The Effects of Moderate Dose

At the time when the attributable risk of alcohol was assessed by Doll and Peto, the impact was considered to be the result only of heavy consumption (233). Heavy consumption has been defined as an average of one or more ounces of ethanol a day or roughly 2 or more drinks a day of a standard-sized alcoholic beverage (204,266). The possible impact of moderate and perhaps even light consumption now merits consideration. Recent estimates define approximately 9% of the adults in the United States as heavy drinkers, 24% as moderate, and a third each as light drinkers and abstainers (204). Moderate consumption has been defined as from 0.22 to 0.99 oz of ethanol a day or, roughly 6.5–30 g (or one-half to two drinks) a day, while light consumption could be defined as one drink a month to one drink every 2 days (266). Breast cancer has been most prominently associated with increased risk at moderate levels of intake (225) and at least one investigator has associated significant risk with light consumption (119). Colon and rectal cancers have also been linked to moderate consumption by several investigators (10,76,203). These two major sites alone require a reassessment of the potential putative effects of alcohol at moderate levels of consumption. Moreover, in addition to the common cancers of the breast and colorectum, it may be valuable to reexamine the effect of moderate consumption on cancers more traditionally associated with heavy consumption—those of the upper aerodigestive tract. Recent detailed studies suggest that there is a statistically significant elevated risk of oral cancer for consumers of moderate levels of alcohol (3,101).

Attributable Risk

The possibility that cancers other than those of the upper aerodigestive tract may be related to alcohol consumption raises the question of the potential attributable risk from alcohol for all cancer. Doll and Peto's often quoted estimate of 3% (233), also suggested by Rothman (123), was based solely on cancers of the mouth, pharynx, larynx, esophagus, and liver, and there was even a portion of this percentage that could not be separated out from the effects of tobacco. If the proportions used by Rothman 10 years ago were to be used for these same cancers today and based on estimates of expected deaths from cancer in 1991 (209), the overall percentage of cancer attributable to alcohol use would still be only 3%, or approximately 16,517 cancer deaths. If, however, cancers of the breast, rectum, and colon are included, and crude approximations of the population attributable fraction are made as was done above, then cancer deaths attributable to alcohol could be as much as 6% and incident cancer as much as 8%. These estimates suggest that the potential public health implications could be substantially greater than appreciated thus far.

Public Health Implications

Although alcohol has been part of the diet of most cultures since the beginning of recorded history and shows no sign of disappearing soon from human societies, there are clearly serious health and social consequences to its use and abuse. Its role in carcinogenesis has been documented for many years for cancer of the upper aerodigestive tract among heavy consumers. The more recent association with cancers of the breast and colorectum at moderate doses has stimulated concern for a possible larger public health role of alcohol in carcinogenesis than previously thought. However, in considering the overall effects of alcohol use at moderate levels, the potential beneficial effects on cardiovascular mortality must also be considered (269). According to some studies, moderate alcohol intake may reduce the risk of heart disease and total mortality (91,121). In 1987, heart diseases caused 35 and 37% of the deaths in the United States for men and women, respectively, while breast cancer causes only 4% and colorectal cancer only 2.5 and 2.8% of deaths for men and women, respectively (209). In view of the current methodologic problems of measurement and other uncertainties of the risk for cancer associated with light or moderate intake of alcohol (269) and the possibility of some beneficial effects for cardiovascular disease, no general public health action seems appropriate. However, women and men with risk factors for breast and colorectal cancer, but not for heart diseases, may benefit by limiting their use of alcoholic beverages.

ACKNOWLEDGMENTS

The comments of Arthur L. Klatsky and Lorraine T. Midanik were appreciated in the preparation of this manuscript.

REFERENCES

1. M. J. Stampfer, G. A. Colditz, and W. C. Willett, Alcohol intake and risk of breast cancer, *Compr. Ther.*, *14*, 8–15 (1988).
2. A. Nomura, J. S. Grove, G. N. Stemmermann, and R. K. Severson. A prospective study of stomach cancer and its relation to diet, cigarettes, and alcohol consumption, *Cancer Res.*, *50*, 627-631 (1990).
3. W. J. Blot, J. K. McLaughlin, D. M. Winn, D. F. Austin, et al., Smoking and drinking in relation to oral and pharyngeal cancer, *Cancer Res.*, *48*, 3282–3287 (1988).
4. J. L. Kelsey, and G. S. Berkowitz. Breast cancer epidemiology, *Cancer Res.*, *48*, 5615–5623 (1988).
5. J. Meara, K. McPherson, and M. Roberts. Alcohol, cigarette smoking and breast cancer, *Br. J. Cancer*, *60*, 70–73 (1989).
6. R. A. Hiatt, A. L. Klatsky, and M. A. Armstrong. Pancreatic cancer, blood glucose and beverage consumption, *Int. J. Cancer*, *41*, 794–797 (1988).
7. H. Yu, R. E. Harris, G. C. Kabat, and E. L. Wynder. Cigarette smoking, alcohol consumption and primary liver cancer: A case-control study in the USA, *Int. J. Cancer*, *42*, 325–328 (1988).
8. F. Clavel, E. Benhamou, and A. Anquier. Coffee, alcohol, smoking and cancer of the pancreas, *Int. J. Cancer*, *43*, 17–21 (1989).
9. C. La Vecchia, and E. Negri. The role of alcohol in oesphageal cancer in non-smokers, and of tobacco in non-drinkers, *Int. J. Cancer*, *43*, 784–785 (1989).
10. A. Wu, A. Paganini-Hill, and R. K. Ross. Alcohol, physical activity and other risk factors for colorectal cancer: A prospective study, *Br. J. Cancer*, *55*, 687–694 (1987).
11. S. Richardson, I. de Vincenzi, and H. Pujol. Alcohol consumption in a case-control study of breast cancer in southern France, *Int. J. Cancer*, *44*, 84–89 (1989).
12. T. E. Rohan, and A. J. McMichael. Alcohol consumption and risk of breast cancerr, *Int. J. Cancer*, *41*, 695–699 (1989).
13. J. Cuzick and A. G. Babiker. Pancreatic cancer, alcohol, diabetes mellitus and gallbladder disease, *Int. J. Cancer*, *43*, 415–421 (1989).
14. H. O. Adami, E. Lund, and R. Bergstrom. Cigarette smoking, alcohol consumption and risk of breast cancer in young women, *Br. J. Cancer*, *58*, 832–837 (1988).
15. P. Toniolo, E. Riboli, and F. Protta. Breast cancer and alcohol consumption: A case-control study in northern Italy, *Cancer Res.*, *49*, 5203–5206 (1989).
16. J. P. Velema, A. M. Walker, and E. B. Gold. Alcohol and pancreatic cancer. Insufficient epidemiologic evidence for a causal relationship, *Epidemiol. Rev.*, *8*, 28–41 (1986).
17. H. Austin, E. Delzell, and S. Grufferman. A case-control study of hepatocellular carcinoma and hepatitis B virus, cigarette smoking, and alcohol consumption, *Cancer Res.*, *46*, 962–966 (1986).
18. S. Kune, G. A. Kune, and L. F. Watson. Case-control study of alcoholic beverages as etiologic factors: The Melbourne Colorectal Cancer Study, *Nutr. Cancer*, *9*, 43–56 (1987).
19. K. Kono, M. Ikeda, and S. Tokudome. Cigarette smoking, alcohol and cancer mortality: A cohort study of male Japanese physicians, *Jpn. J. Cancer Res.*, *78*, 1323–1328 (1987).

20. J. L. Frudenheim, S. Graham, and J. R. Marshall. Lifetime alcohol intake and risk of rectal cancer in western New York, *Nutr. Cancer, 13*, 101–109 (1990).
21. I. Kato, S. Tominaga, and A. Ikari. A case-control study of male colorectal cancer in Aichi Prefecture, Japan: With special reference to occupational activity level, drinking habits and family history, *Jpn. J. Cancer Res., 81*, 115–121 (1990).
22. L. Rosenberg, J. R. Palmer, and D. R. Miller. A case-control study of alcoholic beverage consumption and breast cancer, *Am. J. Epidemiol., 131*, 6–14 (1990).
23. F. La Rosa, A. Cresci, and C. Orpianesi. Esophageal cancer mortality: Relationship with alcohol intake and cigarette smoking in Italy, *Eur. J. Epidemiol., 4*, 93–98 (1988).
24. A. B. Lowenfels, and S. A. Zevola. Alcohol and breast cancer: An overview, *Alcoholism, 13*, 109–111 (1989).
25. K. Tanaka, T. Hirohata, and S. Takeshita, Blood transfusion, alcohol consumption, and cigarette smoking in causation of hepatocellular carcinoma: A case-control study in Fukuoka, Japan, *Jpn. J. Cancer Res., 79*, 1075–1082 (1988).
26. A. J. Garro, and C. S. Lieber. Alcohol and cancer, *Annu. Rev. Pharmacol. Toxicol., 30*, 219–249 (1990).
27. R. T. Falk, L. W. Pickle, and L. M. Brown. Effect of smoking and alcohol consumption on laryngeal cancer risk in coastal Texas, *Cancer Res., 49*, 4024–4029 (1989).
28. M. C. Yu, D. H. Garabrant, and J. M. Peters. Tobacco, alcohol, diet, occupation and carcinoma of the esophagus, *Cancer Res., 48*, 3843–3848 (1988).
29. R. A. Hiatt, A. L. Klatsky, and M. A. Armstrong. Alcohol consumption and the risk of breast cancer in a prepaid health plan, *Cancer Res., 48*, 2284–2287 (1988).
30. D. C. Farrow, and S. Davis. Risk of pancreatic cancer in relation to medical history and the use of tobacco, alcohol and coffee, *Int. J. Cancer, 45*, 816–820 (1990).
31. R. C. Brownson and J. C. Chang. Exposure to alcohol and tobacco and the risk of laryngeal cancer, *Arch. Environ. Health, 42*, 192–196 (1987).
32. M. Jarebinski, H. Vlajinac, and B. Adanja. Biosocial and other characteristics of the large bowel cancer patients in Belgrade (Yugoslavia), *Arch. Geschwulstforsch, 58*, 411–417 (1988).
33. A. H. Wu-Williams, M. C. Yu, and T. M. Mack. Life-style, workplace, and stomach cancer by subsite in young men of Los Angeles County, *Cancer Res., 50*, 2569–2576 (1990).
34. R. R. Watson. Ethanol, immunomodulation and cancer, *Prog. Food Nutr. Sci., 12*, 189–209 (1988).
35. J. L. Lyon, J. W. Gardner, and D. W. West. Cancer risk and life-style: Cancer among Mormons from 1967–1975, *Basic Life Sci., 43*, 137–161 (1988).
36. P. Guenel, H. Moller, and E. Lynge. Incidence of the upper respiratory and digestive tract cancers and consumption of alcohol and tobacco in Denmark, *Scand. J. Soc. Med., 16*, 257–263 (1988).
37. I. Kato, S. Tominaga, and C. Terao. Alcohol consumption and cancers of hormone-related organs in females, *Jpn. J. Clin. Oncol., 19*, 202–207 (1989).
38. P. Boyle, C. C. Hsieh, and P. Maisonneuve. Epidemiology of pancreas cancer (1988), *Int. J. Pancreatol., 5*, 327–346 (1989).

39. D. I. Smith. Relationship between alcohol consumption and breast cancer morbidity rates in western Australia, 1971–1984, *Drug Alcohol Depend.*, *24*, 61–65 (1989).
40. E. Kunze, J. Claude, and R. Frentzel-Beyme. Association of cancer of the lower urinary tract with consumption of alcoholic beverages. A case-control study. *Carcinogenesis*, *7*, 163–165 (1986).
41. D. N. Rao, L., D. Snghvi, and P. B. Desai. Epidemiology of esophageal cancer, *Semin. Surg. Oncol.*, *5*, 351–354 (1989).
42. H. Moller. Changing incidence of cancer of the tongue, oral cavity, and pharynx in Denmark, *J. Oral. Pathol. Med.*, *18*, 224–229 (1989).
43. A. J. Tuyns, E. Riboli, G. Doornbos, and G. Pequignot. Diet and esophageal cancer in Calvados (France), *Nutr. Cancer*, *9*, 81–92 (1987).
44. S. I. Mufti, H. R. Darban, and R. R. Watson, Alcohol, cancer and immunomodulation, *Crit. Rev. Oncol. Hemat.*, *9*, 243–261 (1989).
45. A. J. Tuyns, J. Esteve, and L. Raymond. Cancer of the larynx/hypopharynx, tobacco and alcohol: IARC international case-control study, *Int. J. Cancer*, *41*, 483–491 (1988).
46. J. F. Hu, S. F. Zhang, and E. M. Jia. Diet and cancer of the stomach: A case-control study in China, *Int. J. Cancer*, *41*, 331–335 (1988).
47. E. L. Franco, L. P. Kowalski, and B. V. Olivera. Risk factors for oral cancer in Brazil: A case-control study, *Int. J. Cancer*, *43*, 992–1000 (1989).
48. R. Sankaranarayana, S. W. Duffy, and N. E. Day. A case-control investigation of cancer of the oral tongue and the floor of the mouth in Southern India, *Int. J. Cancer*, *44*, 617–621 (1989).
49. M. A. Rossing, T. L. Vaughan, and B. McKnight. Diet and pharyngeal cancer, *Int. J. Cancer*, *44*, 593–597 (1989).
50. H. Tsukama, T. Hiyana, and A. Oshima. A case-control study of hepatocellular carcinoma in Osaka, Japan, *Int. J. Cancer*, *45*, 231–236 (1990).
51. J. M. Carstensen, L. O. Bygren, and T. Hatschek. Cancer incidence among Swedish brewery workers, *Int. J. Cancer*, *45*, 393–396 (1990).
52. C. Bouchardy, F. Clavel and C. La Vecchia. Alcohol, beer and cancer of the pancreas, *Int. J. Cancer*, *45*, 842–846 (1990).
53. R. Sankaranarayanan, S. W. Duffy, and M. K. Nair. Tobacco and alcohol as risk factors in cancer of the larynx in Kerala, India, *Int. J. Cancer*, *45*, 879–882 (1990).
54. C. La Vecchia, E. Negri, and F. Parazzini. Alcohol and breast cancer: update from an Italian case-control study, *Eur. J. Cancer Clin. Oncol.*, *25*, 1711–1717 (1989).
55. H. Checkoway, G. DiFerdinando, B. Hulka, and D. D. Mickey. Medical, life-style, and occupational risk factors for prostate cancer, *Prostate*, *10*, 79–88 (1987).
56. H. K. Seitz, and U. A. Simanowski. Alcohol and carcinogenesis, *Ann. Rev. Nutr.*, *8*, 99–119 (1988).
57. P. Prior, Long-term cancer risk in alcoholism, *Alcohol Alcohol*, *23*, 163–171 (1988).
58. A. J. McMichael and A. Puzio. Time trends in upper alimentary tract cancer rates and alcohol and tobacco consumption in Australia, *Community Health Stud.*, *12*, 289–295 (1988).
59. M. P. Bravo, J. Del Rey Calero, and M. Conde. Bladder cancer and the consumption of alcoholic beverages in Spain, *Eur. J. Epidemiol.*, *3*, 365–369 (1987).

60. M. F. Bassendine. Aetiolgical factors in hepatocellular cancer, *Baillieres Clinical Gastroenterology, 1*, 1–16 (1987).
61. A. Schatzkin, S. Piantadosi, M. Micozzi, and D. Bartee. Alcohol consumption and breast cancer: a cross-national correlation study, *Int. J. Epidemiol., 18*, 28–31 (1989).
62. K. J. Rothman, C. I. Cann, and M. P. Fried. Carcinogenecity of dark liquor, *A. J. Public Health, 79*, 1516–1520 (1989).
63. A. E. Rogers and M. W. Conner, Alcohol and cancer, *Adv. Exp. Med. Biol., 206*, 473–495 (1986).
64. S. Y. Chu, N. C. Lee, P. A. Wingo, and L. A. Webster. Alcohol consumption and the risk of breast cancer, *Am. J. Epidemiol., 130*, 867–877 (1989).
65. A. S. Whittemore, M. L. Wu, and R. S. Paffenbarger. Personal and environmental characteristics related to epithelial ovarian cancer, *Am. J. Epidemiol., 128*, 1228–1240 (1988).
66. J. Claude, E. Kunze, and R. Frentzel-Beyme. Life-style and occupational risk factors in cancer of the lower urinary tract, *Am. J. Epidemiol., 124*, 578–589 (1986).
67. S. E. Norell, A. Ahlbom, and R. Erwald. Diet and pancreatic cancer: a case-control study, *Am. J. Epidemiol., 124*, 894–902 (1986).
68. R. T. Zagraniski, J. L. Kelsey, and S. D. Walter. Occupational risk factors for laryngeal carcinoma: Connecticut, 1975–1980, *Am. J. Epidemiol., 124*, 167–176 (1986).
69. M. L. Gwinn, L. A. Webster, and N. C. Lee. Alcohol consumption and ovarian cancer risk, *Am. J. Epidemiol., 123*, 759–766 (1986).
70. H. A. Risch, D. Burch, and A. B. Miller. Dietary factors and the incidence of cancer of the urinary bladder, *Am. J. Epidemiol., 127*, 1179–1191 (1988).
71. W. S. Stryker, M. J. Stampfer, and E. A. Stein. Diet, plasma levels of beta-carotine and alpha-tocopherol, and risk of malignant melanoma, *Am. J. Epidemiol., 131*, 597–611 (1990).
72. A. Nomura, L. N. Kolonel, and C. N. Yoshizawa. Smoking, alcohol, occupation, and hair dye use in cancer of the lower urinary tract, *Am. J. Epidemiol., 130*, 1159–1163 (1989).
73. R. C. Brownson, J. C. Chang, and J. R. Davis. Occupation, smoking and alcohol in the epidemiology of bladder cancer, *Am. J. Public Health, 77*, 1298–1300 (1987).
74. P. Van't Veer, F. J. Kok, R. J. J. Hermus, and F. Sturmans. Alcohol dose, frequency and age at first exposure in relation to the risk of breast cancer, *Int. J. Epidemiol., 18*, 511–517 (1989).
75. L. A. Webster and N. S. Weiss. Alcoholic beverage consumption and the risk of endometrial cancer, *Int. J. Epidemiol., 18*, 786–791 (1989).
76. E. S. Pollack, M. Abraham, and Y. Nomura. Prospective study of alcohol consumption and cancer, *N. Engl. J. Med., 310*, 617–621 (1984).
77. R. R. Monson and J. L. Lyon. Proportional mortality among alcoholics, *Cancer, 36*, 1077–1079 (1975).
78. R. R. Williams and J. W. Horm. Interview study from the third national cancer survey: association of cancer sites with tobacco and alcohol consumption and socioeconomic status of patients, *JNCI, 58*, 525–547 (1977).
79. A. Adelstein and G. White. Alcoholism and mortality, *Popul. Trends, 6*, 7–13 (1976).
80. L. Rosenberg. Breast cancer and alcoholic-beverage consumption, *Lancet, 1*, 267–271 (1982).

81. R. A. Hiatt and R. D. Bawol. Alcoholic beverage consumption and breast cancer incidence, *Am. J. Epidemiol., 120*, 676–683 (1984).
82. T. Hakulinen, L. Lehtimaki, M. Lehtonen, and L. Teppo. Cancer mortality among two male cohorts with increased alcohol consumption in Finland, *JNCI, 52*, 1711–1714 (1974).
83. S. Pell and C. A. D'Alonzo. A five-year mortality study of alcoholics, *J. Occup. Med., 15*, 120–125 (1973).
84. W. Schmidt and J. de Lint. Causes of death of alcoholics, *Q. J. Stud. Alcohol., 33*, 171–185 (1972).
85. P. Nicholls, G. Edwards, and E. Kyle. Alcoholics admitted to four hospitals in England, II. General and cause-specific mortality, *Q. J. Stud. Alcohol, 35*, 841–855 (1974).
86. G. Dean, R. MacLennan, H. McLoughlin, and E. Shelley. Causes of death of blue-collar workers at a Dublin brewery, *Br. J. Cancer, 40*, 581–589 (1979).
87. T. Hirayama. Changing patterns of cancer in Japan with special reference to the decrease in stomach cancer mortality, in *Origins of Human Cancer*, Book A, *Incidence of Cancer in Humans* (H. H. Hiatt, J. D. Watson, and J. A. Winsten, eds.), CSH Press, Cold Spring Harbor, NY, 1977, pp. 55–75.
88. O. M. Jensen. Cancer morbidity and causes of death among Danish brewery workers, *Cancer, 23*, 454–463 (1979).
89. O. M. Jensen. Cancer risk among Danish male Seventh-day Adventists and other temperance society members, *JNCI, 70*, 1011–1014 (1983).
90. C. D. Robinette, Z. Hrubec, and J. F. Fraumeni, Jr. Chronic alcoholism and subsequent mortality in World War II veterans, *Am. J. Epidemiol., 109*, 687–700 (1979).
91. A. L. Klatsky, G. D. Friedman, and A. B. Siegelaub. Alcohol and mortality: A ten-year Kaiser-Permanente experience, *Ann. Intern. Med., 95*, 139–145 (1981).
92. W. Schmidt and R. E. Popham. The role of drinking and smoking in mortality from cancer and other causes in male alcoholics, *Cancer, 47*, 1031–1041 (1981).
93. S. Kono, M. Ikeda, and M. Ogata. The relationship between alcohol and mortality among Japanese physicians, *Int. J. Epidemiol., 12*, 437–441 (1983).
94. S. Kono, M. Ikeda, and S. Tokudome. Alcohol and mortality: A cohort study of male Japanese physicians, *Int. J. Epidemiol., 15*, 527–532 (1986).
95. K. J. Rothman and A. Z. Keller. The effect of joint exposure to alcohol and tobacco on risk of cancer of the mouth and pharynx, *J. Chron. Dis., 25*, 711–716 (1972).
96. E. L. Wynder, I. J. Bross, and R. A. Feldman. A study of etiological factors in cancer of the mouth, *Cancer, 10*, 1300–1323 (1957).
97. E. L. Wynder and I. J. Bross. A study of etiologic factors in cancer of the esophagus, *Cancer, 14*, 389–413 (1961).
98. I. Martinez. Factors associated with cancer of the esophagus, mouth and pharynx in Puerto Rico, *JNCI, 42*, 1069–1094 (1969).
99. A. J. Tuyns. Cancer of the esophagus; further evidence of the relation to drinking habits in France, *Int. J. Epidemiol., 5*, 152–156 (1970).
100. P. Cook. Cancer of the oesophagus in Africa, *Br. J. Cancer, 25*, 853–880 (1971).
101. S. Graham, H. Dayal, T. Rohrer, et al. Dentition, diet, tobacco and alcohol in the epidemiology of oral cancer, *JNCI, 59*, 1611–1618 (1977).

102. B. Herity, M. Moriarty, G. J. Bourke, et al. A case-control study of head and neck cancer in the Republic of Ireland, *Br. J. Cancer, 43*, 177–182 (1981).
103. W. D. Flanders and K. J. Rothman. Interaction of alcohol and tobacco in laryngeal cancer, *Am. J. Epidemiol., 115*, 371–379 (1982).
104. E. L. Wynder, L. S. Covey, K. Mabuchi, et al. Environmental factors in cancer of the larynx: A second look, *Cancer, 38*, 1591-1601 (1976).
105. J. G. Feldman and P. Boxer. Relationship of drinking to head and neck cancer, *Prev. Med., 8*, 507–519 (1979).
106. J. M. Elwood, J. C. G. Pearson, D. H. Skippen, et al. Alcohol, smoking, social and occupational factors in the aetiology of cancer of the oral cavity, pharynx and larynx, *Int. J. Cancer, 34*, 603–612 (1984).
107. G. D. McCoy, S. S. Hecht, and E. L. Wynder. The roles of tobacco, alcohol and diet in the etiology of upper alimentary and respiratory tract cancer, *Prev. Med., 9*, 622–629 (1980).
108. K. J. Rothman, C. I. Cann, D. Flanders, and M. P. Fried. Epidemiology of laryngeal cancer, *Epidemiol. Rev., 2*, 195–209 (1980).
109. T. Hirayama. An epidemiologic study of oral and pharyngeal cancer in Central and Southeast Asia, *Bull. World Health Org., 34*, 41–69 (1966).
110. Olsen, J., S. Sabroe, and U. Fasting. Interaction of alcohol and tobacco as risk factors in cancer of the laryngeal region, *J. Epidemiol. Commun. Health, 39*, 165–168 (1985).
111. E. L. Wynder and I. J. Bross. Etiologic factors in mouth cancer. An approach to its prevention, *Br. Med. J., i*, 1137-1143 (1957).
112. M. W. Hinds, L. N. Kolonel, J. Lee, and T. Hirohata. Associations between cancer incidence and alcohol cigarette consumption among five ethnic groups in Hawaii, *Br. J. Cancer, 41*, 929–940 (1980).
113. J. D. Burch, G. R. Howe, A. B. Miller, and R. Semenciw. Tobacco, alcohol, asbestos and nickel in the etiology of cancer of the larynx: A case-control study, *JNCI, 67*, 1219-1224 (1981).
114. U. W. DeJong, N. Breslow, J. Goh Ewe Hong, and et al. Aetiological factors in oesophageal cancer in Singapore Chinese. *Int. J. Cancer, 13*, 291-303 (1974).
115. A. J. Tuyns and G. Masse. Oesophageal cancer in non-smoking drinkers and in non-drinking smokers, *Int. J. Cancer, 32*, 443–444 (1983).
116. L. M. Pottern, L. E. Morris, W. J. Blot et al. Esophageal cancer among black men in Washington, D.C. I. Alcohol, tobacco, and other risk factors, *JNCI, 67*, 777–783 (1981).
117. A. Vassallo, P. Correa, E. De Stefani, et al. Oesophageal cancer in Uruguay: A case-control study, *JNCI, 75*, 1005–1009 (1985).
118. C. G. Victoria, N. Munoz, N. E. Day, et al. Hot beverages and oesophageal cancer in southern Brazil: A case-control study, *Int. J. Cancer, 39*, 710–716 (1987).
119. A. Schatzkin, Y. Jones, R. N. Hoover, et al. Alcohol consumption and breast cancer in the epidemiologic follow-up study of the first National Health and Nutrition Examination Survey, *N. Engl. J. Med., 316*, 1169–1173 (1987).
120. W. C. Willet, M. J. Stampfer, G. A. Colditz, et al. Moderate alcohol consumption and the risk of breast cancer, *N. Engl. J. Med., 316*, 1174–1180 (1987).

121. M. G. Marmot, G. Rose, M. J. Shipley, and B. J. Thomas. Alcohol and mortality: A U-shaped curve, *Lancet, i*, 580–1029 (1981).
122. L. T. Midanik. Validity of self-reported alcohol use: A literature review and assessment, *Br. J. Addict., 83*, 1019–1029 (1988).
123. K. J. Rothman. The proportion of cancer attributable to alcohol consumption, *Prev. Med., 9*, 174–179 (1980).
124. E. L. Wynder, S. Hultberg, F. Jacobsson, and I. J. Bross, Environmental factors in cancer of the upper alimentary tract. A Swedish study with special reference to Plummer-Vinson (Paterson-Kelly) syndrome, *Cancer, 10*, 470–486 (1957).
125. E. L. Wynder. A corner of history, *Prev. Med., 5*, 317–319 (1976).
126. G. D. McCoy and E. L. Wynder. Etiological and preventive implications in alcohol carcinogenesis, *Cancer Res., 39*, 2844–2850 (1979).
127. R. R. Williams. Breast and thyroid cancer and malignant melanoma promoted by alcohol-induced pituitary secretion of prolactin, T.S.H. and M.S.H., *Lancet, 1*, 996–999 (1976).
128. M. P. Longnecker, J. A. Berlin, and M. J. Orza. A meta-analysis of alcohol consumption in relation to risk of breast cancer, *JAMA, 260*, 652–656 (1988).
129. M. J. Stampfer, G. A. Colditz, and W. C. Willett. Alcohol intake and risk of breast cancer, *Compr. Ther., 14*, 8–15 (1988).
130. W. C. Willett, M. J. Stampfer, and G. A. Colditz. Does alcohol consumption influence the risk of developing breast cancer? Two views, *Important Adv. Oncol.*, 267–281 (1989).
131. E. L. Wynder and R. E. Harris. Does alcohol consumption influence the risk of developing breast cancer? Two views, *Important Adv. Oncol.*, 283–293 (1989).
132. A. Schatzkin, C. L. Carter, and S. B. Green. Is alcohol consumption related to breast cancer? Results from the Framingham Heart Study, *JNCI, 81*, 31–35 (1989).
133. R. E. Harris and E. L. Wynder. Breast cancer and alcohol consumption. A study in weak associations. *JAMA, 259*, 2867–2871 (1988).
134. E. B. Harvey, C. Schairer, and L. A. Brinton. Alcohol consumption and breast cancer, *JNCI, 78*, 657–661 (1987).
135. D. L. O'Connell, B. S. Hulka, and L. E. Chambless. Cigarette smoking, alcohol consumption, and breast cancer risk, *JNCI, 78*, 229–234 (1987).
136. C. La Vecchia, A. Decarli, and S. Franceschi. Alcohol consumption and the risk of breast cancer in women, *JNCI, 75*, 61–65 (1985).
137. R. Talamini, C. La Vecchia, and A. Decarli. Social factors, diet and breast cancer in a northern Italian population, *Br. J. Cancer, 49*, 723–729 (1984).
138. M. G. Le, L. H. Moulton, C. Hill, and A. Kramar. Consumption of dairy produce and alcohol in a case-control study of breast cancer, *JNCI, 77*, 633–636 (1986).
139. L. Garfinkel, P. Boffetta, and S. D. Stellman. Alcohol and breast cancer: A cohort study, *Prev. Med., 17*, 686-–693 (1988).
140. C. B. Begg, A. M. Walker, B. Wessen, and M. Zelen. Alcohol consumption and breast cancer, *Lancet, 1*, 293–294 (1983).
141. L. A. Webster, P. A. Wingo, P. M. Layde, and H. W. Ory. Alcohol consumption and risk of breast cancer, *Lancet, 2*, 724–726 (1983).
142. A. Paganini-Hill and R. K. Ross. Breast cancer and alcohol consumption, *Lancet, 2*, 626–627 (1983).

143. T. Byers and D. P. Funch. Alcohol and breast cancer, *Lancet, 1*, 799–800 (1982).
144. J. D. Potter and A. J. McMichael. Diet and cancer of the colon and rectum: A case-control study, *JNCI, 76*, 557–569 (1986).
145. J. K. McLaughlin, G. Gridley, and G. Block. Dietary factors in oral and pharyngeal cancer, *JNCI, 80*, 1237–1243 (1988).
146. J. E. Enstrom. Colorectal cancer and beer drinking, *Br. J. Cancer, 35*, 674–683 (1977).
147. E. L. Wynder, J. Kmet, N. Dungal, and M. Segi. An epidemiological investigation of gastric cancer, *Cancer, 16*, 1461–1496 (1963).
148. W. Haenszel, M. Kurihara, and M. Segi. Stomach cancer among Japanese in Hawaii, *JNCI, 49*, 696–988 (1972).
149. B. MacMahon, S. Yen, and D. Trichopoulos. Coffee and cancer of the pancreas, *N. Engl. J. Med., 304*, 630–633 (1981).
150. I. Heuch, G. Kvale, B. K. Jacobsen, and E. Bjelke. Use of alcohol, tobacco and coffee, and risk of pancreatic cancer, *Br. J. Cancer, 48*, 637–643 (1983).
151. E. L. Wynder, E. L. Hall, and M. Polansky. Epidemiology of coffee and pancreatic cancer, *Cancer Res., 43*, 3900–3906 (1983).
152. E. B. Gold, L. Gordis, and M. D. Diener. Diet and other risk factors for cancer of the pancreas, *Cancer, 55*, 460–467 (1985).
153. T. M. Mack, M. C. Yu, R. Hanisch, and B. E. Henderson. Pancreas cancer and smoking, beverage consumption, and past medical history, *JNCI, 76*, 49–60 (1986).
154. R. S. Lin and I. I. Kessler. A multifactorial model for pancreatic cancer in man (epidemilogic evidence), *JAMA, 245*, 147–152 (1981).
155. G. E. Burch and A. Ansari. Chronic alcoholism and carcinoma of the pancreas. A correlative hypothesis, *Arch. Intern. Med., 122*, 273–275 (1968).
156. J. P. Durbec, G. Chevillotte, and J. M. Bidart. Diet, alcohol, tobacco and risk of cancer of the pancreas: A case control study, *Br. J. Cancer, 47*, 463–470 (1983).
157. S. Graham, W. Schotz, and P. Martino. Alimentary factors in the epidemiology of gastric cancer, *Cancer, 30*, 927–938 (1972).
158. L. Hardell, N. O. Bengtsson, U. Jonsson, et al. Aetiological aspects on primary liver cancer with special regard to alcohol, organic solvents and acute intermittent porphyria—an epidemiologic investigation, *Br. J. Cancer, 50*, 389–397 (1984).
159. J. Higginson. Etiologic factors in gastrointestinal cancer in man, *JNCI, 37*, 527–545 (1966).
160. J. Hoey, C. Montvernay, and R. Lambert. Wine and tobacco: Risk factors for gastric cancer in France, *Am. J. Epidemiol. 113*, 668–674 (1981).
161. K. Ishii, T. Takeuchi, and T. Hirayama. Chronic calcifying pancreatitis and pancreatic carcinoma in Japan, *Digestion, 9*, 429–437 (1973).
162. W. Jedrychowski, J. Wahrendorf, T. Popiela, and J. Rachtan. A case-control study of dietary factors and stomach cancer risk in Poland, *Int. J. Cancer, 37*, 837–842 (1986).
163. G. C. Kabat, C. P. Howson, and E. L. Wynder. Beer consumption and rectal cancer, *Int. J. Epidemiol., 15*, 494–501 (1986).
164. T. Kodama and W. Mori. Morphological lesions of the pancreatic ducts. Significance of pyloric gland metaplasia in carcinogenesis of exocrine and endocrine pancreas, *Acta Pathol. Jpn., 33*, 645–660 (1983).

165. K. C. Lam, M. C. Yu, W. C. Leung, and B. E. Henderson. Hepatitis B virus and cigarette smoking: Risk factors for hepatocellular carcinoma in Hong Kong, *Cancer Res.*, *42*, 5246–5248 (1982).
166. O. Manousos, C. Papadimitriou, D. Trichopoulos, et al. Epidemiologic characteristics and trace elements in pancreatic cancer in Greece, *Cancerr Detect. Prev.*, *4*, 439–442 (1981).
167. A. B. Miller, G. R. Howe, M. Jain, et al. Food items and food groups as risk factors in a case-control study of diet and colo-rectal cancer, *Int. J. Cancerr, 32*, 155–161 (1983).
168. A. Oshima, H. Tsukuma, T. Hiiyama, et al. Follow-up study of HBsAg-positive blood doners with special reference to effect of drinking and smoking on development of liver cancer, *Int. J. Cancer, 34*, 775–779 (1984).
169. D. Schwartz, J. Lellouch, R. Flamant, and P. F. Denoix. Alcohol and cancer. Results of retrospective study (Fr.), *Rev. Fr. Etud. Clin. Biol.*, *7*, 590–604 (1962).
170. A. Shibata, T. Hirohata, H. Toshima, and H. Tashiro. The role of drinking and cigarette smoking in the excess deaths from liver cancer, *Jpn. J. Cancer Res.*, *77*, 287–295 (1986).
171. A. Stemhagen, J. Slade, R. Altman, and J. Bill. Occupational risk factors and liver cancer. A retrospective case-control study of primary liver cancer in New Jersey, *Am. J. Epidemiol.*, *117*, 443–454 (1983).
172. P. Stocks. Cancer incidence in North Wales and Liverpool region in relation to habits an environment, in *Carcinogens and Mutagens in the Environment* (H. F. Stich, ed.), British Empire Cancer Campaign 35th Annual Report, Part II (Suppl.), London, 1957.
173. D. B. Thomas, C. N. Uhl, and P. Hartge. Bladder cancer and alcoholic beverage consumption, *Am. J. Epidemiol.*, *118*, 720–727 (1983).
174. D. Trichopoulos, G. Ouranos, N. E. Day, et al. Diet and cancer of the stomach: A case-control study in Greece, *Int. J. Cancer, 36*, 291–297 (1985).
175. D. Trichopoulos, N. E. Day, E. Kaklamani, et al. Hepatitis B virus, tobacco smoking and ethanol consumption in the etiology of hepatocellular carcinomas, *Int. J. Cancer, 39*, 45–49 (1987).
176. E. L. Wynder and T. Shigematsu. Environmental factors of cancer of the colon and rectum, *Cancer, 20*, 1520–1561 (1967).
177. E. L. Wynder, I. J. Bross, and E. Day. A study of environmental factors in cancer of the larynx, *Cancer, 9*, 86–110 (1956).
178. E. L. Wynder, F. R. Lemon, and I. J. Bross. Cancer and coronary artery disease among Seventh-day Adventists, *Cancer, 12*, 1016–1028 (1959).
179. E. L. Wynder, K. Mabuchi, and W. F. Whitmore, Jr. Epidemiology of cancer of the prostate, *Cancer, 28*, 344–360 (1971).
180. M. C. Yu, T. Mach, R. Hanisch, et al. Hepatitis, alcohol consumption, cigarette smoking, and hepatocellular carcinoma in Los Angeles, *Cancer Res.*, *43*, 6077–6079 (1983).
181. F. R. Lemon, R. T. Walden, and R. W. Woods. Cancer of the lung and mouth in Seventh-day Adventists. Preliminary report on a population study, *Cancer, 17*, 486–497 (1964).

182. J. L. Lyon, M. R. Klauber, J. W. Gardner, and C. R. Smart. Cancer incidence in Mormons and non-Mormons in Utah, *N. Engl. J. Med.*, *294*, 129–133 (1976).
183. J. L. Lyon, J. W. Gardner, and D. W. West. Cancer incidence in Mormons and non-Mormons in Utah during 1967–75, *JNCI*, *65*, 1055–1061 (1980).
184. J. E. Enstrom. Cancer and total mortality among active Mormons, *Cancer*, *4236*, 1943–1951 (1978).
185. J. E. Enstrom. Cancer mortality among Mormons in California during 1968–75, *JNCI*, *65*, 1073–1082 (1980).
186. A. J. McMichael and B. K. Armstrong, Breast cancer in Australia: Occurrence, risk factors, preventability and screening, *Med. J. Aust.*, *148*, 86–88 (1988).
187. A. J. McMichael, J. D. Potter, and B. S. Hetsel. Time trends in colo-rectal cancer mortality in relation to food and alcohol consumption: United States, United Kingdom, Australia and New Zealand, *Int. J. Epidemiol.*, *8*, 295–303 (1979).
188. J. D. Potter, A. J. McMichael, and J. M. Hartshorne. Alcohol and beer consumption in relation to cancer of bowel and lung: An extended correlation analysis, *J. Chron. Dis.*, *35*, 833–842 (1982).
189. C. S. Lieber, A. Garro, M. A. Leo, et al. Alcohol and cancer, *Hepatology*, *6*, 1005–1019 (1986).
190. L. W. Pickle, R. G. Greene, R. G. Ziegler, et al. Colorectal cancer in rural Nebraska, *Cancer Res.*, *44*, 363–369 (1984).
191. S. A. Broitman, Relationship of ethanolic beverages and ethanol to cancer of the digestive tract. In *Vitamins, Nutrition, and Cancer* (K. Prosad, ed.), S. Karger, Basel, 1984.
192. S. Ohnishi, S. Iida, S. Iwama, et al. The effect of chronic habitual alcohol intake on the development of liver cirrhosis and hepatocellular carcinoma: Relation to hepatitis B surface antigen carriage, *Cancer*, *49*, 672 (1982).
193. A. Mashberg, L. Garfinkel, and S. Harris. Alcohol as a primary risk factor in oral squamous carcinoma, *CA*, *31*, 146–155 (1981).
194. R. G. Ziegler, L. E. Morris, W. J. Blot, et al. Esophageal cancer among black men in Washington, D.C. II. Role of nutrition. *JNCI*, *67*, 1199 (1981).
195. Anon., Epidemiologic problems with alcohol, *Lancet*, *1*, 762–763 (1981).
196. M. W. Hinds, D. B. Thomas, and H. P. O'Reilly. Asbestos, dental X-rays, tobacco, and alcohol in the epidemiology of laryngeal cancer. *Cancer*, *44*, 1114–1120 (1979).
197. J. Bulatao-Jayme, E. M. Almero, C. A. Castro Ma, et al. A case-control dietary study of primary liver cancer risk for aflatoxin exposure, *Int. J. Cancer*, *11*, 112–119 (1982).
198. A. Decarli, P. Liati, E. Negri, et al. Vitamin A and other dietary factors in the etiology of esophageal cancer, *Nutr. Cancer*, *10*, 29–37 (1987).
199. A. J. Tuyns, G. Pequignot, M. Gignoux, and A. Valla. Oesophageal cancer and alcohol consumption; importance of type of beverage, *Int. J. Cancer*, *30*, 9–11 (1982).
200. A. J. Tuyns. Alcohol, in *Cancer Epidemiology and Prevention* (D. Schottenfeld, ed.), W. B. Saunders, Philadelphia, 1982, pp. 293–303.
201. E. L. Wynder, T. Kajitani, S. Ishikawa, et al. Environmental factors of cancer

of the colon and rectum. II. Japanese epidemiological data, *Cancer, 23*, 1210–1220 (1969).
202. A. J. Tuyns, R. Kaaks, and M. Haelterman. Colorectal cancer and the consumption of foods: A case-control study in Belgium, *Nutr. Cancer, 11*, 189–204 (1988).
203. A. L. Klatsky, M. A. Armstrong, G. D. Friedman, and R. A. Hiatt. The relations of alcoholic beverage use to colon and rectal cancer, *Am. J. Epidemiol., 128*, 1007–1015 (1988).
204. Committee on Diet and Health, Alcohol, in *Diet and Health* (Committee on Diet and Health, Food and Nutrition Board, Commission of Life Sciences, and National Research Council, eds.), National Academy Press, Washington, DC, 1989, pp. 431–464.
205. A. L. Klatsky, M. A. Armstrong, and H. Kipp. Correlates of alcoholic beverage preference: Traits of persons who choose wine, liquor or beer, *Br. J. Addict., 85*, 1279–1289 (1990).
206. R. Abbe, Cancer of the mouth, *NY Med. J., 102*, 1–2 (1915).
207. C. S. Lieber, H. K. Seitz, A. J. Garro, and T. M. Warner. Alcohol-related diseases and carcinogenesis, *Cancer Res., 39*, 2863–2886 (1979).
208. E. L. Wynder, and S. D. Stellman. Comparative epidemiology of tobacco-related cancers, *Cancer Res., 37*, 4608–4622 (1977).
209. C. C. Boring, T. S. Squires, and T. Tong. Cancer statistics, 1991, *CA, 41*, 19–36 (1991).
210. P. L. Lamy. Statistical clinical study of 134 cases of cancer of the esophagus (Fr.), *Arch. Mal. Appar. Dig., 4*, 451–475 (1910).
211. C. La Vecchia, E. Negri, A. Decarli, et al. A case-control study of diet and gastric cancer in northern Italy, *Int. J. Cancer, 10*, 484–489 (1987).
212. E. Bjelke. Epidemiologic studies of cancerr of the stomach, colon, rectum; with special emphasis on the role of diet, *Scand. J. Gastroenterol.*, (Suppl.) *31*, 42–53 (1974).
213. E. D. Acheson R. Doll. Dietary factors in carcinoma of the stomach: A study of 100 cases and 200 controls, *Gut, 5*, 126–131 (1964).
214. T. Hirayama. Epidemiology of stomach cancer, *Gann, 11*, 3–19 (1971).
215. R. L. Phillips. Cancer among Seventh-day Adventists, *J. Environ. Pathol. Toxicol., 3*, 157–169 (1980).
216. A. J. Tuyns, G. Pequignot, and O. M. Jensen. Le cancer de l'oesphage en Ile-et-Vilaine en function des neveaux de consumation d'alcool et de tabac, *Bull. Cancer, 64*, 45–60 (1977).
217. P. Correa, E. Fontham, L. Pickle, et al. Dietary determinants of gastric cancer in south Louisiana inhabitants, *JNCI, 75*, 645–654 (1985).
218. J. Pernu. An epidemiologic study on cancer of the digestive organs and respiratory system: A study based on 7078 cases, *Ann. Med. Intern. Fenn., 49*, 1–117 (1960).
219. S. Kono and M. Ikeda. Correlation between cancer mortality and alcoholic beverage in Japan, *Br. J. Cancer, 40*, 449–455 (1979).
220. T. Hirayama. Epidemiology of pancreatic cancer in Japan, *Int. J. Pancreatol., 3*, S203–S204 (1988).
221. M. J. Hill. The effect of some factors on the faecal concentration of acid steroids, neutral steroids and urobilins, *J. Pathol., 104*, 239 (1971).

222. B. S. Reddy, J. H. Weisburger, and E. L. Wynder. Faecal bacterial B-glucuronidase: Control by diet, *Science, 183*, 416 (1974).
223. E. Bjelke. Epidemiologic studies of cancer of stomach, colon and rectum; with special emphasis on the role of diet, thesis, University of Minnesota, Vol I IV, University Microfilms, Ann Arbor, MI, 1973.
224. C. Garland, R. B. Shekelle, E. Barett-Connor, et al. Dietary vitamin D and calcium and the risk of colorectal cancer: A 19-year prospective study in men, *Lancet, i*, 307 (1985).
225. R. A. Hiatt. Alcohol consumption and breast cancer, *Med. Oncol. Tumor Pharmacother., 7*, 143–151 (1990).
226. R. L. Phillips, L. Garfinkel, J. W. Kuzman, et al. Mortality among California Seventh-day Adventists for selected cancer sites, *JNCI, 65*, 1097–1107 (1980).
227. C. M. Berlin, Jr. Pharmacologic considerations of drug use in the lactating mother, *Obstet. Gynecol.*, (Suppl) *58*, 17S–23S (1981).
228. J. F. Tomera, P. L. Skipper, J. S. Wishnok, et al. Inhibition of N-nitrosodimethylamine metabolism by ethanol and other inhibitors in the isolated rat liver, *Carcinogenesis, 5*, 113–116 (1984).
229. M. Cohen, M. Lippman, and B. Chabner. Role of pineal gland in aetiology and treatment of breast cancer, *Lancet, 2*, 814–816 (1978).
230. H. B. Moss, L. Tamarkin, E. Majchrowicz, et al. Pineal function during ethanol intoxication, dependence, and withdrawal, *Life Sci., 39*, 2209–2214 (1986).
231. L. Tamarkin, M. Cohen, D. Roselle, et al. Melatonin inhibition and pinealectomy enhancement of 7,12-dimethyl-benx(a)anthracene-induced mammary tumors in the rat, *Cancer Res., 41*, 4432–4436 (1981).
232. H. Seidman, S. D. Stellman, and M. H. Muchinski. A different perspective on breast cancer risk factors: Some implications of the nonattributable risk, *CA, 32*, 301–313 (1982).
233. R. Doll and R. Peto. The causes of cancer: quantitative estimates of avoidable risks of cancer in the United States today, *JNCI, 66*, 1191–1308 (1981).
234. L. M. Brown, W. J. Blot, S. H. Schuman, et al. Environmental factors and high risk of esophageal cancer among men in coastal South Carolina, *JNCI, 80*, 1620–1625 (1988).
235. IARC. IARC Monographs on the Evaluation of Carcinogenic Risks to Humans, Alcohol Drinking, Vol. 44, IARC, Lyon, France, 1988.
236. Committee on Diet, Nutrition and Cancer, Alcohol, in *Diet, Nutrition and Cancer* (Nutrition Committee on Diet, and Cancer, Assembly of Life Sciences, and National Research Council, eds.), National Academy Press, Washington, DC, 1982, pp. 11-1–11-5.
237. P. C. Campanelli, T. E. Dielman, and J. T. Shope. Validity of adolescents' self-reports of alcohol use and misuse using a bogus pipeline procedure, *Adolescence, XXII*, 7–22 (1987).
238. J. C. Duffy and J. J. Waterton. Under-reporting of alcohol consumption in sample surveys. The effect of computer interviewing in fieldwork, *Br. J. Addict., 79*, 303–308 (1984).
239. J. B. Lowe, R. A. Windsor, B. Adams, et al. Use of a bogus pipeline methods to

increase accuracy of self-reported alcohol consumption among pregnant women, *J. Stud. Alcohol, 47*, 173–175 (1986).

240. C. G. Watson, C. Tilleskjor, E. A. Hoodecheck-Schow, et al. Do alcoholics give valid self-reports? *J. Stud. Alcohol, 45*, 344–348 (1984).
241. R. G. Ziegler. Alcohol-nutrient interactions in cancer epidemiology, *Cancer, 58*, 1942–1948 (1986).
242. C. S. Lieber, E. Baroano, M. A. Leo, and A. J. Garro. Metabolism and metabolic effects of ethanol, including interaction with drugs, carcinogens and nutrition, *Mutat. Res., 186*, 201–233 (1987).
243. M. Sato and C. S. Lieber. Hepatic vitamin A depletion after chronic ethanol consumption in baboons and rats, *J. Nutr., 111*, 2015–2023 (1981).
244. M. A. Leo and C. S. Lieber. New pathway for retinol metabolism in liver microsomes, *J. Biol. Chem., 260*, 5228–5231 (1985).
245. V. M. Craddock, A. R. Henderson, and S. Gash. Nature of constitutive and induced mammalian O6-methylguanine DNA repair enzymes, *Biochem. Biophys. Res. Commun., 107*, 546–553 (1982).
246. C. La Vecchia, A. Decarli, M. Fasoli et al. Nutrition and diet in the aetiology of endometrial cancer, *Cancer Res., 57*, 1248–1253 (1986).
247. B. Boland and R. Roizen. Sales sloips and survey responses: new data on the reliability of survey consumption measures, *Drinking Drug Pract. Surv., 8*, 5–10 (1973).
248. R. Flamant, O. Lasserre, R. Lazar, et al. Differences in sex ratio according to cancer site and possible relationship with use of tobacco and alcohol. Review of 65,000 cases, *JNCI, 32*, 1309–1316 (1964).
249. K. W. Kwan. Carcinoma of the esophagus. A statistical study, *Chin. Med. J., 52*, 237–254 (1937).
250. Y. K. Wu and H. H. Louks. Carcinoma of the esophagus or cardia of the stomach: An analysis of 172 cases with 81 reactions, *Ann. Surg., 134*, 946–956 (1951).
251. G. R. Howe, J. D. Burch, A. B. Miller, et al. Tobacco use, occupation, coffee, various nutrients, and bladder cancer, *JNCI, 64*, 701–713 (1980).
252. F. G. Lehmann and G. A. Martini. Incidence of primary liver cell carcinoma in liver cirrhosis: 5 year prospective study, *Digestion, 14*, 530–531 (1976).
253. C. A. Linsell and F. G. Peers. Aflatoxin and liver cell cancer, *Trans. R. Soc. Trop. Med. Hyg., 71*, 471–473 (1977).
254. Y. Nakanuma and G. Ohta. Morphology of cirrhosis and occurrence of hepatocellular carcinoma in alcoholics with and without HBsAg in nonalcoholic HBsAg positive patients. A comparative autopsy study, *Liver, 3*, 231–237 (1983).
255. D. Trichopoulos, B. MacMahon, L. Sparros, and G. Merikas. Smoking and hepatitis B-negative primary hepatocellular carcinoma, *JNCI, 65*, 111–114 (1980).
256. M. G. Filipazzo, E. Aragoma, and C. A. Castro. Assessment of some risk factors for hepatocellular carcinoma: A case control study, *Statist. Med. 4*, 345–351 (1985).
257. M. Gelfand, W. M. Castle, and W. M. Buchanan. Primary carcinoma of the liver in Rhodesia: A clinical study, *S. Afr. Med. J., 46*, 527–532 (1972).
258. J. T. Tu, R. N. Gao, D. H. Zhang, and B. C. Gu. Hepatitis B virus and primary liver cancer on Changming Island, People's Republic of China, *Natl. Cancer Inst. Monogr., 69*, 213–215 (1985).

259. G. Chevilotte, J. P. Durbec, A. Gerolami, et al. Interaction between hepatitis B virus and alcohol consumption in liver cirrhosis, *Gastroenterology, 85*, 141–145 (1983).
260. R. A. Hiatt, A. L. Klatsky, and M. A. Armstrong. Alcohol consumption and smoking and the risk of prostatic cancer in a large health plan cohort, *Am. J. Public Health* (Abstract), 118th Annual Meeting. New York, Sept. 30–Oct. 4, 1990.
261. A. J. Tuyns, Alcohol consumption patterns in the Department of Calvados (France), *Rev. Epidemiol. Sante Publique, 31*, 179–197 (1983).
262. W. C. Willet, M. J. Stampfer, G. A. Colditz, et al. Relation of meat, fat, and fiber intake to the risk of colon cancer in a prospective study among women, *N. Engl. J. Med., 323*, 1664–1672 (1990).
263. G. W. Olsen, J. S. Mandel, R. W. Gibson, et al. A case-control study of pancreatic cancer and cigarettes, alcohol, coffee and diet. *Am. J. Public Health, 79*, 1016–1019 (1989).
264. *The Surgeon General's Report on Nutrition and Health*, USDHHS, PHS, DHHS (PHS) Pub. No. 88-50210, Washington, DC, 1988.
265. J. A. T. Pennington, and H. N. Church. *Bowes and Church's Food Values of Portions Commonly Used*, Harper and Row, New York, 1985.
266. C. A. Schoenborn, and B. H. Cohen. *Trends in Smoking, Alcohol Consumption, and Other Health Practices Among U.S. Adults, 1977 and 1983*, DHHS Publ. No. (PHS) 86-1250, Division of Health Interview Statistics. National Center for Health Statistics, PHS, US DHHS., Hyattsville, MD, 1986.
267. C. D. J. Holman. Thesis dissertation. University of Western Australia, Perth, Australia, 1983.
268. L. T. Midanik, A. L. Klatsky, and M. A. Armstrong. Changes in drinking behavior: Demographic, psychosocial, an biomedical factors. *Int. J. Addict., 25*, 599–619 (1990).
269. P. L. Colser, and R. B. Wallace. Is modest alcohol consumption better than none at all? *Annu. Rev. Public Health, 10*, 203–219 (1989).
270. G. Knupfer. Drinking for health: The daily light drinker myth, *Br. J. Addict., 82*, 547–555 (1987).
271. L. C. Sobell, T. Cellucci, T. D. Nivenberg, et al. Do quantity-frequency data underestimate drinking-related health risks? *Am. J. Public Health, 72*, 823–827 (1982).
272. J. A. Miller and E. C. Miller. Ultimate carcinogens as reactive mutagenic electrophiles. In *Origins of Human Cancer*. (H. H. Hiatt, J. D. Watson, and J. A. Winston, eds.) Cold Spring Harbor, New York, 1977, pp. 605–607.
273. S. Graham, H. Dayal, M. Swanson, et al. Diet in the epidemiology of cancer of the colon and rectum. *JNCI, 61*,709–714 (1978).
274. J. D. Potter, A. J. McMichael, and J. M. Hartshorne, Alcohol and beer consumption in relation to cancer of bowel and lung: an extended correlation analysis. *J. Chron. Dis., 35*, 833–842 (1982).
275. N. E. Breslow and J. E. Enstrom. Geographic correlations between cancer mortality rates and alcohol-tobacco consumption in the United States. *JNCI, 53*, 631–639 (1974).

276. H. A. Skinner and B. A. Allen. Does the computer make a difference? Computerized versus face-to-face self-report assessment of alcohol, drug and tobacco use. *J. Consult. Clin. Psychol.*, *51*, 267–275 (1983).
277. A. B. Lowenfels and S. A. Zevola. Alcohol and breast cancer: an overview. *Alcoholism, 13*, 109–111 (1989).
278. J. C. Licciardone, J. R. Wilkins III, R. C. Brownson, and J. C. Chang. Cigarette smoking and alcohol consumption in the aetiology of uterine cervical cancer. *Int. J. Epidemiol.*, *18*, 533–537 (1989).

11

Serum Albumin and the Risk of Cancer

Richard G. Stevens
Pacific Northwest Laboratory
Richland, Washington

Baruch S. Blumberg
Fox Chase Cancer Center
Philadelphia, Pennsylvania
Balliol College
Oxford, England

INTRODUCTION

Serum albumin has long been used to assess protein-calorie nutritional status (Haider and Haider, 1984; Micozzi et al., 1989). Its half-life of several weeks makes it insensitive to immediate changes in protein intake, but a good indicator of intake in the recent past. Animal and human research on the effect of protein intake on risk of cancer is inconclusive (National Research Council, 1989). The possible effect of protein intake on risk of chronic disease remains uncertain, and the long-term health implications may be quite different for a high protein diet consumed in childhood versus in adulthood (Micozzi, 1985). Dietary intake studies are notoriously difficult to interpret due to the problematic nature of accurately assessing long-term dietary intake patterns. As an alternative, adult height has been used as a test of the hypothesis that early nutrition affects risk of cancer, and again the results vary (Micozzi, 1985, 1987; Albanes et al., 1988; Severson et al., 1988; La Vecchia et al., 1990).

Recent studies of the relationship between serum albumin and subsequent risk of cancer are consistent in showing increased risk with low albumin. The question

Supported by the U.S. Department of Energy under contract DE-AC06-76RL0-1830, and by USPHS grants CA-40737, RR-05895, and CA-06927 from the National Institutes of Health, and an appropriation from the Commonwealth of Pennsylvania.

is how albumin might be involved in the pathogenesis of cancer. In the past, low albumin was believed to be nothing more than a result of the disease process. That low albumin may play some etiologic role in cancer development cannot be so easily dismissed given recent findings from prospective epidemiologic studies.

EPIDEMIOLOGY

There have been a number of published reports of an association of low serum albumin and subsequently increased risk of general mortality, cancer, and cardiovascular disease. In a nested case-control analysis within a prospective study of 2500 aboriginal Solomon Islanders (Stevens et al., 1983), men who died over the 10-year period (~1968–1978) had a mean serum ablumin level of 39.1 g/liter in ~1968, whereas those who survived to 1978 had a mean of 41.5 g/liter ($p = 0.03$). In women the mean serum albumin in those who died and in those who survived was 40.1 and 40.6, respectively, and not significantly different. There were 105 matched pairs (subject who died and age-sex matched control who had not). There was no information on cause of death or smoking status in this study. There was no a priori hypothesis concerning albumin. In the same study it was found that serum ferritin was elevated in those who died. It was suggested that elevated body iron levels (reflected by elevated ferritin) might lead to increased burden of infectious disease and that this might account for the significant difference between those who died (50.4 g/liter) and those who survived (47.5 g/liter) in serum gammaglobulin level.

A second study with an a priori hypothesis was conducted, in part, to test the albumin hypothesis. From a population of 21,000 male government workers followed prospectively from 1975–78 to 1983 in Taiwan (Stevens et al., 1986), the mean serum albumin was 42.0 g/liter in 73 men who developed cancer over the study period and 44.0 in 73 age-HBsAg–matched controls who did not ($p < 0.01$). Serum globulin was higher in men who later died of cancer, though not significantly so.

Another study (Stevens et al., 1988) reported on cancer incidence in the 14,000 subjects in the first National Health and Nutrition Examination Survey (NHANES I) population, a probability sample of the United States population. It showed that serum albumin at enrollment (1971–75) was significantly lower in 242 men who later developed cancer (43.7 g/liter) than in 3355 men who remained free of cancer to 1984 (44.3 g/liter). Cases occurring within 4 years of the albumin determination were excluded from analysis, and adjustment was made for age and smoking. In females there was no significant difference between cases (43.3 g/liter) and controls (43.4 g/liter) except when analysis was restricted to women with high transferrin saturation (>36.7%) at the start of the study (42.5 g/liter vs. 43.6 g/liter).

Phillips et al. (1989) reported on a striking relationship between mortality and serum albumin level determined at least 5 years prior to death. A cohort of 7735 middle-aged British men were followed for an average of 9.2 years. Death rates from both cardiovascular disease and cancer were significantly higher in men with low albumin, and there was a "dose-response" relationship. In their discussion section, the authors stated that although they did not have an a priori hypothesis about serum albumin, the strength of the association rivals that between cigarette smoking and mortality. The relative odds (after exclusion of deaths occurring within 5 years of albumin determination and after adjustment for age, social class, cigarette smoking, serum cholesterol, systolic blood pressure, town of residence, and forced expiratory volume) associated with a one stardard deviation increase in serum albumin (2.55 g/liter) was 0.76 ($p = 0.003$) for cardiovascular disease death, and 0.68 ($p = 0.0002$) for cancer death. Serum albumin was 45 g/liter in never smokers and 44 g/liter in smokers. Lower albumin in smokers has been reported in other studies (Dales et al., 1974; Stram et al., 1990). There is evidence that smoking increases resting metabolic rate, and that both nicotine and the act of inhalation contribute to this effect (Perkins et al., 1989). On this basis, it can be hypothesized that increased metabolic rate may lead to lower serum albumin.

Since Phillips et al. (1989) had smoking information, the association of low serum albumin with mortality may not have been confounded by smoking. It is also possible, however, that part of the association might be attributable to imperfect smoking data and a very strong relation between true smoking behavior and albumin level, in which case albumin levels could be acting as a surrogate for true smoking history. On the other hand, part of the deleterious effect of smoking on health may result from the effect of smoking on biochemical indicators such as serum albumin.

In a letter response to the Phillips et al. (1989) paper, Darne et al. (1990) presented data from a follow-up study of 18,333 men and 9351 women aged 40–59. Average follow-up was 10.5 years. Albumin was strongly and inversely related to death rates from cancer and CV disease over the study period in men, in agreement with the Phillips et al. (1989) study, but not in women. However, when account was taken of globulin as calculated from total serum protein minus albumin, the effect of albumin was not significant. Death rates were significantly and directly related to globulin levels. The authors suggested that the relation of albumin to mortality in the Phillips et al. study was a spurious result arising from a true effect of globulin.

In response to the Darne et al. (1990) letter, Phillips et al. (1990) reported on globulin levels and mortality in their study population. In fact, globulin was not significantly related to mortality after account was taken of albumin. Phillips et al. did not calculate globulin as total protein minus albumin, but rather measured it directly. They pointed out that calculation of globulin by subtraction overestimates the negative correlation of albumin and globulin. The correlation of albumin and globulin in the Darne et al. study was −0.45 in men but only −0.27 in the Phillips et al. study population.

In response to the Phillips et al. (1990) response to Darne et al. (1990), Sweetnam and Yarnell (1990) reported that both low albumin and high globulin were significantly related to mortality within 5 years of assay in a prospective study of 2512 men. They obtained an estimate of serum globulin by subtraction as did Darne et al. (1990).

The studies cited above agree on a strong relationship of serum proteins and risk of cancer and CV disease mortality in men, and they agree with the results reported in the three earlier studies of general mortality (Stevens et al., 1983) and of cancer (Stevens et al., 1986, 1988): Albumin is inversely related to risk, globulin directly related to risk, and the effect is stronger in men than in women.

ALBUMIN STRUCTURE AND FUNCTION

Serum albumin is important for osmotic regulation of blood, and in many transport and regulatory processes (Peters, 1985). It binds an impressive array of substances including fatty acids, heme, calcium, and transition metals such as nickel, copper, and zinc. It also binds tryptophan, thyroxine, and many therapeutic drugs. Despite the fact that serum albumin has been extensively studied for many years, its three-dimensional structure has only recently begun to be elucidated (Carter et al., 1989; Carter and He, 1990).

Human serum albumin is a 67,000 molecular weight protein, made in the liver with 585 amino acid residues, which lacks associated carbohydrate (Peters, 1985). It comprises ~60% of protein in serum. Albumin is acidic, highly soluble, and stable. It can withstand 60°C for 10 hours. During its ~27-day life, albumin travels ~15,000 times through the circulation; it also travels ~15 times through extravascular spaces. It provides ~80% of the colloid osmotic pressure of plasma and is therefore important in keeping fluid inside the blood vessels. Its ability to bind a wide variety of ligands makes it a high capacity reservoir for stabilization of free ligands.

The gene for albumin is on chromosome 4, in the same region as the gene for α-fetoprotein, a protein with which it has a high degree of sequence homology. Albumin contains an odd number of half-cystine residues so that there is a free cysteine which may be important in antioxidant qualities of albumin. Albumin binds strongly to heme, and the product, methemalbumin, often reflects internal hemorrhage. That 10% of serum copper not bound to cerulopasmin is firmly bound to albumin. The binding of these potentially damaging redox cycling agents, heme and copper, provides another mechanism whereby albumin may provide protection from oxidative damage.

Inherited structural differences in the albumin molecule may account for a certain amount of variation in albumin function. They may be of importance in the epidemiologic studies relating albumin with disease outcomes, and provide insights into differences in outcome. There is an extremely rare condition of analbuminemia in which other serum proteins are produced in excess to compensate for the complete lack of circulating albumin.

The known polymorphic variants (alloalbumins) are rare. They are of the order of 1:3,000 to 1:10,000 in most populations. However in some populations the less common allele may reach quite high frequencies. Albumin Naskapi varies from a gene frequency of about 0.05 in several North American Indian populations to 0.13 in the Naskapi Indians of northern Quebec. Very high frequencies of certain alleles are also found in several South American Indian groups, for example, the Yanomamo (Schell and Blumberg, 1977).

There are more known heritable variants of serum albumin than for any other human protein with the exception of hemoglobin. About 80 allotypes have been listed, but many of these are probably the same variant identified electrophoretically by different investigators in different places. Arai et al. (1990) list 26 proven point substitutions which are concentrated in three short segments of the albumin amino acid chain. This includes 585 amino acids in the main chain and an additional 6 in the propeptide, which is ordinarily cleaved before secretion.

No obvious disease associations with the variants have been identified. Homozygotes are known for only a few of the variants (for example, albumin Naskapi), and it is possible that homozygotes for some rare alleles may be lethal and therefore undetected. Differential binding by alloalbumin for warfarin, a plant-derived anticoagulant, has been reported, and this may have some bearing on the response to the medication or to the development of toxicity (Wilding et al., 1977).

The condition "familial dysalbuminemic hyperthyroninemia" is characterized by elevated levels of thyroxine. There is an abnormally high affinity of albumin for thyroxine, but little in the way of symptoms or biochemical abnormalities. This appears to be a variant of albumin for which the amino acid substitution has not been found (Doctor et al., 1981).

The alloalbumins have not, so far, been of significant value in understanding gross pathologic conditions, but may in the future help to explain individual differences related to disease susceptibilities. They have been used to study ancient population affinities, for example, the relation between the Indians of the Americans and the ancestors of current Asian populations using the Naskapi variant as a marker.

ALBUMIN AND DISEASE

It has long been known that the serum albumin level is low in hospital patients (Davidsohn and Henry, 1974). Low albumin results from many disease states including cancer.

Protein-calorie malnutrition (PCM) was once thought to be a problem confined to the nonindustrialized developing countries (Haider and Haider, 1984). It has become clear in the last 20 years that it is also a significant problem for patients hospitalized for cancer, trauma, or surgery in industrialized countries. Consequences of PCM in hospitalized patients include increased incidence and severity of infections, surgical complications, and poor survival. In order to identify PCM, several measures have been utilized in the hospital setting, the most obvious of which is body weight. Body weight, however, may reflect true muscle loss or dehydration, and has different meaning for different people depending on each individual's healthy weight prior to hospital admission. In addition, a patient may be malnourished without showing significant weight loss. Better indications of nutritional status are the levels of the serum proteins, albumin and transferrin. When these are low, prognosis is poorer. The response to nutritional therapy, however, is not immediately apparent when measuring serum albumin due to its long half-life. Transferrin's half-life of approximately 9 days makes it a better indicator of the success or failure of therapy, but its concentration is affected by factors other than protein intake; it rises in iron deficiency, a condition often associated with PCM. Currently, pre-albumin, a 54 kD serum protein with a half-life of only ~2 days, is being suggested as a promising measure of the effectiveness of nutritional therapy, although it may reflect intake rather than nutritional status.

Among the serum proteins, the strongest association with poor prognosis is low serum albumin (Haider and Haider, 1984). In an attempt to explain the poorer prognosis of black women compared to white women, Coates et al. (1990) studied factors affecting prognosis after a diagnosis of breast cancer in 1960 women in the state of Georgia between 1975 and 1979. They found that poorer survival was associated with low serum albumin and low hemoglobin after adjustment for race and stage at diagnosis. High body mass index (BMI) was also strongly associated with poorer survival. Much of the poorer survival of black women could be explained by the fact that they had higher BMI and lower albumin than white women. Analysis of data on 8234 women who participated in the NHANES I showed that serum albumin was significantly lower in heavy women (Micozzi et al., 1989). Coates et al. (1990) offered at least two explanations for the association of low serum albumin with decreased survival: (a) low albumin may result from more serious disease, or occult disease, in apparently healthy individuals, and (b) poor protein nutrition could lead to both low albumin and an impairment of immune function.

Emtage and Blackledge (1990) reported that low serum albumin measured prior to beginning of treatment for prostate cancer was more strongly related to short survival than any other factor, even histologic grade. Chen and Magalhaes (1990) analyzed clinical data on 65 patients with multiple myeloma and concluded that serum albumin was related to extent of myeloma proliferation, and serum albumin below 29.0 g/liter "unequivocally" indicated advanced disease.

BIOLOGICAL MECHANISMS

It is intriguing to ponder (Stevens and Blumberg, 1990) the meaning of the observed associations of serum albumin with subsequent risk of cancer previously observed, and with cardiovascular disease death reported by Phillips et al. (1989). Albumin is important in many facets of human physiology (Peters, 1985). In Stevens et al. (1986, 1988), the effect of albumin on siderophore-mediated iron acquisition was cited as a possible biological mechanism for an association with cancer (Konopka and Neilands, 1984). Excess iron stores may increase cancer risk by at least two possible mechanisms: (a) iron may be a limiting nutrient to a cancer cell (Weinberg, 1984), and (b) iron can catalyze the production of oxygen radicals (Halliwell and Gutteridge, 1984). These two possibilities are reviewed at length in Stevens and Kalkwarf (1990). If albumin affects iron availability, then low albumin may result in more available iron for cancer cells to consume and/or for Fenton chemistry reactions in tissue that might create cancer cells.

Oxidative mechanisms may be a common etiology for both cancer and cardiovascular disease (Cross, 1987). With that in mind, albumin level may affect oxidative stress by another mechanism. Conjugated linoleic acids (CLAs) are derivatives of linoleic acid that contain a conjugated double bond (Pariza, 1988). They are potent antioxidants and are effective anticarcinogens in animals. Ha et al. (1987) treated three groups of mice with 7,12-dimethylbenz(a)anthracene (DMBA), a carcinogen, on the skin. One group also received CLAs at 7 days, 3 days, and 5 minutes before DMBA application. The other two groups received either linoleic acid or acetone in a similar manner. The CLA group developed half the number of tumors of either of the two controls groups, and had significantly lower incidence of tumor.

CLAs are found in human serum, bile, and duodenal juice. The source is unknown. Examples of foods that are high in CLAs are grilled beef (Ha et al., 1987) and processed cheese (Ha et al., 1989). The production of CLAs from linoleic acid requires protein, the most abundant of which in serum is albumin (Cawood et al., 1983; Dormandy and Wickens, 1987). Therefore, albumin may be quantitatively related to CLA production in the body; low albumin may lead to low CLA, which in turn may result in increased oxidative stress and its possible long-term sequelae, cancer and cardiovascular disease. Another possibility is that low serum albumin may reflect a low intake of protein-rich foods that are high in CLAs (which when present in adequate levels may reduce risk of disease) and thereby be indirectly related to cancer and cardiovascular disease mortality.

Apart from the possible effects of albumin on such factors as iron and CLAs, albumin itself may have antioxidant capacity. Halliwell (1988) proposed that the protein may behave as a "sacrificial antioxidant." It is present in such large quantities that small amounts may scavenge radicals, be functionally destroyed, and lower the level of oxidative stress while not significantly affecting the pool of functional albumin.

CONCLUSION

At this time, there is a substantial body of data showing that low serum albumin is associated with cancer. The question is why. Does high protein intake decrease cancer risk? Does low serum albumin confer a risk independent of protein intake? Are the observed associations of low albumin with increased risk of cancer simply due to early disease affecting albumin level? Does low albumin result from the underlying cause of cancer and not have any effect in itself?

The observation of a strong inverse relation of serum albumin and chronic disease mortality is open to a wide variety of interpretations. It is clearly important to investigate this relationship further.

REFERENCES

Albanes, D., Jones, D. Y., Schatzkin, A., Micozzi, M. S., Taylor, P. R. Adult stature and risk of cancer. *Cancer Res. 48*: 1658–1662 (1988).

Arai, K., Madison, J., Shimizu, A., Putnam, F. W. Point substitutions in albumin genetic variants from Asia. *Proc. Natl. Acad. Sci. 87*: 497–501 (1990).

Carter, D. C., He, X-M, Munson, S. H., Twigg, P. D., Gernert, K. M., Broom, B., Miller, T. Y. Three-dimensional structure of human serum albumin. *Science 244*: 1195–1198 (1989).

Carter, D. C., He, X-M. Structure of human serum albumin. *Science 249*: 302–303 (1990).

Cawood, P., Wickens, D. G., Iversen, J. M., Braganza, J. M., Dormandy, T. L. The nature of diene conjugation in human serum, bile, and duodenal juice. *FEBS Lett. 162*: 239–243 (1983).

Chen, Y-H., Hagalhaes, M. C. Hypoalbuminemia in patients with multiple myeloma. *Arch. Intern. Med. 150*: 605–610 (1990).

Coates, R. J., Clark, W. S., Eley, J. W., Greenberg, R. S., Huguley, C. M., Brown, R. L. Race, nutritional status, and survival from breast cancer. *JNCI 82*: 1684–1692 (1990).

Cross, C. E. (moderator). Oxygen radicals and human disease. *Ann. Intern. Med. 107*: 526–545 (1987).

Dales, L. G., Friedman, G. D., Siegelaub, A. B., et al. Cigarette smoking and serum chemistry tests. *J. Chron. Dis. 27*: 293–307 (1974).

Darne, B., Ducimetière, P., Guize, L. Serum albumin and mortality. *Lancet 335*: 350–351 (1990).

Davidsohn, I., Henry, J. B., (eds.). *Clinical Diagnosis by Laboratory Methods*. W. B. Saunders, Co., Philadelphia, 1974.

Docter, R., Bos, G., Krenning, E. P., Fekkes, D., Visser, T. J., Henneman, G. Inherited thyroxine excess: A serum abnormality due to an increased affinity for modified albumin. *Clin. Endocrinol. 15*: 363–371 (1981).

Dormandy, T. L., Wickens, D. G. The experimental and clinical pathology of diene conjugation. *Chem. Phys. Lipids 45*: 353–364 (1987).

Emtage, L. A., Blackledge, G. Association between serum albumin and mortality from prostatic cancer. *Lancet 355*: 482 (1990).

Ha, Y. L., Grimm, N. K., Pariza, M. W. Anticarcinogens from fried beef: Heat-altered derivatives of linoleic acid. *Carcinogenesis 8*: 1881–1887 (1987).

Ha, Y. L., Grimm, N. K., Pariza, M. W. Newly recognized anticarcinogenic fatty acids: Identification and quantification in natural and processed cheeses. *J. Agr. Food Chem. 37*: 75–81 (1989).

Haider, M., Haider, S. Q. Assessment of protein-calorie malnutrition. *Clin. Chem. 30*: 1286–1299 (1984).

Halliwell, B., Gutteridge, J. M. C. Oxygen toxicity, oxygen radicals, transition metals and disease. *Biochem. J. 219*: 1–14 (1984).

Halliwell, B. Albumin—an important extracellular antioxidant? *Biochem. Pharmacol. 37*: 569–571 (1988).

Hasuo, Y., Ueda, K., Fujii, I., Yanai, T., Kiyohara, Y., Wada, J., Kawano, H., Shikata, T., Takeshita, M., Hirota, Y., Omae, T., Fujishima, M. Changes in blood chemical constituents and death in the aged population: The Hisayama study. *Jpn. J. Geriat. 23*: 65–72 (1986).

Konopka, K., Neilands, J. B. Effect of serum albumin on siderophone-mediated utilization of transferrin iron. *Biochemistry 23*: 2122–2127 (1984).

La Vecchia, C., Negri, E., Parazzini, F., Boyle, P., D'Avanzo, B., Levi, F., Gentile, A., Franceschi, S. Height and cancer risk in a network of case-control studies from northern Italy. *Int. J. Cancer 45*: 275–279 (1990).

Micozzi, M. S. Nutrition, body size and breast cancer. *Yearbook of Physical Anthropology 28*: 175–206 (1985).

Micozzi, M. S. Cross-cultural correlations of childhood growth and adult cancer rates. *Am. J. Phys. Anthropol. 73*: 525–537 (1987).

Micozzi, M. S., Albanes, D., Stevens, R. G. Relation of body size and composition to clinical biochemical and hematologic indices in US men and women. *Am. J. Clin. Nutri. 50*: 1276–1281 (1989).

National Research Council. *Diet and Health: Implications for Reducing Chronic Disease Risk*. National Academy Press, Washington, DC, 1989.

Pariza, M. W. Dietary fat and cancer risk. *Ann. Rev. Nutr. 8*: 167–183 (1988).

Perkins, K. A., Epstein, L. H., Stiller, R. L., Marks, B. L., Jacob, R. G. Acute effects of nicotine on resting metabolic rate in cigarette smokers. *Am. J. Clin. Nutri. 50*: 545–550 (1989).

Peters, T. Serum albumin. *Adv. Protein Chem. 37*: 161–245 (1985).

Phillips, A., Shaper, A. G., Whincup, P. H. Association between serum albumin and mortality from cardiovascular disease, cancer, and other causes. *Lancet 2*: 1434–1436 (1989).

Phillips, A., Shaper, A. G., Whincup, P. H. Serum proteins and mortality. *Lancet 335*: 858 (1990).

Schell, L. M., Blumberg, B. S. The genetics of human serum albumin, In *Albumin Structure, Finction and Uses* (Rosenoer, V. M., Oratz, M., Rotschild, M. A., eds.), Pergamon Press, Oxford, 1977, pp. 113–141.

Severson, R. K., Grove, J. S., Nomura, A. M. Y., et al. Body mass and prostatic cancer: A prospective study. *Brit. Med. J. 297*: 713–715 (1988).

Stevens, R. G., Kuvibidila, S., Kapps, M., Friedlaender, J. S., Blumberg, B. S. Iron-binding proteins, hepatitis B virus, and mortality in the Solomon Islands. *Am. J. Epidemiol. 118*: 550–561 (1983).

Stevens, R. G., Beasley, R. P., Blumberg, B. S. Iron-binding proteins and risk of cancer in Taiwan. *JNCI 76*: 605–610 (1986).

Stevens, R. G., Jones, D. Y., Micozzi, M. S., Taylor, P. R. Body iron stores and the risk of cancer. *N. Engl. J. Med. 319*: 1047–1052 (1988).

Stevens, R. G., Kalkwarf, D. R. Iron, radiation, and cancer. *Environ. Health Perspec. 87*: 291–300 (1990).

Stevens, R. G., Blumberg, B. S. Serum albumin and mortality. *Lancet 335*: 351 (1990).

Stram, D. O., Akiba, S., Neriishi, K., Stevens, R. G., Hosoda, Y. Smoking and serum proteins in atomic-bomb survivors in Japan. *Am. J. Epidemiol. 131*: 1038–1045 (1990).

Sweetnam, P. M., Yarnell, J. W. G. Albumin and serum proteins. *Lancet 336*: 128 (1990).

Weinberg, E. D. Iron withholding: A defense against infection and neoplasia. *Physiological Reviews 64*: 65–102 (1984).

Wilding, G., Blumberg, B. S., Vesell, E. S. Reduced warfarin binding of albumin variants. *Science 195*: 991–994 (1977).

12

Dietary Fiber

Elaine Lanza and Sharada Shankar
National Cancer Institute
National Institutes of Health
Bethesda, Maryland

Bruce Trock
Fox Chase Cancer Center
Philadelphia, Pennsylvania

INTRODUCTION

Dietary fiber is now recognized as an important component of our daily diet. It is alleged to influence a host of metabolic functions and to modify physiologic processes in a variety of human diseases. This chapter reviews the evidence for the role of a fiber-rich diet in the prevention of certain types of cancers, especially colon cancer.

While most of the research advances in our knowledge about dietary fiber, including its chemistry, analysis, metabolic functions, and health effects, have been made in the last 15 years, the idea of physiologic benefits deriving from dietary fiber is not new. Hippocrates spoke of the benefits of wheat with bran over refined flour, and medical scientists in the nineteenth and twentieth centuries noted the laxative properties of fiber. Current interest in the role of dietary fiber in the etiology of diseases common in westernized countries can be credited to the observation of Burkitt (1) that diseases such as colon cancer, diverticular disease, gallstones, and ischemic heart disease are rare in most African populations; he hypothesized a link between a diet high in dietary fiber and low risk for these diseases. This seminal paper can be credited with bringing dietary fiber to the attention of professional and lay audiences and labeling dietary fiber as the miracle nutrient of the 1980s.

Since dietary fiber is not a subject that is covered in most medical or nutrition texts it is important to begin this chapter with background on dietary fiber.

DEFINING DIETARY FIBER

Prior to the 1970s the term fiber or roughage was used to describe the components of food not digested by humans. However, little research was done to assess the constitution of these substances, since fiber was considered to have limited physiologic effects. Scientists understood that fiber was not one substance, but a heterogeneous mixture of complex polysaccharides and nonpolysaccharide polymers. Trowell (2) offered the first definition of the term *dietary fiber*, calling it the components of the plant cell wall that resist digestion by secretions of the human alimentary tract. This biological definition grouped together a number of substances including proteins, lipids, and inorganic substances that are resistant to digestion but which are not usually considered to be dietary fiber components. A Canadian government report on dietary fiber (3) proposed the following definition of dietary fiber: "the endogenous components of plant material in the diet which are resistant to digestion by enzymes produced by man. They are predominantly nonstarch polysaccharides and lignin and may incude, in addition, associated substances." This definition attempted to be broad enough to encompass the biological definition and at the same time specific enough to be meaningful to international and health communities. This definition was subsequently used by the more recent Federation of American Societies for Experimental Biology (FASEB) Report on Dietary Fiber and Health (4). While this definition is widely shared by the scientific community, there is still some controversy. Englyst (5) suggested that lignin should not be classified as a dietary fiber and proposed that dietary fiber only include the nonstarch polysaccharides in foods. The problem with defining dietary fiber stems from its heterogeneous nature from both a physiologic and analytic perspective.

A schematic representation of the relation between the major dietary fiber components is given in Fig. 1. Most dietary fibers are polysaccharides and can be classified as either pectin, hemicellulose, or cellulose. The other major fiber class is lignin, which is a nonpolysaccharide, phenylpropane polymer. The structural fibers cellulose, lignin, and some hemicelluloses tend to be nonfermentable by colonic bacteria and less soluble in water, whereas the natural gel-forming fibers, including pectins, gums, mucilages, and the remaining hemicelluloses, are more fermentable and water-soluble.

Cellulose, a simple linear polymer of glucose linked by β-glycosidic bonds, is one of the most abundant molecules in nature and is the principal cell wall structural material. The term hemicellulose was originally applied to polysaccharides which were structurally related and associated with cellulose. The structure of hemicelluloses is quite diverse, with over 250 different known hemicelluloses. These plant polysaccharides consist mostly of branched polymers of pentose and hexose sugars such as mannose, glucose, galactose, xylose, and arabinose. Pectins are a mixture of colloidal polysaccharides present in the cell

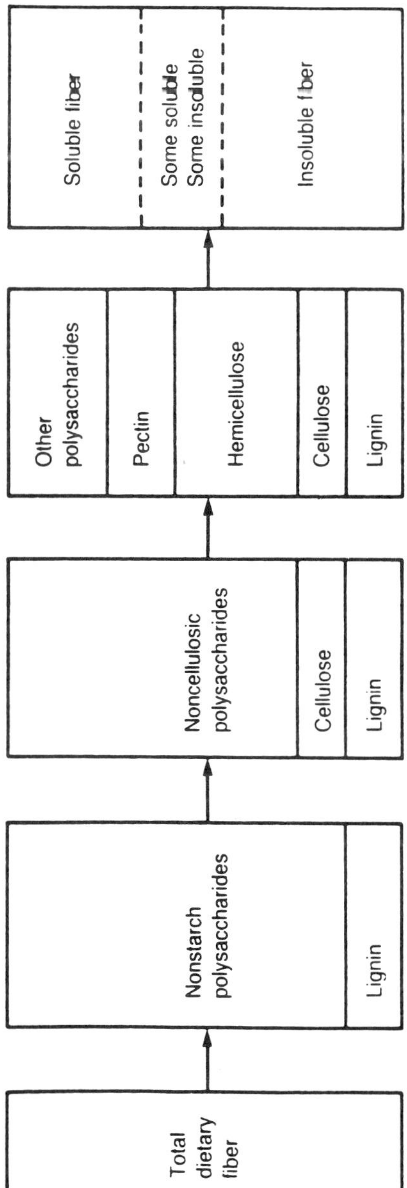

Figure 1 The relationship between the major fiber components.

wall matrix which bind adjacent cell walls. Other polysaccharides include gums, which are found as exudates at the sites of injury to plants, and consist primarily of galactose, glucose, and galacturonic acid; mucilages, which are a mixed group of complex polysaccharides that are not generally part of the cell wall, and are often associated with the endosperm; and algal polysaccharides, which are derived from algae and seaweed and are used as food ingredients. Lignin can be described as three-dimensional networks of phenylpropane units. The precursors of these consist of aromatic alcohols, cinnamyl, coniferyl, *p*-coumaryl, and sinapyl alcohols, which are formed into lignin by a complex polymerization process.

ANALYZING DIETARY FIBER

Even though there is an increased interest in dietary fiber among scientists and the general public, the paucity of analytical data on dietary fiber and the various components of dietary fiber has impeded research on its health effects. Foods differ in both the amount and types of dietary fiber they contain. For example, cereals, except for oats and barley, contain only insoluble fibers and are especially rich in hemicelluloses. Vegetables and fruits tend to be higher in cellulose than most cereals and contain a range of soluble to insoluble fibers. Legumes are a rich source of both total dietary fiber and the highly water-soluble gums. Seaweeds and oats are also rich sources of gums. Pectins are found mostly in fruits, especially apples and citrus fruits. Lignin is highest in fruits with edible seeds or in mature vegetables such as carrots and other root vegetables (6).

Analytic methodology for quantifying total dietary fiber and individual fiber components in foods is complex and time consuming, due to the heterogeneity of the components of dietary fiber, the complexity of the plant material from which fiber is extracted, and controversy over which components actually comprise dietary fiber. Until recently, food composition tables presented data for crude fiber. The method for measuring crude fiber was developed as early as 1800 to analyze animal feed. This procedure utilized the method of treating the food with hot water, strong acids, and bases. This procedure removes as much as 80% of the hemicellulose, 60% of the lignin, and 50% of the cellulose (7). Crude fiber data is of no practical value since it underestimates dietary fiber content by more than 70% (8). The next generation of fiber analysis methods utilized detergents to remove the nonfiber components from animal feeds (9). The neutral detergent fiber (NDF) was later adapted for foods, however, since the detergent solubilized the water-soluble fibers, this procedure could only be used for foods containing insoluble fibers, such as wheat products.

Measurement of fiber has always been approached by quantifying the residue left after all other macronutrients such as starch, protein and fats are removed from the food. Figure 2 shows a general schematic approach to measuring dietary fiber. In general, dietary fiber analysis can be divided into two categories:

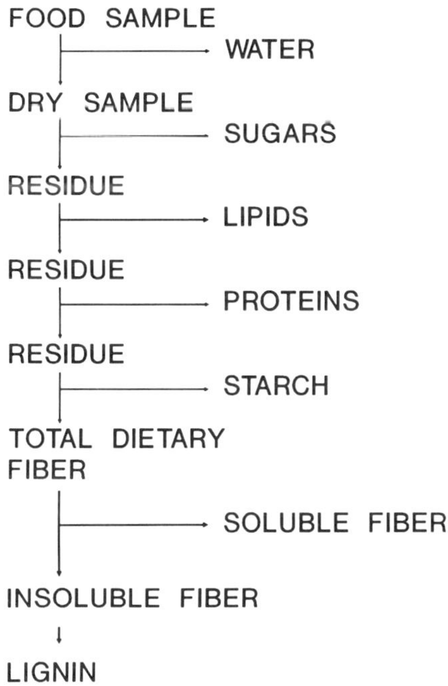

Figure 2 A schematic diagram of the general analytical procedure used for measuring dietary fiber in foods.

gravimetric and chemical analysis (4). In both types of procedures mammalian enzymes are used to remove protein and starch, and thus mimic the separation of these components from indigestible residue as it occurs in the small intestine (10,11). In 1982 the U.S. Food and Drug Administration began a collaborative effort to develop a standard procedure for analyzing total dietary fiber, which led to the now widely used Association of Official Analytical Chemists (AOAC) procedure for dietary fiber (12,13). This procedure measures total dietary fiber gravimetrically in the starch-free residue after corrections for any remaining ash and protein. Since this procedure recovers the solubilized fiber fraction after enzymatic hydrolysis, it accounts for both the insoluble and soluble fibers.

In the chemical procedure the water-insoluble and water-soluble noncellulose polysacharrides, cellulose, and lignin are measured separately. These procedures require acid hydrolysis of the nonstarch polysaccharides, followed by quantification of the resulting sugars by either high pressure liquid chromatography or as their alditol acetates on gas liquid chromatography. This method was first developed by Southgate (14) and further refined by Selvendran and Dupont (15), Theander and Aman (16), and Englyst (17). With the exception of the latter method, a separate procedure is used to determine lignin, which is then added to the total dietary fiber value.

As our knowledge of dietary fiber and its chemistry has expanded, a number of new analytical issues have arisen. One difficulty for all procedures is the complete removal of starch. During food processing, some starch becomes resistant to both enzymatic and chemical removal. This occurs in a variety of foods including corn flakes and potato chips. The current controversy is whether this resistant starch behaves like dietary fiber in the intestine and therefore should be included in the fiber measurement.

Another recent problem is the classification of dietary fiber as either soluble or insoluble, with different procedures yielding quite different results. For most foods, there is no clear distinction between soluble and insoluble dietary fiber fractions, and the ratio of these components is strictly dependent on the pretreatment or the analytical method itself as demonstrated by Graham et al. (18) and Marlett et al. (19). In 1987 the AOAC began a collaborative effort to modify their procedure for total dietary fiber in order to determine soluble and insoluble fiber (20). These modifications, however, did not yield the satisfactory results. At this time grouping dietary fiber according to solubility must be considered a rather arbitrary classification, and data on soluble and insoluble fiber should be used cautiously.

DIETARY FIBER CONSUMPTION

Data on dietary fiber intake in the U.S. population is meager, as there were limited analytic data on the dietary fiber content of foods until the 1980s. Prior to that, food tables only listed crude fiber values, which provide a poor estimate of dietary fiber intake. Data suggest a 29% decrease in crude fiber consumption in the United States from 1901 to 1975 (Table 1) (21). The largest decrease has been in cereal fiber, followed by legumes and potatoes. For other vegetables there has been relatively little change. There has also been a considerable decrease in crude fiber consumption from fruits. The only increase is seen for nut consumption, also a high source of fiber. Even though crude fiber is only a rough estimate of insoluble fiber and measures no soluble fiber, this type of estimation of relative changes across food groups is interesting.

The first estimate of dietary fiber intake in the U.S. population from a cross-sectional national survey found a mean intake of 11.1 g/day of dietary fiber (22). This estimate was derived by examining 24-hour recall data from 11,658 adult respondents in the second National Health and Nutrition Examination Survey (NHANES II, 1976–1980). Dietary fiber values were compiled from literature values using appropriate analytical methodology for estimating total dietary fiber (Lanza and Butrum, 1986). The distribution of dietary fiber intake in the adult

Table 1 U.S. Crude Fiber Consumption, Daily Per Capita Changes 1909–1975

Food group	Changes (%)
Total plant food	−29
Cereals	−55
Legumes	−46
Potatoes	−42
Fruits	−34
Vegetables	− 7
Nuts	+188

Source: Ref. 21.

U.S. population is given in Fig. 3. On any given day, 50% of the population reports dietary fiber intake of < 10 g/day and only approximately 10% consume >20 g/day. This study indicated that dietary fiber consumption is considerably lower than previous estimates, which had suggested intakes close to 20 g/day (24). These earlier estimates were derived either by selecting foods that repre-

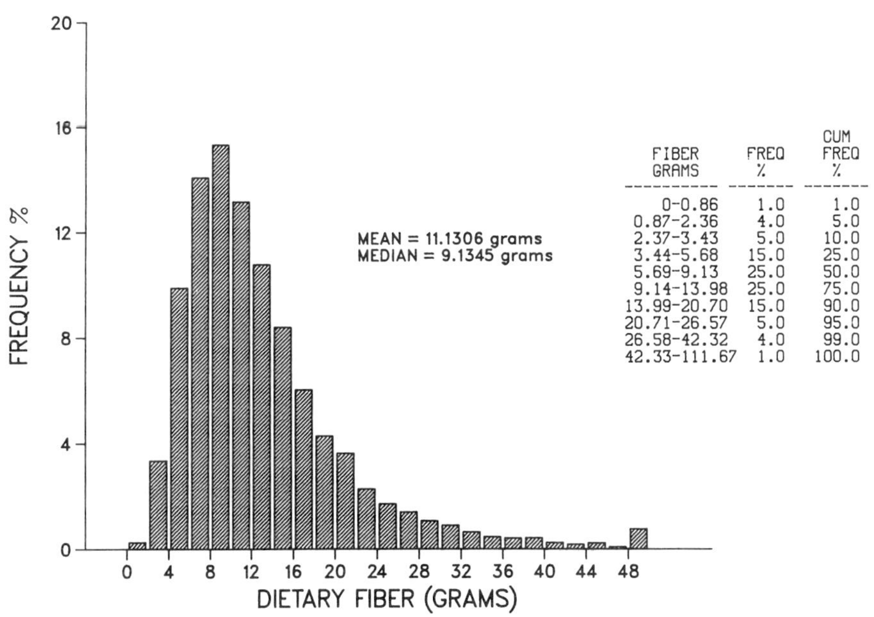

Figure 3 The distribution of dietary fiber intake in the adult U.S. population. (From Ref. 22.)

Table 2 Estimation of Dietary Fiber Intake, U.S. Population

Dietary fiber			
(g/day)	(g/1000 kcal)	Assessment	Ref.
11.2	6.0	NHANES II	22
9.4F	6.5F	NHANES II	22
11.0F	7.0F	CFS II	Personal communication
11.4	5.7	NFCS 77	26

sent an ideal diet (an adequate number of servings from all food groups) (24) or by collecting dietary data from a small segment of the population (25) and then analyzing either of these diets for dietary fiber.

Recent studies have confirmed this low levels of dietary fiber intake in the United States (Table 2). Anderson and colleagues, using the USDA National Food Consumption Survey (NFCS) and analyzing dietary fiber by a modified Southgate procedure, reported a daily intake of 11.4 g (26). In addition the most recent national survey in women, Continuing Food Consumption Survey, Individual Intake, conducted by the USDA reported an intake of 10.9 g/day for women, which is very close to the 9.4 g/day reported by Lanza et al. (22). What is interesting in comparing these recent surveys is the similar values for dietary fiber consumption on a per-1000-kcal basis.

The major source of dietary fiber in the United States and in many Western countries is from vegetables (Table 3). This is an important fact to remember when interpreting epidemiologic association between dietary fiber and cancer. Figure 4 presents the sources of dietary fiber among adults in the NHANES II, aggregated into 10 broad food categories. Vegetables (including potatoes and salads) represent 28% of our dietary fiber intake. If one adds to this the 14% from beans and legumes, a total of 42% of our dietary fiber comes from vegetables.

Table 3 Sources of Dietary Fiber for Various Western Countries

	Cereals (%)	Vegetables (%)	Fruit (%)
Finland	73	17	6
Italy	50	34	16
United Kingdom	31	41	11
Netherlands	32	41	15
Germany	48	32	16
Australia	31	45	23
United States	24	42	17

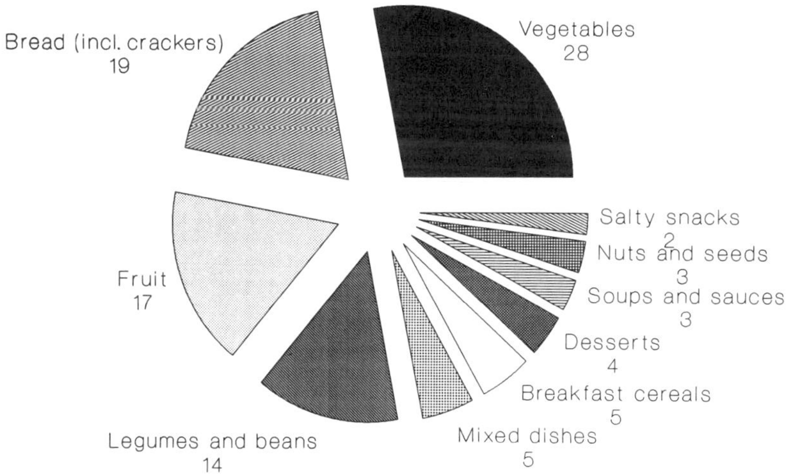

Figure 4 Major sources of dietary fiber among adults in the United States (From Ref. 27.)

This compares to 17% from fruits and only 24% from cereals and grains (19% bread and 5% breakfast cereals) (27). Thus, 59% of our dietary fiber comes from fruits and vegetables, and only 24% from cereals. Legumes, despite their relatively infrequent consumption (approximately 10% of the population on any day), are the fourth most important contributor of dietary fiber by virtue of their high fiber content.

MECHANISMS BY WHICH FIBER MAY AFFECT CANCER RISK

Colon Cancer

One of the reasons that dietary fiber is such an attractive hypothesis is that fiber offers numerous plausible mechanisms by which it could prevent the development of cancer, especially colon cancer. Probably the most widely accepted hypothesis for the development of colon cancer is that fecal bile acids cause small adenomas (with a low malignant potential) to grow to a large size (with a correspondingly high malignant potential) and to become more severely dysplastic (28). Colonic bile acid concentration is thought to increase with a high fat diet (29.30). Colonic bacteria may convert these bile acids to secondary bile acids, primarily lithocholic acid (LA) and deoxycholic acids (DA). These secondary bile acids have been shown in laboratory models to alter the proliferative activity of intestinal crypt cells (31) and to promote tumorigenesis (32). Recent evidence suggested that the LA/DA ratio is most predictive of risk (33). In addition, the amount of fat in the diet directly affects the amount of free fatty acids in the bowel lumen (34), and these free fatty acids have been shown to damage bowel mucosa (35).

Fiber is postulated to reduce these adverse affects of fat and bile acids through several interrelated mechanisms (Table 4). The earliest hypothesis on dietary fiber was related to a reduction of the exposure to carcinogenic agents in the colon by a more rapid transit time of fecal matter and/or dilution of fecal contents by increased fecal bulk of the stools. Figure 5 shows how both insoluble and soluble dietary fibers can increase fecal bulk and reduce transit time. Insoluble dietary fibers tend to be more nonfermentable and therefore add bulk mostly by adsorbing water during their passage in the intestine, which in turn reduces transit time. However, highly fermentable soluble fibers increase bulk by increasing microbial fermentation leading to increased microbial mass, which then also decreases transit time (36).

Newer hypotheses have been proposed that focus on the importance of microbial fermentation in cancer prevention. Colonic bacteria may have an indirect role in colon carcinogenesis through the production of short-chain fatty acids (SCFA), especially butyrate, the reduction of colonic pH, and the decrease in colonic ammonia. Fermentation of carbohydrates by the anaerobic bacteria of the large intestine results in the production of short-chain fatty acids, principally acetate, propionate, and butyrate (37). Butyrate, the principal source of energy of the colonic epithelium (38), has also been shown in cell-free systems to have antineoplastic properties. In vitro studies with human colorectal cell lines have shown that butyrate blocks the cell cycle following mitosis. This results in an increased doubling time and a decrease in saturation densities and cloning efficiencies, and inhibits expression of malignant phenotype, inducing a less neoplastic form of differentiation (39,40). SCFAs also reduce the pH of the colon. Several researchers have suggested that pH could be a key determinant in colon cancer. At a high pH most of the bile acids and acidic lipids which are now widely considered to be tumor promoters (28) are in solution and thus could act as detergents against the colonic mucosa. As the pH is reduced, more of the acids become

Table 4 Hypothesized Effects of Fiber That May Decrease Colon Cancer Risk

1. Altered bile acid concentration
2. Physical dilution of fecal contents
3. Decrease fermentation
4. Microbial fermentation
Production of SCFA, butyrate
Lower pH
Lower ammonia levels

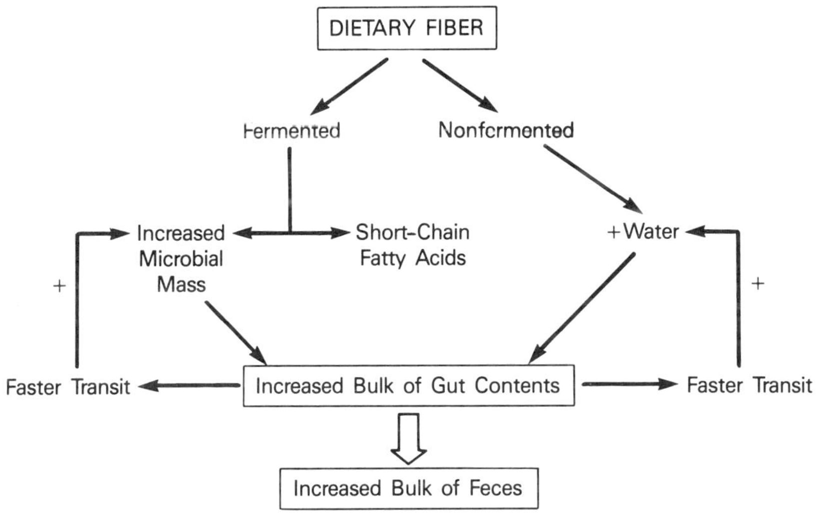

Figure 5 The effect of soluble and insoluble dietary fiber on fecal output.

protonated and thus bind with the calcium and other salts available in the colon (41). In this way reduction of colonic pH could theoretically prevent the colonic mucosa from damage by the bile acids. It is important to note that the pH of the colon is rarely consistent. The pH of the cecum and proximal colon change with the ingestion of fermentable fibers but the pH of the distal colon tends to remain unaltered (37,42). Fermentation in the colon leads to utilization of ammonia, which further leads to a decrease in pH and a decrease of NH_4 (43).

Breast Cancer

Recent evidence suggests that certain types of fibers may modify the biological action of hormones, and thus may reduce the risk of hormone-related cancers, especially breast cancer. The lower plasma prolactin and estradiol levels and higher fecal estrogen levels found in women consuming high fiber diets are generally associated with a lower breast cancer risk. These hormone changes could occur through fiber-mediated changes in the intestinal bacteria which lead to decreased deconjugation of bound estrogens (44,45). An additional mechanism by which dietary fiber may exert its influences is the direct binding of the unconjugated estrogens to fibers (46).

It has been recently reported that in women, dietary fiber intake is directly proportional to the excretion of urinary lignans (47). Lignans, not to be confused with the dietary fiber lignin, can be formed by intestinal bacteria from diphenolic compounds found in grain and other fiber-rich foods, may influence estrogen metabolism (48), and thus offers another explanation for the association of fiber-rich foods with certain types of cancers.

Other Cancers

The mechanism by which fiber might be protective for cancers of the esophagus, oral cavity and pharynx, stomach, and rectum is not known. Over the last decade research has demonstrated that fiber is not merely an inert component of the diet, but one that elicits a variety of physiologic effects. In some studies it is not known whether the protection is due to fiber or other components present in the fiber-rich foods such as carotenoids, vitamin C, micronutrients, or other plant substances such as indoles, flavonoids, lignans, and phytates. In addition, since high fat diets are also usually low in fiber, an indirect protective role for dietary fiber can be accordingly constructed for all cancers positively associated with high fat diets.

EPIDEMIOLOGIC STUDIES

The association between diets rich in fiber and cancer risk has been examined in a large number of observational epidemiologic studies. Although the bulk of this research has focused on colorectal cancer risk, associations with breast cancer have increasingly been the subject of study, while other cancer sites such as stomach, prostate, ovary, and endometrium have also been examined. This research has been conducted in diverse populations, using a variety of study designs and measures of fiber intake. Because of the potential limitations of observational epidemiologic methods, it is necessary to consider not only the magnitude of observed measures of risk, but also the extent to which study results could have been influenced by sources of bias. Some of the more prominent sources of bias will first be discussed below in a general fashion. The potential for bias from these sources will be considered when examining the epidemiologic evidence for risk modification of specific cancers by a fiber-rich diet.

Epidemiologic studies typically estimate dietary fiber intake using questionnaires that assess self-reported consumption frequency and often the usual portion size of individual foods. Some studies assess risk associated with intake frequency of specific foods or food groups without converting these to dietary fiber estimates. Other studies (especially more recent ones) derive dietary fiber estimates from frequency data using databases that list nutrient values for specified amounts of individual foods. These approaches are susceptible to bias from a number of sources. The accuracy of dietary recall exhibits great variability and can be affected by recent disease-related dietary changes or the knowledge that one has a specific disease. Thus, recall problems can give rise to either nondifferential or differential misclassification. The former attenuates the observed dietary association toward the null value, while the latter can produce either risk enhancement or reduction as an artifact (49).

In addition to recall problems, bias may also arise from correlations among dietary fiber, fat, and caloric intake (multicollinearity). Significant correlations among nutrients can result in a loss of power to detect effects of any one of them in a multivariable model (50). Correlations among nutrients can also induce confounding of observed associations with risk, e.g., the positive correlation between dietary fiber and caloric intake can result in apparent excess risk associated with high fiber intake. Furthermore, as Willett and Stampfer have pointed out, the method of controlling for caloric intake can have profound effects on the observed results. For example, use of nutrient density values (nutrient intake divided by caloric intake) for a disease associated with high caloric intake, can produce a spurious inverse association with disease even if the nutrient is not an independent risk factor. This results from the inverse correlation between the nutrient density value and total caloric intake (51).

The precision with which dietary fiber intake can be estimated is also variable. Epidemiologic studies are not based on consumption of individual nutrients, but rather on dietary patterns involving complex interactions among foods, nutrients, and micronutrients. A diet that is high in dietary fiber may be high in vegetables, fruits, or grains, and correspondingly high in other nutrients and micronutrients in addition to fiber; conversely it may be low in fat. Thus, it is difficult if not impossible using current observational data to distinguish a pure dietary fiber effect from effects of other nutrients or dietary patterns (49). This is underscored by the fact that the majority of dietary fiber in Western diets is derived from vegetable sources (27). Furthermore, there is considerable inconsistency across studies in the specific foods that are included in estimates of dietary fiber and in the databases used to derive fiber values. Thus, quantitative estimates of dietary fiber (or components of dietary fiber) may under- or overestimate true intake in any given study, and estimates may not be comparable across studies.

Despite the inability to precisely estimate effects of absolute fiber intake, the data are adequate for ordering individuals into several categories of intake of fiber-containing foods and comparing risk between highest and lowest categories (49). In fact, ranking based on simple food frequency data may often be as food as quantitative estimates of dietary fiber because recall of the usual amount consumed of a given food introduces additional random error (52,49). In addition, risk estimates associated with highest and lowest rank-based quantiles are likely to have greater comparability across studies.

In addition to problems arising from measures of exposure, dietary studies are also subject to bias resulting from the choice of control groups. For example, studies that utilize hospital patients as controls may underestimate effects associated with a high fiber diet if controls include patients with cardiovascular disease or other conditions influenced by diet. Selection bias may also arise if participation rates vary markedly between those eligible to be cases and controls; this could result in overrepresentation of individuals with a healthy lifestyle among the controls and an artifactual protective effect of fiber (49).

STUDIES OF COLORECTAL CANCER

The authors recently completed a detailed quantitative review of all epidemiologic studies of fiber and colorectal cancer published from 1970 to 1988 (49). Results from this review will be summarized below and discussed along with the findings from more recent studies. This review assessed the evidence for a protective effect associated with a fiber-rich diet by considering not only the observed risk estimate from each study, but also the study design and methods, to determine the influence of potential sources of bias. Based on this assessment, each study was classified according to the strength of the evidence for a protective effect. Because of the variety of methods and populations encompassed by this review, emphasis was placed on intake measures that were adequate for ranking individuals according to quantiles of dietary fiber intake. These measures included quantitative dietary fiber estimates, crude fiber estimates, and frequency measures for food groups or specific foods. The review included 23 case-control studies, two cohort studies, one international correlation study, eight intranational correlation studies, and three time-trend analyses. In addition, a meta-analysis was performed on 16 of the case-control studies that provided sufficient data in the published reports to calculate a combined odds ratio.

Colon and rectal cancers will not be distinguished in the discussion which follows. There are many reasons to suspect different etiology for these cancers, including differences in embryonic origin, blood supply, metabolic processes, exposure to fecal matter, and mechanical functions. However, many studies combined data from all large bowel tumors. Furthermore, among those that examined risk separately for colon and rectal tumors, most observed similar results for both sites (results not presented by site below). Finally, classification of a tumor site as colon or rectum is subject to error and interstudy variability, particularly when different ICD coding schemes are used. Therefore, no distinction between these sites is made below; careful study of subsite risk in future studies will be necessary to determine whether dietary risk factors for these sites truly differ.

The evaluation revealed that 21 studies provided strong or moderately strong evidence for a protective effect of high fiber diets, and eight studies were consistent with a protective effect but were deemed to provide equivocal evidence due to inability to rule out potential sources of bias. Conversely, only two studies provided strong evidence of a lack of a protective effect, and six studies provided equivocal evidence for a lack of effect. Although many studies did not adjust for potential confounding effects of other nutrients, it is unlikely that observed protective effects were artifacts of confounding. Among studies that did adjust for intake of other nutrients, adjustment reduced protective effects in only two studies, while protective effects were enhanced in four studies and unchanged in eight. This also suggests that multicollinearity was not a major problem since adjustment for other nutrients did not result in loss of statistical significance (49).

A common criticism of research on the protective effect of dietary fiber has been that the evidence primarily supported an effect associated with vegetable intake but was weak or inconsistent for an effect of dietary fiber per se. As discussed above, the current observational data is not adequate to discrimiante between protective effects associated with the fiber content of vegetables and those due to other nutrients or micronutrients. However, out of 23 case-control studies in the review, 10 provided risk estimates based on vegetable intake, 10 based on estimated dietary fiber intake, and three studies assessed risk using both types of measures. For vegetable intake, seven studies provided strong evidence, two moderately strong, and four equivocal evidence (two consistent with a protective effect, and two consistent with lack of an effect). For fiber intake, five studies provided strong evidence, four moderately strong, two equivocal but consistent with a protective effect, and two strongly supported a lack of effect (49). Thus, the evidence based on vegetable intake was somewhat more compelling than that based on fiber, but the difference was not great.

Evidence for effects from other components of vegetables and fruit was less clear. Eight of nine studies that assessed risk associated with cruciferous vegetables demonstrated protective effects. However, cruciferous vegetable intake is highly correlated with overall vegetable intake; six of the nine studies exhibited protective effects for other vegetables as well. Only four of 12 studies examining fruit intake observed a protective effect, while two of six studies found a protective effect associated with β-carotene, but adjustment for other nutrients eliminated the effect (49).

A meta-analysis was performed using published data from 16 of the case-control studies. The analysis included a test for homogeneity among individual study odds ratios (OR) and calculation of a combined logarithm of the OR as the weighted average of individual log OR, each weighted by the reciprocal of its variance (53). In addition to the analysis of these 16 case-control studies, separate subanalyses were conducted for 10 of the studies which estimated risk associated with fiber intake, and nine studies which assessed effects of vegetable intake (49).

The results were similar for each of the analyses. The chi-square test for homogeneity indicated significant departures from homogeneity of OR across all 16 studies and across each of the subanalyses. However, in each analysis, when studies considered to provide equivocal evidence were excluded, homogeneity could no longer be rejected. Exclusion of these studies resulted in the following combined odds ratios (representing comparisons between highest and lowest intake categories): OR = 0.57 (95% CI 0.50, 0.64) for all 16 studies; OR = 0.58 (95% CI 0.51, 0.66) for studies based on fiber; OR = 0.48 (95% CI 0.41, 0.57) for studies based on vegetables. Furthermore, an analysis of the seven studies which lacked sufficient data to be included in the meta-analysis suggested that exclusion of those studies was unlikely to have changed the combined odds ratio estimate. Thus, the meta-analysis results were consistent with the assessment based on strength of evidence of all epidemiologic studies and suggest that high intake of diets rich in fiber may reduce colorectal cancer risk by approximately 40% (49).

A number of studies of fiber and colorectal cancer have been published since the above-mentioned review was published. These include seven case-control studies (54–60), one cohort study (61), and one case-control study nested in a cohort study (62). The studies have demonstrated results that are very consistent with those in the earlier review. All but one of these studies (57) demonstrated a decrease in risk associated with high intake of fiber, vegetables, or fruits, although the effect was not statistically significant in the cohort study (61). In addition to these studies of fiber and colorectal cancer risk, a recent study examined whether dietary intake influenced survival from the disease. The adjusted risk of death was increased among those in the highest quartile of fiber intake, but the overall effect of fiber was not significant. Risk was significantly reduced among those in the highest quartile of caloric intake. However, participants in the study (who represented only 44% of cases diagnosed in the time interval) demonstrated considerably better prognostic profiles than nonparticipants, so it is difficult to interpret the results (63).

Similar to the results described in the review (49), the recent studies demonstrated little evidence of confounding by other nutrients. Only four studies presented both crude risk estimates and estimates adjusted for other nutrients. In two of those the protective effect was enhanced by adjustment (59,62), while the effect was unchanged in the other two studies (54,58). Two studies compared effects of fiber from fruits and/or vegetables with fiber from grains. One study found the most consistent risk reduction for fruit fiber, although no fiber effects were statistically significant (61). The second study found stronger effects of grain fiber in the colon, but in the rectum, fiber from vegetables and fruit exhibited a greater protective effect (55). Two other studies compared effects of vegetables with estimated dietary fiber; one study found a stronger effect with crude fiber (59), while the other greater evidence for cruciferous vegetables (58). Thus, protective effects in these newer studies are not limited to fruit or vegetable intake, although it is not possible to determine the independent effects of fiber and non-fiber components of vegetables. Taken together, these studies reinforce the earlier evidence that diets high in vegetables, grains, or fruit reduce the risk of colorectal cancer.

BREAST CANCER

Howe and colleagues recently published a pooled analysis of data from 12 case-control studies of diet and breast cancer risk worldwide (64). This will be discussed in some detail since it offers the most complete assessment of dietary fiber and breast cancer risk to date. Unlike the meta-analysis of colorectal cancer studies described above, which utilized published odds ratio measures as aggregates of the data in each study, this analysis obtained the original data on individual cases and controls in each of the 12 studies. These data records were then pooled and analyzed using an approach similar to that appropriate for a large multi-institutional study. The analysis consisted of data on 4427 cases and 6095 controls. Analyses were conducted on all women, and separately on premenopausal and post-menopausal women, due to the different patterns of risk observed in these groups in previous studies (65). All analyses were also stratified on age-group and study, using conditional logistic regression (64).

The analysis, adjusted for total fat intake, revealed a significant decrease in risk among women in the highest quintile of dietary fiber intake compared to the lowest quintile, OR = 0.85, p = 0.001. Similar risk estimates were observed for premenopausal women (OR = 0.89), and postmenopausal women (OR = 0.83), but were statistically significant only for the latter. Significant reductions in risk were also observed among postmenopausal women for vitamin C intake (OR = 0.63), β-carotene (OR = 0.81), and vitamin A (OR = 0.82). None of these nutrients was associated with a significant reduction in risk among premenopausal women, although a nonsignificant effect was observed for vitamin C (OR = 0.84). Power to detect odds ratios of this magnitude among premenopausal women was less than 80% for vitamin C and probably less than 80% for dietary fiber (depending on the proportion of controls with high fiber intake) (66). No nutrient exhibited a statistically significant interaction with menopausal status (64).

All of the nutrients associated with a decrease in risk are highly intercorrelated due to their common correlation with fruit and vegetable intake. Inclusion of all of these nutrients in a multivariable model which also controlled for fat intake revealed a statistically significant protective effect for vitamin C only: OR = 0.73, p = 0.03. A chi-square test of homogeneity of risk estimates for vitamin C (nine studies with vitamin C data, postmenopausal women only) rejected homogeneity. However, after removal of one study which exhibited the strongest protective effect (OR = 0.12), homogeneity could no longer be rejected. Exclusion of this study reduced the protective effect somewhat, OR = 0.82. Only two of the nine studies did not exhibit a protective effect of vitamin C (64).

It is unlikely that these results merely reflect substitution of fruits or vegetables for high fat foods since intake of vitamin C, dietary fiber, and β-carotene were positively correlated with total fat intake in these data (64). Although the data provide stronger support for a diet high in fruits and vegetables than for dietary fiber per se, it is difficult to effectively discriminate among these factors. The loss of statistical significance associated with dietary fiber in the multivariable model may have been influenced by multicollinearity. However, in the published reports from two of the studies included in this pooled analysis, separate intake data were given for grains, pulses, fruits, and vegetables (67,68). Neither of these studies found an association with grains or pulses, but both observed protective effects with vegetable intake; fruit intake was also protective in the former. The published reports from the other studies did not allow such comparisons to be made.

A number of recent studies not included in the pooled analysis have also investigated the association between fiber or fiber-rich foods and breast cancer risk. Two case-control studies observed significant protective effects associated with either cereal intake (69) or vegetables (70) after adjusting for confounders. In both of these studies, the comparison of the highest and lowest intake categories yielded an odds ratio of 0.40. In the former, risk was also reduced in the highest quartile of dietary fiber, β-carotene, fruit, and vegetable intake, but no significant trend was observed. Response bias is a potential problem for this study, due to the considerable differences in response rates among potential cases (80%) and controls (53%). A mailed follow-up questionnaire completed by most responding controls and some of the non-responders indicated that responders more frequently consumed whole grain bread ($p = 0.07$), which may have enhanced the protective effect observed for cereal. However, the two groups did not differ in fat intake, age at first pregnancy, weight or body mass index, suggesting that individuals with a healthy lifestyle were not overrepresented among responders (69).

Two additional studies assessed the association between diet and either high risk mammograhic patterns (71) or breast cancer prognostic factors (72). In the former, dietary intake was associated with mammographic features in a group of healthy women participating in a screening study. High intake of dietary fiber (energy-adjusted) and β-carotene was associated with a decrease in the extent of nodular or homogeneous densities detectable on mammogram. The extent of densities correlates strongly with breast cancer risk (71). Finally, Holm and colleagues (72) observed that breast cancer patients with tumors measuring <20 mm at diagnosis had higher energy-adjusted fiber intake than those with tumors of 20 mm or more, with the odds of a larger tumor decreasing approximately 7% for each one gram increase in fiber per 10 MJ. An association was also seen between higher fiber intake and higher levels of estrogen receptor in the tumor, but this association did not remain after adjustment for other dietary factors (72). Although this study utilized nutrient density measures of fiber, there was no association between energy intake and tumor size, and fiber intake was associated with tumor site independent of energy intake. However, size of the tumor at diagnosis may just represent delay in seeking medical attention. If treatment delay is related to general health habits and knowledge, it is possible that the observed inverse association with fiber could have arisen as an artifact of a more health-conscious lifestyle.

Thus, the data consistently demonstrate an association between decreased risk of breast cancer and diets rich in fruits, vegetables, or grains. Based on the pooled data presented by Howe and colleagues, such a diet may be associated with a decrease in risk of approximately 20%.

OTHER CANCER SITES

Diets high in fiber or fruits and vegetables have been associated with reduced risk for a number of cancers. These associations have been less well studied than those for colorectal cancer or breast cancer. Furthermore, the etiology of most of these other cancer sites is, for the most part, unknown. Thus, it is difficult to rule out confounding by unmeasured factors, particularly with weak associations such as those commonly observed for dietary factors. Nevertheless, the effects of fiber on circulating sex hormone levels suggest that risk for cancers with a probable endocrine component may be modifiable by a diet high in vegetables, grains, or fruit. Etiologic mechanisms for a fiber effect on nonendocrine cancers are less readily apparent. Accordingly, evidence for an association between high fiber diets and other cancers will be briefly discussed.

Ovarian Cancer

Several case-control studies have examined the effect of fiber or fruit and vegetable intake on epithelial ovarian cancer risk. Byers and colleagues observed an increase in risk for women aged 30–49 in the lowest tertile of vitamin A intake from fruits and vegetables, OR = 2.3. The effect remained significant after adjustment for confounding factors. A similar association with low fiber intake was no longer statistically significant in an adjusted analysis. Assessment of potential selection and recall biases suggested that the observed association was not likely to be an artifact of such forms of bias (73). La Vecchia and colleagues also observed significantly lower risk with high intake of green vegetables and whole grain bread or pasta, OR = 0.6 for both after adjustment for confounding factors. No association was observed for fruit, and an association with β-carotene disappeared after adjustment. The low nonresponse rate in both cases and controls (<2%) and similar catchment area for both groups suggests that selection bias was an unlikely explanation for the observed results (74). A more recent case-control study also observed protective effects of β-carotene, OR = 0.5, and both crude and neutral detergent fiber, OR = 0.8 and 0.7, respectively; all OR were adjusted. Only the effect of β-carotene was statistically significant, but the study had only 60% power to detect effects of the observed magnitude (75). A high nonparticipation rate in cases introduced some possibility of selection bias, although the majority of nonresponse was due to disease severity or death or physician refusal (75). It should be noted that none of these studies adjusted for energy intake. However, neither energy intake, fat, or protein was associated with risk in one study (75), fat and protein intake were unrelated to risk in another study (73), and all studies adjusted for body mass index. Thus, the similarity in results among these studies is provocative, but clearly must be regarded as tentative at this point. Larger studies with more comprehensive dietary data and more complete analyses will be required to clarify these associations.

Endometrial Cancer

An inverse association between endometrial cancer risk and high intake of both β-carotene (OR = 0.3), and whole grain bread or pasta (OR = 0.6) has been reported. Both estimates were adjusted for other confounders (including Quetelet index), but only the former was statistically significant (76). However, there were limitations to the study. Energy intake was not determined, and only a limited number of dietary items were included in the questionnaire. Adjustment was not carried out for more than one dietary factor simultaneously. An association with fat was limited to consumption of butter, margarine, and oil; no association with other fat sources was observed. Thus, the study should serve for hypothesis generation, to be investigated in more thorough investigations.

Prostate Cancer

A metabolic epidemiology study among Seventh-day Adventist men revealed significant associations between fiber intake and fecal concentration of sex hormones. Three groups of men were compared: nonvegetarians (NV), lactoovovegetarians (LOV), and vegans (V). Fecal concentration of estrone and estrone plus estradiol were significantly higher among V compared to either LOV or NV. Furthermore, fecal estradiol and testosterone were each higher in V by more than 20%, but the difference was not satistically significant. Among plasma hormones, only prolactin was significantly lower among V than either LOV or NV, and serum prolactin was positively correlated with saturated fat intake. Regression analyses revealed significant correlations between both dietary and crude fiber intake and fecal estrone, estradiol, and testosterone levels among all three groups combined (77). Fecal weight and fecal concentration of fiber components were all significantly higher among V than LOV or NV, and in vitro assays determined that the percentage of bound steroid hormones increased with the dietary concentration of lignin (78). However, it is unclear from the reports whether adjustment was made for body mass index, which was significantly lower in both V and LOV compared to NV, or energy intake, which was significantly higher in V compared to either group.

Only one other epidemiologic study has assessed prostate cancer risk associated with dietary fiber; no effect was observed (79). A number of case-control studies have examined associations with intake of vegetables, vitamin A, or β-carotene. Results have been inconsistent, with several finding excess risk (80–82), while others have found protective effects (83,84,79), and one cohort study has observed both protective and adverse effects according to age (85). None of these studies had adequate adjustment for energy intake, and several of the observed effects were age-dependent but not consistently so (79–82,85). Thus, although an effect of fiber or high fruit and vegetable intake on prostate cancer risk is biologically plausible through an influence on circulating hormone levels, available epidemiologic data are inadequate to determine whether risk modification actually occurs.

Other Cancers

Decreased stomach cancer risk was significantly associated with high dietary fiber intake, adjusted OR = 0.4. Although the study adequately controlled for confounding factors, response rates were low, only 44% for cases and 58% for controls, so selection bias cannot be ruled out (86). Although high intake of "starchy" foods has been associated with increased stomach cancer risk (87), these foods include pastry and other digestible carbohydrates in addition to the nondigestible carbohydrates that contribute to fiber. Furthermore, this study did not adjust for other confounders or dietary factors.

Pancreatic cancer risk has been shown to be inversely correlated with fruit and vegetable intake, with odds ratios of approximately 0.5 for high intake (88–90). All of these effects were significant and adjusted for confounders and other nutrients, but only the latter adjusted for caloric intake. The latter also demonstrated a significant protective effect for fiber from all sources, OR = 0.4, and independent effects of fiber from fuit (OR = 0.4), fiber from vegetables (OR = 0.6), and fiber from cereals (OR = 0.3) in a logistic regression model. Furthermore, simultaneous inclusion of total fiber, fruit, and vegetable intake in a logistic regression model resulted in a significant protective effect only for fiber, suggesting that fiber was not just an indicator of fruit and vegetable intake (90). The studies by Falk et al. and Howe et al. both relied on proxy interviews for at least 50% of the cases, although stratification by proxy status did not appreciably change results. In addition, the latter had a very low response rate among cases (46%) and controls (31%) (90). Thus, these data suggest that pancreatic cancer risk may also be modified by a diet high in fruits, vegetables, and grains, although confirmatory studies less susceptible to recall and selection biases are necessary.

SUMMARY OF EPIDEMIOLOGIC DATA

A very large body of evidence from diverse populations suggests that diets high in vegetables, grains, and fruits may modify risk from several cancers. The strongest evidence to date is for a protective effect on colorectal cancer, although the data for breast cancer is also very consistent. Evidence for other sites, while provocative, is based on only limited investigation and requires larger, methodologically sound confirmatory studies. In particular, clarification of these results will require careful selection of control groups, high response rates, detailed dietary data, and sufficient power to investigate associations among subgroups. The current data do not allow discrimination between effects of dietary fiber per se and nonfiber components of fiber-rich diets. Determination of the specific nutrients or dietary components conferring protection may not be possible with retrospective data.

INTERVENTION STUDIES

While it is generally agreed that a randomized controlled dietary intervention trial would provide the most definitive data in demonstrating a causal relationship between fiber and cancer, the cost and time involved when cancer is the endpoint is enormous. Bruce (41) has estimated that a colon cancer clinical trial would require 100,000 subjects and take from 5 to 10 years. Thus, fiber intervention studies to date have employed only protocols using hypothesized precursor colon cancer lesions as endpoints. These precursors, often referred to as intermediate endpoints, can be divided into two distinct categories: those which produce general changes in the colon such as fecal bile acics, fecal mutagens, and pH, or changes which involve a specific alteration at the organ, tissue, cell or molecular level, such as cell proliferation and adenomatous polyps. Reddy et al. (91) found changes in both the concentration of fecal secondary bile acids and fecal mutagen activity when feeding cellulose and wheat bran, but not with the more fermentable fiber such as oat bran. Two recent studies have examined the effect of wheat bran supplementation on cell proliferation rates in rectal mucosal biopsies. In one study no change in cell proliferation as assayed by thymidine labeling was found in normal healthy volunteers after supplementing their diet for 2 weeks with 30 grams per day of wheat bran fiber (93). The other study found a significant decrease in thymidine labelling in 13 subjects who had previously resected colon cancer after 8 weeks with 13.5 grams per day of wheat bran fiber (93).

It is commonly accepted that most large bowel cancers arise from adenomatous polyps, especially those that are large. These often have a villous growth pattern or show severe dysplasia (94). There are currently three studies examining the effects of fiber on the occurence of adenomatous polyps. A Canadian study comprising 200 participants on a low fat, high cereal fiber supplement has just been completed (95). In an Australian study, the effects of reduced fat intake, a wheat bran fiber supplement, and a β-carotene supplement are being examined in a $2 \times 2 \times 2$ randomized factorial design involving 424 participants (96). This study should be completed in 1991. The third polyp study is just beginning and will involve 2000 subjects from 10 different clinical centers in the United States (97). This trial will randomize participants to either a low fat, high fiber, fruit and vegetable enriched dietary pattern or their usual diet. The change in dietary fiber does not involve a supplement but is, rather, implemented through a change in dietary pattern from the traditional Western diet to one that is considered to be of less risk for colon cancer. Results from this study will not be available until 1997 or later.

Familial adenomatous polyposis, a premalignant autosomal disorder, is characterized by a multitude of adenomatous polyps in the colon and rectum and progression to cancer in almost 100% of patients if not treated (97). In a wheat bran intervention trial of 58 polyposis patients, a limited degree of polyp regression was observed after 6 months in the high fiber group (98). The mean daily intake of fiber for the treatment group was 22.4 grams per day.

PUBLIC HEALTH IMPLICATIONS

Table 5 lists some of the dietary fiber recommendations of a number of organizations in North America since 1977. These recommendations have been for generally good health, disease prevention, and cancer prevention. A step forward was taken by the Canadian Government Expert Advisory Committee on Dietary Fiber (3) when they quantitated the fiber recommendation (double the current intake of dietary fiber). The NCI recommendation is to consume 20–35 grams of dietary fiber per day from a variety of food sources including fruits, vegetables, and cereal products. This level of intake is roughly twice our current dietary fiber intake level of 10–15 grams per day (22). Since the evidence for a protective effect of fiber is generally from an association of dietary patterns in which fiber occurs as a complex mixture with other foods, the extrapolation to the possible beneficial effects from fiber supplements cannot be made at this time. Since totally independent effects of individual dietary components, especially for macronutrients such as dietary fiber, are difficult to establish, recommendations for increasing dietary fiber for cancer prevention should be made in the context of the total diet as suggested by the NCI in their interim dietary guidelines for cancer prevention.

Despite the uncertainties associated with the observations described in this chapter, the possible public health implications of this research are significant. Increasing intake of grains, fruits, and vegetables, while concomitantly decreasing fat intake, has the potential to reduce risk from two of the major causes of cancer (colon and breast) mortality, and possibly from a number of other cancers as well (risk for cancers of the head and neck, which were not discussed here,

Table 5 Dietary Fiber Recommendations

Organization	Recommendations
Dietary Goals-1977 U.S. Government	Increase consumption of vegetables and fruits and whole grains.
National Academy of Science-1980	Consume each day . . . legumes, vegetables, and fruits, and cereals and breads.
National Academy of Science-1982	Include fruits, vegetables, and whole of grain cereal products in the daily diet.
American Cancer Society-1984	Eat more high fiber foods, such as whole grain cereals fruits and vegetables.
Canada-1985	The adult Canadian population should at least double its intake of dietary fibers.
USDA/HHS-1985	Eat foods with adequate starch and fiber.
American Heart Association-1985	Include at least three servings a day of fruits and three servings a day of vegetables.
National Cancer Institute-1986	Eat a variety of foods which provide 20-35 g of of fiber a day.
Federation of American Societies for Experimental Biology-1987	Healthy adults should eat whole grain products, fruits, and vegetables, leading to 20-35 g of fiber a day.
Surgeon General's Report on Nutrition & Health-1988	Complex carbohydrates and fiber: increase consumption of whole grain foods and cereal products, vegetables (including dried beans and peas) and fruits.
National Academy of Science-1989	Every day eat five or more servings of a combination of vegetables and fruits, especially green and yellow vegetables and citrus fruits. Also increase complex carbohydrates by eating six or more daily servings of a combination of breads, cereals, and legumes.

also appears to be reduced by dietary fruit and vegetable intake). Furthermore, such a diet has undeniable cardiovascular benefits and no apparent adverse effects. Thus, even in the absence of detailed knowledge of the etiologic mechanisms, it is likely that meaningful risk reduction can be achieved by dietary modification.

REFERENCES

1. D. P. Burkitt, A. R. P. Walker, and N. S. Painter, *JAMA 229*, 1068 (1974).
2. H. Trowell, *Atherosclerosis, 16*, 138 (1972).

3. Health Protection Branch Health and Welfare Canada, 1985 report on the Expert Advisory Committee on Dietary Fiber, Canada, Minister of National Health and Welfare.
4. S. M. Pilch, *Washington, DC, Life Science Research Office*, 1987.
5. H. Englyst, H. S. Wiggins, and J. H. Cummings, *Analyst, 107*, 307 (1982).
6. J. L. Slavin, *J. Am. Diet. Assoc., 87*, 1164 (1987).
7. P. J. Van Soest and R. W. McQueen, *Proc. Nutr. Soc., 32*, 123 (1973).
8. D. Schaller, *Am. J. Clin. Nutr., 31*, S99 (1978).
9. H. K. Goering and P. J. Van Soest, *U.S. Dept. Agriculture Handbook No. 379*, 1, 1970.
10. N. Asp and G. Johansson, In *Analysis of Dietary Fiber in Foods* (W. T. P. Jones and O. Theander, eds.), Marcel Dekker, New York, 1981, p. 173.
11. I. Fruda, *Cereal Food World, 22*, 252 (1977).
12. L. Prosky, N. Asp, J. Fruda, F. DeVries, T. Schwieizer, and B. Harland. *J. Assoc. Off. Anal. Chem., 68*, 677 (1985).
13. Association of Official Analytical Chemists, In *Official Methods of Analysis*, 15th Ed., Arlington, VA, No. 985.29, 1990.
14. D. A. T. Southgate, *J. Sci. Fd. Agric., 20*, 31 (1969).
15. R. R. Selvendran and M. S. DuPont, *Sci. Food Agric., 31*, 1173 (1980).
16. O. Theander and P. Aman, *J. Sci. Food Agric., 33*, 340 (1982).
17. H. Englyst, H. S. Wiggins, and J. Cummings, *Analyst, 107*, 307 (1982).
18. H. Graham, M-B. G. Rydberg, and P. Aman, *J. Agric. Food Chem., 36*, 494 (1988).
19. J. A. Marlett, J. G. Chesters, M. J. Longacre, and J. J. Bogdanske, *Am. J. Clin. Nutr., 50*, 479 (1990).
20. L. Prosky, N. G. Asp, T. S. Schweizer, J. W. DeVries, and I. Furda, *J. Assoc. Off. Anal. Chem. 71*, 1017 (1988).
21. S. N. Heller and L. R. Hackler, *Am. J. Clin. Nutr., 9*, 1510 (1978).
22. E. Lanza, Y. Jones, G. Block, and L. Kessler, *Am. J. Clin. Nutr., 46*, 790 (1987).
23. E. Lanza and R. Butrum, *Am. J. Diet. Assoc., 86*, 732 (1986).
24. E. H. Ahrens, Jr., and C. A. Boucher, *J. Am. Diet. Assoc., 73*, 613 (1978).
25. J. A. Marlett and R. L. Bokram, *Am. J. Clin. Nutr., 34*, 335 (1981).
26. J. W. Anderson and S. R. Bridges, *Am. J. Clin. Nutr., 47*, 440 (1988).
27. G. Block and E. Lanza, *JNCI, 79*, 83 (1987).
28. M. J. Hill and Fernandez, in *Dietary Fiber* (C.D. Kritchevsky, C. Bonfield, and J. W. Anderson, eds.), Plenum Press, New York, 1990, p. 417.
29. R. M. Kay, *Cancer Res., 41*, 3774 (1981).
30. B. S. Reddy, *Cancer Res., 41*, 3766 (1981).
31. E. E. Deschner, B. I. Cohen, and R. F. Raicht, *Digestion, 21*, 290 (1981).
32. B. S. Reddy, K. Watanabe, and J. Weisburger, *Cancer Res., 37*, 3238 (1977).
33. R. W. Owen, M. H. Thompson, M. J. Hill, M. Willpart, P. Mainguet, and M. Roberfroid, *Nutr. Cancer, 9*, 67 (1987).
34. I. Newmark, M. J. Wargovich, and B. R. Bruce, *JNCI, 76*, 1323 (1984).
35. T. S. Gaginella, V. S. Chadwick, and J. C. Debongnie, *Gastroenterology, 45*, 336 (1977).
36. A. M. Stephen and J. H. Cummings, *J. Med. Microbiol., 13*, 45 (1980).
37. J. H. Cummings, *Gut, 22*, 763 (1981).

38. W. E. W. Roediger, *Gastroenterology, 83*, 424 (1982).
39. Y. S. Kim, D. Taso, A. Marita, et al., *Colonic Carcinogenesis* (R. Malt and R. C. N. Williamson, eds.), MPT Press, Lancaster, UK, 1982, p. 317.
40. J. Kruh, *Mol Cell. Biochem., 42*, 65 (1982).
41. W. R. Bruce, *Cancer Res., 47*, 4237 (1987).
42. J. R. Lupton, D. M. Coder, and L. R. Jacobs, *J. Nutr., 118*, 840 (1988).
43. J. R. Lupton and L. J. Marchant, *J. Nutr., 119*, 235 (1989).
44. B. R. Goldin, H. Adlercruetz, J. Dwyer, et al., *Cancer Res., 41*, 3771 (1981).
45. B. R. Goldin, H. Adlercreutz, S. L. Gorbach, et al., *N. Engl. J. Med., 307*, 1542 (1982).
46. T. D. Schultz and B. J. Howie, *Nutr. Cancer, 8*, 141 (1986).
47. D. P. Rose, *Nutr. Cancer, 13*, 1 (1990).
48. H. Adlercreutz, T. Fotsis, C. Bannwart, et al., *J. Steroid Biochem., 25*, 791, 1986.
49. B. Trock, E. Lanza, and P. Greenwald, *JNCI, 82*, 650 (1990).
50. D. Byar and L. Freedman, Clinical trials in diet and cancer, *Prev. Med., 18*, 203 (1988).
51. W. Willett and M. J. Stampfer, *Am. J. Epidemiol., 124*, 17 (1986).
52. R. L. Prentice, M. Pepe, and S. G. Self, *Cancer Res., 49*, 3147 (1989).
53. J. L. Fleiss, *Statistical Methods for Rates and Proportions*, Wiley, New York, 1981, p. 160.
54. J. L. Freudenheim and S. Graham, *Cancer Res., 50*, 3295 (1990).
55. J. L. Freudenheim, S. Graham, J. R. Marshall, et al., *Am. J. Epidemiol. 131*, 612 (1990).
56. R. K. Peters, D. H. Garabrant, M. C. Yu, et al., *Cancer Res., 49*, 5459 (1989).
57. M. Gerhardsson de Verdier, G. Steineck, U. Hagman, et al., *Int. J. Cancer, 46*, 985 (1990).
58. H. P. Lee, L. Gourley, S. W. Duffy, et al., *Int. J. Cancer, 43*, 1007 (1989).
59. D. W. West, M. L. Slattery, L. M. Robison, et al., *Am. J. Epidemiol., 130*, 883 (1989).
60. A. S. Whittemore, A. H. Wu-Williams, M. Lee, et al., *JNCI, 82*, 915 (1990).
61. W. C. Willett, M. J. Stampfer, G. A. Colditz, et al., *N. Engl. J. Med., 323*, 1664 (1990).
62. L. K. Heilburn, A. Nomura, J. H. Hankin, et al., *Int. J. Cancer, 44*, 1 (1989).
63. M. L. Slattery, T. K. French, M. J. Egger, and J. L. Lyon. *Int. J. Epidemiol., 18*, 792 (1989).
64. G. R. Howe, M. Jain, and A. B. Miller. *Int. J. Cancer, 45*, 604 (1990).
65. J. Kelsey and G. Kerkowitz. *Cancer Res., 48*, 5615 (1988).
66. J. J. Schlesselman, *Case-Control Studies: Design, Conduct, Analysis*, Appendix A, Oxford University Press, New York, 1981.
67. J. M. Iscovich, R. B. Iscovich, G. Howe, et al., *Int. J. Cancer, 44*, 770 (1989).
68. K. Katsouyanni, D. Trichopoulos, P. Boyle, et al., *Int. J. Cancer, 38*, 815 (1986).
69. P. Van 't Veer, C. M. Kolb, P. Verhoef, et al., *Int. J. Cancer, 45*, 825 (1990).
70. C. L. La Vecchia, A. Decarli, S. Franceschi, et al., *Nutr. Cancer, 10*, 205 (1987).
71. J. Brisson, R. Verreault, A. S. Morrison, et al., *Am. J. Epidemiol., 130*, 14 (1989).
72. L. E. Holm, E. Callmer, M. L. Hjalmar, et al., *JNCI, 81*, 1218 (1989).

73. T. Byers, J. Marshall, S. Graham, et al., *JNCI, 71*, 681 (1983).
74. C. L. La Vecchia, A. Decarli, E. Negri, et al., *JNCI, 79*, 663 (1987).
75. M. L. Slattery, K. L. Schuman, D. W. West, et al., *Am. J. Epidemiol., 130*, 497 (1989).
76. C. L. La Vecchia, A. Decalri, M. Fasoli, et al., *Cancer, 57*, 1248 (1986).
77. D. J. Pusateri, W. T. Roth, J. K. Ross, and T. D. Schultz, *Am. J. Clin. Nutr., 51*, 371 (1990).
78. J. K. Ross, D. J. Pusateri, and T. D. Schultz, *Am. J. Clin. Nutr., 51*, 365 (1990).
79. Y. Ohno, O. Yoshida, et al., *Cancer Res., 48*, 1331 (1988).
80. L. N. Kolonel, J. H. Hankin, and C. N. Yoshizawa. *Cancer Res., 47*, 2982 (1987).
81. L. N. Kolonel, C. N. Yishizawa, and J. H. Hankin. *Am. J. Epidemiol., 127*, 999 (1988).
82. M. Y. Heshmat, L. Kaul, et al., *The Prostate, 6*, 7 (1985).
83. R. K. Ross, H. Shimizu, et al., *JNCI, 78*, 5 (1987).
84. C. Mettlin, *Prog. Clin. Biol. Res., 346*, 55 (1990).
85. A. W. Hsing, J. K. McLaughlin, et al., *Cancer Res., 50*, 6836 (1990).
86. H. A. Risch, M. Jain, N. W. Choi, et al., *Am. J. Epidemiol., 122*, 947 (1985).
87. B. Modan, F. Lubin, B. A. Barell, et al., *Cancer, 34*, 2087 (1974).
88. S. E. Norell, A. Ahlbom, R. Erwald, et al., *Am. J. Epidemiol., 124*, 894 (1986).
89. R. T. Falk, L. W. Pickle, E. T. Fontham, et al., *Am. J. Epidemiol., 128*, 324 (1988).
90. G. R. Howe, T. Hirohata, T. G. Hislop, et al., *JNCI, 82*, 561 (1990).
91. B. S. Reddy, A. Engle, S. Katsifis, et al., *Cancer Res., 49*, 4629 (1989).
92. H. S. Stern, R. C. Gregorie, K. S. Young, et al., *Proc. Annu. Meet. Am. Assoc. Cancer Res., 30*, A924 (1989).
93. D. Alberts, W. Buller, J. Einspahr, et al., *Proc. Am. Assoc. Cancer Res., 30*, 258 (1989).
94. B. C. Moreson, *Proc. R. Soc. Med., 67*, 451 (1974).
95. E. Bright-See, G. McKeown, E. A. Jacobson, et al., *Nutr. Cancer, 4*, 211 (1985).
96. R. MacLennan, in *Dietary Fiber* (K. Kritchevesny, C. Bonfield, and J. W. Anderson, eds.), Plenum Press, New York, 1990, p. 481.
97. R. Beart, *Cancer, 33*, 684 (1990).
98. J. J. Decosse, H. Miller, and M. Lesser, *JNCI, 81*, 1290 (1989).

13

Anthropometry, Body Composition, and Cancer

Loïc Le Marchand
Cancer Research Center of Hawaii
University of Hawaii
Honolulu, Hawaii

INTRODUCTION

Epidemiologic investigations have shown great international variations in cancer incidence but, for most common cancer sites, have failed to indicate with certainty the specific factors responsible for these differences. The finding that migrants from low-risk to high-risk countries gradually approach the risk in the new countries implicates the importance of environmental factors. Risk differences among ethnic groups within the same geographical area, as in South Africa, Israel, and Hawaii, support the hypothesis that cultural characteristics are more important than the total environment. As reviewed in other chapters, the suggestion from correlations and animal studies that the risk of most common cancers (cancer of the breast, colon, prostate, endometrium, etc.) is associated with certain aspects of the Western lifestyle (i.e., hypercaloric/high fat diet, low energy expenditure) has received considerable attention. However, case-control and cohort studies have generally been inconclusive for these cancer sites.

One possible explanation for the inconsistency in the epidemiologic evidence is that the methodologies used in these studies were not sensitive enough to discriminate between cases and controls, mainly because of the difficulties

This work was supported in part by grant 5-R29-CA44503 from the National Cancer Institute, N.I.H., D.H.H.S.

involved in measuring the diet and physical activity of free-living individuals. Another possibility is that the relevant period of exposure is not the few years preceding diagnosis, as considered in these studies, but a period that starts earlier in life, possibly during the second or third decade.

In this context, measures of body size and body composition, which are at least in part nutritionally mediated, are important to consider since they present many advantages over diet and physical activity assessments. Their measurements are usually accurate, valid, and reproducible. Recent weight and height can be recalled by individuals with satisfying accuracy (1–3). Moreover, weight and height are often available in a number of existing personal records (e.g., school, military, occupational, medical, insurance, and driver's license records). Thus, misclassification due to measurement error and costs involved in obtaining these data are often minimal.

Furthermore, serial body size measurements taken several years apart reflect nutritional status at different periods of life. Skeletal dimensions reflect nutrition during development. Thus, measures of body size can provide information on past nutritional exposures, as well as changes in nutrition over time. Finally, because of the metabolic functions of adipose tissue, obesity may also play a direct role in the etiology of certain cancers. Since the metabolic activity of adipose tissue varies depending on its anatomic location, the examination of body fat distribution may increase the sensitivity of studies of obesity and cancer.

This chapter reviews the epidemiologic evidence for an association of body size with cancer. The review concentrates on the cancer sites for which strong evidence is available (i.e., endometrial, breast, colorectal, prostate, and kidney cancers). It also attempts to relate the findings of our understandings of the etiology of these diseases. Directions for future research are also suggested.

BREAST CANCER

Adult weight and height, and body mass indices constructed from these measures, are the body size characteristics that have been studied most often in relation to breast cancer. As with other breast cancer risk factors (4), the findings for body weight clearly differ according to menopausal status. They are summarized in Tables 1 and 2 for postmenopausal and premenopausal breast cancer, separately. (Studies that did not classify subjects by menopausal status are listed in Table 1, since they probably included a majority of postmenopausal women.)

As shown in Table 1, most investigators who have examined weight and/or body mass and breast cancer risk in postmenopausal women have found a positive association. This finding has been quite reproducible across populations and study designs and has been attributed to an increase in bioavailable estrogens in these postmenopausal women. The mechanisms proposed include excessive conversion of androstenedione to estrone in adipose tissue (53), lower level of sex-

Table 1 Adult Body Weight and Height in Relation to Postmenopausal Breast Cancer

Ref.	Location	Source of cases/controls	No. of cases	Menopausal status	Results: Weight	Results: BMI	Results: Height	Adjustment variables
			Case-Control and Cross-Sectional Studies					
5	Holland	Hospital	140	All	+			None
6	Athens	Hospital	799	All	+	+	++	Age, parity, SES, marital status
7	Brazil	Hospital	325	Post	++	+	+	Age, education, age at first birth
8	England	Hospital/TB Screening	150	All	0		0	Age
9	Slovenia	Hospital	772	All	+		+	Age
10	Taiwan	Hospital	84	Post	++		0	Age
11	Poland	Hospital	900	Post	++	+	0	Height, age at menarche
12	Finland	Hosp/Screenees	122	All	0	0	0	None
13	Sweden	Population	146	Post	0	0	0	Age
14	Holland	Population	543	Post	++	0	++	Age
15	Canada	Hosp/Population	214	Post	++	++	+	Age
16	Japan	Hospital	167	Post	++		+	Age
17	U.S. (NY)	Hospital	375	Post	0	0	0	Age
18	U.S.	Screenees	405	All	+		0	Age
19	U.S. (CA)	Hospital	1038	Post	+	+	0	Age, race, parity
20	U.S. (CT)	Hospital	284	Post	+		0	All breast cancer risk factors

Continued

Table 1 *Continued*

Ref.	Location	Source of cases/controls	No. of cases	Menopausal status	Results: Weight	Results: BMI	Results: Height	Adjustment variables
21	Canada	Population	55	Post	0		0	Age, education, parity
22	U.S.	Screenees	210	All	+	++	+	Age
23	U.S.	Hospital	706	Post		+		Age
24	U.S.	Hosp/Screenees	255	Post	+	+	0	All breast cancer risk factors
25	Italy	Hospital	279	Post		+		Occupation, parity, education
26	Israel	Hosp/Population	664	Post		++		All breast cancer risk factors
27	Canada	Pop'n/Neighbors	198	Post	+	0	0	Age
28	Hawaii	Pop'n/Neighbors	138 Japanese	Post	0	0	0	All breast cancer risk factors
			142 White	Post	0	0	0	All breast cancer risk factors
29	U.S.	Hospital	310	Post		++		All breast cancer risk factors
30	Beijing	Pop'n/Neighbors	206	Post	+	0		All breast cancer risk factors
31	Denmark	Population	484	Post	0	0	0	Age, neighborhood
32	Australia	Hosp/Population	109	All	0	0	0	Age, neighborhood
33	Italy	Population	250	All		+		All breast cancer risk factors
34	U.S.	Screenees	2128	Post	+	+	+	All breast cancer risk factors
35	Italy	Hospital	2137	Post	+	+	−	All breast cancer risk factors

Prospective Studies								
36	Holland	General Practice	70	All	++	0	++	Age
37	U.S. (HI)	Population	728	All	+		+	Age, race
38	U.S.	Population		All	++			Age
39	Iceland	Population	147	All	+	0	+	Age
40	U.S.	College Alumni	69	All	0	0	0	Age
41	U.S. (HI)	Population	280	Post	+	+	0	Age at first birth, SES, parity
42	U.S.	Population	121	All	0	0	++	All breast cancer risk factors
43	U.S. (CA)	Population	215	All		+		All breast cancer risk factors
44	Norway	TB Screening	5122	Post	+	+	+	Age
45	U.S.	Nurses	420	Post (<60 yr)	0	0	0	All breast cancer risk factors
46	U.S. (IA)	Population	229	Post	0	0	0	All breast cancer risk factors

0: No association.
+: Increased risk, magnitude small ($1.0 < RR < 2.0$).
++: Increased risk, magnitude large ($RR \geq 2.0$).
−: Decreased risk, magnitude small ($0.5 < RR < 1.0$).
Blank indicates that the information was not reported.

hormone-binding globulin (54), and increased 2- versus 16-hydroxylation of estradiol (55).

However, it is notable that, despite this plausible mechanism, 25% of the studies in Table 1 failed to find an association. One possible reason is that some of these "negative" studies included proportionally fewer women over age 60 or with advanced tumors, among whom this association is more clearly observed (41,42,44,45). This age effect may reflect the increase in estrogen production capacity of adipose tissue observed with aging (56–58). The stage effect suggests that obesity may preferentially affect the later stage of carcinogenesis, as also indicated by the inverse association of obesity with breast cancer survival after adjustment for stage (59).

It is also noteworthy in Table 1 that weight-corrected-for-height indices, such as the Quetelet index, which are thought to be better measures of adiposity than body weight, did not better discriminate between cases and controls than weight alone. Moreover, among the studies which found a positive association with weight or body mass and looked for a dose-gradient, about half found a dose reponse and half did not. These observations suggest that the obesity–postmenopausal breast cancer association may reflect more than one mechanism.

Recent studies have been very consistent in finding a direct, dose-dependent relationship between adult weight gain and risk of postmenopausal breast cancer (19,26,32,41,46,60). This association with weight gain appears to be independent of the current obesity level (41,46,60). Thus, net energy balance, or factors related to it (caloric intake, metabolic efficiency, or physical activity), may play a separate role in the etiology of postmenopausal breast cancer.

The lack of consistency in the weight data could also be due to variation in fat patterning in the populations examined. Three recent studies have found an association between abdominal adiposity and postmenopausal breast cancer which was independent of the degree of obesity (46,61,62). This is consistent with some data suggesting that women with upper-body obesity may have a greater increase in biologically active estrogens than women with lower-body obesity (63,64).

The evidence for a role of adult obesity in premenopausal breast cancer is much less convincing, since most studies showed no association (Table 2). However, about a third of the studies in Table 2 found a negative association. It has been proposed that such an excess risk among lean, premenopausal women could be explained by the easier and, thus, earlier diagnosis of breast tumors in such women, since thin women are more likely to be diagnosed with smaller tumors (32,34,45,50). The studies that found a negative association were conducted in populations with high level of medical care and health awareness (Table 2) and, thus, may have been subject to a diagnosis bias. However, it seems unlikely that earlier detection could entirely explain the sometimes strong inverse association of body weight with premenopausal breast cancer found in these studies (34,45,50). If this negative association is confirmed, it would be consistent with the hypothesis of Key and Pike (65) that the total number of ovulatory menstrual cycles and the accompanying mitoses of breast tissue increases breast cancer risk, since obese women are known to have irregular cycles more frequently.

Because many risk factors for breast cancer are determined early in life (e.g., family history of breast cancer, first pregnancy before age 20, age at menarche, and residence in the United States, as compared to residence in Asia or Mexico), and because at least the latter two factors are related to nutrition, interest has also focused on early dietary exposures, as reflected in stature and adolescent body mass. It has been hypothesized that overnutrition during childhood increases breast cancer risk.

Height has been positively associated with pre- and postmenopausal breast cancer in a number of studies. However, as shown in Tables 1 and 2, the results are far from being consistent, as the majority of studies found no association. The positive associations with height observed in some studies were probably not due to the possible confounding effect of weight (which was generally not adjusted for), since several of these studies did not find a concomitant association with weight. To explain the inconsistency in the height data, it has been proposed that, unlike for rodents, caloric restriction in early life would need to be sufficiently severe as to stunt growth in order to decrease breast cancer risk in humans (66,69). Accordingly, an association with height would primarily be seen in countries where people could have experienced a substantial energy deprivation during childhood. The geographical information given in Tables 1 and 2 does not entirely fit with such a pattern. However, the reports of a positive association with height in a cohort of U.S. women in which underprivileged women were overrepresented (42) and in a cohort of Norwegians who were adolescent during a period of national food restriction (51) have recently given support for this hypothesis.

Another possible explanation for the inconsistency in the height and breast cancer data is that nutrition is only a minor determinant of adult height. It has been suggested that other measures of skeletal size (e.g., sitting height, biacromial and biiliac dimensions) may constitute more sensitive markers of early maturity and adolescent nutrition (67). In an international comparison, biacromial width was found to correlate better with breast cancer incidence than adult height (68). The correlation coefficient for biacromial width was 0.84, compared to 0.68 for height. Moreover, in an early case-control study of anthropometry and breast cancer, biacromial dimension and biacromial-biiliac ratio were positively associated with risk, whereas height was not (8). However, after adjustment for the marked age-difference between cases and controls in this study, no association was observed with sitting height. This latter finding is consistent with the much weaker association with breast cancer noted for the sitting height component of stature than for leg length in the NHANES Follow-Up Study (69).

Adolescent obesity has been most often investigated by asking breast cancer patients and controls to recall their weight at early ages. Adolescent weight or

Table 2 Adult Body Weight and Height in Relation to Premenopausal Breast Cancer

Ref.	Location	Source of cases/controls	No. of cases	Results: Weight	Results: BMI	Results: Height	Adjustment variables
			Case-Control Studies				
5	Holland	Hospital	60	0			None
7	Brazil	Hospital	211	0	0	0	Age, education, age at first birth
10	Taiwan	Hospital	125	+		0	Age
47	U.S. (CA)	Hospital	452	–		0	Age
11	Poland	Hospital		0	0	++	Weight, age at menarche
13	Sweden	Population	30	0	0	0	Age
14	Holland	Population	191	0	0	0	Age
15	Canada	Hosp./Population	88	—	—	—	Age
16	Japan	Hospital	233	0			Age
17	U.S. (NY)	Hospital	409	0	0	0	Age
19	U.S. (CA)	Hospital	274	—	—	+	Age, race, parity
20	U.S. (CT)	Hospital	48	--		0	All breast cancer risk factors
48	U.S. (WA)	Population	112	0	0	+	Age
23	U.S.	Hospital	478		--		Age
24	U.S. (MA)	Hosp./Screenees	104	0	0	0	All breast cancer risk factors

25	Italy	Hospital	89		0		SES, parity
26	Israel	Hosp./Population	363	—		0	All breast cancer risk factcrs
27	Canada	Pop./Neighbors	313	0	0	0	Age
29	U.S.	Hospital	221		0		All breast cancer risk factors
30	Beijing	Pop./Neighbors	288	0	0		All breast cancer risk factors
31	Denmark	Population	639	0	0	0	Age, neighborhood
49	U.S. (UT)	Population	99		--		All breast cancer risk factors
34	U.S.	Screenees	1484	0	0	+	All breast cancer risk factors
35	Italy	Hospital	1110	0	0	0	All breast cancer risk factors
			Prospective Studies				
50	U.S.	Nurses	561	—	—	0	All breast cancer risk factors
41	U.S. (HI)	Population	289	0	0	0	Age, age at first birth, parity, SES
44	Norway	TB Screening	3305	—	—	+	Age
51,52	Norway	Screenes	137		--	+	Age

0: No association.
+: Increased risk, magnitude small (1.0 < RR < 2.0).
–: Decreased risk, magnitude small (0.5 < RR < 1.0).
--: Decreased risk, magnitude large (RR ≤ 0.5).
Blank indicates that the information was not reported.

body mass has usually not been associated with postmenopausal breast cancer (15,19,26–28,45,46). However, adolescent body mass was found to be inversely related to premenopausal breast cancer in four (15,19,27,50) of the five studies (15,19,27,49,50) that reported on this issue. The questionable validity of weight information recalled from a distant past may cast some doubt on these findings. However, supportive evidence for this negative association of adolescent body mass with premenopausal breast cancer came from a prospective study in Hawaii, which used historically recorded data on adolescent weight and height (41). In this study, a dose-dependent negative association was found between body mass at peri-pubertal age and premenopausal breast cancer. This association was observed in each of the five ethnic groups included in the cohort. Albeit consistent across populations, these findings are in conflict with the observation that obese girls have their menarche at a younger age than lean adolescent, a characteristic which should increase, not decrease, their breast cancer risk.

Finally, because there is some evidence that pre- or postnatal factors, in particular nutrition, could play a role in mammary carcinogenesis (71,72), weight at birth (71) and during early childhood (41) were also investigated in relation to breast cancer risk. No association was found in these studies.

In conclusion, the associations between body size and breast cancer described above probably involve different mechanisms. Obesity appears to increase breast cancer risk in older women (particularly after age 60 and in women with upper-body obesity) through a direct hormonal mechanism (increase in circulating levels of bioavailable estrogens). The associaton of obesity and, more specifically, adult weight gain with postmenopausal breast cancer may also be indirect and reflect an association with sustained positive energy balance. This is consistent with the well-established protective effect of energy restriction, which is obtained in animal models whether caloric restriction is initiated during early life or after growth completion (72,73) and by apparent inhibition of the initiation as well as the promotion stage (74). In humans, early-age energy restriction would need to be severe in order to affect breast cancer risk and, thus, would not provide a practical approach to the prevention of this disease. Indeed, less severe caloric restriction during growth may even be harmful if the apparent inverse relationship of adolescent body mass to premenopausal breast cancerr is confirmed.

However, humans could be more sensitive to the effect of energy balance during adulthood. Although the increase in breast cancer risk is only twofold among older obese women, the high prevalence of obesity in our society suggests that the recommendations made to the public to avoid overweight, if successful, could significantly reduce the morbidity and mortality due to this disease after the menopause.

ENDOMETRIAL CANCER

Endometrial cancer is probably the cancer for which an association with body weight has been best established. There is now convincing evidence from the epidemiologic literature that adult obesity increases risk of postmenopausal endometrial cancer (38,75–84). There is some evidence, although more limited, that weight is also associated with endometrial cancer in premenopausal women (78–80).

The elevated risk of endometrial cancer among obese women has been attributed to their increased peripheral conversion of precursors to circulating estrogens (53) and lower levels of sex-hormone-binding globulin (54). After the menopause, obese women are known to have higher levels of circulating estrogens than nonobese women. In women with functioning ovaries, the contribution from adipose tissue to the overall estrogen production is small, and estrogen levels are not greater in the obese. However, in both pre- and postmenopausal women, the proportion of estradiol which is unbound and, thus, bioavailable has been shown to be greater in obese than in nonobese women (85), explaining perhaps the association of obesity with premenopausal endometrial cancer. The precise mechanism by which increased circulating estrogens produce endometrial cancer is unclear but could involve their growth-stimulating effect on the endometrium that would present a greater opportunity for abnormal cells to arise.

Other aspects of obesity or body size have rarely been considered in relation to endometrial cancer. For example, we are not aware of any report on adult weight gain and this cancer. Positive energy balance could be associated with risk since both a high-fat diet (86,87) and physical inactivity (88) have been associated with endometrial cancer. There is also a lack of data addressing the issue of when in a woman's life the development of obesity is most important. The possible modifying effect of body fat distribution on endometrial cancer risk has also received little attention. However, two recent small studies observed no difference in risk between upper-body and lower-body obesity (84,89).

Similarly, few studies have investigated the effect of early-age obesity on endometrial cancer risk. Blitzer et al. (76) compared the lifetime prevalence of this cancer among 56,111 members of TOPS Club, Inc. (Take Off Pounds Sensibly) by levels of adolescent and current body mass. They found a positive association with maximal weight at age 10–20 years, independent of the current obesity level. However, in a case-control study of endometrial cancer among young women aged 45 years or less, Henderson et al. (79) found no association with weight at age 18.

Similar to the lack of agreement in the data on adolescent obesity and endometrial cancer is the lack of consistency in the height data. Approximately equal numbers of studies found (69,75,83) and did not find (76,77,81) an association between height and endometrial cancer. Thus, although several nutrition-related risk factors for this disease are determined early in life (age at menarche and residence from an early age in the United States, as compared with migration from Asia later in life), the role of early nutrition in the etiology of endometrial cancer remains obscure.

COLORECTAL CANCER

As for the previous cancer sites, adult weight and height have been the body size characteristics most frequently examined in relation to colorectal cancer. However, unlike for the other sites, findings for colorectal cancer have been more inconsistent in case-control studies than in prospective studies. Thus, past studies are summarized in Tables 3 and 4 separately by type of design.

As shown in Table 3, case-control studies that were hospital-based generally failed to show an association with body weight. In contrast, obesity was found positively associated with colorectal cancer in most studies that were population-based. This discrepancy may reflect the fact that obesity is related to many diseases. Thus, selection of controls among hospitalized patients may have biased the hospital-based studies. However, it is unclear why such a bias did not seem to have plagued hospital-based case-control studies of weight and breast cancer (Table 1). In line with the population-based case-control studies, the prospective studies of colorectal cancer (Table 4) have been fairly consistent in finding a positive association with weight or body mass.

Although fewer studies have been conducted in women, the positive association with weight has been more consistently shown in males than in females. The reasons for this difference are unclear, but it does not seem to result from the known sex-difference in subsite distribution for colonic tumors, since the weight association appears not to be limited to any subsite of the large bowel.

Several mechanisms may be involved in explaining the obesity-colorectal association. Although not entirely consistent, the animal and epidemiologic data point to a high-fat, hypercaloric diet as a risk factor for colorectal cancer (108,109). More recently, lack of physical activity has been consistently associated with an increased colon cancer risk. This suggests that net energy balance, as reflected in weight change, could be more relevant than obesity per se.

Few authors have reported on adult weight gain and colorectal cancer. In a cohort study of Japanese men in Hawaii, Nomura et al. (104) found a positive association between adult weight gain and colon cancer among men aged 55 or older. In this study, a similar association was found with baseline weight, but not with weight at age 25 years. However, these findings are difficult to interpret because the independence of these associations was not tested.

Only a small proportion of the studies in Tables 3 and 4 reported on height. Those that did usually did not find any association with this variable. Similarly, studies that considered early-age body mass did not find any association between

Table 3 Case-Control Studies of Adult Body Size and Colorectal Cancer

Ref.	Location	Source of cases/controls	No. of cases	Weight	BMI	Height	Adjustment variables	Comments
90	U.S. (KS)	Hospital	340	0		0	Age	
91	U.S. (NY)	Hospital	791	+			Age	
92	Japan	Hospital	157	0			Age	
93	U.S. (CA)	Hospital	280	0		0	Age	
94	Canada	Pop'n/Neighbor	542	0			Age	
95	U.S. (NE)	Pop'n/Hospital	86	+	+		Age	Colon cancer studied only
96	U.S. (NY)	Pop'n/Neighbor	428		++		Age, education	Association observed in both sexes for all subsites
97	U.S. (UT)	Population	231		++		Age, diet, physical activity	Association observed for both subsites of the colon
98	Australia	Population	715		+		Age, diet	Association observed in males with rectal cancer only
99	Majorca	Population	286	+			Age	
100	U.S. (NY)	Pop'n/Neighbor	422	0	0	0	Age	Rectal cancer studied only
101	Italy	Hospital	910			0		
102	U.S./ Canada	Population	473		+	0	Age, diet, physical activity	Association with BMI at age 40 for colon cancer only. In North America, association observed in females only.
	China	Population	432		++	0		

0, +, ++: See footnotes to Table 1.

Table 4 Prospective Studies of Adult Body Size and Colorectal Cancer

Ref.	Location	Source of subject	No. of cases	Weight	BMI	Height	Adjustment variables	Comments
38	U.S.	Population		+			Age	Association observed in males only
103	U.S. (CA)	Population	182	++			Age, diet	Association observed in males and younger females only
104	U.S. (HI)	Japanese	164		+		Age	Male Japanese cohort. Association limited to older men (age ≥55)
105	U.S. (IL)	Western Electric Co.	49		+		Age	Male cohort
40	U.S.	College alumni	303		0		Age	Male cohort
106	U.S. (CA)	H.M.O.	245		0		Age	
107	U.S. (CA)	Retirement community	126		++		Age, diet physical activity	Association observed in males only, and for both subsites of the colon
69	U.S.	Population	129			+	Age	Association observed in males only

0, +, ++: See footnotes to Table 1.

body mass in the third decade of life and colorectal cancer (40,91,102,104). Although still limited, the available data suggest no or little role for early nutrition in the etiology of colorectal cancer. This is consistent with the rapid upward drift of colon cancer incidence rates observed among Japanese who migrated to the United States (110).

PROSTATE CANCER

Prostate cancer has been less often studied epidemiologically than the other cancer sites reviewed above. Thus, the evidence is still limited and does not allow for firm conclusions to be drawn on a possible association of prostate cancer with body size. The available results regarding adult body weight and height have differed for case-control and prospective studies. The two types of studies are reviewed separately in Table 5.

All past case-control studies of prostate cancer (111,112,114–117) except one (113) found no association with adult weight (Table 5). Although most of these studies were hospital-based, the three studies that were population-based also found no association with weight, suggesting that selection bias is not an explanation for the lack of association with weight in retrospective studies. The results of the prospective studies are more supportive of a positive association with weight or body mass, since this association was observed in four out of six cohort studies (Table 5). In case-control studies, there is the possibility that the disease process may affect the weight of cancer patients, reducing the chances of finding a positive association. Thus, more importance should probably be given to the results of follow-up studies in which weight is assessed several years before diagnosis.

Although little is known of the etiology of prostate cancer, a high-fat diet has been rather consistently associated with an increased risk of this disease (112,114–116,118). Thus, an association of prostate cancer with body mass may indirectly reflect a relation with high fat intake. However, an association with body mass may not necessarily be related to obesity, since body mass reflects lean tissue as well as body fat (122). Severson et al. (119) have recently proposed that this association might be accounted for more by muscle mass than by fat tissue. They found in their cohort of Japanese-Americans that risk of prostate cancer was significantly *decreased* for men in the lower tertile of arm muscle area, as estimated from triceps skinfold thickness and arm circumference. No relation was found with arm fat area. These results are consistent with two recent studies suggesting a positive association between prostate cancer and physical activity (123,124).

None of the studies of prostate cancer that reported on height found an association with this variable (Table 4). Few studies reported on early age obesity. However, two prospective studies found no relation between prostate cancer and body mass at college physical examination (40,125). In contrast, in their cohort

Table 5 Adult Body Weight and Height in Relation to Prostate Cancer

Ref.	Location	Source of cases/controls	No. of cases	Weight	BMI	Height	Adjustment variables
			Case-Control Studies				
111	U.S. (NY)	Hospital	300	0		0	Age
112	U.S. (NY)	Hospital	260		0		Age
113	Italy	Hospital	166	++	++	0	Age, marital status, diet
114	U.S. (CA)	Pop'n/Neighbors	142 Blacks	0	0	0	Age
		Retirement community	142 Whites	0	0	0	Age
115	U.S. (HI)	Population	452	0	0	0	Age, ethnicity
116	U.S. (NY)	Hospital	371	0		0	Age
117	Italy	Hospital	80			0	Age
			Prospective Studies				
38	U.S.	Population		+			Age
118	U.S. (CA)	Population	84	++			Age, diet
40	U.S.	College alumni	243	0	0		Age
104	U.S. (HI)	Japanese pop'n	96		0		Age
69	U.S.	Population	95			0	Age
119	U.S. (HI)	Japanese pop'n	174	0	+	0	Age
120	U.S. (LA)	Population	180		0		Age
121	U.S. (CA)	Population	100		+		Age, CHD risk factors

0, +, ++: See footnotes to Table 1.

of Japanese men in Hawaii, Nomura et al. (104) found a weak positive association between prostate cancer incidence and body mass at age 25.

KIDNEY CANCER

Although investigations of renal cell cancer have been few, past studies have been very consistent in finding an association between weight or body mass index and this cancer (38,40,126–129). This association appears to be stronger in females (38,126–128), suggesting a role for hormonal factors such as increased levels of endogenous estrogens. When women were asked to recall their weight at an early age, the association was also present for weight at age 20 in the study by Yu et al. (128) and at college examination in the historical cohort study by Whittemore et al. (40). Thus, obesity may play a role in the early, as well as late, stage of the development of renal cell tumors.

FUTURE DIRECTIONS

As mentioned earlier, the field of anthropometry and cancer appears promising (see Chapter 6). However, its contribution has as yet been relatively limited. Only the associations of adult obesity with endometrial and postmenopausal breast cancers are now well established and have furthered our understanding of these diseases. Other associations have not been consistent or, if they have been, are difficult to interpret.

One problem is the lack of specificity or sensitivity of some of the measurements commonly used in the past. For example, the body mass index is known to correlate not only with adiposity but also with lean body mass. Adult height is mainly under genetic influence and is not a good marker of energy intake during growth for most populations. Total adiposity is probably less relevant to the risk of breast and endometrial cancers than abdominal and visceral adiposity.

Several recently proposed measures offer some interesting prospects for future research. Biacromial and biiliac diameters, and/or other measures of adult frame size, may constitute better indices of childhood energy balance (67,68). New methods to measure body fat distribution and total adipose tissue, which have been developed for clinical use, may be applicable to epidemiologic settings. However, the validity of these new methods has not yet been demonstrated in the populations most relevant to cancer epidemiology (elderly and minority populations). For example, present prediction equations for body composition using anthropometric and bioelectric variables were developed from young and middle-aged white adults (130). They are not likely to be valid when applied to elderly subjects and other ethnic or racial groups (130).

Another difficulty arises from the fact that it is not always clear whether some of the body size–cancer associations reflect direct or indirect mechanisms.

Although indirect associations can further our understanding of the disease process, they usually do not lead readily to preventive measures. For example, the association of postmenopausal breast cancer with adult weight gain, and probably that of body mass with colorectal cancer, point to a role for positive energy balance. However, although the animal data suggest that energy balance per se is important (131), it is not clear what the relevant factors are in humans. Excessive caloric intake or lack of physical activity, or even increased metabolic efficiency, could be as important. Resolving this question will require improving our current methods for assessing diet and physical activity. However, this knowledge is necessary in order to design intervention methods specifically tailored to high risk groups.

REFERENCES

1. A. J. Stunkard and J. M. Albaum, *Am. J. Clin. Nutr., 34*, 1593 (1981).
2. A. L. Steward, *J. Chron. Dis., 35*, 295 (1982).
3. L. Le Marchand, C. N. Yoshizawa, and A. M. Y. Nomura, *Am. J. Epidemiol., 128*, 874 (1988).
4. D. E. Anderson, in *Current Controversies in Breast Cancer* (F.C. Ames, G. R. Blumenschein, and E. D. Montague, eds.), University of Texas Press, 1984, p. 34.
5. F. De Waard, E. A. Baanders-van Halewijn, and J. Huizinga, *Cancer, 17*, 141 (1964).
6. V. G. Valaoras, B. MacMahon, D. Trichopoulos, and A. Polychronopoulou, *Int. J. Cancer, 4*, 350 (1969).
7. A. P. Mirra, P. Cole, and B. MacMahon, *Cancer Res., 31*, 77 (1971).
8. D. Brinkley, R. G. Carpenter, and J. L. Haybittle, *Brit. J. Prev. Med., 25*, 65 (1971).
9. B. Ravnihar, B. MacMahon, and J. Lindtner, *Europ. J. Cancer, 7*, 295 (1971).
10. T. M. Lin, K. P. Chen, and B. MacMahon, *Cancer, 27*, 1497 (1971).
11. J. Staszewski, *Prev. Med., 6*, 410 (1977).
12. I. Soini, *Int. J. Epidemiol., 6*, 365 (1977).
13. H. O. Adami, A. Rimsten, B. Stenkvist, and V. Vegelius, *Br. J. Cancer, 36*, 787 (1977).
14. F. De Waard, J. P. Cornelis, K. Aoki, and M. Yoshida, *Cancer, 40*, 1269 (1977).
15. N. W. Choi, G. R. Howe, A. B. Miller, et al., *Am. J. Epidemiol., 107*, 510 (1978).
16. T. Hirayama, *Prev. Med., 7*, 173 (1978).
17. E. L. Wynder, F. A. MacCornack, and S. D. Stellman, *Cancer, 41*, 2341 (1978).
18. L. A. Brinton, R. R. Williams, R. N. Hoover, et al., *JNCI, 62*, 37 (1979).
19. R. S. Paffenbarger, J. B. Kampert, and H-G Chang, *Am. J. Epidemiol., 112*, 258 (1980).
20. J. L. Kelsey, D. B. Fisher, T. R. Holford, et al., *JNCI, 67*, 327 (1981).
21. J. D. Burch, G. R. Howe, and A. B. Miller, *Can. Med. Ass. J., 124*, 1326 (1981).
22. L. A. Brinton, R. Hoover, and J. F. Fraumeni, *JAMA, 249*, 483 (1983).
23. S. P. Helmrich, S. Shapiro, L. Rosenberg, et al., *Am. J. Epidemiol., 117*, 35 (1983).
24. J. Brisson, A. S. Morrison, D. S. Kopans, et al., *Am. J. Epidemiol., 119*, 371 (1984).
25. R. Talamini, C. La Vecchia, A. Decarli, et al., *Br. J. Cancer, 49*, 723 (1984).

26. F. Lubin, A. M. Ruder, Y., Wax, and B. Modan, *Am. J. Epidemiol.*, *122*, 579 (1985).
27. T. G. Hislop, A. J. Goldman, J. M. Elwood, et al., *Cancer Detection Prev.*, *9*, 47 (1986).
28. L. N. Kolonel, A. M. Y. Nomura, J. Lee, and T. Hirohata, *Nutr. Cancer*, *8*, 247 (1986).
29. A. Schatzkin, J. R. Palmer, L. Rosenberg, S. P. Helmrich, et al., *JNCI*, *78*, 213 (1987).
30. S. C. Tao, M. C. Yu, R. K. Ross, and K. W. Xiu, *Int. J. Cancer*, *42*, 495 (1988).
31. M. Ewertz, *Int. J. Cancer*, *42*, 832 (1988).
32. D. Ingram, E. Nottage, S. Ng, et al., *Cancer*, *64*, 1049 (1989).
33. P. Toniolo, E. Riboli, F. Protta, et al., *Cancer Res.*, *49*, 5203 (1989).
34. C. A. Swanson, L. A. Brinton, P. R. Taylor, et al., *Am. J. Epidemiol.*, *130*, 1133 (1989).
35. F. Parazzini, C. LaVechhia, E. Negri, et al., *Int. J. Cancer*, *45*, 397 (1990).
36. F. De Waard and E. A. Baanders-van Halewijn, *Int. J. Cancer*, *14*, 153 (1974).
37. M. N. Rashad, S. M. Onizuka, and M. P. Mi, *Proc. First Int. Cong. Auxology*, 65 (1977).
38. E. A. Lew and L. Garfinkel, *J. Chron. Dis.*, *32*, 563 (1979).
39. H. Tulinius, N. Sigfusson, H. Sigvaldason, and N. E. Day, In *Diet and Human Carcinogenesis* (J. V. Joossens, ed.), Elsevier, Holland, 1985, p. 173.
40. A. S. Whittemore, R. S. Paffenberager, K. Anderson, and J. E. Lee, *JNCI*, *74*, 43 (1985).
41. L. Le Marchand, L. N. Kolonel, M. E. Earle, and M. P. Mi, *Am. J. Epidemiol.*, *128*, 137 (1988).
42. M. S. Micozzi. Childhood nutrition, growth and development: Relation to the long term risk of breast cancer in human populations. Ph.D. dissertation. Ann Arbor, MI, University Microfilms International, 1986.
43. P. K. Mills, W. L. Beeson, R. L. Phillips, et al., *Cancer*, *64*, 582 (1989).
44. S. Tretli, *Int. J. Cancer*, *44*, 23 (1989).
45. S. J. London, G. A. Colditz, M. J. Stampfer, et al., *JAMA*, *262*, 2853 (1989).
46. A. R. Folsom, S. A. Kaye, R. D. Prineas, et al., *Am. J. Epidemiol.*, *131*, 794 (1990).
47. E. Fasal, and R. S. Paffenbarger. *JNCI*, *55*, 767 (1975).
48. N. V. Harris, N. S. Weiss, A. M. Francis, and L. Polisar, *Am. J. Epidemiol.*, *116*, 643 (1982).
49. M. Pryor, M. L. Slattery, L. M. Robison, and M. Egger, *Cancer Res.*, *49*, 2161 (1989).
50. W. C. Willett, M. L. Browne, C. Bain, et al., *Am. J. Epidemiol.*, *122*, 731 (1985).
51. L. J. Vatten and S. Kvinnsland, *Int. J. Cancer*, *45*, 440 (1990).
52. L. J. Vatten and S. K. Kvinnsland, *Br. J. Cancer*, *61*, 881 (1990).
53. P. C. MacDonald, C. D. Edman, D. L. Hemsell, et al., *Am. J. Obstet. Gynecol.*, *130*, 448 (1978).
54. J. A. Nisker, G. L. Hammond, B. J. Davidson, et al., *Am. J. Obstet. Gynecol.*, *138*, 637 (1980).
55. J. Schneider, H. L. Bradlow, G. Strain, et al., *J. Clin. Endocrinol. Metab.*, *56*, 973 (1983).

56. D. L. Hemsell, J. M. Grodin, P. F. Breuner, et al., *J. Clin. Endocrinol. Metab.*, *38*, 476 (1974).
57. E. R. Simpson and C. R. Mendelson, *Am. J. Clin. Nutr.*, *45*, 290 (1987).
58. J. A. Nisker, G. L. Hammond, B. J. Davidson, et al., *Am. J. Obstet. Gynecol.*, *138*, 637 (1980).
59. L. Le Marchand, *Breast Cancer Res. Treat.*, (in press).
60. R. Ballard-Barbash, A. Schatzkin, P. R. Taylor, and L. L. Kahle, *Cancer Res.*, *50*, 2152 (1990).
61. D. V. Schapira, B. K. Nagi, G. H. Lyman, et al., *Ann. Int. Med.*, *112*, 182 (1990).
62. R. Ballard-Barbash, A. Schatzkin, C. L. Carter, et al., *JNCI*, *82*, 286 (1990).
63. P. F. Bruning, *J. Steroid Biochem.*, *27*, 487 (1987).
64. M. A. Kirschner, E. Samojlik, E. Szmal, et al., *J. Clin. Endocrinol., Metab.*, *70*, 473 (1990).
65. T. J. A. Key and M. C. Pike. *Eur. J. Cancer Clin. Oncol.*, *24*, 29 (1980).
66. W. C. Willett, *Am. J. Clin. Nutr.*, *45*, 354 (1987).
67. M. S. Micozzi, *Yearbook Phys. Anthropology*, *28*, 175 (1985).
68. M. S. Micozzi, *Am. J. Phys. Anthropology*, *73*, 525 (1987).
69. D. Albanes, D. Y. Jones, A. Schatzkin, M. S. Micozzi, and P. R. Taylor, *Cancer Res.*, *48*, 1658 (1988).
70. L. Le Marchand, L. N. Kolonel, B. C. Myers, and M. P. Mi, *Br. J. Cancer*, *57*, 437 (1988).
71. D. Trichopoulos, *Lancet*, *335*, 939 (1990).
72. M. H. Ross and G. Bras, *JNCI*, *47*, 1095 (1971).
73. J. R. Weindzuch and R. L. Walford, *Science*, *215*, 1415 (1982).
74. D. Kritchevsky, M. M. Weber, and D. M. Klurfeld, *Cancer Res.*, *44*, 3174 (1984).
75. E. L. Wynder, G. C. Escher, and N. Mantel. *Cancer*, *19*, 489 (1966).
76. P. H. Blitzer, E. Crawford-Blitzer, and A. A. Rimm, *Prev. Med.*, *5*, 20 (1976).
77. J. M. Elwood, P. Cole, K. J. Rothman, and S. D. Kaplan, *JNCI*, *59*, 1055 (1977).
78. J. L. Kelsey, V. A. Livolsi, T. R. Holford, et al., *Am. J. Epidemiol.*, *116*, 333 (1982).
79. B. E. Henderson, J. T. Casagrande, M. C. Pike, T. Mack, I. Rosario, and A. Duke, *Br. J. Cancer*, *47*, 749 (1984).
80. C. La Vecchia, S. Francheschi, A. Decarli, G. Galuus, and G. Tognomi, *JNCI*, *73*, 667 (1984).
81. M. Ewertz, S. G. Machado, J. D. Boice, Jr., and O. M. Jensen, *Br. J. Cancer*, *50*, 687 (1984).
82. C. Lawrence, I. Tessaro, S. Durgerian, et al., *Cancer*, *59*, 1665 (1987).
83. Y. Koumantaki, A. Tzonou, E. Koumantakis, D. Aravantinos, and D. Trichopoulos, *Int. J. Cancer*, *43*, 795 (1989).
84. A. R. Folson, S. A. Kaye, J. D. Potter, and R. J. Prineas, *Cancer Res.*, *49*, 6828 (1989).
85. J. W. Moore, T. J. A. Key, R. D. Bulbrook, et al., *Br. J. Cancer*, *56*, 661 (1987).
86. B. K. Armstrong, J. B. Brown, H. T. Clarke, et al., *JNCI*, *67*, 761 (1981).
87. C. La Vecchia, A. Decarli, M. Fasoli, et al., *Cancer*, *47*, 1248 (1986).
88. R. E. Frisch, G. Wyshak, N. L. Albright, et al., *Br. J. Cancer*, *52*, 885 (1985).
89. L. Lapidus, O. Helgesson, C. Merck, and P. Bjorntop, *Int. J. Obesity*, *12*, 361 (1988).

90. J. Higginson, *JNCI, 37*, 527 (1966).
91. E. L. Wynder and T. Shigematsu, *Cancer, 20*, 1520 (1967).
92. E. L. Wynder, T. Kajitani, S. Ishikawa, H. Dodo, and A. Takano, *Cancer, 23*, 1210 (1969).
93. L. G. Dales, G. D. Friedman, H. K. Ury, S. Grossman, and S. R. Williams, *Am. J. Epidemiol., 109*, 132 (1979).
94. M. Jain, G. M. Cook, F. G. Davis, M. G. Grace, G. R. Howe, and A. B. Miller, *Int. J. Cancer, 26*, 757 (1980).
95. L. W. Pickle, M. H. Greene, R. G. Ziegler, A. Toledo, R. Hoover, H. T. Lynch, and J. F. Fraumeni, Jr., *Cancer Res., 44*, 363 (1984).
96. S. Graham, J. Marshall, B. Haughey, A. Mittelman, M. Swanson, M. Zielezny, T. Byers, G. Wilkinson, and D. West, *Am. J. Epidemiol., 128*, 490 (1988).
97. D. West, M. L. Slattery, L. M. Robinson, K. L. Schuman, M. H. Ford, A. W. Mahoney, J. L. Lyon, and A. W. Sorenson, *Am. J. Epidemiol., 130*, 8883 (1989).
98. G. A. Kune, S. Kune, and L. F. Watson. *Nutr. Cancer, 13*, 9 (1990).
99. E. Benito, A. Obrador, A. Stiggelbout, F. X. Bosch, M. Mulet, N. Munoz, and J. Kaldor, *Int. J. Cancer, 45*, 69 (1990).
100. J. L. Freudenheim, S. Graham, J. R. Marshall, B. P. Haughey, and G. Wilkinson, *Am. J. Epidemiol., 131*, 612 (1990).
101. C. La Vecchia, E. Negri, F. Parazzini, P. Boyle, B. D'Avanzo, F. Levi, A. Gentile, and S. Franceschi, *Int. J. Cancer, 45*, 275 (1990).
102. A. S. Whittemore, A. H. Wu-Williams, M. Lee, Z. Shu, R. P. Gallagher, J. Dengao, Z. Lun, W. Xianghui, C. Kun, D. Jung, C. Teh, L. Chengde, X. J. Yao, R. S. Paffenbarger, and B. E. Henderson, *JNCI, 82*, 915 (1990).
103. R. L. Philips and D. A. Snowdon, *JNCI, 74*, 307 (1985).
104. A. Nomura, L. K. Heilbrun, and G. N. Stemmermenn, *JNCI, 74*, 319 (1985).
105. C. Garland, E. Barrett-Connor, A. H. Rossof, R. B. Shekclle, M. H. Criqui, and O. Paul, *Lancet, i*, 307 (1985).
106. S. Sidney, G. F. Friedman, and R. A. Hiatt, *Am. J. Epidemiol. 124*, 33 (1986).
107. A. H. Wu, A. Paganini-Hill, R. K. Ross, and B. E. Henderson, *Br. J. Cancer, 55*, 687 (1987).
108. L. N. Kolonel, and L. Le Marchand, In *Progress in Clinical and Biological Research*, vol. 222: *Dietary Fat and Cancer* (C. Ip, A. Rogers, D. Birt, C. Mettlin, eds.), Alan R. Liss, Inc., New York, 1986, p. 69.
109. W. Willett, *Nature, 338*, 389 (1989).
110. L. N. Kolonel, In *Genetics and Environmental Factors in Experimental and Human Cancer* (H. V. Gelboin et al., eds.), Japan Sci. Soc. Press, Tokyo, 1980, p. 327.
111. E. L. Wynder, K. Mabuchi, and W. F. Whitmore, Jr., *Cancer, 28*, 344 (1971).
112. S. Graham, B. Haughey, J. Marshall, R. Priore, T. Byers, T. Rzepka, C. Mettlin, and J. E. Pontes, *JNCI, 70*, 687 (1983).
113. R. Talamini, C. La Vecchia, A. Decarli, E. Negri, and S. Franceschi, *Br. J. Cancer, 53*, 817 (1986).
114. R. K. Ross, H. Shimizu, A. Paganini-Hill, G. Honda, and B. E. Henderson, *JNCI, 78*, 869 (1987).
115. L. N. Kolonel, C. N. Yoshizawa, and J. H. Hankin, *Am. J. Epidemiol., 127*, 999 (1988).

116. C. Mettlin, S. Selenskas, N. Natarajan, and R. Huben, *Cancer, 64*, 605 (1989).
117. C. La Vecchia, E. Negri, F. Parazzini, P. Boyle, B. D'Avanzo, F. Levi, A. Gentile, and S. Franceschi, *Int. J. Cancer, 45*, 275 (1990).
118. D. A. Snowdon, R. L. Phillips, and W. Choi, *Am. J. Epidemiol., 120*, 244 (1984).
119. R. K. Severson, J. S. Grove, A. M. Y. Nomura, and G. N. Stemmermann, *Br. J. Cancer, 297*, 713 (1988).
120. P. K. Mills, W. L. Beeson, R. L. Phillips, and G. E. Fraser, *Cancer, 64*, 598 (1989).
121. M. M. Thompson, C. Garland, E. Barrett-Connor, K. Kahaw, N. J. Friedlander, and D. L. Wingard, *Am. J. Epidemiol., 129*, 511 (1989).
122. S. M. Garn, W. R. Leonard, and V. M. Hawthorne, *Am. J. Clin. Nutr., 44*, 996 (1986).
123. R. S. Paffenbarger, R. T. Hyde, and A. L. Wing, *Am. J. Clin. Nutr., 45*, 312 (1987).
124. L. Le Marchand, L. N. Kolonel, and C. N. Yoshizawa, *Am. J. Epidemiol., 133*, 103 (1991).
125. P. Greenwald, A. Damon, V. Kirmss, and A. K. Polan, *JNCI, 53*, 341 (1974).
126. E. L. Wynder, K. Mabuchi, and W. F. Whitmore, *JNCI, 53*, 1619 (1974).
127. J. K. McLaughlin, J. S. Mandel, W. J. Blot, L. M. Schuman, E. S. Mehl, and J. F. Fraumeni, J., *JNCI, 72*, 275 (1984).
128. M. C. Yu, T. M. Mack, R. Hanisch, C. Cicioni, and B. E. Henderson, *JNCI, 77*, 351 (1986).
129. M. T. Goodman, H. Morgenstern, and E. L. Wynder, *Am. J. Epidemiol., 124*, 926 (1986).
130. W. C. Chumlea and R. N. Baumgartner, *Am. J. Clin. Nutr., 50*, 1158 (1989).
131. D. Albanes, *Cancer Res., 47*, 1987 (1987).

14

Metabolic Effects and Micronutrient Interactions

David Kritchevsky
The Wistar Institute
Philadelphia, Pennsylvania

INTRODUCTION

The role of nutrition in the etiology of cancer is an area of intensive research and vigorous debate. Vogel and McPherson (1) have reviewed the limitations to which human studies are subject. There is still no universally acceptable means of assessing past diet; for instance, case-control studies may be hampered by difficulties in dietary recall (2) and a possible inability to pinpoint specific nutrients (3). Consider the fact that studies of the influence of dietary fiber on risk of colon cancer conducted in Australian cities about 400 miles apart yielded quite different conclusions (4,5).

Animal (usually rat) studies have some utility, but they are carried out in a number of different strains of rat and under different conditions of diet (semipurified vs. commercial diet, for instance). The laboratory rat resembles an overweight, indolent human subject. Caloric restriction has been shown to inhibit spontaneous or induced tumorigenesis in rats and mice regardless of dietary regimen (6–9). Caloric restriction is carried out by limiting availability of macronutrients. There are no data relating to variation of the micronutrient content of calorically restricted diets.

Experimental studies of diet and cancer are usually designed to study effects of single variables, and experiments are not tuned to interactions among nutrients. Despite the long history of experimental and epidemiologic research in cancer, we may not yet have enough of a database to seek interactions among nutrients. The data relating macronutrients to cancer risk are not yet consistent. Take, for example, the effect of fat or meat consumption on risk of colorectal cancer. The earliest study, reported in 1933, by Stocks and Karn (10) found dairy products to be a negative risk factor in an English population. Almost half a century later Jensen et al. (11) reported saturated fatty acids to be a negative risk factor and meats, fats, and oils to have no significant effect in Scandinavians. Meat consumption or fat intake were found to correlate positively with colorectal cancer in Japan (12) but not in the United States (13,14) or Israel (15). Recently Willett et al. (16) have reported that animal fat (as meat) presented a risk for colorectal cancer but animal fat (dairy) did not. A puzzling finding was that animal protein was negatively (but not significantly) correlated with risk. Except for cases where foods are examined as a paradigm for micronutrients such as vitamins, our data on effects of diet on cancer are still concerned with major components of the diet, with much of the emphasis being on fat and fiber. Wattenberg (17) and Davis (18) have summarized inhibitors of chemically induced tumors and anticarcinogens in foods, respectively. Wattenberg (17) lists three general categories of inhibition, namely, blocking agents, suppressing agents, and compounds that prevent conversion of a precursor into a carcinogen (Table 1). A number of these substances occur in foods. Davis (18) divides the area into inhibitors of covalent DNA binding, inhibitors of promotion, inducers of biotransformation, and compounds that reduce absorption (Table 2). Most of the substances listed in the two tables are lipid-soluble.

FATS

Studies of the influence of dietary fat on incidence of spontaneous and induced cancer have been concerned primarily with levels of fat (as percentage of energy) but there is also a large body of data relating to type of fat: saturated or unsaturated. Animal studies have shown generally that the incidence of chemically induced tumors is greater when the test animals are fed diets high in unsaturated fat (19). Ip et al. (20) have shown that linoleic acid is responsible for the tumor-enhancing effect of unsaturated fat. Increasing the linoleic acid content of the diet leads to increased incidence of tumors until its concentration reaches 5% of the diet after which no further enhancement of tumorigenicity is observed. Increasing the polyunsaturated fatty acid (PUFA) content of the diet increases the level of PUFA found in membranes, which, in turn, affects the induction of membrane-bound enzymes such as epoxide hydratase and the mixed function oxidase system. The latter enzyme system is involved in the activation of carcinogens. This phenomenon has been discussed in depth by Gower (21).

The plasma lipids, whose level and composition can be influenced by amount and type of dietary fat, are the vehicle for many of the subsances listed in

Table 1 Inhibitors of Chemically Induced Tumorigenesis

Inhibitors of conversion of precursor to carcinogen	Blocking agents	Suppressing agents
Reducing acids	Phenols	Retinoids
Tocopherols	Indoles	Carotenoids
Phenols	Aromatic isothiocyanates	Selenium salts
	Coumarins	Protease inhibitors
	Flavones	Arachidonic acid metabolism inhibitors
	Dithiothiones	Cyanates
	Diterpenes	Isothiocyantes
	Dithiocarbamates	Phenols
	Phenothiazines	Plant sterols
	Barbiturates	Methylated xanthines
	Trimethylquinolines	

Source: From Ref. 17.

Tables 1 and 2. This includes the fat-soluble vitamins A, D, and E, all of which have been implicated as having anticancer activity.

Vitamin A: Carotenoids

Vitamin A compounds (retinoids or carotenoids) have been the most widely studied. Vitamin A appears in the diet in the form of retinol or retinyl esters (usually present in foods of animal origin) or as β-carotene (usually present in green or yellow leafy vegetables). There is a large body of literature concerning the influence of carotenoids on tumorigenesis. The data are not uniform, which may be due to differences in assessment of vitamin A status—as vitamin A in plasma or as carotene in plasma and/or food. Another problem inherent in all assessments of the effects of single nutrients on cancer is that they are ingested as part of a diverse diet. The effect of the rest of the diet on their absorption or utilization is rarely addressed. Furthermore, studies that measure level of intake in quartiles or quintiles seldom ask what nutrients have been displaced at highest levels of intake of the food or food component under investigation.

Carotenoids have been studied for their influence on more types of cancer than virtually any other micronutrient. In studies of correlation between serum or plasma carotenoids (usually measured as β-carotene) and cancer, findings range from no correlation (22) to define negative associations with lung cancer (23,24). There have been a number of retrospective studies of the association between

Table 2 Anticarcinogens in Foods

Action/Substance	Source
Inhibit covalent DNA binding:	
Phenyl isothiocyanate	Broccoli, cabbage
Ellagic acid	Fruits, nuts, berries
Flavonoids	Fruits, vegetables
Inhibit tumor promotion:	
Retinol	Green/Yellow vegetables, fruits
Tocopherol	Nuts, wheat germ
β-Carotene	Green/Yellow vegetables, fruits
Ascorbic acid	Vegetables, fruits
Organosulfur compounds	Garlic, onions
Curcumin	Tumeric/Curry
Capsaicin	Chili peppers
Induce biotransformation:	
Indole-3-carbinol	Cruciferous vegetables
Selenium	Garlic, seafood
Reduce absorption of carcinogens:	
Fiber	Grains, fruits, vegetables
Riboflavin	Fruits, vegetables

Source: From Ref. 18.

dietary carotenoids and lung cancer and, as detailed in the prior volume (25), almost all the studies show a negative correlation. Correlations of dietary carotenoids with other types of cancer are suggestive of an effect but less convincing (25).

Stahelin (26) has recently summarized data from a prospective study carried out in Switzerland and found a strong inverse relationship between β-carotene and all cancers, especially lung cancer and stomach cancer. A significant inverse relationship was also seen for vitamin A and cancer mortality. Le Marchand et al. (27) found no clear association between retinol, vitamin C, folic acid, iron, fiber, or fruits and lung cancer. Vegetable intake showed a stronger inverse correlation with risk than β-carotene. De Wet (28) has concluded that high carotene intake affects cancer incidence either by itself or after conversion to retinol. Several mechanisms have been suggested to explain the anticancer activity of retinol and β-carotene. Retinol may exert its effect at the level of the cell nucleus by influencing the processing of genetic information (29–31). The participation of retinol in glycosylation reactions (32) also suggests the possibility that retinoids can affect cell-cell interactions and thus influence cellular proliferation (33). Another effect arising from the involvement of retinoids in glycosylation phenomena may be enhancement of immune function (34,35).

Carotenoids are known to have antioxidant properties. β-Carotene can react with "singlet oxygen," a highly reactive form of oxygen which can alter or destroy DNA as well as other cellular components (36). β-Carotene also protects cellular membranes from the damaging effects of free radicals (37,38). The different properties of β-carotene and retinoids may act alone or in concert. Mathews-Roth (39) established skin tumors in mice using three different kinds of carcinogen—ultraviolet light, croton oil, 7,12-dimethylbenz(a)anthracene (DMBA) administration—and also administered carotenoids with or without vitamin A activity. Vitamin A activity was necessary to inhibit the action of the two chemical carcinogens. Similarly, Stich et al. (40) showed the canthaxanthin, a carotenoid without vitamin A activity, could not lower the number of cells with micronuclei observed in exfoliated oral mucosa taken from betel nut chewers, whereas β-carotene and retinol were effective.

The foregoing may explain the discrepancies between action of retinol or β-carotene in certain types of induced tumors. It may also explain the dichotomies in some of the epidemiologic data. Actually, the differences might be used to tell us more about the origins of the tumor being studied. Vitamin E has been implicated as a possible anticancer nutrient for almost half a century (41). There is evidence that increased vitamin E intake may be associated with reduced risk of colon cancer, but the association is not robust (14,42–44). There are no data supporting any connection between vitamin E intake and risk of breast (45–47) or lung (48) cancer. A recent study links high vitamin E intake with low risk of cervical cancer (49). Investigators have found reduced levels of vitamin E in sera of subjects with colorectal cancer (22,50,51), breast cancer (23,52,53), and lung cancer (50,54).

Vitamin E

Like vitamin A, vitamin E exerts a number of effects. It is an antioxidant and free radical scavenger (55), stimulates the immune system (56,57), and protects against cell injury (58). Which of these functions is the most important in mediating the anticancer effects of vitamin E is not known.

High intake or high plasma levels of carotenoids, vitamin A, and vitamin E have been found in some cases to reduce the risk of cancers of different types. Which of the inherent properties of these substances accounts for the basis of this protection is unelucidated at this writing.

FIBER

Another macronutrient which by interactions with micronutrients may affect the course of cancer is dietary fiber. Dietary fiber is the subject of another chapter in this volume, so no attempt will be made to describe the many types of dietary fiber and their physiologic roles. The possibility that the fiber content of their diet might play a role in the protection of African blacks from colon cancer was first articulated by Higginson and Oettle (59) in 1960 and crystallized into a hypothesis by Burkitt (60) about 10 years later. The effects of dietary fiber in the human colon are summarized in Table 3.

Effects of fiber on transit time and fecal weight have not been associated with level of colon cancer risk in studies from Hawaii (61) or Scandinavia (11). Dilution of colonic contents could influence colon cancer in several ways. It would dilute the amount of carcinogen or procarcinogen that came into contact with the colonic mucosa and reduce risk in that way. Dilution of cocarcinogens would be another way in which fiber exerted an effect. Hill et al. (62) have reported that the concentration of bile acids [promoters of chemically induced colon cancer (63)] in the feces of Western populations with high incidence of colon cancer (England, Scotland, United States) is 10 times that of Uganda, Japan, and India, which have a low incidence of cancer (6.15 ± 0.66 mg/g vs. 0.61 ± 0.13 mg/g). Studies from Hong Kong (64), Scandinavia (11), and the United States (65) all show higher concentrations of fecal bile acids in population groups with higher incidence of colon cancer.

Dietary fiber binds bile acids and bile salts in vitro, the extent of binding depending on both the substrate and the fiber (66,67). Fiber may also bind carcinogens (68). Any protective phenomenon may also depend on excretion of the bile acid–fiber complex. Fiber also affects the morphology of the bowel mucosa of rats, the extent of abnormality increasing as binding affinity increases (69). The deviation from normality is due to the bile acid (70). Nigro et al. (71) found that cholestyramine, a very potent binder of bile acids, greatly enhanced carcinogenesis when fed to rats that had been given any one of three colon carcinogens.

The liver produces cholic and chenodeoxycholic acids (the primary bile acids), and these are dehydroxylated at the 7 position to yield deoxycholic and lithocholic acids (the secondary bile acids). The ratio of fecal anaerobic to aerobic bacteria is higher in countries with a high incidence of colon cancer (62), and, generally,

Table 3 Effects of Dietary Fiber in the Human Colon

Increased fecal weight
Increased frequency of defecation
Decreased transit time
Dilution of colonic contents
Increased microbial growth
Altered energy metabolism
Absorption of organic and inorganic substances
Decreased dehydroxylation of bile acids
Production of H_2, CH_4, CO_2 and short-chain fatty acids

anaerobic bacteria are more active metabolically. Secondary bile acids have been shown to posses cocarcinogenic or comutagenic activity (72).

Dietary fiber (with the exception of lignin) is fermented in the colon to yield short-chain fatty acids (SCFA), principally acetic, propionic, and butyric. SCFA can influence intestinal or fecal pH, and McDonald et al. (73) have shown that subjects with large bowel cancer exhibit higher fecal pH than controls. The fecal pH of South African populations increased with increasing susceptibility to colon cancer (74). Butyrate has been shown to suppress differentiation and to alter properties of human colon cells in vitro (75,76).

Finally, dietary fiber has been shown to enhance fecal energy loss (77,78). Caloric restriction will inhibit the growth of spontaneous, induced, or transplanted tumors in rats and mice (6–9,79). A recent epidemiologic study of colon cancer incidence in human subjects found a strong positive correlation with energy intake (80). In a recent discussion of nutritional epidemiology (81), Willett states: "The measurement of total energy intake and its control in analyses in epidemiologic studies are essential for interpreting data on intake of specific nutrients." He goes on to suggest that the primary presentation of nutrient data is best done in the form of energy-adjusted intakes. The effect of high fiber in a normally low caloric diet would be greater than in a Western diet.

The interaction among nutrients requires further research. Lee et al. (82) found a strong negative correlation between colon cancer risk and a low ratio of meat to vegetables. Human epidemiologic data are based on comparisons of foods high or low in specific nutrients. Thus, fiber-rich foods may be protective, but the effect is usually associated with vegetable or fruit consumption (83). Vegetables contain vitamins, indoles, phenols, tannins and other substances, which, in isolated form, have reduced the incidence of experimentally induced tumors (84).

We have established a large database regarding dietary effects on tumorigenesis. The data are usually adduced from studies of the specific dietary component(s) of interest to the individual investigators. We must now begin to examine the effects of interactions among the various components. This type of study will require ingenuity.

ACKNOWLEDGMENT

Supported, in part, by a grant (CA43856) and a Research Career Award (HL00734) from the National Institutes of Health and by funds from the Commonwealth of Pennsylvania.

REFERENCES

1. V. G. Vogel and R. D. McPherson, *Hematology/Oncology Clinics of No. America, 3*, 35 (1989).

2. G. E. McKeown-Eyssen, K. S. Yeung, and E. Bright-See, *Am. J. Epidemiol.*, *124*, 94 (1986).
3. G. R. Howe, *Cancer Res.*, *41*, 3731 (1981).
4. J. D. Potter and A. J. McMichael, *JNCI*, *76*, 557 (1986).
5. S. Kune, G. A. Kune, and L. F. Watson, *Nutr. Cancer*, *9*, 21 (1987).
6. P. S. Lavik and C. A. Baumann, *Cancer Res.*, *3*, 749 (1943).
7. A. Tannenbaum, *Cancer Res.*, *5*, 609 (1945).
8. D. Kritchevsky and D. M. Klurfeld, *Adv. Exp. Med. Biol.*, *206*, 55 (1986).
9. D. Albanes, *Cancer Res.*, *47*, 1987 (1987).
10. P. Stocks and M. K. Karn, *Ann. Eugen. (London)*, *5*, 237 (1933).
11. O. M. Jensen, R. MacLennan, and J. Wahrendorf, *Nutr. Cancer*, *4*, 5 (1982).
12. W. Haenszel, F. B. Locke, and M. Segi, *JNCI*, *64*, 17 (1980).
13. S. Graham, H. Dayal, M. Swanson, A. Mittelman, and G. Wilkinson, *JNCI*, *61*, 709 (1978).
14. J. Higginson, *JNCI*, *37*, 527 (1966).
15. B. Modan, V. Barell, F. Lubin, M. Modan, R. Greenberg, and S. Graham, *JNCI*, *55*, 15 (1975).
16. W. C. Willett, M. J. Stampfer, G. A. Colditz, B. A. Rosner, and F.E. Speizer, *N. Engl. J. Med.*, *232*, 1664 (1990).
17. L. W. Wattenberg, *Cancer Res.*, *45*, 1 (1985).
18. D. L. Davis, *Environmental Res.*, *50*, 322 (1989).
19. K. K. Carroll and H. T. Khor, *Lipids*, *6*, 415 (1971).
20. C. Ip, C. A. Carter, and M. M. Ip, *Cancer Res.*, *45*, 1997 (1985).
21. J. D. Gower, *Free Radical Biol. Med.*, *5*, 95 (1988).
22. W. C. Willett, B. F. Polk, B. A. Underwood, M. J. Stampfer, S. Pressel, B. Rosner, J. O. Taylor, K. Schneider, and C. G. Hames, *N. Engl. J. Med.*, *310*, 430 (1984).
23. H. B. Stahelin, F. Rosel, E. Buess, and G. Brubacher, *JNCI*, *73*, 1463 (1984).
24. A. M. Y. Nomura, G. N. Stemmerman, L. K. Heilbrun, R. M. Salkeld, and J. P. Vuilleumier, *Cancer Res.*, *45*, 2369 (1985).
25. M. S. Micozzi, In *Nutrition and Cancer Prevention: Investigating the Role of Micronutrients* (T. Moon and M. S. Micozzi, eds.), Marcel Dekker, New York, 1989.
26. H. B. Stahelin, *Soz. Praeventivmed.*, *34*, 75 (1989).
27. L. Le Marchand, C. N. Yoshizawa, L. N. Kolonel, J. H. Hawkin, and M. T. Goodman, *JNCI*, *81*, 1158 (1989).
28. H. C. W. De Wet, *Anticancer Res.*, *9*, 145 (1989).
29. R. Lotan, *Biochem. Biophys. Acta*, *605*, 33 (1980).
30. M. B. Sporn and A. B. Roberts, *Cancer Res.*, *43*, 3034 (1983).
31. M. B. Sporn and A. B. Roberts, *JNCI*, *73*, 1381 (1984).
32. S. S. Shapiro and D. J. Mott, *Ann. N.Y. Acad. Sci.*, *359*, 306 (1981).
33. D. J. Morre, K. E. Creek, D. M. Morre, and C. L. Richardson, *Ann. N.Y. Acad. Sci.*, *359*, 367 (1981).
34. E. L. Felix, M. H. Cohen, and B. C. Lloyd, *J. Surg. Res.*, *21*, 307 (1976).
35. T. H. Maugh, *Science*, *186*, 1198 (1974).
36. C. S. Foote, R. W. Denny, L. Weaver, Y. Chong, and J. Peters, *Ann. N.Y. Acad. Sci.*, *171*, 139 (1970).

37. N. I. Krinsky and S. M. Deneke, *JNCI, 69*, 205 (1982).
38. G. W. Burton and K. U. Ingold, *Science, 224*, 569 (1984).
39. M. M. Mathews-Roth, *Oncology, 39*, 33 (1982).
40. H. F. Stich, W. Stich, M. P. Rosen, and M. O. Vallejera, *Int. J. Cancer, 34*, 745 (1984).
41. W. Jaffe, *Exp. Med. Surg., 4*, 278 (1946).
42. M. Jain, G. M. Cook, F. G. Davis, M. G. Grace, G. R. Howe, and A. B. Miller, *Int. J. Cancer, 23*, 454 (1980).
43. G. N. Stemmerman, A. M. Y. Nomura, and L. K. Heilbrun, *Cancer Res., 44*, 4633 (1984).
44. G. Macquart-Moulins, E. Riboli, J. Cornee, B. Charnay, P. Berthezene, and N. Day, *Int. J. Cancer, 38*, 183 (1986).
45. A. B. Miller, A. Kelly, N. W. Choi, V. Matthews, R. W. Morgan, L. Munan, J. D. Burch, J. Feather, G. R. Howe, and M. Jain, *Am. J. Epidemiol., 107*, 499 (1978).
46. T. Hirohata, A. M. Y. Nomura, J. H. Hankin, L. N. Kolonel, and J. Lee, *JNCI, 78*, 595 (1987).
47. W. C. Willett, M. J. Stampfer, G. A. Colditz, B. A. Rosner, C. H. Hennekens, and F. E. Speizer, *N. Engl. J. Med., 316*, 22 (1987).
48. T. E. Byers, S. Graham, B. P. Haughey, J. R. Marshall, and M. K. Swanson, Am. J. Epidemiol., 122, 41 (1987).
49. R. Verreault, J. Chu, M. Mandelson, and K. Shy, *Int. J. Cancer, 43*, 1050 (1989).
50. N. J. Wald, S. G. Thompson, J. W. Densem, J. Boreham, and A. Bailey, *Br. J. Cancer, 55*, 69 (1987).
51. P. Knekt, A. Aromaa, J. Maatela, G. Alfthan, R-K. Aaran, L. Teppo, and M. Hakama, *Int. J. Cancer, 42*, 846 (1988).
52. N. Wald, J. Boreham, J. L. Hayward, and R. D. Bulbrooke, *Br. J. Cancer, 49*, 321 (1984).
53. M. Gerber, S. Richardson, P. Crastes de Paulet, H. Pujol, and A. Crastes de Paulet, *Cancer, 64*, 2347 (1989).
54. J. T. Salonen, R. Salonen, R. Lappetelainen, P. H. Maenpaa, G. Alfthan, and P. Puska, *Br. J. Cancer, 290*, 417 (1985).
55. K. N. Prasda, *Prog. Clin. Biol. Res., 259*, 363 (1988).
56. M. P. Carpenter, in *Vitamins and Cancer* (F. L. Meyskens, Jr., and K. N. Prasad, eds.), Humana Press, Clifton, NJ, 1986, p. 199.
57. R. R. Watson, in *Vitamins and Cancer* (F. L. Meyskens, Jr., and K. N. Prasad, eds.), Humana Press, Clifton, NJ, 1986, p. 439.
58. G. A. Pascoe, K. Olafsdotter, and D. J. Reed, *Arch. Biochem. Biophys., 256*, 150 (1987).
59. J. Higginson and A. G. Oettle, *JNCI, 24*, 589 (1960).
60. D. P. Burkitt, *Cancer, 28*, 3 (1971).
61. G. A. Glober, A. Nomura, S. Kamiyama, A. Shimoda, and B. C. Abba, *Lancet, 2*, 110 (1977).
62. M. J. Hill, B. S. Drasar, V. C. Aries, J. C. Crowther, G. Hawksworth, and R. E. O. Williams, *Lancet, 1*, 95 (1971).
63. L. F. Narisawa, N. E. Magadia, J. A. Weisburger, and E. L. Wynder, *JNCI, 55*, 1093 (1975).

64. J. S. Crowther, B. S. Drasar, M. J. Hill, R. MacLennan, D. Magnin, S. Peck, and C. H. Teah-Chaun, *Br. J. Cancer, 34*, 191 (1976).
65. N. Turjman, C. Guidry, B. Jaeger, A. I. Mendeloff, B. Caulkins, and P. P. Nair, in *Colon and Nutrition* (H. Kaspar and H. Goebell, eds.), MTP Press Ltd., Lancaster, U.K., 1982, p. 291.
66. M. A. Eastwood and D. Hamilton, *Biochim. Biophys. Acta, 152*, 165 (1968).
67. J. A. Story and D. Kritchevsky, *J. Nutr., 106*, 1292 (1976).
68. P. Smith-Barbaro, D. Hansen, and B. Reddy, *JNCI, 67*, 495 (1981).
69. M. M. Cassidy, F. G. Lightfoot, L. E. Grun, J. A. Story, D. Kritchevsky, and G. V. Vahouny, *Am. J. Clin. Nutr., 34*, 218 (1981).
70. G. V. Vahouny, S. Satchithanandan, F. Lightfoot, L. Grau, S. Haas-Smith, D. Kritchevsky, and M. M. Cassidy, *Dig. Dis. Sci., 29*, 432 (1984).
71. N. D. Nigro, N. Bhadrochari, and C. Chomchai, *Dis. Colon Rectum, 16*, 428 (1973).
72. M. J. Hill, in *Dietary Fiber in Health and Disease* (G. V. Vahouny and D. Kritchevsky, eds.), Plenum Press, New York, 1982, p. 299.
73. I. A. MacDonald, G. R. Webb, and D. E. Mahony, *Am. J. Clin. Nutr., 31*, S233 (1978).
74. A. R. P. Walker, B. F. Walker, and A. J. Walker, *Br. J. Cncer, 53*, 489 (1986).
75. H. K. Hagopian, M. G. Riggs, L. A. Swartz, and V. M. Ingram, *Cell, 12*, 855 (1977).
76. Y. S. Kim, D. Tsao, A. Morita, and A. Bella, in *Colon Carcinogenesis* (R. A. Malt and R. C. N. Williamson, eds.), MTP Press Ltd., Lancaster, U.K., 1982, p. 317.
77. D. A. T. Southgate and J. V. G. A. Durnin, *Br. J. Nutr., 24*, 517 (1970).
78. K. W. Heaton, P. M. Emmett, C. L. Henry, J. R. Thornton, A. Manhire, and M. Hartog, *Human Nutr. Clin. Nutr., 37C*, 31 (1983).
79. D. Kritchevsky, *Proc. Soc. Exp. Biol. Med., 193*, 35–38 (1990).
80. J. L. Lyon, A. W. Mahoney, D. W. West, J. W. Gardner, K. R. Smith, A. W. Sorenson, and W. Stanish, *JNCI, 78*, 853 (1987).
81. W. C. Willett, *Int. J. Cancer, 46*, 770 (1990).
82. H. P. Lee, L. Gourley, S. W. Duffy, J. Esteve, J. Lee, and N. E. Day, *Int. J. Cancer, 43*, 1007 (1989).
83. M. L. Slattery, A. W. Sorenson, A. W. Mahoney, T. K. French, D. Kritchevsky, and J. C. Street, *JNCI, 80*, 1974 (1988).
84. L. W. Wattenberg, *Proc. Nutr. Soc., 49*, 173 (1990).

part four

CLINICAL TRIALS ON MACRONUTRIENTS AND CANCER

15

Rationale, Feasibility, and Design of a Low Fat Diet Intervention Trial Among Postmenopausal Women

Ross L. Prentice
Fred Hutchinson Cancer Research Center
Seattle, Washington

INTRODUCTION

In 1983 the National Cancer Institute (NCI) approved in concept the conduct of a randomized clinical trial to determine whether a reduction in dietary fat among middle-aged women would reduce subsequent breast cancer incidence. A feasibility phase of this Women's Health Trial (WHT) was initiated in 1984. Randomization into a "full-scale" trial began in early 1986, following the successful completion of the feasibility phase (1,2) that included 303 women randomized to either a low fat diet intervention (60%) or to a control (40%). The decision as to whether or not to proceed with the full trial, involving the randomization of 32,000 women (3), was much debated during 1987. In the meanwhile, an additional 1761 women were randomized to a refined and streamlined dietary intervention protocol (40%) or to control (60%). A recommendation (4) against proceeding further with the WHT as proposed at that time was made in early 1988 and accepted by the NCI. The principal reason given concerned the strength of evidence in support of a dietary fat and breast cancer hypothesis (see Refs. 5 and 6 for discussion). WHT investigators then set out to conduct further studies of relevance to the fat and breast cancer hypothesis and to consider design changes that may lead to a strengthened and more efficient trial. As a result a trial proposed under the acronym DIET FIT (Dietary Fat Intervention Trial for Disease Prevention in Women) was submitted to the NIH by a group of cancer and cardiovascular disease researchers for possible funding as an investigator-initiated research grant in late 1988. The proposal involved a focus on a combined cancer endpoint, consisting of breast, colon, rectum, ovary, and endometrium cancer among women aged 55–69, as well as a focus on coronary heart disease incidence and on total mortality. It included certain changes in eligibility criteria and trial duration that implied an approximate 25% reduction in projected cost. This proposal was site visited in the usual peer review fashion in mid-1989 and recommended for approval with a fundable priority score. However, in late 1989 the NCI's National Cancer Advisory Board chose to make an exception of this grant request and recommended that it not be funded from the regular research grant pool, primarily on the basis of cost. As this recommendation was being entertained, the Board of Scientific Counsellors (BSC) of NCI's Division of Cancer Prevention and Control conducted a workshop on research strategies for the prevention of breast cancer. The DIET FIT concept received substantial support from the BSC. In part to follow-up on BSC's interest in this proposal, the NCI and National Heart, Lung and Blood Institute (NHLBI) jointly convened a workshop in mid-1990 entitled "Research Designs for Studying the Health Consequences of Dietary Modification Among Women." The report (7) of this workshop recommends that the two institutes mount a substantial program of research on the possible effects of diet on disease incidence and mortality, including basic, clinical, and epidemiologic research and that a long-term field trial on the effects of a reduced fat diet on human health services as the central enterprise of this research program. The NCI has subsequently (10/90) approved the concept of a new Women's Health Trial, evidently clearing the way for a trial to begin within the next few months. The concept, like the DIET FIT proposal, involves the randomization of 24,000 middle-aged and older women to either an intervention program (40%) that emphasizes fat reduction or control, at approximately 12 clinical units, with an average follow-up time in excess of 10 years.

Even though some further refinement of trial design can be anticipated, it seems timely to review the rationale, feasibility, and design of the type of trial that is intended. (See Chapter 9 for a comprehensive review of data pertinent to the relationship between dietary fat and cancer risk.)

TRIAL RATIONALE

Aggregate Data Studies

We have recently presented (8) an analysis of the incidence rates of selected cancers in relation to the per capita disappearance of fat, using cancer incidence data from *Cancer Incidence in Five Continents* (9), and dietary fat from the Food and Agriculture Organization of the United Nations (10) for 21 countries thought to have cancer incidence data representative of the country as a whole. Ordinary linear regression analysis of log-incidence rates on per capita grams of fat disappearance yielded relative risk estimates (95% confidence intervals) for a 50% reduction from U.S. levels of total fat (Table 1) as follows: 0.39(0.27,0.55), 0.33(0.18,0.61), 0.71(0.51,0.97), 0.39(0.26,0.60), and 0.26(0.17,0.40) for cancers of the breast, colon, rectum, ovary, and endometrium, respectively, among women in the age range 55–69, and 0.37(0.21,0.65), 0.64(0.45,0.91), and 0.17(0.09,0.32) for cancers of the colon, rectum, and prostate among men of ages 55–69. Among a younger age group (ages 30–44) the corresponding relative risk estimates tended to be much closer to unity, with only those for breast, ovary, and endometrium cancer suggesting an association with relative risk estimates (95% CI) of 0.53(0.37,0.78), 0.57(0.38,0.85), and 0.57(0.30,1.11), respectively. Furthermore, the suggested associations with fat intake were remarkably robust to the inclusion of a range of other dietary and nondietary factors in the regression. Relative risk estimates for a 50% reduction from U.S. levels in percent calories from fat (i.e., 41.7–20.9%), rather than grams of fat, were almost identical to those listed above (11). These analyses suggest that a 50% reduction in fat from U.S. levels may eventually reduce total cancer incidence by about 33% among U.S. women of ages 55–69 and by about 17% among U.S. men of ages 55–69.

Regression analyses of the type just mentioned were also conducted for several other cancer sites. Some results, which we have not previously reported, for kidney, bladder, pancreas, and lung cancer are given in Table 1. A 50% reduction from U.S. levels in per capita fat disappearance is associated with an approximate threefold reduction in kidney cancer in either sex in both the 55–69 and 30–44 age ranges. Per capita fat disappearance provides an explanation for about 50% of the international variation in the incidence rates for this tumor. Similarly, fat disappearance provides an explanation for about 30–40% of the international variation in bladder cancer rates among females and males in the age range 55–69, but only a small fraction of the variation among persons in the 30–44 age range.

Per capita fat disappearance provides an explanation for only a small fraction of the variation in the rates of pancreatic and lung cancer. However, a major difficulty in the interpretation of Table 1 arises from the possibility of confounding by cigarette smoking. As a partial accommodation of such potential confounding, the regression analyses were repeated including per capita cigarettes per day in 1958 (12). Following such inclusion there is no hint of association between per capita fat disappearance and lung or pancreatic cancer. For example, among females and males of ages 55–69 the relative risks (95% CI) associated with a 50% reduction from U.S. levels in per capita fat are, respectively, 1.18(0.44,3.17) and 0.81(0.45,1.43). The corresponding cigarette smoking-adjusted relative risk estimates and confidence intervals for kidney cancer among females and males of ages 55–69 are 0.31(0.18,0.51) and 0.19(0.10,0.36), respectively, and

Table 1 Estimated Relative Risks (RR) from International Regression Analyses for a 50% Reduction from the U.S. Value in Per Capita Fat Disappearance

	Cancer site			
	Kidney	Bladder	Pancreas	Lung
		Females, Ages 55–69		
RR	0.38	0.43	0.71	0.69
95% CI	(0.24,0.59)	(0.25,0.75)	(0.45,1.13)	(0.29,1.68)
r^2(%)[a]	49	32	10	3
		Males, Ages 55–69		
RR	0.26	0.49	0.78	0.66
95% CI	(0.15,0.46)	(0.33,0.72)	(0.53,1.14)	(0.41,1.07)
r^2(%)[a]	54	41	8	13
		Females, Ages 30–44		
RR	0.43	0.54	0.91	0.56
95% CI	(0.29,0.64)	(0.16,1.78)	(0.47,1.78)	(0.27,1.17)
r^2(%)[a]	49	5	<1	7
		Males, Ages 30–44		
RR	0.34	0.55	1.26	0.84
95% CI	(0.24,0.50)	(0.30,1.01)	(0.73,2.17)	(0.46,1.54)
r^2(%)[a]	65	18	4	2

[a]Percentage of variation in log-incidence rates explained by fat disappearance.

among females and males of ages 30–44 are 0.35(0.21,0.55) and 0.27(0.19,0.39), respectively. For bladder cancer among females and males 55–69 the corresponding rates are 0.48(0.24,0.95) and 0.47(0.29,0.76), while for females and males 30–44 they are 0.97(0.24,3.97) and 0.64(0.31,1.33). Although a more thorough control for the distribution of cigarette smoking exposures among the 21 countries would be desirable, these analyses suggest that fat consumption may be an important risk factor for kidney cancer and for bladder cancer in the older age range. These results were affected little by the inclusion of various other dietary and nondietary factors in the regression equation, though the kidney cancer relative risks were somewhat closer to unity upon including per capita gross national product.

Regression analyses of changes in the logarithm of cancer incidence rates between the mid-1960s and 1980 in relation to corresponding lagged changes in nutrient disappearance were also conducted (8) for cancers of the breast, colon, rectum, ovary, and endometrium in women, and cancers of the colon, rectum, and prostate among men. Even though based on only 10 countries, these analyses were rather consistent with those mentioned above. For example, the relative risk estimates (95% CI) for a 50% reduction from U.S. levels in per capita fat were 0.23(0.13,0.40) and 0.40(0.21,0.76) for female breast cancer in the age ranges 55–69 and 30–44, respectively. Among females and males in the age range 55–69 the corresponding colon cancer relative risk estimates were 0.38(0.22,0.67) and 0.26(0.16,0.41), with little evidence for association in the younger age group. The corresponding rectal cancer relative risk estimates were 0.38(0.21,0.61) and 0.23(0.14,0.39), notably smaller than from the international comparisons, again with little indication for a fat association among younger persons. Among men of ages 55–69 the prostate cancer relative risk estimate was 0.24(0.12,0.49), while the relative risk estimates for ovarian cancer and endometrial cancer were 0.57(0.30,1.09) and 0.36(0.20,0.66) among women 55–69.

The regression analysis of international variations in cancer rates was extended to consider fat disappearance by degree of saturation. Polyunsaturated and saturated, but not monounsaturated, fat disappearance appeared to be related to cancer incidence in the 55–69 age range. There was a suggestion of a particularly important role for polyunsaturated fat in relation to female breast cancer in both the 55–69 and 30–44 age groups and for saturated fat in relation to colon cancer among men and women of ages 55–69. Also, both polyunsaturated and saturated, but not monounsaturated, fat disappearance appeared to be related to kidney cancer incidence in both the 55–69 and 30–44 age ranges and to bladder cancer incidence in the 55–69 age range.

In summary, both international comparisons and time-trends sugget associations between per capita fat disappearance and cancers of the breast, colon, rectum, ovary, endometrium, and prostate among persons in the age range 55–69, and for breast, and possibly ovarian, cancer among younger women. International comparisons also suggest a relationship between per capita fat disappearance and kidney cancer among older and younger persons and bladder cancer among older persons. Subsequent subsections consider the consistency of these strong international associations with the results of various other types of studies, including case-control and cohort studies, migrant studies, studies of time-trends in U.S. cancer rates, and cholesterol-lowering trials.

Analytic Epidemiologic Studies

A rather large number of case-control studies have examined the relationship between estimates of individual fat consumption and the incidence of selected cancers, particularly cancers of the breast, colon, and prostate. Recently Howe et al. (13) presented an analysis of the raw data from 12 case-control studies of breast cancer. Among postmenopausal women this analysis indicated a highly significant ($p < 0.0001$) association with relative risk estimates of 1, 1.20, 1.24, 1.24, and 1.46 across fat intake quintiles defined by a Canadian study (14). At first glance a relative risk gradient of this magnitude seems smaller than would be consistent with the relative risk of 0.39 for a 50% fat reduction arising in the international regression analysis. However, after noting the typical narrow range of fat intakes within countries as compared to between countries, and upon making a sensible accommodation for random measurement error in individual dietary assessment using data from the excellent validation study of Willett and colleagues (15), the international regression analyses project a relative risk gradient of 1, 1.07, 1.15, 1.26, and 1.53 across these quintiles (see Ref. 8 for details). Hence international regression analyses and case-control studies seem quite consistent in suggesting an important role for dietary fat in determining the risk of postmenopausal breast cancer. Among premenopausal women, the analysis of Howe et al. (13) estimates a nonsignificant relative risk of 1.13 between extreme quintiles of fat intake, smaller than the 1.32 projected from our analysis (8) of international variations in breast cancer rates. Also, the cohort study of Willett et al. (16), with 601 breast cancer cases, approximately 200 of whom were postmenopausal, failed to identify an association between fat intake and breast cancer risk, as did the study of Jones et al. (17), based on a total of only 99 breast cancer cases.

The state of the epidemiologic data for colon and rectal cancer seems rather similar to that for breast cancer. The strong associations for persons 55–69 years of age suggested by international regression analyses were projected onto the dietary fat categories used in seven case-control studies (8). Observed relative risk gradients were quite variable but generally agreed with those projected for colon cancer, and were somewhat larger than those projected for rectal cancer. The one published cohort study (18) that reported quantitative estimates of fat intake suggests that saturated fat may relate positively to rectal cancer incidence and negatively to colon cancer incidence, based on only 59 and 106 cases, respectively. A preliminary report (19) from the Nurses Health Study evidently suggests a positive association between colon cancer and total fat that is considerably stronger than would be expected based on international regression analyses.

The observed dietary fat relative risk gradients for prostate cancer were likewise similar to, but overall somewhat smaller than, those projected from international comparisons, based on five case-control and two cohort studies (8). The observed relative risk gradient across fat intake categories in four case-control studies of epithelial ovarian cancer also appeared to be quite consistent with projections from international regressions.

Some insight into the rather variable results obtained in case-control and cohort studies is obtained by consideration of the results of the validation study (15) of 173 Boston area nurses who completed four 7-day food records over the course of a one-year period, and a food frequency questionnaire that was intended to retrospectively assess typical diets over the same time period. The 28 days of food records represent unusually precise dietary information, at least over the one-year period, while the food frequency instrument provided the basis for dietary information in the various reports (e.g., 16,19) from the Nurses Health Study cohort. While the food record percent calories from fat quintiles in the validation study (15) were 32, 36, 39, 41, and 44, the estimated food record percent calories from fat averages, across food frequency percent calories from fat quintiles are, respectively, 35.6, 37.2, 38.4, 40.4, and 40.8. Hence if the food records can be regarded as essentially without error, one only expects a 5% range in percent calories from fat across the fat intake categories used in the Nurses Health Study. This is rather like trying to study the relationship between cigarette smoking and lung or bladder cancer in a cohort in which everyone smokes between 36 and 41 cigarettes per day.

Possible differential effects of various types of fat may also affect the reliability and interpretation of specific analytic studies. For example, our analysis of international variations and time-trends in disease rates suggest that polyunsaturated fat may have a particular role in enhancing breast cancer risk, as is also the suggestion from experimental studies of mammary carcinogenesis in rodents (see Ref. 20 for a recent review). As an exercise (see Ref. 11 for details) suppose that the breast cancer relative risk is 1, 1.25, 1.5, 1.75, and 2.0 across percent calories from polyunsaturated fat quintiles in the population of U.S. nurses studied by Willett et al. (16). Again taking the 28 days of food records (15) as a "gold-standard" and assuming other types of fat do not affect breast cancer risk, one can estimate the breast cancer relative risk across food frequency percent calories from fat qunitiles to be 1, 1.11, 1.07, 1.08, and 1.02. It seems clear that this population, with the food frequency dietary assessment instrument used in Ref. 16, is not suited to detecting even a major association between polyunsaturated fat and breast cancer. In comparison, if the risk of a disease depends on saturated fat but not other types of fat, with relative risks of 1, 1.25, 1.5, 1.75, and 2.0 across percent calories from saturated fat quintiles, then the estimated relative risks are 1, 1.09, 1.18, 1.32, and 1.38 across food frequency percent calories from fat quintiles. The apparent contrast between the ability of the Willett food frequency instrument to assess associations with polyunsaturated versus saturated fat may help to explain the differing breast and colon cancer results (16,19) from the nurses cohort. More generally, however, the range of nutrient intakes in a study population and the measurement properties of the dietary instruments can be expected to have a major influence on the results, interpretation, and reliability of cohort and case-control studies. Much more work on methods for accommodating random measurement errors in dietary assessment is crucial to assessing the potential of analytic epidemiologic studies for reliable inference in the diet and cancer research area.

Migrant Studies, U.S. Time-Trends, and Cholesterol-Lowering Trials

It is interesting to consider also the implications of the major associations between dietary fat and cancer suggested by international comparisons of disease rates in respect to various data sources additional to the analytic epidemiologic studies discussed above. For example, Tominaga (21) presents cancer incidence data on Japanese migrants (first and later generations) to the United States. Among women relative risks (i.e., ratios of age-adjusted cancer incidence rates) for Japanese in the United States versus Japanese in Japan were 3.5, 3.2, 1.5, 2.9, and 11.3 for breast, colon, rectum, ovary, and endometrium cancers, respectively. In comparison, upon making a sensible assumption (8) concerning the change in dietary fat following migration our international regression analysis for the age range 55–69 predict corresponding relative risks of 2.9, 3.5, 1.5, 2.9, and 4.6. Among men the observed relative risk estimates for colon, rectum, and prostate cancer are 3.5, 2.3, and 5.7 as compared to projected values of 3.0, 1.6, and 7.2 from international regression analyses. Hence dietary fat provides a possible explanation for a large fraction of the increased rates of prominent cancers experienced by Japanese migrants to the United States, as compared to Japanese in Japan.

At the 1990 annual meeting of the American Society of Preventive Oncology, NCI Director Dr. Samuel Broder challenged the cancer prevention community to provide explanations for important U.S. trends in the incidence and mortality of various cancers. Such trends for the time period 1947–50 to 1983–84 are documented in Devesa et al. (22).

In order to use the results of international regression analyses of dietary fat and cancer to predict changes in U.S. cancer incidence rates, one can note (23) that the per capita daily disappearance of polyunsaturated, saturated, and monounsaturated fat in the United States was 17, 59, and 54 grams, respectively, in 1945, as compared to 31, 58, and 63 grams in 1980. Note the remarkable 82% increase in polyunsaturated fat disappearance over this time period. Table 2 shows relative risk projections for the age range 55–69 that result from inserting these changes in fat disappearance into the international regression analyses of cancer incidence rates on the per capita disappearance of polyunsaturated, saturated, and monounsaturated fat. In agreement with observed incidence rate changes, this exercise predicts substantial increases in breast and prostate cancer incidence, with more modest increases in the incidence of colon, rectum, ovary, and endometrium cancer. In order to reduce the influence of exogenous steroids, the observed and projected relative risks for ovarian and endometrial cancer are based on changes in the food supply between 1945 and 1965 and changes in cancer incidence between 1947–50 and 1969–71. It seems evident that changing patterns of fat consumption, particularly the well-documented major increase in polyunsaturated fat consumption, provide a possible explanation for important increases in the rates of certain cancers in the United States.

It is also interesting to note that changes in per capita food disappearance between 1945 and 1980 predict noteworthy reductions in blood cholesterol concentration and coronary heart disease risk. In particular, the per capita disappearance of total calories increased from 3300 in 1945 to 3400 in 1980, while the

Table 2 Projected Changes in Cancer Incidence Rates from Changes in U.S. Food Supply, 1945-1980

	Projected relative risk					
	Breast	Colon	Rectum	Ovary[a]	Endo-metrium[a]	Prostate
Females, ages 55-69	1.47	1.10	1.20	1.15	1.24	
Males, ages 55-69		1.19	1.06			1.69
	Observed Relative Risk (1947-50 to 1983-84)					
	Breast	Colon	Rectum	Ovary[a]	Endo-metrium[a]	Prostate
Females, ages 55-69	1.42	1.06	0.83	0.95	1.20	
Males, ages 55-69		1.50	0.95			1.94

[a]Based on changes in food supply 1945-1965 and changes in cancer incidence 1947-50 to 1969-71.

disappearance of dietary cholesterol declined from 610 mg per day to 500 mg (23). These values, along with the change in fat disappearance noted above predict, via the Key's equation (24), a reduction in total blood cholesterol of 9.0 mg/dl between 1945 and 1980 for persons consuming an average U.S. diet. Such a reduction, in turn, would predict a reduction in the vicinity of 10% in coronary heart disease incidence. It may be that advice over past decades to reduce saturated fat and dietary cholesterol for the purpose of reducing heart disease risk has primarily led to a shift in dietary composition, with increased ratios of unsaturated to saturated fat, but without much reduction in total fat. If so, the heart disease benefits achieved may have been at the expense of increasing the risk of certain cancers. This type of thinking argues strongly for a primary emphasis on total fat reduction in a dietary fat intervention trial and in attempts to encourage population changes in dietary habits.

Finally it is of interest to project cancer relative risks, using our international regression analysis of cancer incidence rates on per capita fat disappearance, in randomized trials of cholesterol lowering via diet. Two such trials (25,26) provided enough information on dietary intakes in the intervention and control groups to permit such projects. The Oslo trial (25) involved the 5-year follow-up of 1232 men aged 40–49 years who were at high risk for coronary heart disease and an intervention diet in which saturated and monounsaturated fat were considerably reduced with little change in polyunsaturated fat (Table 3). Average daily consumption of total fat was 39% lower among intervention group men than control group men. Upon rescaling per capita fat disappearance so that the U.S. value agrees with the control group average total fat in this trial, our international regression analyses for men of ages 55–69 project intervention versus control group

Table 3 Projected Cancer Relative Risks in Trials of Cholesterol Lowering via Diet

	Dietary factors[a]				Projected cancer relative risks (I VS C)			Observed cancer relative risks (total)
	Total fat (g)	S	P	M	Colon	Rectum	Prostate	
Oslo Study (25)								
Intervention	69.7	20.5	20.7	28.5	0.46	0.70	0.25	5/8 = 0.625
Control	114.2	47.4	18.4	48.4				(cancer deaths)
VA Domiciliary Study (26)[b]								
Intervention	107.9	32.6	42.6	32.6	0.97	1.09	3.11	57/35 = 1.63
Control	111.2	50.1	11.1	50.1				

[a]S, P, and M denote daily grams of saturated, polyunsaturated, and monounsaturated fat.
[b]Average grams of saturated and monounsaturated fat assumed to be equal.

relative risk estimates of 0.46, 0.70, and 0.25 for colon, rectum, and prostate cancer, respectively. The intervention in this trial also involved cigarette smoking cessation efforts, but such efforts are unlikely to effect the incidence rates for the three cancers listed. Five cancer deaths were observed (25) among intervention men as compared to eight among control men. Cancer incidence data were not provided.

The dietary intervention in the Veterans' Administration Domiciliary Study (26) of 846 men of average age in the mid-60s was similar to the Oslo study in giving rise to a major increase in the ratio of polyunsaturated to saturated fat intake, but different in having very little effect on average fat intake. Intervention activities in both trials give rise to marked reductions in blood cholesterol by about 13% on average. However, the implications for cancer risk are quite different. As shown in Table 3, upon assuming average consumptions of saturated and monounsaturated fat to be equal and rescaling the per capita disappearance of total fat so that the U.S. value agrees with the control group average (26), one obtains projected relative risks from the international regression analyses of 0.97 for colon cancer, 1.08 for rectal cancer, and 3.11 for prostatic cancer. These projections appear to be consistent with the observed total (excluding skin) cancer relative risk of 1.63, based on 57 intervention group cancers and 35 control group cancers during the 8-year intervention phase of this pure dietary intervention trial. Hence patterns of cancer occurrence in these dietary cholesterol lowering trials, which have been regarded by some as anomalous (e.g., 27), may be partially explainable on the basis of patterns of fat consumption.

Conceptually, migrant studies have considerable potential to provide information on the time period between dietary change and change in cancer risk. However, few studies are in possession of data that allow disease rates to be calculated as a function of time since migration, and most studies have little information on the dietary and lifestyle habits of the migrants themselves. As an exception the mortality experience of various migrant groups to Australia has been examined as a function of time from migration (28), and the dietary habits of some such migrant groups have been studied (29). For example, Italian migrants to Australia have been shown to adopt high fat eating patterns and to have age-adjusted breast cancer mortality rates that are 43, 60, and 105% of Australian rates among women who are 0–6, 7–18, and 18+ years from migration, respectively, based on a dataset including 149 breast cancer deaths among women of ages 40 or older. Upon allowance for a period of time until dietary acculturation and a lag between incidence and mortality rate changes, these data seem consistent with the notion that cancer risk may be primarily influenced by dietary and other lifestyle factors over the preceding decade. It would be valuable to have additional study of such topics, including a study of migrants from countries with a high fat consumption to countries with low fat dietary patterns.

Other Studies

There has been substantial experimental study of dietary factors and carcinogenesis. Rodent mammary carcinogenesis experiments were initially interpreted as indicating calorie intake to be important with little or no specific effect of fat (e.g., 30). A recent careful meta-analysis (31), however, shows fat reduction to have an important specific effect in reducing mammary cancer incidence, beyond the well-established risk reduction due to calorie restriction. Risk reduction by type of fat was not examined in these overviews. Similarly a recent meta-analysis of rat colon carcinogenesis (32) suggests that both saturated fat and polyunsaturated fat relate to risk, though results were somewhat inconsistent between Sprague-Dawley and Fischer rats. (See Ref. 20 for a review of the experimental evidence in the nutritional prevention of cancer.)

A number of lines of evidence strongly suggest that hormonal factors are important in determining the risk of various human neoplasms. For example, breast cancer risk has been shown to depend on the timing of major hormone-dependent events in a woman's life, estrogen-blocking agents such as tamoxifen have an important place in breast cancer treatment, and there is supportive data from animal studies. The use of sequential and combined oral contraceptives have been shown to effect the rates of cancers of the endometrium and ovary as well as cancers of certain other sites (see Ref. 33 for review). It is then of particular interest to note that plasma estradiol concentrations among postmenopausal intervention women not taking exogenous estrogens were found in the Women's Health Trial (34) to drop by an average of 17% ($p < 0.001$) within a few weeks after undertaking a low fat diet. A reduction by this amount appears to provide an explanation for a major component of the international variation in breast cancer rates

(34) and may be important for certain other cancers. Similarly, Boyar et al. (35) reported a significant reduction in total estradiol at 5–6 months after beginning a low fat diet intervention among postmenopausal women with Stage II breast cancer, while Rose et al. (36) report reduction in estradiol and other hormone concentrations after 3 months of a low fat diet intervention among premenopausal women with cystic breast disease. These studies add to the biological plausibility of the hypotheses that dietary fat reduction can reduce the risk of such diseases as breast, ovary and endometrium cancers. To the extent that fat consumption may increase pertinent hormone concentrations by interfering with the binding of gonadal steroids to serum binding proteins, polyunsaturated fats and short-chain saturated fats may be specifically implicated (37).

Firmness of the Evidence

In spite of evidence from a wide variety of sources supporting the hypothesis that dietary fat reduction can reduce the risk of prominent cancers, there is no denying that such hypotheses are by no means proven. In fact, prominent nutritional epidemiologists have recently assessed the epidemiologic data in support of an association between dietary fat and breast and colon cancers as unpromising (38) and inconsistent (39), respectively. The discussions (11,40–42) following our review (8) of the epidemiologic data on dietary fat and selected cancers illustrates some reasons for varied attitudes to these hypotheses. Moreover, it seems unlikely that any of the data sources or study types discussed above can yield definitive and reliable tests of these hypotheses. Because of limited exposure heterogeneity in populations available for study and the potentially dominating influences of random measurement error, it is unclear whether analytic epidemiologic study methods, so successful for the study of the disease consequences of many other exposures, can yield reliable tests of association between fat consumption and the risk of specific cancers. Certainly such methods are unlikely to ever provide tests of cancer prevention hypotheses associated with fat reduction during, for example, the middle decades of life. Such hypotheses have major public health potential and most likely can only be reliably tested by means of a randomized clinical trial. The next section discusses aspects of the feasibility of such a trial.

TRIAL FEASIBILITY

Dietary Change

The impact of trial activities on dietary behavior in the Women's Health Trial Vanguard Study has recently been reported in considerably detail (1,2). Briefly, this study involved the randomization of 303 women in the age range 45–69 who were at increased breast cancer risk, to either an intensive dietary intervention

(60%) or control (40%). Intervention women were organized into small groups with an average of eight members. Each group met with a particular nutritionist for eight weekly sessions, four bimonthly sessions, and subsequent monthly sessions. The nutritionist served as educator, facilitator, and dietary counselor. Nutritional and behavioral sciences knowledge and skills were integrated throughout the intervention modules. Each study subject developed an individualized and flexible plan to achieve dietary goals (20% of calories from fat). Fat-reduction strategies involved food selection, food preparation, and portion size selection.

Based on 4-day food records, average daily grams of fat among intervention women were 75.8 at baseline vs. 30.7 at 6 months, 31.3 at 12 months, and 34.1 at 24 months from randomization. As a percent of calories intervention women averaged 39.1, 20.9, 21.6, and 22.6 at baseline, 6, 12, and 24 months from randomization. In comparison, daily grams of fat in the control group averaged 74.5, 66.7, 66.2, and 66.8 at baseline, 6, 12, and 24 months, and percent calories from fat averaged 38.9, 38.1, 37.3, and 36.8. The ratios of polyunsaturated and monounsaturated fat to saturated fat differed little between intervention and control subjects. Average intakes of other nutrients examined were fairly similar between intervention and control subjects (1), with the exception of dietary cholesterol, which was nearly 50% lower for intervention as compared to control women, and carbohydrate intake, which was somewhat higher for intervention than for control women.

Evidence in support of the food record information includes the reasonable nature of the reported nutrient changes within food groups among intervention women and agreement between observed and expected intervention minus control group difference in average plasma total cholesterol (2). Specifically, at 12 months from randomization the observed plasma cholesterol difference was 13.1 + 4.6 mg/dl as compared to an expected 15.1 + 1.1 mg/dl based on the Key's equation (24). At 24 months the observed difference was 15.5 + 4.3 mg/dl as compared to an expected difference of 12.0 + 1.2 mg/dl. The agreement between the reported caloric intake and study subject weight is more difficult to assess. With due allowance for the time course to the achievement of dietary goals (1), the average 3.2 kg of weight loss experienced by intervention women 6 months from randomization is consistent with expectation, whereas no suitable model for predicting longer-term weight loss seems to be available, especially in view of the frequent use of prescription medicines (2) that have weight-altering capabilities in both intervention and control groups. In the absence of such a model, one cannot rule out the possibility that the food records present more accurate data for percent calories from fat, as used in the Key's equation, than for absolute fat. Food record percent calories from fat averages for the intervention group were about 2% lower than corresponding food frequency estimates, using the instrument of Block and colleagues (43). This difference is most likely attributable to the inability of an instrument of the frequency type to fully capture a woman's low fat eating pattern, for example, in respect to portion sizes, but differential dietary composition on the days of food recording could also contribute. In summary, however, the WHT Vanguard Study demonstrates that women assigned to dietary intervention can make substantial dietary changes and maintain these changes at least over a 2-year period, hence supporting the feasibility of a full-scale intervention trial.

As mentioned in the introduction, an additional 1761 women were randomized to either a streamlined dietary intervention (40%) or to control (60%) while the advisability of proceeding with the WHT was under discussion. These women achieved equally good dietary intervention results. For example, the 73 postmenopausal women not taking exogenous estrogens who participated in the study of plasma hormone changes mentioned above (34) experienced an average 12 mg/dl reduction in total plasma cholesterol ($p < 0.001$) and an average weight loss of 3.4 kg ($p < 0.001$) following 10–22 weeks of participation in a low fat diet intervention. Moreover, the plasma cholesterol reduction evidently pertained primarily to low density lipoprotein cholesterol as the concentration of high density lipoprotein cholesterol was not significantly altered by intervention activities.

Study Recruitment

The experience of the three clinical units active in WHT feasibility studies (Cincinnati, Houston, and Seattle) allowed valuable information to be assembled regarding study subject recruitment strategies and expectations. Women were recruited from a variety of sources including a health maintenance organization, an earlier breast cancer detection and demonstration clinic roster, mammographic screening units, medical insurance subscriber lists, and general population mailing lists. The experience with broadly based lists indicated that about 3% of age-eligible women could be expected to meet additional eligibility and exclusionary criteria and to agree to participate in a rigorous long-term trial. This meant that a clinic in a city of about 1 million persons could be expected to randomize about 2000 women over a 2.5-year period without undue logistical difficulties, even if the actual recruitment rate turned out to be 2% rather than 3%. Even with a key dependence on clinic microcomputers for eligibility determination, projected recruitment costs in a full-scale trial are substantial and may affect protocol decisions, for example, concerning eligibility criteria. Cost considerations will be discussed further below.

ASPECTS OF TRIAL DESIGN

Design Assumptions and Power Calculations

This section discusses design exercises conducted for the DIET FIT trial proposal, which, as mentioned above, received favorable peer review but was not funded. It is now anticipated that the NCI, in collaboration with the NHLBI, will initiate within the upcoming months a dietary intervention trial under the name Women's Health Trial. The design of this WHT is likely to be similar to the DIET FIT design discussed here.

For reasons elaborated below, the DIET FIT proposal called for the randomization of 24,000 women in the age range 55–69, approximately 2000 at each of 12 specified clinical units. Study subjects were to meet a simple eligibility criterion in addition to age—namely, that their food frequency percent calories from fat exceed the population median of 38%—and to satisfy a short list of exclusionary criterion that were intended to exclude women for whom a special diet is indicated or who may be unwilling or unable to meet protocol requirements. Study subjects were to be enrolled over a 2.5-year period and to have an average follow-up of 10 years. The primary cancer endpoint was defined to be the occurrence of breast, colon, rectum, ovary, and endometrium cancer, with specific cancers serving as secondary endpoints. Other primary endpoints consisted of coronary heart disease incidence, defined as nonfatal myocardial infarction or CHD death, and total mortality, a key consideration for the evaluation of any primary prevention maneuver.

One set of design exercises was cast in terms of absolute fat intakes. As noted above, intervention group women in the WHT Vanguard Study reported an average 60% reduction in daily grams of fat by 6 months from randomization. The regression analysis of international variations in cancer rates were then used to specify a full compliance relative risk estimate of 0.5 for the combined cancer primary endpoint, with full compliance defined as a 60% reduction in daily grams of fat. In fact, the international regression analyses described above predict a full compliance relative risk of about 0.25 for this combined cancer endpoint, so that our design assumption makes a provision for possible confounding in the international data and for the possibility that more than 10 years may be required for the hypothesized risk reduction to be complete. It is worth noting that this provision, though seemingly modest, affects trial sample size by a factor of about four. The basic relative risk assumption is completed by assuming the relative risk for a fully compliant intervention woman, versus a control woman who does not change diet, to drop linearly from unity at baseline to 0.5 at 10 years from randomization, without change thereafter. Relative risk assumptions of the same form were also assumed for the specific cancers in the combined cancer endpoint, which together constitute about 54% of total cancer incidence in the age range in question. The 10-year full compliance relative risk assumptions for breast, colon, rectum, ovary, and endometrium cancer were 0.45, 0.52, 0.67, 0.53, and 0.45, respectively. In relation to the relative risks for dietary fat listed earlier, the colon cancer assumption made a specific provision for possible confounding of the dietary fat relative risk estimate by protein intake.

Age-specific cancer incidence rates for women with the average daily fat consumption reported at baseline in the WHT Vanguard Study were assumed equal to SEER rates for white females in 1978–81 with the exception of endometrial cancer where a downward adjustment was made to accommodate an elevated hysterectomy rate in the study population. The assumed rates are listed in Table 4.

Average daily grams of fat in the intervention group was assumed to adhere to the WHT Vanguard Study experience described above up to 24 months from randomization, and to drift up linearly to 40 grams per day at 10 years from randomization. Similarly, average daily grams of fat in the control group was assumed to agree with Vanguard Study results up to 24 months and to drift downward to 60.5 grams per day at 10 years from randomization. Overall these assumptions allow over 50% of the well-documented early intervention versus control group difference in daily grams of fat to dissipate over the follow-up course of the trial.

Competing risk mortality rates were taken to be equal to the age-specific mortality rates for U.S. white women in 1978–81 multiplied by two thirds to allow for a healthy volunteer effect. Study subject accrual was assumed to be uniform over a 2.5-year follow-up period.

These assumptions were then combined using a model in which cancer risk depends linearly on integrated grams of fat over the preceding decade, in a manner completely analogous to that detailed in Ref. 13, in order to calculate cumulative cancer incidence probabilities for the intervention and control groups over the trial follow-up period. As shown in Table 5, one obtains a projected probability of 4.77% for the combined cancer endpoint in the intervention group versus a projected probability of 5.83% in the control group. Hence the projected ratio of incidence of the combined cancer endpoint in the intervention versus the control group is 0.82. The corresponding statistical power for a two-sided 5% test of hypothesis, based on the distribution of the odds ratios (proportion test),

Table 4 Age-Specific Cancer Incidence Rates ($\times 10^5$)

Endpoint	55–59	60–64	65–69	70–74	75–79	80–84	85+
Cancer incidence[a]							
Breast	216.8	265.9	301.5	326.4	344.4	343.2	384.1
Colon	54.0	89.4	132.7	194.1	259.9	334.5	367.9
Rectum	25.2	39.4	49.9	70.0	88.1	97.0	110.4
Ovary	36.8	44.8	48.4	49.3	56.6	48.5	43.0
Endometrium[b]	71.0	102.3	97.2	88.7	81.3	64.9	50.2
CHD incidence[c]	300.0	550.0	1000.0	1775.0	3050.0	3050.0[d]	3050.0[d]
Total mortality[e]	716.5	1143.4	1628.2	2612.5	4564.3	7606.7	14079.0

[a]White females 1978–81, from SEER Cancer Institute and Mortality in the USA, 1973–81.
[b]Population rates reduced by 15% to adjust for increased prevalence of hysterectomy in study population.
[c]CHD mortality rates in white U.S. women during 1984 divided by 0.4.
[d]Data extrapolated from age group 75–79.

Table 5 Projected Disease Probabilities and Estimated Power for Various Endpoints

		Event probability			Estimated power (%)	
Endpoint	Full compliance[a] relative risk	Intervention P_i (×100)	Control P_c (×100)	P_i/P_c	Proportions test	Weighted log-rank
Combined cancer occurrence (breast, colon, rectum, ovary, endometrium)	0.50	4.77	5.83	0.82	94	98
Cancer incidence						
Breast	0.49	2.31	2.82	0.82	68	79
Colorectal	0.55	1.43	1.73	0.83	44	50
Ovary/endometrium	0.47	1.13	1.39	0.82	40	47
CHD incidence[b]	0.80	5.92	6.66	0.89	63	66
	0.75	5.70	6.62	0.86	82	86
	0.70	5.47	6.58	0.83	94	96
Total mortality[b]	0.85	10.62	11.27	0.94	35	40
	0.825	10.49	11.26	0.93	46	51
	0.80	10.38	11.24	0.92	56	61
	0.75	10.13	11.22	0.90	76	81

[a]Tabled relative risk is relative risk assumed to be achieved after 10 years of perfect compliance to the low-fat diet for cancer and total mortality endpoints. For CHD endpoint, the tabled relative risk is assumed to be achieved after 5 years of perfect compliance.
[b]Event rate used is 2/3 times the rate in Table 2 to accommodate a healthy volunteer effect.

then gives a power of 94% for rejecting the null hypothesis for the combined cancer endpoint. Table 5 also lists the trial power of 98% for the null hypothesis, under the same design assumptions, but using the weighted logrank statistic that was proposed for trial evaluation. The weights in this statistic are simply time from randomization. Table 5 also lists projected disease incidence rates and power for breast, colorectal, and ovary/endometrium cancer. The desire to have a projected power in the vicinity of 80% for breast cancer alone was one of the considerations in proposing a sample size of 24,000.

The coronary heart disease incidence rates listed in Table 4 were obtained by dividing CHD mortality rates in 1984 by 0.4 and multiplying the resulting rate by two thirds to acknowledge a healthy volunteer effect. The total mortality rates were likewise national rates for white women (44) multiplied by two thirds. Table 5 lists three possible full compliance relative risk assumptions for CHD incidence, which was assumed to be realizable by 5, rather than 10, years from randomization. For example, the average total plasma cholesterol intervention group of 210.0 as compared to 225.2 in the control group at 2 years from randomization in the WHT Vanguard Study (2), if applied to the CHD mortality experience of 356,222 MRFIT screenees (45), would predict a intervention versus control relative risk of about 0.82. Upon acknowledging for some lack of compliance to intervention and control group drift, and upon noting that the slope of the MRFIT screenees risk function is likely to be attenuated by a factor of about two thirds owing to the random measurement error in a single blood cholesterol measurement, one could hypothesize a CHD full compliance relative risk of 0.70, leading under the other assumptions listed to projected powers for CHD incidence of 94% and 96% for the odds ratio and weighted logrank statistics, respectively. On the other hand, a rule of thumb in cholesterol-lowering trials is that the approximate 6% intervention versus control group difference on bood cholesterol observed in the WHT Vanguard study would imply an approximate 12% difference in CHD incidence. The average follow-up periods in key cholesterol-lowering trials (e.g., 46) have been in the 7-year range, so that under our hypothesized CHD relative risk form, in conjunction with the above rule of thumb, one might predict an intervention versus control group difference in CHD incidence of about 14%, with corresponding projected power of 82% and 86% for the two test statistics previously described. Even these power figures may be optimistic if the baseline CHD incidence rates have been overestimated, or if exclusionary criteria beyond the simple ones included in the DIET FIT proposal are implemented.

Finally, Table 5 indicates that the proposed trial has a power of about 80% for detecting a 10% intervention versus control group difference in total mortality rate. However, the mortality rates listed in Table 4 may be too high if stringent exclusionary criteria are imposed, since an adjustment factor less than our assumed two thirds would be required to acknowledge the good health of trial enrollees.

It is worth commenting that the power calculations given in Table 5 can be equally well justified if the basic relative risk assumption and the compliance assumptions are expressed in terms of percent calories from fat rather than grams of fat, as was done in our initial WHT design proposal (33). In fact, for the breast cancer endpoint the DIET FIT design preserves the 80% power projected in Ref. 3 while reducing the sample size from 32,000 to 24,000 by replacing a breast cancer risk factor eligibility criteria by a narrowing of the age range from 45–69 to 55–69 and by extending the average follow-up period from 8.5 to 10 years. These changes had a beneficial effect on the power for each of the other trial endpoints discussed above, while allowing trial cost to be reduced by nearly 25%.

Cost Containment

Detailed projections of trial costs played a key role in protocol decisions and design choices in formulating the DIET FIT proposal. As detailed in Urban et al. (47), the staff time requirements associated with each trial phase (e.g., recruitment, dietary intervention, data collection) were carefully estimated from WHT feasibility study experience and were used to develop clinic staffing requirements and clinic variable costs. Fixed costs associated with clinic activities were also estimated, as were the fixed and variable costs associated with coordinating activities. These basic data were then used to project total trial direct costs while varying such design choices as eligibility criteria, duration of follow-up, randomization fraction, and number of clinics, and varying other such protocol choices as sampling fractions for the collection, coding and analysis of food records and for the analysis of stored blood samples. Design choices thought to merit specific evaluation varied by as much as 50% in projected direct costs, with that outlined above having the minimum projected total direct cost of $72 million, corresponding to a total projected cost of about $100 million (1989 dollars). (See Ref. 48 for additional discussion of opportunities for reducing prevention trial costs.)

Ancillary Studies

The availability of a trial cohort for a range of ancillary studies adds to the motivation for embarking on a large and expensive disease prevention trial. Potential ancillary studies associated with the type of low fat intervention trial discussed above include the study of fat reduction in relation to cancer of the colon, rectum, and prostate among the partners of trial enrollees. Preliminary study of spouses of WHT Vanguard women suggested that these men also make a dietary change, with the dietary fat reduction about one-half that of the women. The colon and rectum cancer experience of trial enrollees and their partners may even usefully be jointly analyzed. Another important ancillary study could involve the relationship of fat reduction to blood hormones, and an examination of the extent to which hormonal effects may be able to explain intervention versus control differences in disease rates. The trial cohort would also allow study of additional biomarkers of a low fat diet, which may help to document compliance to a low fat diet or may serve as surrogate endpoints in subsequent dietary intervention trials. A randomized trial would also permit study of the effect of low fat intervention program on other diseases, such as benign tumors or diabetes. Trial enrollees would also constitute a rather unique cohort study with longitudinal dietary information for a range of other diet and cancer topics, for example, concerning vitamins and fiber consumption in relation to selected cancers. Assuming women remained active in the trial following the diagnosis of cancer or CHD, the trial would also allow valuable study of patient survival in relation to previous and current dietary fat consumption.

CONCLUSION

The above presentation indicates that a dietary intervention trial that emphasizes fat reduction is well motivated by a variety of data sources. An extensively field-tested intervention program appears to be able to induce a major dietary change with good maintenance results at least up to 2 years. Trial designs are available that are feasible in terms of study subject recruitment and total trial cost. Trial results should give support for, or modification of, existing dietary guidelines. Furthermore, under the trial design assumption mentioned above and full population penetration of the dietary change in question, total cancer incidence rates would eventually decline by about 25%, coronary heart disease incidence rates would eventually decline by 15–20%, and total mortality rates would also experience major reductions among middle-aged and older women. There are few existing practical maneuvers having as much public health potential. It is encouraging that the NIH evidently intends to embark on this important effort.

ACKNOWLEDGMENTS

This work was supported by grants GM-24472/CA-53996. The author would like to acknowledge the contribution of a number of colleagues in the work described above. Dr. Steven Self played a major role in the DIET FIT design work. Lianne Sheppard contributed actively to the aggregate data studies. Drs. Maureen Henderson, Donovan Thompson, Curt Furburg, and Nicole Urban contributed extensively to the DIET FIT proposal and to its many presentations and discussions. The efforts of a long list of other DIET FIT collaborators are also gratefully acknowledged.

REFERENCES

1. W. Insull, M. M. Henderson, R. L. Prentice, et al., *Arch. Intern. Med., 150*, 421–427 (1990).

2. M. M. Henderson, L. H. Kushi, D. J. Thompson, et al., *Prev. Med., 19*, 115–133 (1990).
3. S. G. Self, R. L. Prentice, D. Iverson, et al., *Controlled Clin. Trials, 9*, 119–136 (1988).
4. Subcommittee for the Women's Health Trial, Bethesda, Maryland, Board of Scientific Counsellors, Division of Cancer Prevention and Control, National Cancer Institute, January 1988.
5. P. Greenwald, *JNCI, 80*, 788–790 (1988).
6. R. L. Prentice, F. Kakar, S. Hursting, et al., *JNCI, 80*, 802–814 (1988).
7. Final report of workshop on Research Strategies for Studying the Health Consequences of Dietary Modification among Women, July 9–10, 1990, Bethesda, Maryland, Presented to the Board of Scientific Counsellors, Division of Cancer Prevention and Control, National Cancer Institute, October 1990.
8. R. L. Prentice and L. Sheppard, *Cancer Causes and Control, 1*, 81–97 (1990).
9. C. Muir, J. Waterhouse, T. Mack, et al. (eds.), *Cancer Incidence in Five Continents V*, IARC, Lyon, 1987.
10. Food and Agriculture Organization of the United Nations, *Food Balance Sheets 1975–77 Average*, FAO, Rome, 1980.
11. R. L. Prentice and L. Sheppard, *Cancer Causes and Control, 2*, 53–58 (1991).
12. Food and Agriculture Organization of the United Nations, *Trade Yearbook 1959*, 13, FAO, Rome, 1960, pp. 173–175; and *Production Yearbook 1959*, 13, FAO, Rome, 1960, pp. 13–15, 135–137.
13. G. R. Howe, T. Hirohota, G. Hislop, et al., *JNCI, 82*, 561–569 (1990).
14. A. B. Miller, A. Kelly, and N. W. Choi, *Am. J. Epidemiol., 107*, 499–509 (1989).
15. W. C. Willett, L. Sampson, M. J. Stampfer, et al., *Am. J. Epidemiol., 122*, 51–65 (1985).
16. W. C. Willett, M. J. Stampfer, G. A. Colditz, et al., *N. Engl. J. Med., 316*, 22–28 (1987).
17. D. Y. Jones, A. Schatzkin, S. B. Green, et al., *JNCI, 79*, 465–471 (1987).
18. G. N. Stemmerman, A. M. Y. Namura, and L. K. Heilbrun, *Cancer Res., 44*, 4633–4637 (1984).
19. W. C. Willett, M. J. Stampfer, G. A. Colditz, et al., (Abstract), *Am. J. Epidemiol., 130*, 820 (1989).
20. P. M. Newberne, T. E. Shrager, and M. W. Conner, in *Nutrition and Cancer Prevention: Investigating the Role of Micronutrients* (T. E. Moon and M. S. Micozzi, eds.), Marcel Dekker, New York, 1989, pp. 33–82.
21. S. Tominaga, *Natl. Cancer Inst. Monogr., 69*, 83–92 (1985).
22. S. S. Devesa, D. T. Silverman, J. L. Young, et al., *JNCI, 79*, 701–770 (1987).
23. United States Department of Agriculture, *Nutrient Content of the U.S. Food Supply*, Hyattsville, Maryland, Human Nutrition Information Service Admin. Report 299-21, 1988, pp. 8–9.
24. A. Keys, *Am. J. Clin. Nutr., 40*, 351–359 (1984).
25. I. Hjermann, I. Holme, K. Velve Byre, et al., *Lancet, ii*, 1303–1310 (1981).
26. M. L. Pearce and S. Dayton, *Lancet, ii*, 464–471 (1971).
27. F. Ederer, P. Leren, O. Turpeinen, et al., *Lancet, ii*, 203–206 (1971).

28. B. K. Armstrong, T. L. Woodings, N. S. Stenhouse, et al., *Mortality from Cancer in Migrants to Australia—1962 to 1971*, The University of Western Australia, Perth, 1983.
29. B. M. Margetts, S. M. Hopkins, C. W. Binns, et al., *Food Nutr.*, *38*, 7–10 (1981).
30. D. Albanes, *Cancer Res.*, *47*, 1987–1992 (1987).
31. L. S. Freedman, C. Clifford, and M. Messina, *Cancer Res.*, *50*,5710–5719 (1990).
32. L. P. Zhao, L. H. Kushi, R. Klein, et al., *Nutr. Cancer*, in press (1990).
33. R. L. Prentice and D. B. Thomas, *Adv. Cancer Res.*, *49*, 285–401 (1987).
34. R. L. Prentice, D. J. Thompson, C. Clifford, et al., *JNCI, 82*, 129–134 (1990).
35. A. P. Boyar, D. P. Rose, J. R. Loughridge, et al., *Nutr. Cancer, 11*, 93–99 (1988).
36. D. P. Rose, A. P. Boyar, C. Cohen, et al., *JNCI, 78*, 623–626 (1987).
37. C. Street, R. J. S. Howell, L. Perry, et al., *Acta Endocrinologia, 120*, 175–179 (1989).
38. W. Willett, *Nutritional Epidemiology*, Oxford University Press, New York, 1990, Chapter 14.
39. L. Kolonel, *Am. J. Clin. Nutr.*, *45*, 336–341 (1987).
40. G. Howe, *Cancer Causes and Control, 1*, 99–100 (1990).
41. J. E. Hiller and A. McMichael, *Cancer Causes and Control, 1*, 101–102 (1990).
42. W. Willett and M. J. Stampfer, *Cancer Causes and Control, 1*, 103–109 (1990).
43. G. Block, A. M. Hartmann, C. M. Dresser, et al., *Am. J. Epidemiol.*, *124*, 453–459 (1986).
44. *Vital Statistics of the United States*, Vol. II—*Mortality*, Part A, National Center for Health Statistics, Hyattsville, Maryland, 1980.
45. J. Stamler, D. Wentworth, J. D. Neaton, et al., *J. Am. Med. Assoc.*, *256*, 2823–2828 (1986).
46. Lipids Research Clinics Prgram, *J. Am. Med. Assoc.*, *251*, 351–374 (1984).
47. N. Urban, S. Self, L. Kessler, et al., *Contr. Clin. Trials, 11*, 129–146 (1990).
48. R. L. Prentice, *Statist. Med.*, *9*, 161–172 (1990).

16

Clinical Trials on Breast Cancer

Richard R. Love
The University of Wisconsin
Madison, Wisconsin

INTRODUCTION

In the United States the incidence of breast cancer has been increasing at rates of 1–2% per year, with apparent recent acceleration of the annual increases (1). Most of the overall increase has been due to age-specific increases in incidence in older women (1). While a fraction of the increased incidence may be due to more widespread screening, some real increases in incidence are generally believed to be occurring. The reasons for these increases are mostly unknown. Dietary patterns, oral contraceptive use, and alcohol consumption are possible factors. Only the changing pattern of child-bearing later in life offers a partial, generally accepted explanation (2). Were the numerically most significant initiating factors (other than unspecified age-related factors) in breast cancer development clearly identified, then removal of these or chemo*prevention* by interference with these might be proposed rationally as breast cancer control strategies. At present, however, both factors important in and interventions to modify promotion are better understood, and thus the possibility of chemo*suppression* of preclinical breast malignancies holds greater immediate promise.

Mortality from breast cancer has changed little over the last three decades. Some favorable impact from increasing use of effective adjuvant therapies is now expected to become evident in population-based data. Detection of breast malignancies, particularly in postmenopausal women, consequent to more widespread use of screening mammography, should also have a measurable and favorable impact on stage at diagnosis and, over time, on mortality rates. Thus, absent any new technological breakthroughs, some future decreases in breast cancer mortality can be expected from technology transfer of current strategies.

Because of the age-specific incidence increases and the aging of the American population, the societal burden of breast cancer is anticipated to increase significantly over the next 20 years (3). Any possibility of altering the level of this burden thus bears serious consideration.

An ideal intervention to prevent the appearance of clinical breast cancer would have three general characteristics:

1. The biological *rationale* for the intervention should be well understood and convincing.
2. The full spectrum of *biologic effects* on all major organ systems should be understood, and these should be found to be nontoxic.
3. The *symptoms effects* of the intervention should be well understood and minimal.

To date, adequate comprehensive data have been developed for only two proposed interventions to justify proposals for clinical trials with primary breast cancer prevention as the major endpoint: dietary fat reduction and hormone replacement therapy (HRT) with the antiestrogen tamoxifen citrate. Other chapters in this volume have developed well the rationale for a dietary fat reduction trial. Thus in this chapter the major focus initially will be biological rationale and biological and symptomatic effects of tamoxifen. Following this detailed discussion, attention will be directed to various logistical issues involved in developing a clinical trial that is feasible and thus likely to test successfully hypotheses about an intervention to prevent clinical breast cancer.

HORMONE REPLACEMENT THERAPY AND BREAST CANCER

Hormone replacement therapy is employed by approximately one-third of American women age 40–79 who have stopped menstruating (4). When first used, estrogen replacement therapy (ERT) was prescribed for relief of estrogen-deficiency conditions of postmenopausal women: vasomotor symptoms such as "hot flashes" and urogenital complaints such as vaginal dryness. More recently, because of suggested favorable effects on rates of coronary heart disease (CHD) (5) and demonstrated benefits in preserving bone mineral density (6), thereby reducing rates of osseous fractures (7), ERT is often prescribed for these reasons, absent significant reported symptoms. The effect of estrogen replacement therapy on risk of breast cancer is unknown. Several epidemiologic studies have failed to demonstrate increased risk to estrogen users, although theoretical considerations and limited data suggest that some modest increased risk is associated with long-term ERT (8). It is generally agreed that ERT is associated with increased risk of uterine endometrial cancer (9). Continuous ERT is associated with the development of endometrial hyperplasia at annual rates of 7–15% (10). U.S. SEER data from 1973–1986 (a period of increased use of ERT) demonstrate no changes in rates of primary hepatocellular carcinoma in older women (11). Cost-effectiveness analyses of ERT, using the preceding general conclusions have suggested significant benefits to populations of women using ERT (12,13). These analyses, however, are based on interpretation of the benefits and risks of ERT from studies which may be biased by self-selection of ERT subjects. The overall health benefits of ERT have not been demonstrated in a randomized clinical trial, although it has been suggested that a breast cancer prevention or a hormone replacement health trial should evaluate ERT (14). Two among several possible logistical considerations suggest that this would be difficult. First, widespread use and prescription of ERT would create a disincentive to participation or would increase the likelihood of other participants "dropping into" the trial by taking ERT. A second more significant barrier is that, in the context of a clinical trial, breast cancer incidence would have to be a major endpoint, and a governing hypothesis would be, based on current data, that ERT did (or did not) *increase* the risk of breast cancer. Designing a trial to disprove an adverse and very serious complication of ERT has limited appeal. In particular, the process of eliciting informed consent from participants in such a clinical trial would be likely to uncover significant reticence among potential participants. A randomized placebo-controlled clinical trial to evaluate biological effects of ERT (and three other estrogen-progestin combinations) is currently (1990) accruing subjects (The Postmenopausal Estrogen/Progestin Intervention (PEPI) Trial).

In this context, hormone replacement treatment with tamoxifen may be a rational, long-term health-preserving alternative to ERT. Because tamoxifen use in healthy women is currently limited, rigorous evaluation of long-term benefits in a clinical trial may actually be feasible. In particular, a tamoxifen health trial may be feasible because no major numerically significant long-term consequences are suspected.

Combination hormone replacement therapy with the addition of progestin to estrogen came into widespread use in the United States in the late 1970s when data on increased incidence of endometrial cancerr in unopposed ERT users emerged (9). While the use of progestin may make the postmenopausal hormonal milieu more physiologic, the benefits and risks of its use have been assessed in only limited ways. Some women with uterus intact find reestablishment of menstrual cycles undesirable. The effects of added progestin on cardiovascular risk factors have not been quantified. These and other effects are the endpoints of the PEPI study. Despite the significant uncertainties about biological and disease effects of combination estrogen/progestin treatment, in the United States in 1985 approximately 2% of women aged 40–79 were taking this therapy (4).

THE BIOLOGICAL RATIONALE FOR A BREAST CANCER PREVENTION TRIAL WITH TAMOXIFEN

Breast Cancer Effects of Tamoxifen

Tamoxifen citrate is a synthetic antiestrogen with antifertility (15) and antitumor (16) properties in laboratory animals. Antiestrogens are effective in controlling some metastatic breast cancers (17), and over the last 20 years tamoxifen has come to play an increasingly useful role in the management of all stages of breast cancer (18,19).

Tamoxifen is believed to act primarily by binding to the estrogen receptor in breast cancer cells (20). This binding appears to prevent estrogen-stimulated cell division and block breast cancer cells at the G1 phase of the cell cycle, possibly modulating stimulatory and inhibitory growth factors (21). In addition a number of non-estrogen receptor–mediated effects have been described that could also modulate breast cancer cell replication (22).

There is persuasive evidence from rodent models that tamoxifen can prevent mammary carcinogenesis (23–26). Long-term tamoxifen therapy appears to be the optimal strategy to prevent the development of tumors after the initiation of carcinogenesis in rat models (27) or to inhibit the growth of human hormone-responsive breast cancer inoculated into immune deficient (athymic) mice (28). However, if therapy is stopped, tumor growth recurs. Tamoxifen appears to act as a tumoristatic agent to suppress the growth of tumor cells (29).

In the treatment of women with primary breast cancer where tamoxifen is employed as adjuvant therapy, when the primary breast tumor exhibits positive levels of estrogen receptor and/or progesterone receptor proteins, benefits in terms of prolongation of the diverse-free survival are usually seen (30). In some studies prolongation of overall survival has been seen, and an overview analysis has concluded that tamoxifen does confer survival benefit in postmenopausal node-positive patients (31). Data from these adjuvant trials indicate that some subjects with estrogen receptor–negative tumors may also benefit from tamoxifen adjuvant therapy (30). Further, there is a suggestion that when the body burden of tumor cells is smallest, the use of tamoxifen results in approximately a halving of the recurrence rates (32). The absence of survival benefits from adjuvant tamoxifen in many individual studies may be because only short-term therapy (1–3 years) was administered (30,31). Based on the animal studies (27) more recent studies are evaluating longer-term or indefinite adjuvant tamoxifen treatment (33–36).

Fifty to 65% of breast cancers in postmenopausal women are estrogen receptor–positive at the time of diagnosis (37). The major tumor-suppressing effect of tamoxifen in rodent cancer model systems compared to its more modest effects in controlling or suppressing established clinical breast cancers in women suggests an hypothesis about the development of breast malignancies. It is possible that breast tumors begin as clones of estrogen receptor–positive cells, which in the course of replication produce estrogen receptor–negative daughter cells. If estrogen is required for these cell divisions, then application of tamoxifen earlier in the natural history of the development of these clones, prior to usual clinical detection, might be expected to have a greater impact on tumor appearance than on the suppression of growth of established clones of estrogen receptor–positive and –negative cells.

Possibly contradicting this hypothesis are limited data showing significant variations in the percentages of estrogen receptor positive straining ductal cells in normal breast tissue (38).

Observations of the rates of second primary breast cancers in adjuvant tamoxifen treatment trials have supported the prediction that tamoxifen can effectively suppress preclinical breast cancer. In four trials the rates of second primary or contralateral breast cancers have been approximately half of those seen in the control or placebo groups (34,39–41). The previous observations suggest that clearly the duration of tamoxifen treatment and the points in time when the comparisons of rates of second breast tumors are made would be expected to influence the results significantly.

The impact of tamoxifen therapy in women with histologic evidence of "premalignancy" (e.g., atypical epithelial hyperplasia) has not been evaluated because of significant logistical barriers.

Overall the laboratory and clinical studies support the hypothesis that continuous treatment with tamoxifen might be expected to suppress preclinical breast cancers in postmenopausal women by up to 50%. In considering how to test this hypothesis, the biological and symptomatic effects of tamoxifen on other tissues and organs in women become critical. The effects of tamoxifen on hormone levels in premenopausal women are less completely understood and possibly unfavorable, and in these women the biological effects and detailed symptomatic effects have received only limited investigation (27). The majority of premenopausal women continue to have menses during tamoxifen therapy. Those with ovulatory cycles are clearly at risk for pregnancy. However, tamoxifen should not be administered during pregnancy to avoid the possibility of teratogenesis (although this effect has not been documented). Thus, the current considerations of a clinical trial concern only postmenopausal women.

In postmenopausal women tamoxifen causes minor increases in circulating estrogens, significant decreases in elevated levels of FSH and LH, no changes in progesterone and prolectin, and significant increases in sex hormone–binding globulin (SHBG) (19,30). With the exception of the increases in SHBG, which may contribute to tamoxifen's therapeutic effect by removing free estrogen from the circulation (42,43), these changes would not be expected to result in any long-term favorable or adverse effects.

Cardiovascular Effects of Tamoxifen

In the United States, mortality from myocardial infarction in women begins to exceed that from breast cancer in the sixth decade of life (i.e., between ages 55 and 60), and thereafter the mortality rates rise very rapidly. Tamoxifen has major effects on established risk factors for coronary heart disease (CHD) and stroke.

Total cholesterol and LDL cholesterol levels in plasma are lowered by tamoxifen treatment. In the Wisconsin Tamoxifen Study, a randomized, placebo-controlled, double-blind toxicity trial, total cholesterol was lowered by 26 mg/dl (12%, $p = 0.0001$) from 216 mg/dl at baseline to 190 mg/dl at 3 months (43). LDL cholesterol was lowered by 20% ($p = 0.0001$) from 138 mg/dl at baseline to 110 mg/dl at follow-up. These changes were sustained through 2 years of treatment without any waning of the effects. Minor increases in triglycerides and decreases in HDL cholesterol were seen, each of borderline or no statistical significance depending on the time point (43). The total cholesterol/LDL cholesterol and the HDL/LDL cholesterol ratios in tamoxifen-treated subjects in this study were statistically improved at all study timepoints.

Small longitudinal studies by Powles (44), Bruning (45), Bertelli (46), Sedlacek (47), Bagdade (48), and Schapira (49) each show similar findings with respect to lowering of LDL and total cholesterol by tamoxifen. No certain picture of tamoxifen's effects on HDL cholesterol has emerged from these studies. There is one case report of an individual who has experienced very high increases in triglycerides with tamoxifen therapy (50).

With tamoxifen treatment, fibrinogen levels were found to decrease from a baseline of 320 mg/dl to 268 mg/dl at 6 months (−52 mg/dl, $p = 0.0003$) in the Wisconsin Tamoxifen Study (51). Powles has also reported data suggesting decreases in fibrinogen levels with tamoxifen treatment (44). In the ongoing PEPI Study, fibrinogen is considered to be a major CHD risk factor and is one of the major study endpoints.

In the Wisconsin Tamoxifen Study, evaluations of systolic and diastolic blood pressure changes over one year showed no differences in the tamoxifen and placebo groups. This study had 95% power to detect an average change of 10 mmHg in stystolic blood pressure, and 90% power to detect a change of 5 mmHg in diastolic blood pressure should such changes have occurred with tamoxifen treatment. Similarly, in the same study, no differences in weight or reported exercise, work activity, or smoking habits developed between the two groups (R. R. Love, L. Cameron, and H. Leventhal, unpublished data). In this study fasting plasma glucose levels were unchanged after 12 months of tamoxifen treatment (R. R. Love and D. A. Wiebe, unpublished data).

Subfraction HDL and apolipoprotein data or changes in waist, hip, and thigh girth or ratios of these with tamoxifen treatment are not available. Each of these has been suggested to be related to CHD incidence.

The impact that these lipid and fibrinogen changes might have on rates of CHD in postmenopausal women is uncertain but likely favorable. Triglyceride levels are not considered to be a major independent risk factor for cardiovascular disease (52,53). Population studies have demonstrated a relationship between fibrinogen levels, myocardial infarction, and stroke, with lower levels associated with lower cardiovascular risk (54). In the Framingham study, coronary heart disease incidence in women was lower with lower fibrinogen levels (55). Extrapolations from nine lipid-lowering trials in men with hypercholesterolemia suggest that lowering of total cholesterol by 12% seen with tamoxifen might be associated with decreases of 20% in CHD incidence, and 20% decreases in LDL seen with tamoxifen might be associated with decreases of 30% in CHD incidence (56). Data in women suggest that a 20% decrease in LDL may result in a 6% decrease in CHD (57). There are data to suggest that greater benefit follows from a fixed percentage lowering of cholesterol when the initial level is high, compared to low (58), and that elevated lipid levels are more important in older than younger individuals (57).

In sum, the directions of changes in total cholesterol, LDL cholesterol, lipoprotein ratios, and fibrinogen all *suggest* a favorable impact on CHD risk with tamoxifen treatment. Any stated level of favorable impact, however, can only be speculation. Further data on tamoxifen's effects on apolipoproteins, total and HDL subfractions, blood pressure, and body girth changes are needed in healthy women to better predict likely effects on CHD rates. Further data on the significance of each of these suggested CHD risk factors in older women are also needed. In some large controlled adjuvant studies such as NSABP B14 (40), follow-up of subjects may allow analyses for cardiovascular disease endpoints. In a preliminary report from one study, the Scottish Trial, among postmenopausal axillary node-negative women there were 18 acute noncancer deaths in 373 control subjects and 5 in 374 long-term tamoxifen recipients (59).

As a companion study integral to the first phases of a tamoxifen trial, further data on the major intermediary factors important in CHD in women should be obtained, specifically on systolic and diastolic blood pressure, HDL cholesterol, fibrinogen, fasting glucose, and insulin. Such data are needed because, as reviewed above, *none* are available in healthy non-breast cancer–afflicted women, and those in disease-free women are limited. Since small changes in these risk factors could have major impact on occurrence of CHD and the frequency of CHD endpoints in a full-scale tamoxifen trial, detailed information on these is critical to a refined design for such a tamoxifen trial.

Bone Effects of Tamoxifen

Skeletal fractures are a major cause of morbidity in postmenopausal women over age 55. As measured by number of hospitalizations, fractures are equivalent to breast cancer, with days per hospitalization threefold those for breast cancer (60).

Animal and in vitro laboratory studies indicate that tamoxifen decreases rates of resorption of trabecular bone, with resultant net preservation of bone density (61–64). In humans, two retrospective studies have suggested no differences in radial and lumbar spine bone density in tamoxifen-treated and untreated women (65,66). Limited prospective studies have suggested increased bone mineral density in two investigations (67,68) and no differences in four others (44,69–71). In the Wisconsin Tamoxifen Study, with only limited incomplete data, a statistically significant preservation of bone density was found in the lumbar spine and a trend to preservation of bone density was found in the radius. In addition, in this study osteocalcin levels at 12 and 24 months fell in the tamoxifen-treated group, and alkaline phosphatase levels fell at 6 months, findings consistent with an estrogenlike, bone density–preserving effect of tamoxifen (R. R. Love, R. Mazess, S. Epstein, and D. Wiebe, unpublished data).

Over time the decreases in trabecular bone loss with tamoxifen strongly suggested by the above data would be expected to be reflected in 25% lower fracture rates in a manner similar to the effects from estrogen (7). Analyses for these possible changes in fracture rates and of effects of tamoxifen on bone density in other bony sites such as the femoral neck are warranted and should be proposed in companion studies and in a full-scale tamoxifen study.

Carcinogenic Effects of Tamoxifen

Carcinogenic effects of long-term tamoxifen therapy on the liver and uterus have been suggested.

Liver Carcinogenicity

Rodent carcinogenicity studies have demonstrated the development of liver tumors in tamoxifen-treated animals at even low doses (72,73). Mutagenicity studies have all been negative (73). Recent rodent studies suggest that tamoxifen is a hepatocellular carcinoma promoter, but has a potency somewhat higher than that of phenobarbital but only 1/100 that of mestranol (74,75). Phenobarbital is not a cause of hepatocellular carcinoma in humans (76). Mestranol has been found to be associated with the development of benign and possibly malignant neoplasms of the liver, both at extremely low rates (77).

The ages and strains of animals used in the reported experiments, the routes and vehicles used in drug administration, and the metabolic and other differences among species make the relevance of these results for humans uncertain. In particular, for example, the half-life of tamoxifen in the rat is 5 hours, whereas it is 5–7 days in the human. In addition, the Pitot data suggest the possibility that the usual human dose is at or below the threshold for promotional effect (74). Animal studies in progress should be helpful in further clarifying this issue.

Despite widespread use of postmenopausal estrogen replacement therapy, SEER data do not show any significant increase in the very low liver neoplasm rates in women over the 1973–1986 period (11). Another analysis of SEER data does not show any changes in rates of second primary liver neoplasms in women with breast cancer given hormonal, presumably often tamoxifen, treatment (R. Curtis, personal communication). These findings for ERT and tamoxifen are in contrast to findngs for oral contraceptives, where small case-control studies have implicated oral contraceptives as a risk factor for cancer (78–80). A recent study of the relationship of development of liver tumors to both oral contraceptive and hepatitis exposures has shown no synergistic effects (81). Reports from several large tamoxifen adjuvant trials have not shown increased numbers of liver neoplasms in treated subjects, but it must be noted the numbers of subjects are small and durations of treatment and follow-up in even these studies are relatively short (82).

In sum, the animal data suggest that like other steroid hormones, tamoxifen is a weak promoter of hepatocellular carcinomas. The limited data in humans suggest that long-term tamoxifen therapy is unlikely to be a cause of liver cancers. Further, because of the extremely low absolute rates of hepatocellular cancer, were a cohort of 8000 women aged 50–69 treated with tamoxifen for 5 years, during which time the relative risk of liver cancer was increased to 10, two to three, instead of less than one case of hepatocellular cancer might be expected. Thus, even in a large prevention study, a major increase in risk of liver cancer with tamoxifen would likely prove difficult to demonstrate. In addition, there are no sensitive and low-cost serologic or radiologic means of monitoring for this possible complication. Serum transaminase and α-fetoprotein levels could be monitored serially, but low "abnormal" cut-off values would require further evaluations of many subjects with hepatic ultrasound. Abnormal ultrasound and/or subsequent scan findings would lead to liver biopsy, with associated morbidity and rare mortality. Because of concerns about this issue, however, some monitoring may be necessary.

Endometrial Carcinogenicity

There are reports that steroid receptor-positive human endometrial carcinomas will grow rapidly in athymic mice during tamoxifen therapy (83). It has been demonstrated that in athymic mice bi-transplanted with human endometrial and breast tumors, tamoxifen will control the growth of the breast tumor but stimulate the growth of endometrial tumor (84,85). Three reports from Sweden have suggested increased rates of endometrial cancer in women treated with tamoxifen. Two of these reports are retrospective epidemiologic studies (86,87), and the third comes from a randomized clinical tiral (41). The clinical trial is remarkable in that the rates of endometrial cancer are very high and the dose of tamoxifen was 40 mg instead of the more commonly used 20-mg daily dose (41). In contrast, increases in endometrial cancer have not been seen in several other adjuvant trials (82). If it does prove to be the case that tamoxifen is carcinogenic to the uterine endometrium, there is every reason to assume that, as in the case of estrogen-induced uterine endometrial neoplasms, the canceers will be superficial, detected early, and have very high cure rates. In addition, it should be noted that for up to possibly 40% of tamoxifen recipients the concern is irrelevant, as this the approximate prevalence of hysterectomy in some postmenopausal populations. In sum, if uterine endometrial cancer is a complication of long-term tamoxifen therapy, it is likely to be rare, less frequent than for estrogen replacement therapy alone, and highly curable. To minimize risk of this possible complication in a tamoxifen prevention study, only subjects with a normal gynecologic evaluation should be eligible, and subjects should be examined annually and questioned repeatedly about the cardinal sign of endometrial malignancy—vaginal bleeding.

Ovarian Cancer

In a summary of types of second primary cancers occurring in adjuvant trials, ovarian cancers appeared to be *less* frequent with tamoxifen treatment (12 cases in controls, 6 in tamoxifen recipients) (82).

Other Biological Effects of Tamoxifen

Other serious biological side effects of tamoxifen treatment have been suggested, but are of such low frequencies, or occur on background rates in normal individuals, such as to preclude conclusions about their causative relationships to tamoxifen treatment.

Thrombophlebitis

Thrombophlebitis *may* occur at an excess rate of 1/800 women-years over control or placebo rates (40). Whether this postulated complication occurs more frequently in individuals with a previous history of this condition, or other risk factors is unknown. Investigations of antithrombin III levels have shown some depression of this protein (88), but in the Wisconsin Tamoxifen Study, no single subject had a level fall to a clinically significant level (51). Platelet levels fall 7–9% with tamoxifen treatment; again in the Wisconsin study no single subject of 70 had depression of the count to below 145,000/mm^3 (51). The effects of tamoxifen in lowering fibrinogen, antithrombin III, and possibly thrombopoetin all appear to be effects in liver synthesis of these proteins.

To minimize the postulated increase risk of thrombophlebitis from tamoxifen, women with a history of this condition should not be eligible for a tamoxifen prevention study.

Eye Changes

There are reports of ophthalmologic changes with high dose (89) and occasionally usual dose tamoxifen treatment (90). With usual dose treatment it is unclear whether the tamoxifen can be implicated because of the frequency of corneal and lens changes seen in aging women (91). Animal toxicity studies have shown increased cataract formation with tamoxifen (73), and other cationic amphophilic compounds like tamoxifen have been implicated in cataract formation. Because a controlled study (91) has not been able to demonstrate any ocular changes following tamoxifen treatment in usual doses, in a prevention study subjects should be carefully questioned about the development of eye disease only, and these responses should be carefully monitored.

Other Changes

Long-term estrogen treatment may be associated with decreased bile secretion and increased biliary tract disease from gallstone formation (92). The estrogenic effects of tamoxifen on lipids and lipoproteins suggest that it might also have a similar effect on secretion of bile and gallstone formation. The occurrence of biliary tract disease should be monitored in a tamoxifen trial.

Symptomatic Effects of Tamoxifen

Major symptomatic effects from tamoxifen treatment are of four types: vasomotor symptoms, gynecologic symptoms, depression, and nausea. While tamoxifen is very acceptable therapy for women in adjuvant studies where approximately only 4% drop out because of side effects (30,93), the seriousness of the side effects and the morbidity would warrant particular attention in a study of healthy women.

Depression, which can be very serious and insidious in onset, occurs in 1% or more of treated postmenopausal women (93). It is possible that a previous history of postpartum or postmenopausal depression predicts for this complication.

Nausea is said to be an occasional complication of treatment. However, in the Wisconsin Tamoxifen Study no single treated subject complained of nausea, and self-reported scores for upset stomach were identical in placebo and tamoxifen-trerated women (94). Powles has also found no significant nausea associated with tamoxifen therapy (41).

Vasomotor symptoms—hot flashes, flushed face, episodes of sweaty palms, and racing heart—are increased in frequency and severity in postmenopausal women treated with tamoxifen. After 6 months of treatment, an additional 17% of tamoxifen-treated subjects over placebo reported moderate or greater hot flashes in the Wisconin Tamoxifen Study (94). Treatment for these symptoms is currently limited.

Gynecologic symptoms of increased vaginal discharge, vaginal-external genitalia irritation, or vaginal bleeding complicate tamoxifen therapy. Approximately 4%

of postmenopausal women will complain of moderate or greater such symptoms after 6 months of treatment (94). Evaluation and treatment algorithms have received limited attention.

Because estrogens favorably effect pelvic muscle and urinary sphincter tone, tamoxifen's effects on these tissues warrant attention. An adverse effect might lead to increased risks of urinary tract infection or incontinence.

On careful questioning, 35–48% of treated postmenopausal subjects will consistently complain of moderate or greater symptomatic side effects over the first several months of tamoxifen therapy (94). Treated women with these symptoms develop heightened anxiety about trial participation and increased worry about cancer (94). Long-term compliance with treatment might be expected to be compromised in the presence of these side effects. Because greater symptomatology may accompany treatment in women who are in the years immediately following menopause, it is reasonable to select for a clinical trial women who are remote from menopause. Because of these symptomatic effects of tamoxifen, which in some circumstances may have major adverse consequences on quality of life, limited but careful monitoring of these should take place in a tamoxifen prevention study and clinical study staff vigilance should be stressed to seek out and assist in limiting these effects.

Tamoxifen: Dose Effects

Adjuvant studies with tamoxifen have used doses of 20 mg (usually 10 mg b.i.d.), 30 mg, and 40 mg daily without evidence of greater efficacy for recurrence of breast cancer at any of these doses (30,31). Whether a 10-mg dose would be equally effective as a breast cancer adjuvant treatment or chemosuppressive agent is not known and can only be determined by means of large clinical trials. In addition, the current data concerning cardiovascular intermediary effects and bone-preserving effects of tamoxifen are for the 20-mg dose of tamoxifen. Concerns that the 20-mg dose exceeds the threshold for promotion of hepatocellular carcinomas and that a lower dose might be associated with fewer and less intense symptomatic side effects, which in turn might further compromise compliance, prompt consideration of evaluation of a lower dose. It would seem that a 20-mg daily dose would be reasonable.

MAJOR ISSUES IN BREAST CANCER PREVENTION CLINIC TRIAL DESIGN

Several issues deserve particular attention in breast cancer prevention trials; these will be considered here in the context of considering a tamoxifen prevention trial in postmenopausal women.

Population

Several issues are worthy of consideration in the choice of a study population for a prevention trial: the specific biologic question or questions to be addressed and the generalizability of the results, the event rate(s) in the populations, the total pool of potential study volunteers, the size of study needed to answer the critical question(s), the feasibility of the entire study, and the total costs—considering all resources needed. The ethical concerns about safety for subject volunteers would apply equally to any population. Two general *post*menopausal populations should be considered for study:

1. Women 50–69 at increased risk because of (a) a family history of breast cancer in at least one first-degree relative (95–105), (b) two or more surgical breast biopsies (105); (c) nulliparity or age 30 or greater at first full-term pregnancy (106).
2. "Normal" risk healthy women aged 55–69.

Unfortunately, the relative risk of breast cancer in these increased risk populations averages 2 or less (95–108). The population of women with higher relative risks for breast cancer, which are well agreed on, are small and/or complex and costly to identify.

Critical considerations pertaining to these populations are the following:

Generalization

A successful study with one or both populations will be generalizable to large segments of the American population of postmenopausal women.

Event Rates

The incidence of breast cancer in these populations is predictable and will depend on the specific mixture of age and risk factors in actual volunteering study subjects. First, specifically, the newest SEER data on incidence of breast cancer (11), combined with projected incidence increases through the coming years can be used to estimate a possible breast cancer incidence figure (see below). Second, published data on the relative risks associated with each of the specific named "increased risk" factors, as well as data on incidence of breast cancer in multiple risk factor subjects from BCDDP (105), can be used to estimate breast cancer incidence in high risk women. While practically all of these data are for white populations, it is reasonable to assume that most risk factors apply to black and other minority populations.

Finally, the actual risk factor profile of volunteering subjects (age, risk factors) can be combined with the frequently observed "healthy volunteer" effect (which results in an actual event rate of 0.75 compared to predicted in similar studies) to predict a likely breast cancer incidence in a full scale trial. Table 1

Table 1 Projected Breast Cancer Incidence in Breast Cancer Prevention Study Populations

	Age-specific incidence/1000		Estimated incidence/1000 in increased risk group[c]
	1982–1986[a]	1991[b]	
50–54	2.0	2.3	4.1
55–59	2.5	2.9	5.0
60–64	3.1	3.5	6.3
65–69	3.5	4.0	7.2
Average rate[d]		3.5	5.7
"Healthy" volunteer rate[e]		2.6	4.3

[a]From Ref. 11.
[b]Projected figures, based on 15% increase.
[c]Three increased risk groups: (1) Family history in a first degree relative; estimated relative risk (ERR) 2.1(95–105), e.g., in BCDDP 2.1 (100). (2) Two or more surgical breast biopsies; estimated relative risk 1.6 (105) (−BCDDP). (3) Nulliparity or ≥30 at first pregnancy; estimated relative risk 1.5-(nulliparity (105); 1.9 (≥30) (105). Nulliparous women outnumber ≥30 in ratio 2:1 (107). Based on these data and on availability of women in each of these groups, an ERR of 1.8 is assigned to the increased risk group.
[d]For increased risk group aged 50–69; for normal risk group aged 55–69.
[e]Estimated for prevention studies to be 0.75 of "predicted" rate.

shows projected actual breast cancer incidence rates in two large postmenopausal female populations.

In BCDDP, after screening out prevalent cancers, the actual rates of breast cancer did remain elevated in high risk subjects (1056) although the magnitude of risk is small. In the large Canadian National Breast Cancer Screening Study, however, in the same circumstances, the rates of breast cancer in high risk women were only slightly higher than in those women at "normal risk" (A. B. Miller, personal communication).

Total Pool of Populations

In 1990, the total population of women aged 50–69 in the United States was about 23 million (108), and by 1995 this figure is projected to be 24 million; in 1990 the pool 55–69 is *16* million. Based on published case-control studies of breast cancer risk factors, the population prevalence of having a first-degree relative with breast cancer is 7.8% (109). Thus an estimated 1.8 million women aged 50–69 will have a family history of breast cancer, mostly sisters. Almost 20% of women 60 years of age have undergone surgical (not needle aspiration) breast biopsy (109). In BCDDP, of women who underwent biopsies, one fourth to one third had two or more biopsies (105). Thus 5–7% of all women in a postmenopausal study's age group may have had two or more biopsies at maximum, or 1.15–1.61 million women. Twelve percent of women 55–64 years of age were reported in the NHIS-CEC health survey in 1987 to have no full-term pregnancies; an additional 6.3% underwent first full-term pregnancy at 30 or more years (4). These data suggest that 4.14 million American women fall into this risk category.

Thus the total U.S. pool of 50–69-year-old women at increased risk for breast cancer because of a family history, two or more breast biopsies, or nulliparity or age at first birth ≥30 appears at maximum to be 7.3 million (1.8 + 1.4 + 4.14) (obviously some women may be in more than one of these groups and thus the actual figure must be lower).

Feasibility of Acquiring Adequate Numbers of Subjects in These Populations

If the actual total pool of increased risk women is 7.3 million, and the full-scale breast cancer prevention study size required 16,000 *total* subjects (this depends on a number of statistical considerations), then one in every 456 women in the United States would need to be entered on a high risk only woman study. Geographic dispersion, interest, and eligibility restrictions combined with other logistical considerations suggest that these numbers would present a major barrier to complete accrual.

That these population estimates accurately reflect what is feasible at the regional investigator level is supported by experience in the feasibility of the Women's Health Trial (WHT). In brief, complete accrual of very high risk women (basically women with two of the three named risk factors listed above) in the WHT at Seattle was only achieved with great difficulty and was not achieved at all in two other centers. These accrual difficulties led to a decision in the later feasibility phases of the study to target an increased risk women population like that suggested above. Subsequently, given multiple endpoints (other cancers besides breast, and CHD endpoints), the much discussed low fat diet trial population is now suggested to be older women *without* any breast cancer risk factors.

In addition, an analysis of Puget Sound SEER tumor registry data determined that sisters of women with breast cancer were geographically dispersed and hard to contact (E. White, personal communication).

In Pittsburgh, for a study of hormones and risk factors for breast cancer, sisters of postmenopausal breast cancer cases were sought using the Pennsylvania Cancer Registry. Nine hundred and fifty cases yielded 70 (7.3%) sisters recruited (L. Kuller, personal communication). Case refusal or noncooperation, subject sister refusal or illness, and geographic dispersal, in order, were the barriers to recruitment. Unfortunately, for any intervention/prevention study with additional eligibility restrictions, this yield may genuinely represent what is possible with sister recruiting, even when special efforts are made to address the major barriers. In sum, these experiences suggest that recruitment of women at increased risk for breast cancer *in large numbers* is difficult.

The three groups of increased risk women suggested above have been chosen because their identification by women themselves is straightforward and usually accurate. Confirmation of family history or actual occurrence of breast biopsy is not necessary. Unfortunately, other risk factors are rare, of even lower impact, or require extensive confirmation. For example, a proliferative histologic change on breast biopsy identifies a high risk woman, but the pathologic interpretation likely requires review, and the logistics of obtaining slides and conducting this review are expensive. In addition, in the United States finding these women may be difficult and costly to begin with.

There are no easy, inexpensive logistical approaches to rapidly identifying and accruing a high *fraction* of the total pool of the high risk women. While working through affected sisters is logical, it is likely to be very inefficient. Lists of high risk women are dispersed if they exist at all. Since direct contact with potential subjects is the most efficient way to recruit, the absence of readily available mechanisms to identify such subjects presents a major barrier.

The data from Pittsburgh suggest that in using cases to find subjects, a clinical center for a breast cancer prevention trial would need a base of 3000 postmenopausal breast cancer cases to recruit 200 sisters. Such centers would usually have to be in major population centers.

In contrast for "normal risk" women (some authors feel that all American women are at "high risk" because the vast majority of breast cancers occur *absent* any identifiable risk factors), identification and successful recruitment of adequate numbers of subjects appears achievable based on population approaches used in other prevention studies. Because incidence increases with age and the total numbers of normal risk women are large, a slightly older age group of normal risk women (starting at 55 instead of 50) is suggested. Recent studies have suggested that a high waist-to-hip ratio may identify women at increased risk for breast cancer *and* heart disease (110–112). Data on this variable might be obtained on all study subjects and refinement of study design could be explored pending further confirmatory data.

Total Costs of Recruitment and Compliance Facilitation

The foregoing discussion presents a challenge: how to plan a full-scale breast cancer prevention trial likely to succeed because of adequate recruitment and high compliance, but efficient in use of all resources. Detailed cost analysis of the proposed Women's Health Trial specifically concluded that because

> "establishing and maintaining a clinical center represents a significant proportion of the clinical center's costs, use of a smaller number of larger clinical centers offers important cost savings. Because restrictive eligibility requirements reduce the recruitment potential of each clinical center, use of high-risk participants may not improve the efficiency of a prevention trial; its favorable

impact on sample size may fail to compensate for its cost in terms of additional clinical centers and higher recruitment costs." (113).

Summary of Appropriate Populations for Study

The foregoing discussion suggests that a reasonable general strategy for a breast cancer prevention trial might be to *target the high risk populations named for priority recruitment*. The first-phase recruitment experience should optimally be one that is efficient in financial and time costs *and* likely to reproducible over time in the same and other sites.

Minority populations and members of lower socioeconomic groups should be targeted also whenever possible. It must be recognized that there are trade-offs in ability to address major study objectives when different populations are recruited. Higher risk groups may be more compliant than lower risk ones; minority groups may be less compliant, and may have lower incidence of breast cancer. On the other hand, minority group mortality from breast cancer is high. To the maximal degree possible it seems reasonable that clinical centers should recruit high risk subjects to meet their accrual/time goals. However, given the constraints on available and eligible high risk subjects, it is anticipated that to achieve complete accrual for a prevention trial, within a short time frame and on a limited budget, centers will be able to accrue 40–50% high risk subjects. In this circumstance an actual study population would be like that which volunteered for BCDDP (105).

Feasibility Study

The advantages of a specific feasibility study for a breast cancer prevention trial deserve consideration. A breast cancer prevention trial will likely involve 12,000–16,000 total volunteer subjects and require considerable financial resources (114). Prior to committing the study subjects to the possible risks and loss of financial resources, there must be developed convincing feasibility data in several areas.

It is crucial to demonstrate first that it is logistically possible to recruit subjects in a timely manner and that they will comply with the study protocol. Consideration of the following issues makes this rationale clearer. The possible risks that must be described in study informed consent materials may represent a major barrier to recruitment. As an example, in recent FDA hearings and in writing to their members, some womens' health groups have expressed serious opposition to a tamoxifen study in healthy women. The available alternatives of estrogen or combination hormone replacement therapies may be significantly more attractive to women so as to prevent adequate recruitment. The side effects of tamoxifen and the requirements of study participation may lead to high rates of study dropout. In NSABP B14, 16.8% of tamoxifen recipients and 15% of placebo subjects had dropped out by 29 months median follow-up (40), while in Powles's prevention first phase almost 30% of healthy women had stopped treatment by 2 years (44). Dropout rates of this magnitude are not surprising, but would mandate significantly increased study sample sizes in a full-scale tamoxifen trial. Thus careful evaluation to determine optimal means to assure the highest possible recruitment and compliance rates *before* attempting recruitment for a full-scale trial are logical (116).

In addition to demonstrating feasibility of a full-scale trial, a feasibility study will allow piloting of materials (recruitment and compliance) and refinement of trial operations mechanisms so that a full-scale trial can be more *efficiently* conducted.

A feasibility study in which the critical demographic characteristics of actual subjects (age, risk factors for disease) are demonstrated allows for refinement of study design, e.g., likely needed sample size. It is impossible to predict the characteristics of the volunteer group in advance.

Finally, with respect to feasibility, it is not known which types of patient systems can be used most efficiently to recruit subjects for particular prevention trials—HMOs, community hospitals, screening clinics, or CCOPS. Clearly in a full-scale trial the most efficient systems should be the first used. A feasibility study can have different sites and develop needed data on this issue.

The second area in which further data may be important to justify a full-scale trial is safety. In general, many questions about harmful consequences of a long-term intervention treatment may only be addressable through special mechanisms; in the case of tamoxifen these include meta-analyses of adjuvant studies or postmarketing surveys, because the postulated adverse consequences are apparently very rare. However, both postulated beneficial and adverse effects of an intervention can be carefully monitored in a "vanguard" group of subjects whose time on treatment is 2 years ahead and larger than that of a full-scale trial study group. This can help to limit adverse consequences and maximize benefits to the larger full-scale trial population. Healthy women in any significant numbers may not have been treated with the intervention, and some assurance that when carefully monitored a cohort of such women show no serious adverse effects is needed.

The third area in which a feasibility study can provide additional data to justify an efficiently designed, full-scale trial is biological risk factor effects. Tamoxifen studies have not been done in healthy women, and further confirmatory data as well as data on less common effects on cardiovascular risk factors are needed. For example, blood pressure, HDL cholesterol, and glucose intolerance are important associates of heart disease risk in older women. Before exposing a very large cohort of healthy women to possible risks because of adverse changes in these parameters, large numbers of women need to be carefully evaluated to assess these parameters.

All of the data—feasibility, safety, and biological—will allow refinement of the study design of a full-scale trial as well as of a cost-effectiveness analysis of the intervention, which will facilitate the most rigorous possible analysis of the costs and benefits of conducting a full-scale trial.

Run-In

A run-in period should be considered and evaluated in the first phases of a breast cancer intervention trial. The rationale for this is as follows. High compliance with an intervention over long periods is essential to the success of a prevention trial because as compliance falls, the sample size necessary to demonstrate a benefit of the intervention with high power rises dramatically (114). In previous prevention trials, a major fraction of individuals who become noncompliant or dropped out of the trial did this in the first few months. In the Physician's Health Trial, one third of physicians initially enrolled dropped out prior to randomization during a run-in period (116). The power of the trial was increased by having a smaller number of very compliant subjects. In colon polyp prevention trials from 3 to 7% of subjects became noncompliant during a placebo run-in period (117). In the PEPI Study a 10-week placebo run-in period was used (10).

In a tamoxifen study an active agent, i.e., tamoxifen, run-in period might possibly identify and cause to become noncompliant an even greater percentage of subjects than a placebo-run-in period would. This would be due to the added fraction of subjects who would have tamoxifen-induced side effects. However, such a procedure would likely create problems with different compliance rates in tamoxifen and placebo groups after randomization because different fractions of these groups would then perceive themselves to be taking or not taking tamoxifen. In addition, companion studies of biological effects of tamoxifen on cardiovascular risks and bone could not be conducted with such an active agent run-in design.

Thus in the feasibility phase of a prevention trial, a run-in should be used. Interim analysis of the fraction of subjects dropped out during this run-in and correlates of compliance with the protocol should be conducted so that should this run-in not be necessary or of limited benefit, it can be dropped early in the trial program.

Eligibility Restrictions

Eligibility restrictions for a breast cancer prevention trial are of two types: those designed to increase the safety of the intervention by excluding individuals more likely to suffer complications and those designed to maximize the likelihood that the objectives of the study can be reached. These later restrictions include those designed to increase the chances that a study participant will not have any major medical problems during the planned duration of the study and will be likely to comply with the intervention completely for the entire study duration.

Endpoint Assessment

Definitive assessment of a diagnosis of breast cancer can only be made by means of pathologic diagnosis. This seemingly unarguable dictum, however, has significant implications when dealing with breast cancer. First, it is possible to make a diagnosis of breast cancer prior to the usual time of diagnosis (following clinical symptoms or signs) by use of mammography or periodic breast palpation. Because the signs of preclinical breast cancer can be subtle, the quality of these examinations can affect their accuracy and thus the point in time when a diagnosis is made. Second, since "preclinical" disease (early disease) is actively sought and screening should be a part of breast cancer prevention trial, atypical lesions, noninvasive, borderline, or minimally invasive breast cancers will be diagnosed in a significant percentage of all cases. The pathologic interpretation of these lesions is difficult. In sum because the times of diagnosis and type of diagnoses in a breast cancer prevention trial depend significantly on the quality of screening—mammography services and the quality of pathology—some quality assurance activities and panel reviews of mammograms and breast pathology, in addition to use of certified/professional practitioners in all clinical units are desirable. The argument is sometimes made that randomization will make these issues less important because it is assumed they will affect each randomized group equally. This is, however, a potentially dangerous assumption. For example, in a tamoxifen prevention trial diminution of radiologic dysplasia may occur with active therapy rendering earlier recognition of signs of malignancy possible, and the pathologic characteristics of small breast cancers occurring in the face of tamoxifen treatment may differ significantly.

Statistical Considerations

Elegant discussions of considerations of sample size methods are presented in Lachin (118) and Friedman et al. (119). It is important for clinical investigators, however, to be sensitive to potentially very major determinants of adequate sample size, the most important being compliance with the intervention. There are two types of noncompliance (119). The first and most obvious is noncompliance of intervention subjects who "drop out" of being treated with the intervention. These subjects may completely cease participation in the study or may be partially compliant in adopting the intervention. The other type of noncompliance, initially less obvious, is "drop in," the situation in which subjects in the control, no intervention, or standard treatment group begin to take or adopt the "active" intervention. The net result of either type of noncompliance is to dilute the investigated and sought-after difference between the randomized groups. The major strategy that has been used to compensate for noncompliance is to increase the study sample size. Depending on critical assumptions about other variables, for breast cancer prevention trials, increasing sample sizes by 50–60% becomes necessary when compliance falls to 80%. This observation makes it obvious that several factors which bear on "dropout" and "drop-in" rates must receive careful attention in the planning and conduct of breast cancer prevention trials. The use of a run-in period previously discussed is one strategy. The timing of the conduct of a prevention trial is a second: A trial needs to be conducted in the narrow window of time between when the scientific community (and thus the subject community) believes the intervention is reasonable and safe and thus when subjects are likely to comply with the intervention, and the time when the communities come to believe that the intervention works and the control subjects begin adopting the intervention (as "drop-ins").

Other statistical issues are worthy of attention, but each usually has less overall impact than the noncompliance issue (119).

Costs and Benefits of Clinical Trials to Prevent Breast Cancer

Clinical trials testing either the diet-fat hypothesis or tamoxifen to prevent breast cancer have been estimated to cost $60–100 million in direct costs, primarily because of their sizes (10–20,000 subjects) and durations (5–10 years). Scientists in other research areas may find these possible expenditures great for their perceived return. Several observations are worthwhile. Historically, large clinical trials have been found to be cost-effective investments despite their large costs (120). This is because their impact can be enormous: The widespread application (or nonapplication in the case of an intervention found useless) involving millions of individuals over long periods of time of a costly intervention (e.g., tamoxifen currently costs the consumer about $750 a year for a 20-mg daily dose) involves billions and trillions of dollars. The cost-effectiveness of prevention trials—public health trials—under consideration for breast cancer–dietary fat reduction or tamoxifen are further enhanced because in each case prevention of other chronic diseases such as heart disease and other malignancies are also postulated. An example of the consequences of *not* testing an intervention for overall health benefit with uncertain but costly consequences is the use of estrogen or other hormone replacement therapy described earlier. While cost-effectiveness analyses considering benefits in heart and bone disease for estrogen alone have been favorable, these have assumed *no* increased risk of breast cancer (12,13). Thus, the use of estrogen after menopause by about 16% of American women (4), now of uncertain *overall* benefit, may represent a very costly public health practice.

Unrelated to the cost directly, the development of clinical trials in breast cancer prevention can be viewed as the setting up of programs in women's health (121). Such trials will foster a myriad of ancillary studies, both biological and social scientific, from which, if past experience is repeated, much of significance will be learned. As an example, much about the national history of cervical cancer was learned from screening programs. Even if the primary hypotheses of such trials are not supported (although as indicated above this would be very useful information), the program yields will likely be very great. Women's health in general has received less attention than men's, and thus the emphasis in these trials in fact will correct an imbalance in past public health efforts.

CONCLUSION

Clinical trials of interventions to prevent breast cancer—dietary fat reduction, tamoxifen, or other—are extraordinarily complex and costly undertakings, with, however, major potential public health benefit, which appear to easily justify the efforts. Such clinical trials should be viewed broadly as the foundations for progress in women's health from which unexpected knew knowledge will inevitably arise.

ACKNOWLEDGMENTS

Drs. D. L. DeMets, C. Furberg, V. C. Jordan, P. A. Newcomb, and R. Prentice, in addition to my colleagues of the Tamoxifen Health Trial Group have contributed ideas and partial reviews of the text presented here. During the period over which these ideas were developed the author has been supported by grants PDT 302A and B from the American Cancer Society, by grants from ICI Pharma Division of ICI Americas, Inc., by Public Health Service grants CA-14520 and CA-50243 from the National Cancer Institute, the National Institutes of Health, Department of Health and Human Services.

REFERENCES

1. S. S. Devesa, D. T. Silverman, J. L. Young, Jr., et al., Cancer incidence and mortality trends among whites in the United States, 1974–84, *JNCI, 79*(4), 701 (1987).
2. E. White, Projected changes in breast cancer incidence due to the trend toward delayed childbearing, *Am. J. Public Health, 77*, 495–497 (1987).
3. Anonymous, Premature mortality due to breast cancer—United States, *JAMA, 258*, 3229–3231 (1987).
4. D. A. Dawson and G. B. Thompson, Breast cancer risk factors and screening: United States 1987, National Center for Health Statistics, *Vital Health Statistics, 10*, 172 (1989).
5. B. E. Henderson, R. K. Ross, A. Paganini-Hill, and T. M. Mack, Estrogen use and cardiovascular disease, *Am. J. Obstet. Gynecol., 154*, 1181–1186 (1986).

6. J. DeQueker, E. Muylder, and J. Ferin, The effect of long-term lynestrenol treatment of bone mass in cyclic women, *Contraception, 15*, 717 (1972).
7. N. J. Weiss, C. L. Ure, J. H. Ballard, et al., Decreased risk of fractures of the hip and lower forearm with post-menopausal use of estrogen. *N. Engl. J. Med., 303*, 1195 (1980).
8. B. S. Hulka, Hormone replacement therapy and the risk of breast cancer, *CA, 40*, 289–296 (1990).
9. R. Hoover, J. F. Fraumeni, Jr., R. Everson, and M. H. Myers, Cancer of the uterine corpus after hormonal treatment for breast cancer. *Lancet, ii*, 885–887 (1976).
10. Anonymous, Protocol for the postmenopausal estrogen/progestin intervention trial, (PEPI) p. 3.
11. E. J. Sondik, *Cancer Statistics Review*, 1973–1986, USDHHS/PHS, NIH Publication #89-2789, 1989.
12. M. C. Weinstein, Estrogen use in postmenopausal women—costs, risks and benefits, *N. Engl. J. Med., 303*, 308–316 (1980).
13. B. E. Hillner, J. P. Hollenberg, and S. G. Pauker, Postmenopausal estrogens in prevention of osteoporosis. Benefit virtually without risk if cardiovascular effects are considered, *Am. J. Med., 80*, 1115–1127 (1986).
14. M. C. Pike, Breast cancer and hormone replacement therapy, *Lancet, 1*, 297 (1990).
15. M. J. K. Harper, and A. L. Walpole, A new derivative of triphenylethylene: Effects on implantation and mode of action in rats, *J. Reprod. Fertil., 13*, 101–119 (1967).
16. V. C. Jordan, Antiestrogenic and antitumor properties of tamoxifen in laboratory animals, *Cancer Treat. Rep., 60*, 1409–1419 (1976).
17. S. S. Legha and S. K. Carter, Antiestrogens in the treatment of breast cancer, *Cancer Treat. Rev., 3*, 205–216 (1976).
18. L. J. Lerner and V. C. Jordan, Development of antiestrogens and their use in breast cancer: Eighth Cain Memorial Award Lecture. *Cancer Res., 50*, 4177–4189 (1990).
19. B. J. A. Furr and V. C. Jordan, The pharmacology and clinical use of tamoxifen, *Pharm. Thera., 25*, 127–205 (1984).
20. V. C. Jordan, Biochemical pharmacology of antiestrogen action, *Pharm. Rev., 36*, 245–276 (1984).
21. R. B. Dickson and M. E. Lippman, Estrogenic regulation of growth and polypeptide growth factor secretion in human breast carcinoma, *Endo. Rev., 8*, 29–56 (1987).
22. V. C. Jordan and C. S. Murphy, Endocrine pharmacology of antiestrogens as antitumor agents, *Endo. Rev.*, (in press).
23. V. C. Jordan, Effect of tamoxifen (ICI46,474) on initiation and growth of DMBA-induced rat mammary carcinomata, *Eur. J. Cancer, 12*, 419–422 (1976).
24. C. W. Welsch, M. Goodrich-Smith, C. K. Brown, et al., Effect of an estrogen antagonist (tamoxifen) on the initiation and progression of radiation-induced mammary tumors in female Sprague-Dawley rats, *Eur. J. Cancer, 17*, 1255–1258 (1981).
25. V. C. Jordan, M. K. Lababidi, and D. M. Mirecki, The antiestrogenic and antitumor properties of prolonged tamoxifen therapy in C3H/OUJ mice, *Eur. J. Cancer, 26*, 718–721 (1990).
26. H. M. Lemon, P. F. Pradeep, Peterson, C., et al., Inhibition of radiogenic

mammory carcinoma in rats by estriol or tamoxifen, *Cancer, 63*, 1685–1692 (1989).

27. V. C. Jordan, Laboratory studies to develop general principles for the adjuvant treatment of breast cancer with antiestrogens: Problems and potential for future clinical applications. *Breast Cancer Res. Treat. 3*(Suppl), 73–86 (1983).
28. C. K. Osborne, K. Hobbs, and C. M. Clark, Effects of estrogens and antiestrogens on growth of human breast cancer cells in athymic mice, *Cancer Res., 45*, 584–590 (1985).
29. V. C. Jordan, Chemosuppression of breast cancer with tamoxifen—laboratory evidence and future clinical investigations, *Cancer Invest., 6*, 589–595 (1988).
30. R. R. Love, Tamoxifen therapy in primary breast cancer: Biology, efficacy and side effects, *J. Clin. Oncol., 7*, 803–815 (1989).
31. Early Breast Cancer Trialists Collaborative Group. The effects of adjuvant tamoxifen and of cytotoxic therapy on mortality in early breast cancer: An overview of 61 randomized trials among 28,896 women, *N. Engl. J. Med., 319*, 1681–1692 (1988).
32. B. Fisher, C. Redmond, D. L. Wickerham, et al., Systemic therapy in patients with node negative breast cancer. *Ann. Int. Med., 111*, 703–712 (1989).
33. B. Fisher, A. Brown, N. Wolmark, et al., Prolonging tamoxifen therapy for primary breast cancer. Findings from the National Surgical Adjuvant Breast and Bowel Project clinical trial, *Ann. Int. Med., 106*, 649–654 (1987).
34. Breast Cancer Trials Committee, Scottish Cancer Trials Office (MRC): Adjuvant tamoxifen in the management of operable breast cancer: The Scottish trial, *Lancet, i*, 171–75 (1987).
35. H. C. Falkson, R. Gray, W. H. Wolbert, et al., Adjuvant trial of twelve cycles of CMFPT followed by observation or continuous tamoxifen versus four cycles of CMFPT in postmenopausal women with breast cancer. An ECOG Phase III study, *J. Clin. Oncol., 8*, 599–607 (1990).
36. F. Boccardo, A. Rubagotti, P. Bruzzi, et al., Chemotherapy versus tamoxifen versus chemotherapy plus tamoxifen in node positive estrogen receptor positive breast cancer patients: Results of a multicentric Italian study, *J. Clin. Oncol., 8*, 1310–1320 (1990).
37. J. R. Harris, S. Hellman, G. P. Canellos, and B. Fisher, Cancer of the breast, In *Cancer Principles and Practice of Oncology*, 2nd ed. (DeVita, V. T., Jr., Hellman, S., Rosenberg, S. A., eds.), J. B. Lippincott Company, Philadelphia, 1985, p. 1150.
38. K. J. Walker, M. Price-Thomas, W. Candlish, W., and R. I. Nicholson. Does tamoxifen have a direct effect on the normal human breast? Relevance to prophylactic therapy, *Brit. J. Cancer, 62*(Suppl. II), Oct. 1990, p. 3 (Abstract #4).
39. J. Cuzick and M. Baum, Tamoxifen and contralateral breast cancer, *Lancet, ii*, 282 (1985).
40. B. Fisher, J. Constantino, C. Redmond, et al., A randomized clinical trial evaluating tamoxifen in the treatment of patients with node negative breast cancer who have estrogen receptor positive tumors, *N. Engl. J. Med., 32*, 479–484 (1989).
41. T. Fornander, B. Cedarmark, A. Mattson, et al., Adjuvant tamoxifen in early breast cancer: Occurrence of new primary cancers, *Lancet, i*, 117–119 (1989).

42. V. C. Jordan, N. F. Fritz, and D. C. Tormey, Long-term adjuvant therapy with tamoxifen: Effects on sex hormone-binding globulin and antithrombin III, *Cancer Res.*, *47*, 4517–4519 (1987).
43. R. R. Love, P. A. Newcomb, D. L. Wiebe, et al., Lipid and lipoprotein effects of tamoxifen therapy in postmenopausal women with node-negative breast cancer. *JNCI*, *82*, 1327–1332 (1990).
44. T. J. Powles, Hardy, Jr., S. E. Ashley, et al., A pilot trial to evaluate the acute toxicity and feasibility of tamoxifen for prevention of breast cancer, *Br. J. Cancer*, *60*, 126–131 (1989).
45. P. F. Bruning, J. M. G. Bonfrer, A. A. M. Hart, et al., Tamoxifen, serum lipoproteins and cardiovascular risk, *Brit. J. Cancer*, *58*, 497–499 (1988).
46. G. Bertelli, P. Pronzato, D. Amoroso, et al., Adjuvant tamoxifen in primary breast cancer: influence on plasma lipids and antithrombin III levels. *Breast Cancer Res. Treat.*, *52*, 339–346 (1988).
47. S. Sedlacek, Estrogenic properties of tamoxifen on serum lipids in postmenopausal women with breast cancer, *Breast Cancer Res. Treat.*, (abstract) *14*, 153 (1989).
48. J. D. Bagdade, J. Wolter, P. R. Subbaiah, and W. Ryan, Effects of tamoxifen treatment on plasma lipids and lipoprotein lipid composition, *J. Cin. Endo. Metab.*, *70*, 1132–1135 (1990).
49. D. Schapira, M. Kumar, and G. H. Lyman. The effect of tamoxifen therapy on serum cholesterol. *Proc. Am. Soc. Clin. Onc.*, *9*, 49 (1990).
50. L. D. Brun, C. Gagne, C. Rousseau, et al., Severe lipemia induced by tamoxifen, *Cancer*, *57*, 2123–2126 (1986).
51. R. R. Love, T. S. Surawicz, and E. C. Williams, Antithrombin III, fibrinogen and platelet number changes with tamoxifen therapy in postmenopausal women (submitted manuscript).
52. S. B. Hulley, R. H. Rosenman, R. D. Bawol, and R. J. Brand. Epidemiology as a guide to clinical decisions. The association between triglyceride and coronary heart disease, *N. Engl. J. Med.*, *302*, 1383–1389 (1980).
53. M. A. Austin, Plasma triglyceride as a risk factor for coronary heart disease. The epidemiolgic evidence and beyond, *Am. J. Epidemiol.*, *129*, 249–259 (1989).
54. M. B. Hultin, Fibrinogen and factor VII as risk factors in vascular disease, *Prog. Hemost. Thrombo*, *10*, 215–241 (1991).
55. W. B. Kannel, P. A. Wolf, W. P. Castelli, R. B. D'Agostino, Fibrinogen and risk of cardiovascular disease, *JAMA*, *258*, 1183–1186 (1987).
56. Lipid Research Clinics Program: The Lipid Research Clinics Coronary Prevention Trial results II, The relationship of reduction in incidence of coronary heart disease to cholesterol lowering, *JAMA*, *251*, 365–374 (1984).
57. T. Bush, L. P. Fried, and E. Barrett-Connor, Cholesterol, lipoprotein, and coronary heart disease in women, *Clin. Chem.*, *34*, 60–70 (1988).
58. J. Stamler, D. Wentworth, and J. D. Meaton, Is relationship between serum cholesterol and risk of premature death from coronary heart disease continuous and graded? *JAMA*, *256*, 2823–2828 (1986).
59. H. Stewart, Data presented at Consensus Conference on Adjuvant Therapy in Node

Negative Breast Cancer, Washington, DC, June 18, 1990.
60. E. Barrett-Connor, Postmenopausal estrogen, cancer and other considerations, *Womens Health*, 179–195 (1986).
61. V. C. Jordan, E. Phelps, and J. U. Lingren, Effect of antiestrogens on bone in castrated and intact female rates, *Breast Cancer Res. Treat.*, *10*, 31–35 (1987).
62. R. T. Turner, G. K. Wakely, K. S. Hannon, and N. A. Bell, Tamoxifen prevents the skeletal effects of ovarian hormone deficiency in rats, *J. Bone. Min. Res.*, *2*, 449–456 (1987).
63. R. T. Turner, G. K. Wakely, K. S. Hannon, and N. A. Bell, Tamoxifen inhibits osteoclast mediated resportion of trabecular bone in ovarian hormone deficient rats, *Endocrinology*, *122*, 1146–1150 (1988).
64. G. K. Wakely, K. S. Hannon, N. A. Bell, and R. T. Turner, The effects of tamoxifen on the osteopenia induced by sciatic neurotomy in the rat: Histomorphometric study, *Calcif. Tissue Int.*, *43*, 383–388 (1988).
65. R. R. Love, R. B. Mazess, D. C. Tormey, et al., Bone mineral density in women with breast cancer treated with adjuvant tamoxifen for at least two years, *Breast Cancer Res. Treat*, *12*, 297–301 (1988).
66. T. Fornander, L. E. Rutquist, H. E. Sjoberg, et al., Long term adjuvant tamoxifen in early breast cancer: Effect in bone mineral density in postmenopausal women, *J. Clin. Oncol.*, *8*, 1019–1024 (1990).
67. J. Wolter, W. G. Ryan, V. Subbaiah, et al., Apparent beneficial effects of tamoxifen on serum lipoprotein subfractions and bone mineral content in patients with breast cancer, *Proc. Am. Soc. Clin. Oncol.*, *7*, 10(A-34) (1988).
68. S. Turken, E. Siris, D. Seldin, et al. Effects of tamoxifen on spinal bone density in women with breast cancer, *JNCI*, *81*, 1086–1088 (1989).
69. A Gotfredsen, C. Christiansen, and T. Palshof, The effect of tamoxifen on bone mineral content in premenopausal women with breast cancer, *Cancer*, *53*, 853–857 (1984).
70. I. S. Fentiman, M. Calelfi, A. Rodin, et al., Bone mineral content of women receiving tamoxifen for mastalgia, *Br. J. Cancer*, *60*, 262–264 (1989).
71. P. J. D. K. Daves, A. Wilson, and A. MacKenzie, Bone mineral content following administration of adjuvant tamoxifen to women aged between 37 and 59 years, *Brit. J. Cancer*, *62*(Suppl. II), 34 (Abstract #52) (1990).
72. C. Maltoni, Long-term bioassays on the toxic, carcinogenic and tumor chemoprevention effects of tamoxifen on Sprague-Dawley rats: ongoing studies and early results, Presentation at Tamoxifen Health Trial Network meeting, Madison, WI, June 3, 1990.
73. J. C. Topham, Presented data before FDA, Washington, DC, June 29, 1990.
74. Y. P. Dragan, Y. Hu, and H. C. Pitot, Tumor promotion as a target for estrogen/antiestrogen effects in rat hepatocarcinogenesis. *Prev. Med.*, *20*(1), 15–26, (1991).
75. J. D. Yager and Y. E. Shi, Synthetic estrogen and tamoxifen as promoters of hepatocarcinogenesis, *Prev. Med.*, *20*(1), 27–37 (1991).
76. J. Clemmesen, Statistical studies in malignant neoplasms V. Trends and risks (suppl 261), *Acta Pathologica et Microbiologica Scandinavica*, 38–50 (1977).

77. J. R. Palmer, L. Rosenberg, and D. W. Kaufman, Oral contraceptive use and liver cancer, *Am. J. Epidemiol.*, *130*, 878-882 (1989).
78. D. Forman, R. Doll, and R. Peto, Trends in mortality from carcinoma of the liver and the use of oral contraceptives, *Br. J. Cancer, 48*, 349-354 (1983).
79. B. E. Henderson, S. Preston-Martin, H. A. Edmondson, R. J. Peters, and M. C. Pike, Hepatocellular carcinoma and oral contraceptives, *Br. J. Cancer, 48*, 437-440 (1983).
80. J. Neuberger, D. Forman, R. Doll, and R. Williams, Oral contraceptives and hepatocellular carcinoma, *Br. J. Cancer, 292*, 1355-1357 (1986).
81. WHO Collaborative Study Group, Combined oral contraceptives and liver cancer, *J. Cancer, 43*, 254-259 (1989).
82. P. Plourde, Presentation before FDA, Washington, DC, June 29, 1990.
83. P. G. Satyaswroop, R. J. Zaino, and R. Mortel, Estrogen-like effects of tamoxifen on human endometrial carcinoma transplanted into nude mice. *Cancer Res.*, *44*, 4006-4010 (1984).
84. C. L. Clark and P. G. Satyaswaroop. Photoaffinity labelling of the progesterone receptor from human endometrial carcinoma, *Cancer Res.*, *45*, 5417-5420 (1985).
85. M. M. Gottardis, S. P. Robinson, P. G. Satyaswaroop, and V. C. Jordan, Contrasting actions of tamoxifen on endometrial and breast tumor growth in the athymic mouse, *Cancer Res.*, *48*, 812-815 (1988).
86. K. Hardell, Tamoxifen as risk factor for carcinoma of corpus uteri, *Lancet, 2*, 563 (1988).
87. K. Hardell. Pelvic irradiation and tamoxifen as risk factors in corpus uteri, *Lancet, 11*, 1432 (1988).
88. V. C. Jordan, N. F. Fritz, and D. C. Tormey, Long-term adjuvant therapy with tamoxifen: Effects on sex hormone-binding globulin and antithrombin III, *Cancer Res.*, *47*, 4517-4519 (1987).
89. M. I. Kaiser-Kupfer and M. E. Lippman, Tamoxifen retinopathy, *CAncer Treat. Rep.*, *62*, 315-320 (1978).
90. A. R. Ashford, I. Donev, R. P. Tiwari, et al., Reversible ocular toxicity related to tamoxifen therapy, *Cancer, 61*, 33-35 (1988).
91. S. Longstaff, H. Sigurdsson, M. O'Keeffe, et al. A controlled study of the ocular effects of tamoxifen in conventional dosage in the treatment of breast carcinoma. *Europ. J. Cancer Clin. Onc.*, *25*, 1805-1809 (1989).
92. Boston Collaborative Drug Surveillance Program, Surgical confirmed gallbladder disease, Venias thromboembolism and breast tumors in ? to postmenopausal estrogen treatment, *N. Engl. J. Med.*, *290*, 15-19 (1974).
93. Nolvadex Adjuvant Trial Organization, Controlled trial of tamoxifen as a single adjuvant agent in the management of early breast cancer, *Br. J. Cancer, 57*, 608-611 (1988).
94. R. R. Love, L. Cameron, B. O'Connor, and H. Leventhal, Symptoms associated with tamoxifen treatment in postmenopausal women (unpublished manuscript).
95. H. O. Adami, J. Hansen, B. Jung, et al. Familiarity in breast cancer: A case-control study in a Swedish population, *Br. J. Cancer, 42*, 71-77 (1980).

96. E. Negri, C. La Vecchia, P. Bruzzi, et al. Risk factors for breast cancer: Pooled results from three Italian case-control studies, *Am. J. Epidemiol.*, *128*, 1207–1215 (1988).
97. R. W. Sattin, G. L. Rubin, L. A. Webster, et al., Family history and risk of breast cancer, *JAMA*, *253*, 1908–1913 (1985).
98. R. Ottman, M. C. Pike, M. C. King, et al., Familial breast cancer in a population-based series, *Am. J. Epidemiol.*, *123*, 15–21 (1986).
99. C. Bain, F. E. Speizer, B. Rosner, et al., Family history of breast cancer as a risk indicator for the disease, *Am. J. Epidemiol.*, *111*, 301–308 (1980).
100. L. A. Brinton, R. Hoover, and J. F. Fraumeni, Interaction of familial and hormonal risk factors for breast cancer, *JNCI*, *69*, 817–822 (1982).
101. N. Duban, B. S. Pasternack, and P. Strax. Epidemiology of breast cancer in a screened population, *Cancer Detect. Pre.*, *7*, 87–102 (1984).
102. T. G. Hislop, A. J. Coldman, J. M. Edward, et al. Relationship between risk factors for breast cancer and hormonal status, *Int. J. Epidemiol.*, *15*, 469–476 (1986).
103. C. Mettlin, I. Crogham, M. Hatarajen, W. Lane, The association of age and family risk in a case control study of breast cancer, *Am. J. Epidemiol.*, *131*, 973–983 (1990).
104. E. B. Claus, M. J. Risch, W. D. Thompson, Age at onset as an indicator of familial risk of breast cancer, *Am. J. Epidemiol.*, *131*, 961–972 (1990).
105. M. H. Gail, L. A. Brinton, D. P. Byar, et al., Projecting individualized probabilities developing breast cancer for white females who are being examined annually, *JNCI*, *81*, 1879–1886 (1989).
106. L. A. Brinton, R. Hoover, and J. F. Fraumeni, Jr., Reproductive factors in the etiology of breast cancer, *Br. J. Cancer*, *47*, 757–762 (1983).
107. U.S. Bureau of Census, Current Population Reports, Series P25. Publication Number N1018, p. 15. U.S. Government Printing Office, Washington, DC, 1989.
108. V. G. Vogel, High risk populations as targets for breast cancer prevention trials, *Prev. Med.* Vo. 20, no. 1, Jan. 1991, pp. 86–100.
109. L. Lapidus, C. Bengtsson, B. Larsson, et al., Distribution of adipose tissue and risk of cardiovascular disease and death: A 12 year follow up of participants in the population study of women in Golenberg, Sweden, *Br. Med. J.*, *289*, 1257–1261 (1984).
110. D. V. Schapiro, N. B. Kumar, G. H. Lyman, and C. E. Cox, Abdominal obesity and breast cancer risk, *Ann. Int. Med.*, *112*, 182–186 (1990).
111. R. Ballard-Barbash, A. Schatzbin, C. L. Carter, et al., Body fat distribution and breast cancer in the Framingham study, *JNCI*, *82*, 286–290 (1990).
112. A. R. Fulsom, S. A. Kay, R. J. Prineas, et al., Increased incidence of carcinoma of the breast associated with abdominal adiposity in postmenopausal women, *Am. J. Epidemiol.*, *131*, 794–803 (1990).
113. M. Urban, S. Self, L. Kessler, et al., Analysis of costs of a large prevention trial *Controlled Clin. Trials*, *11*, 129–146 (1990).
114. D. L. DeMets, P. A. Newcomb, and P. Carey, Design issues for a breast cancer chemoprevention trial, *Prev. Med.* Vol. 20, no. 1, Jan. 1991, pp. 101–108.

115. R. L. Prentice, Editorial: Tamoxifen as a potential preventive agent in healthy postmenopausal women, *JNCI, 82*, 1310–1311 (1990).
116. C. H. Hennekens, M. J. Stampfer, and W. Willett, Micronutrients and cancer chemoprevention, *Cancer Detect. Prev., 7*, 147–158 (1984).
117. M. Stevens, E. R. Greenberg, and J. A. Baron, Practical aspects of cancer prevention trials, In *Nutrition and Cancer Prevention—Investigating the Role of Micronutrients*, (T. Moon and M. S. Micozzi, eds.), Marcel Dekker, Inc., New York, 1989, pp. 513–532.
118. J. M. Lachin, Introduction to sample size determination and power analysis for clinical trials, *Controlled Clinical Trials, 2*, 93–113 (1981).
119. L. Friedman, C. Furberg, and D. DeMets, *Fundamental of Clinical Trials*, 2nd ed. John Wright-PSG Inc., Littleton, MA, 1985.
120. A. S. Detsky, Are clinical trials a cost effective investment? *JAMA, 262*, 1795–1800 (1989).
121. C. Furberg, Organizing multicenter trials: Lessons from cardiovascular prevention trials, *Prev. Med., 20*(1), 158–161, (1991).

17

Clinical Trials on Colorectal Cancer

Perla A. Vargas and David S. Alberts
The University of Arizona Health Sciences Center
Tucson, Arizona

INTRODUCTION

Colorectal cancer is the third most common malignant neoplasm worldwide (1), and the second leading cause of cancer deaths in the United States (2). In spite of advances in surgery and chemotherapy the 5 year survival rate of patients with advanced colon cancer at the time of diagnosis has shown little change (3). As a result, it is probable that preventive measures will provide the primary means for significantly decreasing the high mortality rates from this disease in the United States.

The causes of colon cancer have not yet been identified fully. Evidence from epidemiologic (4–6), experimental (7–9), and genetic (10,11) studies suggests that colon cancer genesis may be the product of complex interactions of genetic susceptibility, carcinogens, promoters, and inhibitors. Environmental and dietary factors are considered to be responsible for up to 85–90% of all cases. Dietary factors—the affluent Western diet in particular—have been linked consistently to increased colon cancer incidence. According to Doll and Peto (12), dietary factors may account for about 30% of attributable risk. Among the dietary components suggested as colon cancer promoters are excess fat and excess calories, whereas

This work was supported in part by Grant CA-41108 from the National Institutes of Health, Bethesda, Maryland.

high intakes of fiber, calcium, and other micronutrients have been suggested as colon cancer inhibitors (13–17). A proposed hypothesis about induction of colorectal cancer suggests that fats and other steroids (bile acids and bile salts) are metabolized in the gut to secondary carcinogens (deoxycholic and lithocholic), which promote the growth of adenomas and subsequently invasive cancer. Thus, limiting the intake of fat may reduce the quantity of these carcinogens. On the other hand, by increasing consumption of dietary fiber or calcium, colonic exposure to these carcinogens may be reduced.

The suggested mechanism by which dietary fibers reduce carcinogen exposure involves increased fecal bulk and decreased concentration in stool of mutagenic compounds. The proposed hypothesis about the protective role of calcium suggests that ionized calcium can inhibit the effects of both fatty and bile acids by binding with these lipids to form insoluble calcium soaps (15–19). It has been observed that dietary fibers absorb calcium. Such interactions could nullify or modify the protective effect of calcium (20,21).

Despite the vigorous research activity in this area, current evidence from epidemiologic case-control and animal studies does not conclusively support any *single* dietary component as protective against colorectal cancer. Interactions among individual dietary components are complex; dietary intakes are often multicollinear, and it has been difficult to separate the effects of individual variables (22).

ENDPOINTS IN CLINICAL TRIALS

There is growing experimental evidence showing that colorectal carcinogenesis is not an irreversible process. To the contrary, dietary changes (e.g., fat reduction, calcium or fiber supplementation) or the systematic incorporation of into the diet of certain anticarcinogenic agents (e.g., piroxicam, omega-3 fatty acids, difluoro-methylornithine) seem to reduce colon cancer risk in various rat tumor models.

It has become apparent that most human cancers have precursors and/or biologic markers that are identifiable and may function as indicators of high cancer risk or risk reduction. These intermediate markers serve as highly valued endpoints in preventive clinical trials. Recent findings support the hypothesis that most (i.e., up to 95%) colorectal cancers arise from adenomatous polyps (23,24). Fifteen to more than 50% of patients who have a polyp removed will have polyp recurrence one or more years after the initial polypectomy (25–29). These studies have led to the adoption of adenomatous polyps as a preneoplastic endpoint for colon cancer.

In many precancerous conditions the epithelial cells involved enter a hyperproliferation state that may function as subclinical or microscopic manifestations of carcinogenesis. Indices of cell proliferation, such as the rate of DNA synthesis in rectal mucosa, have been correlated with the onset and advancement of these precancerous stages as they progress toward frank expression of cancer. Lipkin and collaborators (30,31) have pointed out that a major application of these markers is to evaluate the effect of possible chemopreventive agents. The advantage of this approach lies in reducing the time required to evaluate the efficacy of an intervention and in providing a logical rationale for further studies that ultimately would evaluate cancer incidence. However, it is important to keep in mind that there is not a one-to-one correspondence between the occurrence of adenomatous polyps and high rates of cell proliferation and invasive cancer. In some cases such precancerous conditions may revert to normal or never progress regardless of treatment (32).

A cancer endpoint is clear and readily interpretable; however, it also bears virtually insurmountable drawbacks: (a) a prolong duration of follow-up is required before sufficient number of cases or deaths can be observed, (b) the large size of such studies requires a huge clinical trials staff, and (c) the cost associated with running a colon cancer prevention trial with cancer recurrence or mortality as endpoint can be prohibitive.

FAT CONSUMPTION AND COLON CANCER RISK

Of the possible dietary alternatives to prevent colon cancer, fat reduction and fiber supplementation seem to be the most attractive approaches, since both are considered major risk factors in the genesis of this disease. Dietary modification by a low fat diet has been advocated for several years for prevention of cardiovascular disease (33) and breast cancer (34). A major limitation of this approach, however, is that it requires personalized diet counseling and intensive follow-ups, similar to interventions in well-programmed weight-reduction clinics. Drastic changes in long-established eating behaviors are extremely difficult to accomplish (35), as illustrated by the high attrition (20–80%) and low long-term success rate (less than 5%) of weight-management programs (36).

Subject adherence determines the ultimate success of any regimen, an issue of particular importance to a colon cancer preventive intervention aimed at lowering fat intake in the general population. On the other hand, lowering fat consumption does not automatically translate into a significant increase in fiber intake. For example, milk drinkers can easily reduce fat intake by 10% by switching to low fat products; similarly those who eat red meat regularly can reduce fat by eating leaner cuts without a meaningful increase in fiber consumption.

In general, evidence from epidemiologic and laboratory studies support the role of dietary fat, particularly animal fat, in the etiology of colon carcinogenesis (37–47). High correlations between per capita intake of dietary fat and colon cancer have been reported (38,39,48). High fat intake has been shown to increase the incidence of induced colon tumors in laboratory animals (49–54). Diets high in fat also have been associated with increased bile acid excretion in humans (54,55) and laboratory animals (49,55). However, the findings have not been totally consistent (53,56–61). Some population and case-control studies have documented lower colorectal cancer incidence rates in populations with high intakes of fat and fiber as compared to populations with high intakes of fat, but low levels of fiber consumption (13,14,17,62). For example, in a 15-year prospective study, Stemmerman and collaborators (63) found a negative association between saturated fat and colon cancer.

Recently, Willet et al. (37) in a 6-year prospective study among 88,751 women (the Nurses Trial) reported a positive association between consumption of red meat and animal fat and colon cancer incidence, independent of total energy intake. No association was observed for vegetable fat. A protective effect of high intake of fruits was also observed, however, this negative association was neither significant nor independent of meat intake.

Inconsistencies in the literature may reflect the fact that often researchers have not taken into account the possible modulating effect of other nutrients (e.g., dietary fiber, calcium, selenium, etc.). On the other hand, they might also reflect the difficulties of interpreting the data from epidemiologic studies due to "concurrent" dietary factors. Two such concurrent factors, for example, are the high consumption of fat which is usually accompanied by an equally high consumption of animal protein, particularly red meat (37,64).

Although the current evidence is inconclusive regarding the role of dietary fat in the etiology of colorectal cancer, an interaction effect between fat consumption, colon cancer risk, and other dietary factors is strongly suggested.

At the present time, there have been few publications of intervention studies in human examining the effect of dietary fat on indices of colon carcinogenesis. However, there are at least two clinical trials underway. The Australian Polyp Prevention Project (65) involves a 2-year trial using a $2 \times 2 \times 2$ randomized factorial design to test the efficacy of reducing fat intake (30% total energy), wheat bran supplementation (25 g/day), and β-carotene supplementation (20 mg/day) on the recurrence rate of colorectal adenomatous polyps. The study was completed in May 1990, and data analyses are currently underway. The second is a multiinstitutional clinical trial sponsored by the NCI Division of Cancer Prevention and Control aimed to evaluate the effect of a low fat, high fiber, high fruit and vegetable dietary intervention on polyp recurrence. Secondary endpoints of this study include [^{3}H]-thymidine crypt epithelial cell labeling and ornithine decarboxylase activity (ODC) in biopsies of rectal mucosa. Participants will continue the intervention for up to 5 years. Repeat colonoscopies are to be performed at the end of the first and third study years. The results of these studies should help to determine the effect of fat reduction on colonic pre-cancerous lesions and provide the basis for future research.

DIETARY SUPPLEMENTS AND HEALTH PROMOTION

Dietary supplementation (e.g., iodine, iron, calcium, vitamins A and D) has long been used by nutritionists to ensure adequate intake of certain components for populations at high risk. This approach is comparatively less demanding than is a radical change in food habits. Additionally, dietary supplementation by familiar food items presents a workable alternative, with expected good adherence. Supplementation by dietary fiber (66,67) and calcium (31,68,69) especially have been studied in recent clinical trials.

DIETARY FIBER AND COLON CANCER RISK

There is considerable evidence from human and animal studies suggesting a protective effect of dietary fiber on colon carcinogenesis, although it is acknowledged that further research is needed regarding human colonic physiology and underlying mechanisms (9,13,14,17,47,48,70–77). However, there are several well-designed animal studies (78–80) and a few epidemiologic studies (41,81) which suggest that dietary fiber might even promote colon tumor growth. Comparative studies of Finns and Americans (14,17) suggest that dietary fat intake may be a risk factor, particularly when intake of dietary fiber is low. These studies documented similar consumption levels of dietary fat and animal protein by Finns in Kuopio to that of Americans in New York. However, the Finns consumed more than twice the fiber of their American counterparts (mainly as a dark, hard rye bread), and their incidence of colon cancer was only one third that of New Yorkers. In the United States, cereal (grain) fiber has been the mainstay of a diet high in fiber.

Although fruits and green vegetables contain fiber, much larger quantities of these food groups are required to provide sufficient amounts of fiber in the daily diet (82). Thus, cereal supplementation seems to be the easiest way to increase significantly the fiber intake of North Americans.

But not all dietary fibers seem to have the same protective effect. Studies in laboratory animals have shown that different types of fiber have different effects on colon carcinogenesis (7,83–88). According to Reddy and collaborators (8) dietary cellulose and wheat bran are the most effective fibers to protect against chemically induced colon cancer, whereas corn and oat brans have no such protective effect.

Wheat bran fiber has received special attention as a potential daily supplement. In a 4-year randomized trial, DeCosse and coworkers (66) studied the effect of high fiber supplementation plus vitamins C and E (22.5 g/day, 4 g/day, and 400 mg/day, respectively) compared to low fiber plus vitamins (2.2 g/day, 4 g/day, and 400 mg/day, respectively) and to low fiber placebo (2.2 g/day) in 58 patients with familial adenomatous polyposis. Although compliance to the supplementation decreased significantly throughout the trial ($p < 0.005$), the investigators found that an excess of 11 g/day of wheat fiber supplementation was associated with a reduced incidence of polyp recurrence, whereas the vitamin supplementation had no beneficial effect. Additionally, Alberts et al. (67) supplemented the diets of disease-free patients with a history of resected colon or rectal cancer with 13.5 g/day of wheat bran cereal for 2 months. Results of this study showed an overall significant ($p < 0.001$) decrease of 22% in 24-hour outgrowth [^{3}H]-thymidine labeling indices in rectal mucosal biopsies obtained at study termination in the entire group of patients.

Examining the effect of 10 g/day of wheat bran, cellulose, and oat bran fiber on fecal mutagenicity in healthy humans, Reddy et al. (8) documented decreased fecal mutagenic activity in subjects on wheat bran fiber and cellulose supplementation, whereas no measurable inhibition was observed during oat bran supplementation. The results of this study also indicated that wheat bran and cellulose fiber caused a decrease in the concentration of fecal secondary bile acids (shown to have a tumor-promoting effect in the large bowel). No such effect was observed during oat fiber supplementation; to the contrary, total and secondary bile acid fecal excretion increased during this intervention. In a previous study, Reddy et al. (89) documented similar reductions in both mutagenetic activity and bile acid concentrations following dietary supplementation of healthy subjects with 11 g/day of whole grain cereal fiber (whole wheat and rye) in the form of bread.

Investigators at the University of Arizona Cancer Center currently are analyzing the results of a phase II randomized double-binded polyp trial conducted in Sun City, Arizona. In this sample of 100 resected colorectal adenoma patients, a high fiber supplement in the form of cereal plus calcium (13.5 g/day of wheat bran, 250 mg of elemental calcium) was compared to a low fiber supplement plus calcium (2 g/day, 250 mg, respectively). The endpoints of this study included (a) inhibition of [^{3}H]-thymidine labeling in rectal mucosa crypts and 24-hour outgrowth cultures of unaffected flat rectal mucosal biopsy samples, and (b) lowering of fecal bile acid concentrations, specifically deoxycholic acid. The high fiber cereal was associated with good overall compliance ($\geq$75%) with an average rate of 93.3% for the one-year trial. The supplement was associated with excellent gastrointestinal tolerance among this sample of older adults. Only a few cases of mild gastrointestinal toxicity were reported. The most common side effect reported was an increase in flatus (2%) and a change in bowel habits (3%), considered acceptable to most patients. Similar toxicity levels were observed with respect to toxicity in blood and urine samples. Regarding the DNA-labeling index technique, the University of Arizona investigators have just started a study to compared [^{3}H]-thymidine to bromodeoxyuridine (BrdU) indices, an alternative method to be used in colonic proliferation studies. Preliminary results have revealed a high correlation between them ($r = 0.78$), suggesting that BrdU may be a feasible alternative, even though BrdU indices were somewhat lower than those obtained by [^{3}H]-thymidine labeling (90).

We also initiated recently a phase III randomized, placebo-controlled trial to evaluate the efficacy of supplemental wheat bran fiber in the prevention of colon polyp recurrence. This trial is evaluating the activity of a 13.5-g wheat bran supplement in patients with a history of at least one resected adenomatous polyp. As a secondary endpoint, this study will analyze the epithelial cell proliferation rates of rectal mucosal crypts in a subsample of 250 patients, utilizing BrdU assays. The recruitment goal of the study is 950 patients, and it is expected to achieve full accrual within 3 years. Biopsies are to be performed at study entry and at the end of years 1, 3, and 5. Dietary intakes, toxicity, and compliance levels are monitored throughout the study.

SUPPLEMENTAL CALCIUM AND COLORECTAL CANCER PREVENTION

Intracellular calcium plays a vital role in many cellular processes; it is certainly essential in the regulation of cellular proliferation (91). Recent laboratory studies in humans (31,92) and animals (93–95) suggest a protective effect of dietary calcium in colon cancer etiology. Two clinical studies have demonstrated than an excess of 1250 mg/day of dietary calcium lowered the rectal crypt LI of patients with familial colon cancer (31,68). In a laboratory study, Buset and collaborators (92) found a decrease in the LI of patients with familial polyposis, adenomas, and colon cancer after a 4–8 week period of 1500 mg/day of calcium supplementation. Similar decrements in LI were observed in patients with sporadic adenomas after 10 weeks of calcium glutonate-lactate supplementation (68). A study in laboratory animals has documented that reducing the calcium intake in the diets of rodents from 0.5% (rodent RDA) to 0.1% (human RDA) increased rectal epithelial cell proliferation when exposed to 0.5% cholic acid (96). In a similar study, Bird and Stamp (93) found that cell proliferation decreased monotonically with increasing calcium supplementation (0.1 to 1.0%), in both experimental and control groups. The groups fed 0.1% calcium plus 0.25% cholic acid showed significantly ($p \leq 0.05$) higher values for LI and position of the uppermost labelled cells, compared to those associated with the 1.0% calcium plus 0.25% cholic acid.

There are a limited number of epidemiologic studies investigating the association between calcium and cancer risk (19). Even though the evidence is not striking, it suggests an inverse relationship between calcium intake and colon cancer incidence. Slattery et al. (15) observed this inverse association in a study conducted in Utah with members of the Church of Jesus of Latter-day Saints (JCL) and Seventh-day Adventists (SDA) as compared to the U.S. population. Both groups had calcium intake—mainly milk—higher than the national average and abstained from alcohol, tea, coffee, and cigarettes; however, the JCLs had a similar consumption of meats and fats to that of the U.S. population. Similar associations were observed in Scandinavia when colon cancer incidence and calcium intake of a rural area of Finland was compared to Copenhagen, Denmark—an urban area (97). Rural Finns had higher calcium intakes and a lower incidence of colon cancer than urban Danes. However, other studies from the region have documented a higher consumption of dietary fiber by rural Finns (14,17) as compared to the urban Danes (98), which suggests the possibility of confounding factors.

Similar findings regarding calcium intake and colorectal cancer mortality rates were reported in an ecological study comparing 24 counties in Sweden (62). However, in this study the associations between fat and fiber intakes and colon cancer risk were also evaluated. An inverse association between fiber and colon cancer risk was documented. No association between fat consumption and cancer was found, suggesting that the protective effect of calcium and fiber prevail despite high consumption of fat. In the Melbourne case-control colorectal study (46), a low intake of milk drinks was identified as a colon cancer risk factor for both males and females, whereas in similar case-control studies (99,100) no relationship between calcium intake and colon cancer risk was observed. Negri et al. (100) suggest that the average range of calcium intake consumed in Italy and most Western countries (0.5–1.5 g/day) has no significant impact on colon cancer risk. Higginson (101), studying 340 cases and 1020 controls, observed higher consumption of milk and milk products among controls than cases, however, no statistical difference was obtained. Although further research is needed, preliminary data suggest that the hypothesized relationship between calcium and colon cancer risk should be further investigated. Some clinical trials evaluating such possible links are being conducted presently in the United States. Dr. John Potter of the University of Minnesota is conducting a phase II double-blinded randomized placebo controlled trial of 1 vs. 2 g of elemental calcium (carbonate) per day in adenomatous polyp patients. Proliferate compartment labeling indices in rectal mucosal crypts serve as the endpoint for this study. Rectal mucosal biopsies are obtained at entry and again at months 1, 2, and 6 (102). Additionally, Dr. John Baron of Dartmouth University is coordinating a multiinstitutional clinical trial with the same objective, the examination of the role of calcium in the prevention of colon polyp recurrence. After a 3-month run-in period, patients are randomized to either 1200 mg of elemental calcium (carbonate) per day or placebo for a 4-year period. Colonoscopies are performed at entry and subsequently in years 1 and 4 to document the presence or absence of polyp recurrence. According to Dr. Baron, this study has accrued approximately three quarters of the necessary number with a goal of 850 evaluable participants (103). Finally, we have completed recently a randomized phase II trial of 1500 mg/day elemental calcium (carbonate) vs. wheat bran fiber (13.5 g/day), vs. the combination of fiber plus calcium, vs. placebo in 100 patients with adenomatous polyps. The [^{3}H]-thymidine labeling index and fecal bile acid concentration data from this study currently are undergoing final analysis.

VITAMIN D IN THE PREVENTION OF COLON CANCER

The role of calcium and other cofactors which facilitate its transport, such as vitamin D, is important to the understanding of the molecular processes of tumorigenesis. Little is known about the potential impact of vitamin D on cancer risk; however, preliminary laboratory—in vitro and animal—studies suggest that vitamin D might be a promising cancer preventive agent. Studies of cell cultures have shown antiproliferative and differentiation effects for this vitamin in HS695T melanoma cells (104), breast cancer cells (105), and leukemic cells (106–108). Likewise, topical application of $1\alpha,25(OH)_2D_3$ was shown to inhibit induction of ODC (109,110) and tumor production (111,112) in rodent skin, stomach, colon, and liver tissues (113). However, Kuroki et al. (114) found that $1\alpha,25(OH)_2D_3$ was also involved in tumor promotion in some cell culture studies. This discrepancy suggests that further investigation is required. In a 19-year cohort study with 1954 men, Garland and associates (115) found colorectal cancer to be inversely correlated to vitamin D ($p < 0.05$) and calcium ($p < 0.05$). The association remained significant after adjusting for age, smoking, alcohol consumption, body mass, and percentage of calories obtained from fat. Nevertheless, human epidemiologic and intervention studies of the cancer prevention effect of vitamin D are yet to be developed. At the present time vitamin D seems like an interesting new agent that should be pursued.

CONCLUSIONS

Evidence from laboratory studies show that alterations in normal cells induced by carcinogenic exposure at the initiation stage are irreversible; however, there is increasing evidence suggesting that the process of promotion may be reversed by removing or neutralizing the chemical insult. The results of recent epidemiologic and clinical studies of the effects of dietary factors on the promotion or prevention of colorectal cancer suggest that high consumption of fat may promote the carcinogenic process, whereas dietary fiber and intakes of supplemental calcium and cofactors facilitating its transport, such as vitamin D, may slow the process.

Up to the present time, epidemiologic and laboratory studies have provided inconclusive observations regarding the role of dietary factors in cancer prevention, suggesting that this question may only be resolved conclusively by intervention trials. Dietary clinical trials for colon cancer prevention have been undertaken recently. Only a few, relatively small, phase II and phase III trials have been completed thus far. The methodologic strategies that underlie the design of these trials are being developed at the same time that the investigations are being run. The novelty of these trials has presented numerous challenges and difficulties to the multidisciplinary teams of investigators involved in their completion. New approaches are continuing to be developed to deal with these methodologic issues.

One of the most innovative cancer prevention strategies is the use of precancerous lesions as study endpoints. Monitoring precancerous manifestations has the advantage of requiring a relatively small number of subjects and producing results more rapidly. However, even if a significant finding is documented, we can only speculate about its effect on cancer incidence and/or mortality.

There continue to be a number of methodologic issues related to the successful completion of cancer prevention clinical trials. First, there is an immediate need for more specific and precise intermediate markers of cancer risk (e.g., bromodeoxyuridine, labeling index in rectal mucosal crypts). The identification and availability of such markers and/or precursor lesions enables investigators to pursue cost-effective research, testing hypotheses and developing new strategies for cancer prevention. Thus, development of more specific, less complex, and easily reproduced intermediate marker assays is an important research goal for the future.

A second issue under debate is the development of prevention strategies using specific single nutrients in lieu of food groups or a combination of nutrients. Unfortunately, the complexity and variety of the human diet and the problems investigators have faced evaluating it have weakened the single-nutrient perspective. Researchers (116,117) argue in favor of testing the effect of more complex variables (i.e., combinations of nutrients, food groups, or foods) to be able to examine potential synergistic effects of various dietary components. On the other hand, it is not clear from the current data whether a single dietary change (e.g., increase in fiber consumption) can produce a long-lasting alteration required to prevent colon cancer in healthy populations. A better understanding is needed concerning the interaction between the multiple nutrients that have preventive activities.

Dietary assessment as analyzed by Block and Hartman (118) is a third controversial issue. Discovering relationships between dietary factors and cancer depends primarily on our ability to accurately assess dietary patterns. Currently, all dietary assessment methods are flawed to some degree by errors due to imprecision and misclassification. It is clear that the field has improved, but further work remains to reduce error and to improve the accuracy of the instruments available. Finally, a better understanding is also needed concerning the biological, biochemical, and pharmacologic mechanisms by which nutrients interact and affect human colorectal physiology.

A fourth important barrier to the successful completion of prevention trials involves participant adherence. Some features common to these studies that could have an adverse impact on adherence include: (a) a requirement for dietary changes of long-term duration (usually one or more years); (b) the consumption of food products available to the general public (i.e., vitamins, minerals, cereals, breads, etc.) leading to the possibility of trial contamination; and (c) the need for a strict protocol involving multiple clinic visits, interviews, questionnaires, record keeping, and clinical tests and/or biopsies. Unfortunately, this area of research has tended to be neglected and many questions regarding patient adherence to interventions remain unanswered. It should not be forgotten that the level of adherence can affect the appraisal of the efficacy and safety of a dietary regimen, and it can make or brake the power and validity of a study (119–121). Greater emphasis and resources need to be committed to study this critical area of behavioral research.

As mentioned earlier, the National Cancer Institute is currently sponsoring several cancer prevention trials to evaluate the effects of dietary component interventions (e.g., fat reduction, vegetable and fiber increases, and calcium and/or fiber supplementation) utilizing as endpoints human rectal mucosal proliferation rates or recurrence rates of premalignant lesions such as adenomas. The results of such studies should help to determine the potential importance of such dietary interventions in the reduction of colorectal cancer risk. However, the goal of cancer prevention is the reduction of cancer incidence and mortality, and the achievement of such a goal will be the ultimate test of each particular dietary intervention.

REFERENCES

1. M. Shike, S. J. Winawer, P. H. Greenwald, A. Bloch, M. J. Hill, and S. V. Swaroop. *Bull. World Health Organ., 68*, 377-385 (1990).
2. American Cancer Society, *Cancer Facts and Figures*, American Cancer Society, New York, 1990.
3. Gastrointestinal Tumor Study Group, *N. Engl. J. Med., 310*, 737–743 (1984).
4. P. Correa, W. Haenszel, in *Advances in Cancer Research* (G. Klein and S. Weinhouse, eds.), Academic Press, New York, 1978, p. 26.
5. D. P. Burkitt, in *Colorectal Cancer: Prevention, Epidemiology and Screening* (S. Winawer, D. Schottenfeld, and P. Sherlock, eds.) Raven Press, New York, 1980, pp. 13–18.
6. E. L. Wynder and B. S. Reddy, *Semin. Oncol., 10*, 264-272 (1983).
7. H. J. Freeman, G. A. Spiller, and Y. S. Kim, *Cancer Res., 38*, 2912 (1978).
8. B. S. Reddy, A. Engle, S. Katsifis, et al., *Cancer Res., 49*, 4629–4635 (1989).
9. B. S. Reddy, in *Dietary Fiber in Health and Disease* (G. V. Vahouny and D. Kritchevsky, eds.), Plenum Press, New York, 1982, pp. 265-286.

10. W. Willet, *Nature, 338*, 389-394 (1989).
11. L. A. Cannon-Albright, M. H. Skolnick, D. T. Bishop, R. G. Lee, and R. W. Burt, *N. Engl. J. Med., 19*, 533-537 (1988).
12. R. Doll and R. Peto, *JNCI, 66*, 1191-1308 (1981).
13. B. S. Reddy, A. Hedges, K. Laakso, and E. L. Wynder, *Cancer, 42*, 2832-2838 (1978).
14. B. S. Reddy, A. Hedges, K. Laakso, and E. L. Wynder, *Cancer Lett., 4*, 217-222 (1978).
15. M. L. Slattery, A. W. Sorenson, and M. H. Ford, *Am. J. Epidemiol., 128*, 504-514 (1988).
16. M. L. Slattery, A. W. Sorenson, A. W. Mahoney, T. K. French, D. Kritchevsky, and J. C. Street, *JNCI, 80*, 1474-1480 (1988).
17. D. W. West, in *Banbury Report 4: Cancer Incidence in Defined Populations* (J. Cairns, J. L. Lyon, M. Skolnick, eds.), Cold Spring Harbor Laboratory, Cold Spring Harbor, NY, 1980, pp. 31-49.
18. H. L. Newmark, M. J. Wargovich, and W. R. Bruce. *JNCI, 72*, 1323-1325 (1984).
19. A. W. Sorenson, M. L. Slattery, and M. H. Ford, *Nutr. Cancer, 11*, 135-145 (1988).
20. L. R. Jacobs, in *Essential Nutrients in Carcinogenesis* (L. A. Poirier, P. M. Newberne, M. W. Pariza, eds.), Plenum Press, New York, 1986, pp. 1320-1329.
21. D. M. Klurferd and D. Kritchevsky, in *Essential Nutrients in Carcinogenesis* (L. A. Poirier, P. M. Newberne, M. W. Pariza, eds.), Plenum Press, New York, 1986, pp. 119-136.
22. V. G. Vogel and R. S. McPherson, *Hematol. Oncol. Clin. North Am., 3*, 35-63 (1989).
23. B. C. Morson, *Proc. R. Soc. Med., 67*, 454 (1974).
24. B. Vogelstein, E. R. Fearon, and S. R. Hamilton. *N. Engl. J. Med., 319*, 525 (1988).
25. S. J. Winawer, L. S. Gottlief, E. T. Stewart, A. Zauber, and B. Diaz, *Gastrointest. Endosc., 30*, 147 (abstr) (1984).
26. D. A. Gilbert, S. L. Shaneyfelt, F. E. Silverstein, A. K. Mahler, A. P. Hallstrom, and 674 members of the ASGE, *Gastrointest. Endosc., 30*, 143 (1984).
27. F. A. Macrae and C. B. Williams, *Gastrointest. Endosc., 28*, 138 (1982).
28. H. Nava, G. Carlsson, N. J. Petrelli, L. Herrera, and A. Mittelman, *Dis. Colon Rectum, 30*, 465-468 (1987).
29. A. J. Holtzman, J. B. Poulard, S. Bank, L. R. Levin, G. W. Flint, R. J. Strauss, and I. B. Margolis, *Dis. Colon Rectum, 30*, 185-188 (1987).
30. M. Lipkin, W. A. Blatter, J. F. Fraumeni, H. T. Lynch, E. E. Deschner, and S. Winawer, *Cancer Res., 43*, 1899-1904 (1983).
31. M. Lipkin and H. L. Newmark, *N. Engl. J. Med., 313*, 1381-1384 (1985).
32. B. H. Patterson and S. Piantadosi, in *Nutrition and Cancer Prevention: Investigating the Role of Micronutrients* (T. E. Moon and M. S. Micozzi, eds.), Marcel Dekker, New York, 1989, p. 491-512.
33. American Heart Association, *Circulation, 69*, 1065A-1069A (1984).
34. A. P. Boyar, D. P. Rose, and E. L. Wynder, *Am. J. Clin. Nutr., 48*, 896S-900S (1988).
35. A. J. Stunkard, in *Eating and Weight Disorders: Advances in Treatment and Research* (R. K. Goldstein, ed.), Springer Press, New York, 1983.

36. J. M. Dunbar and A. Stunkard, in *Nutrition, Lipids and Coronary Heart Disease* (R. Levy, B. Rifkin, B. Dennis, and N. Ernst, eds.), Raven Press, New York, 1979, pp. 391–423.
37. W. C. Willett, M. J. Stampfer, G. A. Colditz, B. A. Rosner, and F. E. Speizer, *N. Engl. J. Med.*, *323*, 1664–1672 (1990).
38. B. Armstrong and R. Doll, *Int. J. Cancer, 15*, 617–631 (1975).
39. D. P. Rose, A. P. Boyar, and E. L. Wynder, *Cancer, 58*, 2363–2371 (1986).
40. M. Jain, G. M. Cook, F. G. Davis, M. G. Grace, G. R. Howe, and A. B. Miller, *Int. J. Cancer, 26*, 757–768 (1980).
41. J. D. Potter and A. J. McMichael, *JNCI, 76*, 557–569 (1986).
42. J. L. Lyon, A. W. Mahoney, D. W. West, et al., *JNCI, 78*, 853–861 (1987).
43. S. Graham, J. Marshall, B. Haughey, et al., *Am. J. Epidemiol.*, *128*, 490–503 (1988).
44. J. B. Bristol, P. M. Emmett, K. W. Heaton, and R. C. N. Williamson, *BMJ, 291*, 1467–1470 (1985).
45. G. A. Kune and S. Kune, *Nutr. Cancer, 9*, 1–4 (1987).
46. G. A. Kune, S. Kune, and L. F. Watson, *Br. J. Surg.*, *74*, 1064–1065 (1987).
47. S. Kune, G. A. Kune, and L. F. Watson, *Nutr. Cancer, 9*, 21–42 (1987).
48. E. G. Knox, *Br. J. Prev. Soc. Med.*, *31*, 71 (1977).
49. B. S. Reddy, T. Narisawa, D. Vukusich, J. H. Weisburger, and E. L. Wynder, *Proc. Soc. Exp. Biol. Med.*, *151*, 237–239 (1976).
50. B. S. Reddy, S. Mangat, A. Sheinfil, J. H. Weisburger, and E. L. Wynder, *Cancer Res.*, *37*, 2132–2137 (1977).
51. N. D. Nigro, D. V. Singh, R. L. Campbell, and M. Sook, *JNCI, 54*, 439–442 (1975).
52. S. A. Broitman, J. J. Vitale, E. Vavrousek-Jakuba, and L. S. Gottlieb, *Cancer, 40*, 2455–2463 (1977).
53. K. M. Nauss, M. Locniskar, and P. M. Newberne, *Cancer Res.*, *43*, 4083–4090 (1983).
54. M. J. Hill, in *Origins of Human Cancer* (H. H. Hiatt, J. D. Watson, J. A. Winsten, eds.), Cold Spring Harbor, New York, 1977, pp. 1627–1640.
55. B. S. Reddy, *Cancer Res.*, *41*, 3766–3768 (1981).
56. G. Macquart-Moulin, R. Fiboli, J. Cornee, B. Charnay, P. Bertherene, and N. Dan, *Int. J. Cancer, 38*, 183–191 (1986).
57. J. L. Berta, T. Coste, J. Rautureau, M. Guilloud-Bataille, and G. Pequignot, *Gastroenterol. Clin. Biol.*, *9*, 348–353 (1985).
58. A. J. Tuyns, M. Haelterman, and R. Kaaks, *Nutr. Cancer, 10*, 181–196 (1987).
59. J. L. Lyon and A. W. Sorenson, *Am. J. Clin. Nutr.*, *31*, S227 (1978).
60. S. Bingham, D. R. Williams, T. J. Cole, and W. P. T. James, *Br. J. Cancer, 40*, 456 (1979).
61. L. N. Kolonel and L. L. Marchand, in *Dietary Fat and Cancer* (C. Ip et al., eds.), Alan R. Liss, New York, 1986.
62. M. Rosen, L. Nystrom, and S. Wall, *Am. J. Epidemiol.*, *127*, 42–49 (1988).
63. G. N. Stemmerman, A. M. Y. Nomura, and L. Heilbrun, *Cancer Res.*, *44*, 4633–4637 (1984).
64. Committee on Diet, Nutrition and Cancer, Assembly of Life Sciences, National Research Council, *Diet Nutrition and Cancer*, National Academy Press, Washington, DC, 1982, pp. 5–22.

65. C. Bain, R. MacLennan, M. Ward, M. Wahlqvist, F. Macrae, P. Gaffney, J. Lambert, H. Gratten, D. Battistutta, and K. Goulson, *Proc. Nutr. Aust.*, 80-87 (1990).
66. J. J. DeCosse, H. H. Miller, and M. L. Lesser, *JNCI, 81*, 1290–1297 (1989).
67. D. S. Alberts, J. Einspahr, S. Rees-McGee, P. Ramanujam, M. K. Buller, L. Clark, C. Ritenbaugh, J. Atwood, P. Pethigal, D. Earnest, H. Villar, J. Phelps, M. Lipkin, M. Wargovich, and F. L. Meyskens. *JNCI, 82*, 1280–1285 (1990).
68. P. Rozen, Z. Fireman, N. Fine, Y. Wax, and E. Ron, *Gut, 30*, 650 (1989).
69. G. Isbell, P-J Hu, F. Lanza, et al., *Gastroenterology, 96*, A228 (1989).
70. M. L. Clark and T. B. Hernandez, in *Summary of Literature Review of Epidemiologic and Metabolic Studies in Humans* (JWK, ed.), prepared for the Diet and Cancer Branch, Division of Cancer Prevention and Control, National Cancer Institute, 1984.
71. P. Greenwald. *Dietary Fiber and Lower Colon Cancer Risk: A Statement from the Director's Office*, Division of Cancer Prevention and Control, National Cancer Institute, 1984.
72. P. Greenwald, E. Lanza, and G. A. Eddy, *J. Am. Diet. Assoc., 87*, 1178–1188 (1987).
73. P. Greenwald and K. M. Witkin, *JNCI, 81*, 1272-1273 (1989).
74. D. W. Heitman, V. A. Ord, K. E. Hunter, and I. L. Cameron, *Cancer Res., 49*, 5581–5585 (1989).
75. G. E. McKeown-Eyssen, and E. Bright-See, *Nutr. Cancer, 6*, 160–170 (1984).
76. B. S. Reddy, A. Engle, S. Katsifis, B. Simi, H-P. Bartram, P. Perrino, and C. Mahan, *Cancer Res., 49*, 4629–4635 (1989).
77. A. J. Tuyns, R. Kaaks, and M. Haelterman, *Nutr. Cancer, 11*, 189-204 (1988).
78. L. R. Jacobs, *Cancer Res., 44*, 2458 (1984).
79. L. R. Jacobs, *Cancer Res., 43*, 4057 (1983).
80. L. R. Jacobs and J. R. Lupton, *Am. J. Physiol., 246*, G378–G385 (1984).
81. J. D. Potter, A. J. McMichael, and A. Z. Bonett, *Proc. Nutr. Soc. Aust.*, 117, 123 (1982).
82. J. W. Tollison and J. W. Griffin, *Am. Fam. Phys., 22*, 121–125 (1988).
83. H. J. Freeman, *Clin. Res., 29*, 32A (1981).
84. H. J. Freeman, G. A. Spiller and Y. S. Kim, *Cancer Res., 40*, 2661-2665 (1980).
85. H. J. Freeman, *Clin. Res., 29*, 32A (1981).
86. B. S. Reddy and H. Mori, *Carcinogenesis, 2*, 21-25 (1981).
87. B. S. Reddy, H. Mori, and M. Nicolais, *Cancer Inst., 66*, 553-557 (1981).
88. P. Smith-Barbaro, D. Hansen, and B. S. Reddy, *JNCI, 67*, 495–497 (1981).
89. B. S. Reddy, C. Sharma, B. Darby Simi, et al., *Cancer Res., 47*, 644–648 (1987).
90. J. Einsphar, J. Hixson, D. S. Alberts, D. Durbin, K. Pennie, J. Davison, D. McGee, and H. Garewall, AGA/AASLD Abstracts. New Orleans, LA, May 19–22, 1991.
91. H. Hennings, D. Michael, C. Cheng, P. Steinert, K. Holbrook, and S. H. Yuspa, *Cell, 19*, 245 (1980).
92. M. Buset, M. Lipkin, S. Winawer, S. Swaroop, and E. Friedman, *Cancer Res., 46*, 5426–5430 (1986).
93. R. P. Bird and D. Stamp, *Cancer Lett., 31*, 61-67 (1986).
94. M. J. Wargovich, V. W. S. Eng, and H. L. Newmark, *Cancer, 23*, 253–258 (1984).
95. M. J. Wargovich, V. W. S. Eng, H. L. Newmark, and W. R. Bruce, *Carcinogenesis, 9*, 1205–1207 (1983).

96. M. J. Wargovich and A. R. Baer, *Prev. Med.*, *18*, 672–679 (1989).
97. O. M. Jensen, R. McLennan, and J. Wahrendork, *Nutr. Cancer*, *4*, 5–19 (1982).
98. R. McLennan, O. M. Jensen, J. Mosbech, and H. Vuori, *Am. J. Clin. Nutr.*, *31*, S239–242 (1978).
99. O. Manousos, N. E. Day, D. Trichopoulos, et al., *Int. J. Cancer*, *32*, 1–5 (1983).
100. E. Negri, C. LaVecchia, B. D'Avanzo, and S. Franceschi, *Nutr. Cancer*, *13*, 255–262 (1990).
101. J. Higginson, *JNCI*, *37*, 527–545 (1966).
102. J. D. Potter, personal communication, March 1991.
103. J. Baron, personal communication, February 1991.
104. K. Colston, M. J. Colston, and D. Feldman, *Endocrinology*, 108, 1083 (1981).
105. J. A. Eisman, I. McIntyre, T. Martin, and J. M. Moseley, *Lancet*, *2*, 1335 (1979).
106. E. Abe, H. Miyaura, M. Sakagami, K. Takeda, T. Konno, S. Yamasaki, S. Yoshiki, and T. Suda, *Proc. Natl. Acad. Sci. USA*, *78*, 4990 (1981).
107. R. Munsker, A. Norman, and H. P. Koeffler, *J. Clin. Invest.*, *78*, 424 (1986).
108. C. Miyaura, E. Abe, T. Kuribayashi, H. Tanaka, K. Honno, Y. Nishii, and T. Suda, *Biochem. Biophys. Res. Commun.*, *102*, 937–943 (1981).
109. K. Chida, H. Hashiba, T. Suda, and T. Kuroki, *Cancere Res.*, *44*, 1387–1391 (1984).
110. K. Chida, H. Hashiba, M. Fukushima, T. Suda, and T. Kuroki, *Cancer Res.*, *45*, 5426 (1985).
111. A. W. Wood, R. L. Chang, M. T. Huang, M. Uskokovic, and A. H. Conney, *Biochem. Biophys. Res. Commun.*, *116*, 605 (1983).
112. A. W. Wood, R. L. Chang, M. T. Huang, E. Baggiolini, J. J. Partridge, M. Uskokovic, and A. H. Conney, *Biochem. Biophys. Res. Commun.*, *130*, 924 (1985).
113. H. Hashiba, M. Fukushima, K. Chida, and T. Kuroki, *Cancer Res.*, *47*, 5031–5035 (1987).
114. T. Kuroki, K. Chida, H. Hashiba, J. Hosoi, J. Hosomi, K. Sasaki, E. Abe, and T. Suda, *Carcinogenesis*, *10*, 275–286 (1985).
115. C. Garland, R. B. Shekelle, E. Barrett-Connor, M. H. Criqui, A. H. Rossof, and O. Paul, *Lancet*, *1*, 307–309 (1985).
116. F. L. Meyskens, in *Nutrition and Cancer Prevention: Investigating the Role of Micronutrients* (T. E. Moon and M. S. Micozzi, eds.), Marcel Dekker, New York, 1989, pp. 569–576.
117. M. S. Micozzi, in *Nutrition and Cancer Prevention: Investigating the Role of Micronutrients* (T. E. Moon and M. S. Micozzi, eds.). Marcel Dekker, New York, 1989, pp. 213–242.
118. G. Block, A. M. Hartman, in *Nutrition and Cancer Prevention: Investigating the Role of Micronutrients* (T. E. Moon and M. S. Micozzi, eds.), Marcel Dekker, New York, 1989, pp. 159–180.
119. T. E. Moon, *Stat. in Med.*, *5*, 435 (1986).
120. T. Pullar, S. Kumar, and M. Feely, *J. Rheum. Dis.*, *48*, 871–875 (1989).
121. A. R. Feinstein, in *Compliance with Therapeutic Regins* (D. L. Sackett and R. B. Haynes, eds.), John Hopkins University Press, Baltimore, MD, 1976.

18

Dietary Intervention Trials on Prostate Cancer

Laurence N. Kolonel
University of Hawaii
Honolulu, Hawaii

Abraham M. Y. Nomura
Kuakini Medical Center
and University of Hawaii
Honolulu, Hawaii

INTRODUCTION

Prostate cancer is the second leading cancer in incidence among U.S. men (1). It is estimated that 122,000 men will be diagnosed with this disease in 1991, and that 32,000 men will die from it (2). The incidence appears to be increasing, although this may be a diagnostic artifact related to increased surgical intervention (transurethral resection or prostatectomy) for benign prostatic hypertrophy (3). As a consequence of the morbidity and mortality associated with this very high incidence, substantial medical and psychosocial costs can be attributed to this cancer. Thus, control of prostate cancer, especially through primary prevention, would have a significant impact on the overall burden of cancer among U.S. men. Logically, practical measures for primary prevention would best follow from a clear knowledge of the causal factors for the disease.

Unfortunately, the etiology of this cancer is unknown. Although a growing body of evidence points to a role of diet, especially among older men (see below), the inconclusiveness of this evidence precludes the implementation of any meaningful public health control measures at present. This chapter considers the evidence regarding diet and prostate cancer, factors that need to be considered in determining the appropriateness of a dietary intervention trial, and whether such a trial at this time would likely clarify the role of diet, particularly macronutrients, in the etiology of this cancer.

OVERVIEW OF EPIDEMIOLOGIC EVIDENCE ON DIETARY AND RELATED RISK FACTORS FOR PROSTATE CANCER

Dietary Fat

The epidemiologic data on dietary fat and prostate cancer are discussed in detail in Chapter 10 and are summarized in Table 1. The data from ecologic and case-control studies (4–15) are very consistent in supporting a role of dietary fat. The only exception is the study by Ohno and colleagues (12), which was conducted in Japan, a country where fat intake is very much lower than in the United States and Europe. While most studies did not identify the specific type of fat responsible for the observed effect, the available data point to animal and saturated fats rather than vegetable or unsaturated fats (see Table 1).

Data from five cohort studies (16–20) have been reported, and the numbers of cases are generally fewer than those for the case-control studies. The data related to dietary fat, however, are not so convincing in these reports as in the case-control studies. The studies of Hirayama (16), Hsing and colleagues (20), and Severson et al. (18) show no association with meat or fat intake, although the report of Severson does show a borderline positive association with intake of butter/margarine/cheese and eggs. Although the two studies among Seventh-day Adventists (17,19) show positive relationships for meat and dairy products, the relative risks are not statistically significant. The lack of highly supportive data from cohort studies, although based on few reports as yet, tempers somewhat the conclusion on dietary fat from the case-control studies.

It should be noted that hormonal factors have also been associated with prostate cancer and may be related to the etiology of the disease (21). Since androgen and estrogen levels in men appear to be influenced by alterations in the level of fat in the diet (22–23), these two putative risk factors may be closely related.

Vitamin A/Carotenoids

The second major area of interest in diet and prostate cancer pertains to vitamin A and related compounds. The findings from both case-control studies (7–15,24–26) and cohort studies (17–20,27–29) are summarized in Table 2 and are altogether inconsistent. Some reports have suggested that retinol and/or carotenoids (especially β-carotene) increase the risk of prostate cancer (8,9,20,24,27), especially among men aged 70 and above (8,24,27). Such an effect, if real, would be a basis for concern, since these compounds in general have been highlighted as potential cancer preventive agents. However, other reports have shown protective effects against prostate cancer from intake of β-carotene or foods high in carotenoid content (7,11,12,14), although the age relationships are inconsistent among studies.

It is possible that the protective effect of β-carotene emerges only among men with a relatively low dietary fat intake (11). It is also possible that the adverse effect is not due to β-carotene but to some other constituent of fruits, as suggested by the study of Le Marchand et al. (30) and by the fact that β-carotene estimated from fruits alone showed a positive association with prostate cancer in the study of Ohno and colleagues in Japan (12). Thus, at present it is premature to state that vitamin A and/or particular carotenoids either increase or decrease the risk of prostate cancer.

Cadmium

Although there is much interest in the role of cadmium in the etiology of prostate cancer, the data on dietary intake of cadmium and this cancer are fragmentary at the present time. Kolonel and Winkelstein (31) found that an index of cadmium exposure (based on cadmium exposure from cigarette smoking, diet, and occupational inhalation) was somewhat higher in prostate cancer cases than controls, but dietary exposure alone was not higher in the cases. A recent report of a study among Mormons in Utah (32) also showed a borderline significant increase in risk of prostate cancer for any of these same three sources of exposure and a nonsignificant increase when diet alone was considered. Nevertheless, some studies based solely on occupational exposure to cadmium have suggested a positive association (33). The plausibility of this relationship is increased by the evidence of carcinogenicity of cadmium in laboratory animals (33) and by the observation that in humans cadmium concentrates heavily in the prostate gland, where it may act as an antagonist of zinc (34).

Other Dietary Factors

Epidemiologic evidence for other dietary factors and prostate cancer is meager. Vitamin C was positively associated with risk in one case-control study (8), but not another (13). Similarly, zinc intake was positively associated with prostate cancer in one case-control study (13), but not another (15). In a cohort study among Japanese men in Hawaii, prostate cancer was positively associated with consumption of seaweed, and inversely associated with consumption of rice/tofu and black tea (18,35). In a cohort of Seventh-day Adventist men (19), there was an inverse association of prostate cancer with frequency of intake of beans, lentils, and peas.

Summary

The role of diet in the etiology of prostate cancer is not yet clear. The strongest evidence pertains to dietary fat, especially saturated fat. The data are not entirely consistent, however, and somewhat troublesome is the lack of strong support from cohort studies. Dietary fat may act as a prostate carcinogen by influencing serum and tissue androgen levels.

Table 1 Epidemiologic Studies of Dietary Fat and Prostate Cancer

Investigator, year (Ref.)	Location	No. of subjects	Major findings[a]
		Ecologic Studies	
Howell, 1974 (4)	International	Correlations among 41 countries	Positive association of mortality with per capita intake of meat, milk, and fats ($r = 0.7$).
Blair and Fraumeni, 1978 (5)	U.S.	Correlations among 4 regions	Positive association of mortality with average household consumption of high fat foods.
Kolonel et al., 1981 (6)	Hawaii	Correlations among 5 ethnic groups	Positive association of incidence with age-specific intakes of animal and saturated fat ($r = 0.9$).
		Case-Control Studies	
Schuman et al., 1982 (7)	Minneapolis–St. Paul, Minnesota	223 cases 223 neighborhood controls	No association with meat; suggested positive association with ice cream and eggs.
Graham et al., 1983 (8)	Buffalo, NY	262 cases 259 hospital controls	Positive association in men ≥ 70 years with total fat (RR = 1.9, linear trend NS), and animal fat (RR = 3.2, linear trend $p < 0.05$).
Heshmat et al., 1985 (9)	Washington, DC	180 cases 180 hospital controls	Positive association with total and saturated fat (especially consumption at ages 30–49, $p < 0.10$).
Talamini et al., 1986 (10)	Pordenone, Italy	166 cases 202 hospital controls	Positive association with meat (RR = 1.7, $p = 0.05$), milk/dairy products (RR = 2.5, $p < 0.05$).
Ross et al., 1987 (11)	Los Angeles, CA	142 black and 142 white cases 142 black and 142 white population controls	Positive association with fat (RR = 1.9, $p < 0.05$ for blacks; RR = 1.6, NS for whites).
Ohno et al., 1988 (12)	Kyoto, Japan	100 cases 100 hospital controls	No association with fat (RR = 0.8, NS).

Kolonel et al., 1988 (13)	Oahu, HI	452 cases 899 population controls	Positive association in men ≥70 years with total fat (RR = 1.5, NS), saturated fat (RR = 1.7, $p = 0.05$) and cholesterol (RR = 1.6, $p = 0.05$).
Mettlin et al., 1989 (14)	Buffalo, NY	371 cases 371 hospital controls	Positive association, especially in men <69 years, with animal fat (RR = 1.5, NS), and whole milk (RR = 3.1, $p < 0.05$).
West et al., 1991 (15)	Utah	358 cases 679 population controls	Positive association for aggressive tumors in men 68–74 years with total fat (RR = 2.9, $p = 0.05$), saturated fat (RR = 2.2, NS), monounsaturated fat (RR = 3.6, $p < 0.05$), and polyunsaturated fat (RR = 2.7, $p < 0.05$).
		Cohort Studies	
Hirayama, 1979 (16)	Japan	122,261 men (63 fatal cases)	No association with intake of meat (RR = 0.8[b]).
Snowdon et al., 1984 (17)	California	6,763 Adventist men (99 fatal cases)	Positive association with meat (RR = 1.3, NS) milk (RR = 1.5, NS), cheese (RR = 1.4, NS) and eggs (RR = 1.3, NS).
Severson et al., 1989 (18)	Oahu, HI	7999 Japanese men (174 cases)	No association with total fat (RR = 0.9, NS), saturated fat (RR = 1.0, NS), or meat (RR = 1.0, NS). Positive association with butter/margarine/cheese (RR = 1.5, $p = 0.05$) and eggs (RR = 1.6, $p = 0.05$).
Mills et al., 1989 (19)	California	14,000 Adventist men (180 cases)	Positive association with meat and % calories from animal fat (RR = 1.4, NS).
Hsing et al., 1990 (20)	Minnesota and northeastern U.S.	17,633 Lutheran men (149 cases)	No association with intake of meat (RR = 0.8, NS), eggs (RR = 0.9, NS), or dairy products (RR = 1.0, NS).

[a]Based on extreme quantiles
[b]Estimated from the data
RR = relative risk; NS = not statistically significant.

Although the data on possible protective effects of carotenoids or vitamin A are inconsistent, there is a suggestion of a possible adverse effect. Data on other dietary risk factors for prostate cancer are very limited and weak, and offer no basis for their consideration in intervention trials at this time.

PROSPECTS FOR AN INTERVENTION TRIAL OF DIET AND PROSTATE CANCER

Considerations Favoring a Trial

A number of arguments can be offered for the timeliness and appropriateness of a dietary intervention trial for prostate cancer:

1. As reviewed above, a substantial body of epidemiologic evidence suggests a role of dietary fat as a risk factor for prostate cancer. (Relative risks for total and saturated fat in the case-control studies with positive findings were about 2.0.) Ultimate proof of a causal association, especially when relative risks are low, cannot be obtained from case-control and cohort data alone. Since the results from an intervention trial are closer to experimental evidence, they are thus more conclusive.

In general, an intervention trial would be considered when the evidence from other analytic studies was quite strong and consistent, so that the high costs associated with such a trial could be justified. The intent of the trial would be to provide unequivocal support for the association, so that public health measures to prevent the disease could then be promoted. (Certain other considerations for such a trial are noted below.)

2. The impact of the disease is great. The overall incidence among men in the United States is very high, but among blacks is especially remarkable. The reduced morbidity, medical care costs, and psychosocial dislocation that would attend the primary prevention of prostate cancer would be substantial.

3. The dietary fat hypothesis is plausible and supported by laboratory data, although animal models for the study of fat and prostate cancer are limited (36). Fat could promote prostate carcinogenesis through several potential pathways, such as effects on cellular membrane composition, hormonal balances, and prostaglandin synthesis (33).

4. A trial among elderly adults can be rationalized, since animal data suggest that dietary fat acts as a promoting agent. This is important, since an intervention necessitating implementation at an early age would not be practical, unless some very early marker of the disease were available.

5. The risk: benefit ratio for such a trial would seem to be very favorable. Although there would be little apparent risk from dietary fat reduction itself, atttention would have to be given to maintaining proper balance of other nutrients, since men in the older age groups often have marginal intakes of certain

Table 2 Epidemiologic Studies of Vitamin A/Carotenoids and Prostate Cancer

Investigator, year (Ref.)	Location	No. of subjects	Major findings[a]
		Case-Control Studies	
Schuman et al., 1982 (7)	Minneapolis–St. Paul, Minnesota	223 cases 223 neighborhood controls	Inverse association with carrots (RR = 2.2, NS), tomatoes (RR = 1.4, NS) and peas (RR = 1.5, NS).
Graham et al., 1983 (8)	Buffalo, NY	262 cases 259 hospital controls	Positive association with vitamin A index especially in men ≥70 years (RR = 2.0, linear trend $p < 0.05$).
Heshmat et al., 1985 (9)	Washington, DC	180 cases 180 hospital controls	Positive association with vitamin A (especially consumption at ages 30–49, $p < 0.01$).
Talamini et al., 1986 (10)	Pordenone, Italy	166 cases 202 hospital controls	Positive association with green vegetables (RR = 1.2, NS).
Midleton et al., 1986 (26)	Buffalo, NY	219 cases 1,238 hospital controls	Positive association with vitamin A index (RR = 1.3, NS).
Ross et al., 1987 (11)	Los Angeles, CA	142 black and 142 white cases 142 black and 142 white population controls	Inverse association with β-carotene intake, especially in presence of high fat intake (RR = 1.9–2.0)
Ohno et al., 1988 (12)	Kyoto, Japan	100 cases 100 hospital controls	Inverse association with β-carotene intake (RR = 2.9, $p < 0.05$), especially for men ≥70 years. Inverse association with β-carotene intake from green/yellow vegetables (RR = 2.2, $p < 0.05$). Positive association with β-carotene intake from fruits (RR = 2.0, $p < 0.05$).

Continued

Table 2 *Continued*

Investigator, year (Ref.)	Location	No. of subjects	Major findings[a]
Kolonel et al., 1988 (24)	Oahu, HI	452 cases 899 population controls	Positive association in men ≥70 years with total vitamin A (RR = 2.0, $p < 0.05$), β-carotene (RR = 1.5, NS), and other carotenes (RR = 1.6, $p = 0.05$).
Hayes et al., 1988 (25)	Rotterdam, The Netherlands	134 cases 130 hospital controls	Inverse association with serum retinol (RR = 2.4, $p = 0.04$), and β-carotene (RR = 1.3, NS).
Mettlin et al., 1989 (14)	Buffalo, NY	371 cases 371 hospital controls	Inverse association in men <69 years with β-carotene index (RR = 3.3, $p < 0.05$).
West et al., 1991 (15)	Utah	358 cases 679 population controls	Positive association in men 68–74 years with vitamin A (RR = 1.6, NS for all tumors; RR = 1.4, NS for aggressive tumors) and β-carotene (RR = 1.4, NS for all tumors; RR = 1.0 for aggressive tumors).
		Cohort Studies	
Snowdon et al., 1984 (17)	California	6,763 Adventist men (99 fatal cases)	No association with vegetable or fruit intake (data not shown).
Hirayama, 1986 (27)	Japan	122,201 men (183 fatal cases)	Inverse association with green-yellow vegetables (GYV) in men <75 years (RR = 1.8). Suggestive positive association with GYV in men ≥75 years.

Paganini-Hill et al., 1987 (28)	Laguna Hills, CA	11,538 men (93 cases)	No association with β-carotene intake (RR = 1.0). Positive association with total vitamin A intake (RR = 1.4, NS).
Severson et al., 1989 (18)	Oahu, HI	7,999 Japanese men (174 cases)	Positive association with fruit (RR = 1.6, NS).
Mills et al., 1989 (19)	California	14,000 Adventist men (180 cases)	No association with fruit index. Inverse association with dried fruits (RR = 0.6, NS), and tomatoes (RR = 0.6, p = 0.02).
Reichman et al., 1990 (29)	U.S.	2,440 men (84 cases)	Inverse association with serum vitamin A (RR = 2.2, $p < 0.05$).
Hsing et al., 1990 (20)	Minnesota and northeastern U.S.	17,633 Lutheran men (149 cases)	Positive association in men <75 years with total vitamin A (RR = 2.8, $p < 0.05$) and β-carotene (RR = 1.9, $p = 0.05$). Inverse association in men ≥75 years with total vitamin A (RR = 0.4, $p < 0.05$) and β-carotene (RR = 0.2, $p < 0.05$).

[a]Based on extreme quantiles
RR = relative risk; NS = not statistically significant.

micronutrients (37). The potential benefits would be substantial. Not only might prostate cancer incidence be reduced, but other cancers for which dietary fat is suspected to play a role (e.g., colorectal cancer) might be reduced as well. In addition, risk of coronary heart disease would be expected to be lowered in the group who received the intervention. It is unlikely that the risk from any cancer or other disease would be increased by such a fat-lowering trial (33).

6. Means other than primary prevention for effectively dealing with the public health burden of this disease have not been established. Screening for this cancer has not yet been demonstrated to be effective (38), and such measures as are available (digital rectal examination, transrectal ultrasonography, and prostate specific antigen) are relatively costly to implement on a mass basis. In any regard, primary prevention is the ultimate goal of any risk reduction program, and this generally requires the initial establishment of etiology.

7. Such a trial could be feasible. Certain high risk groups can be identified (e.g., adult black and white men, men above age 70, men with a diet currently high in fat, etc.), and, as noted above, fat may be a late-stage promoter, making reasonable the conduct of the study among elderly men. Furthermore, there is growing evidence that adults can modify their diets and maintain a low fat intake (39).

Considerations Opposing a Trial

1. As summarized in the previous section of this chapter, the level of consistency of the data on dietary fat and prostate cancer at present is not as high as would be desirable. While the data from ecologic and case-control studies would suggest that an intervention trial should be the next step in establishing the dietary fat association, the lack of sufficient supportive data from cohort studies tempers this conclusion. It would seem prudent, as a first step, to examine the data from published cohorts further to address this apparent discrepancy. It would also be helpful if data from other ongoing cohorts could be made available to address this issue more thoroughly.

2. Even if sufficient consistency were found on such further analysis, plans for a trial would require careful decisions regarding the amount and duration of fat reduction in the diet. The dose-response curve for the effect of dietary fat has not been characterized, and the level of fat in the diet that would produce an optimal reduction in risk has not been determined.

3. The conflicting data on carotenoids/vitamin A are a concern. While the evidence that retinol or carotenoids may be risk-enhancing factors seems to be weakening (30), this issue has not been resolved, and the possibility of a protective effect of these agents or other constituents of foods is far from clear. Resolution of this ambiguity should be sought first, so that other dietary protective factors could be incorporated into a fat-reduction intervention trial.

4. Since the magnitude of the relative risk relating dietary fat to prostate cancer is not very great, an intervention trial would require large numbers of subjects to generate meaningful results. Some gain in cost-effectiveness could be achieved by restricting the study to a high risk group for prostate cancer. Although U.S. blacks and whites, age 70 or older, comprise such a high risk population, it would be desirable to identify other high risk factors that could be incorporated into the design of the trial.

5. Although methods to monitor compliance with a low fat regimen, such as self-reported dietary changes and measurement of serum cholesterol levels (40), are available, these methods are limited. A dietary intervention trial essentially involves a lifestyle modification; differences among participants in the degree of adherence to the recommendations need to be sensitively monitored.

6. The sample size requirements of such an undertaking would almost certainly necessitate that the trial be multicentered, which would contribute significantly to its cost. In addition, the need to incorporate behavior modification methods into the study (to increase the likelihood that the subjects in the intervention arm would adhere to their recommended diet) would also be a significant cost factor (41). Data are insufficient at this time for a meaningful assessment of benefit to society relative to cost of a prostate cancer dietary intervention trial.

7. Other issues relevant to a dietary intervention trial, such as the potential problem of control drift and its impact on the projected sample size requirements for the study, could also be considered as potentially dissuasive (42).

Other Considerations

In any intervention trial, it is important that similar methods of determining outcome be applied to both the intervention and the control groups. A distinctive feature of prostate cancer is that among elderly subjects there is a high prevalence of latent tumors (defined as unsuspected malignant lesions, usually localized and found incidentally at autopsy or after surgical removal of prostatic tissue for clinically benign hypertrophy). Autopsy studies in different countries, including the United States, have detected latent prostate cancer in 13–37% of necropsy subjects (43), whereas the lifetime risk of death due to prostate cancer is about 2–3% in U.S. men (44).

Because of this high prevalence of latent cancer, groups subjected to different levels of diagnostic effort could easily appear to differ in their incidence rates (45). In one study (46), 33% of the incident cases of prostate cancerr were discovered as incidental lesions, leading the authors to conclude that unsuspected cancers are a highly variable component of the reported incidence of prostate cancer. For this reason, it would be important to record the stage of incident cancers in the intervention and control groups of an intervention trial. Although mortality due to prostate cancer may be a more reliable endpoint than incidence in this regard, mortality as the principal outcome measure would necessarily require a larger sample size for the study.

CONCLUSION AND RECOMMENDATIONS

Conclusion

While there are several persuasive arguments for the planning of a fat-reduction intervention trial for prostate cancer among U.S. men, certain issues require resolution before such an undertaking can be justified. These pertain primarily to the lack of supportive data on fat from cohort studies and the role of retinol, carotenoids, or other constituents of fruits and vegetables as either risk-enhancing or protective factors. Clarification of these issues would enable investigators to better plan a trial with a successful outcome.

Recommendations

1. Additional data on dietary fat and prostate cancer should be available from new and existing cohort studies over the next few years. These data should not only clarify the role of fat as a risk factor for prostate cancer, but also help to establish which component(s) of fat may be responsible for the effect. It will be important to note the interval between the dietary assessment and the occurrence of the disease. This will be important in resolving the discrepancies in the current reports from cohort studies, as well as in establishing the appropriateness of intervening late in adult life for any future intervention trial (and ultimately for communitywide cancer control efforts).
2. It would be useful to have more data that could support a particular optimal level of fat reduction for such a trial. A fat level of 25% of total calories would be easier to achieve than one which was lower, but if only a miminal (or no) effect could be expected to be demonstrated at this level, it would not be an appropriate choice.
3. More refined analyses of existing or new datasets might help to clarify the vitamin A/carotenoid issue. It might also help identify other constituents of foods that are protective against prostate cancer. As noted above, this information could be incorporated into the design of the intervention trial.
4. Better methods of monitoring fat intake in trial subjects should be developed. Although self-reports of dietary intake and measurements of serum cholesterol have been useful, more sensitive and reliable measures of compliance are needed.
5. The role of hormones in relation to diet should be investigated further, as this could have an impact on the design of such a trial. For example, if men with a particular androgen profile form a subgroup who are at increased risk from high fat intake in adult life, this would make possible the identification of an

optimal study group for the trial and increase the likelihood of demonstrating statistically meaningful differences between the trial arms.

REFERENCES

1. C. Muir, J. Waterhouse, T. Mack, J. Powell, and S. Whelan, eds., *Cancer Incidence in Five Continents* IARC Scientific Publication No. 88, International Agency for Research on Cancer, Lyon, 1987.
2. C. C. Boring, T. S. Squires, and T. Tong, *CA, 41*, 19 (1991).
3. A. L. Potosky, *JNCI, 82*, 1624 (1990).
4. M. A. Howell, *Br. J. Cancer, 29*, 328 (1974).
5. A. Blair and J. F. Fraumeni, Jr., *JNCI, 61*, 1379 (1978).
6. L. N. Kolonel, J. H. Hankin, J. Lee, S. Y. Chu, A. M. Y. Nomura, and M. Hinds, *Br. J. Cancer, 44*, 332 (1981).
7. L. M. Schuman, J. S. Mandel, A. Radke, U. Seal, and F. Halberg, in *Trends in Cancer Incidence: Causes and Implications* (K. Magnus, ed.), Hemisphere Publishing Corp., Washington, DC, 1982, p. 345.
8. S. Graham, B. Haughey, J. Marshall, R. Priore, T. Byers, T. Rzepka, C. Mettlin, and J. E. Pontes, *JNCI, 70*, 687 (1983).
9. M. Y. Heshmat, L. Kaul, J. Kovi, M. A. Jackson, A. G. Jackson, G. W. Jones, M. Edson, J. P. Enterline, R. G. Worrell, and S. L. Perry, *The Prostate, 6*, 7 (1985).
10. R. Talamini, C. La Vecchia, A. Decarli, E. Negri, and S. Franceschi, *Br. J. Cancer, 53*, 817 (1986).
11. R. K. Ross, H. Shimizu, A. Paganini-Hill, G. Honda, and B. E. Henderson, *JNCI, 78*, 869 (1987).
12. Y. Ohno, O. Yoshida, K. Oishi, K. Okada, H. Yamabe, and F. H. Schroeder, *Cancer Res., 48*, 1331 (1988).
13. L. N. Kolonel, C. N. Yoshizawa, and J. H. Hankin, *Am. J. Epidemiol., 127*, 999 (1988).
14. C. Mettlin, S. Selenskas, N. Natarajan, and R. Huben, *Cancer, 64*, 605 (1989).
15. D. W. West, M. L. Slattery, L. M. Robison, T. K. French, and A. W. Mahoney, *Cancer Causes and Control 2*, 85 (1991).
16. T. Hirayama, *Natl. Cancer Inst. Monogr., 53*, 149 (1979).
17. D. A. Snowdon, R. L. Phillips,and W. Choi, *Am. J. Epidemiol., 120*, 244 (1984).
18. R. K. Severson, A. M. Y. Nomura, J. S. Grove, and G. N. Stemmerman, *Cancer Res., 49*, 1857 (1989).
19. P. K. Mills, W. L. Beeson, R. L. Phillips, and G. E. Fraser, *Cancer, 64*, 598 (1989).
20. A. W. Hsing, J. K. McLaughlin, L. M. Schuman, E. Bjelke, G. Gridley, S. Wacholder, H. T. Co Chien, and W. J. Blot, *Cancer Res., 50*, 6836 (1990).
21. R. K. Ross, A. Paganini-Hill, and B. E. Henderson, *The Prostate, 4*, 333 (1983).
22. P. Hill, E. L. Wynder, L. Garbaczewski, and A. R. P. Walker, *Cancer Res., 42*, 3864 (1982).
23. B. J. Howie and T. D. Schultz, *Am. J. Clin. Nutr., 42*, 127 (1985).
24. L. N. Kolonel, J. H. Hankin, and C. N. Yoshizawa, *Cancer Res., 47*, 2982 (1987).
25. R. B. Hayes, J. F. A. T. Bogdanovicz, F. H. Schroeder, A. De Bruijn, J. W. Raatgever, P. J. Van Der Maas, K. Oishi, and O. Yoshida, *Cancer, 62*, 2021 (1988).

26. B. Middleton, T. Byers, J. Marshall, and S. Graham, *Nutr. Cancer, 8*, 107 (1986).
27. T. Hirayama, in *Diet, Nutrition and Cancer* (Y. Hayashi et al., eds.), Japan Scientific Societies Press, Tokyo, 1986, p. 41.
28. A. Paganini-Hill, A. Chao, R. K. Ross, and B. E. Henderson, *JNCI, 79*, 443 (1987).
29. M. E. Reichman, R. B. Hayes, R. G. Ziegler, A. Schatzkin, P. R. Taylor, L. L. Kahle, and J. F. Fraumeni, Jr., *Cancer Res., 50*, 2311 (1990).
30. L. Le Marchand, J. H. Hankin, L. N. Kolonel, and L. R. Wilkens. *Am. J. Epidemiol. 133*, 215 (1991).
31. L. Kolonel and W. Winkelstein, Jr., *Lancet, 2*, 566 (1977).
32. N. Abd Elghany, M. C. Schumacher, M. L. Slattery, D. W. West, and J. S. Lee, *Epidemiology, 1*, 107 (1990).
33. National Research Council, Committee on Diet and Health, *Diet and Health*, National Academy Press, Washington, DC 1989.
34. S. A. Gunn, T. C. Gould, and W. A. D. Anderson, *Acta Endocrinologica, 37*, 24 (1961).
35. L. K. Heilbrun, A. Nomura, and G. N. Stemmermann, *Br. J. Cancer, 54*, 677 (1986).
36. D. P. Rose, in *Dietary Fat and Cancer* (C. Ip, D. F. Birt, A. E. Rogers, and C. Mettlin, eds.), Alan R. Liss, Inc., New York, 1986, p. 43.
37. P. M. Suter and R. M. Russell, *Am. J. Clin. Nutr. 45*, 501 (1987).
38. P. T. Scardino, *Adv. in Urologic Ultrasound, 16*, 635 (1989).
39. S. L. Gorbach, A. Morrill-LaBrode, M. N. Woods, J. T. Dwyer, W. D. Selles, M. Henderson, W. Insull, Jr., S. Goldman, D. Thompson, C. Clifford, and L. Sheppard, *J. Am. Diet. Assoc., 90*, 802 (1990).
40. M. M. Henderson, L. H. Kushi, D. J. Thompson, S. L. Gorbach, C. K. Clifford, W. Insull, Jr., M. Moskowitz, and R. S. Thompson, *Prev. Med., 19*, 115 (1990).
41. D. P. Byar and L. S. Freedman, *Prev. Med., 18*, 203 (1989).
42. Multiple Risk Factor Intervention Trial Research Group, *JAMA, 248*, 1465 (1982).
43. R. Yatani, I. Kusano, T. Shiraishi, T. Hayashi, and G. N. Stemmermann, *Jpn. J. Clin. Oncol., 19*, 319 (1989).
44. American Cancer Society, *Cancer Facts and Figures—1989*, New York, 1989, p. 12.
45. D. G. Zaridze, P. Boyle, and M. Smans, *Int. J. Cancer, 33*, 223 (1984).
46. M. Beckner, J. W. Berg, and L. W. Franz, *J. Chron. Dis., 38*, 225 (1985).

19

Participation in Macronutrient Trials

Barbara K. Rimer* and Paul F. Engstrom
Fox Chase Cancer Center
Cheltenham, Pennsylvania

INTRODUCTION

The cancer prevention horizon is expanding. A previous volume discusses the role of micronutrients in reducing cancer risk (Moon and Micozzi, 1989). Earlier chapters in this volume discuss the specific mechanisms by which risk may be reduced through modification of macronutrient intake. Doll and Peto (1981) concluded that as much as 35% of cancer mortality might be avoided by "practicable dietary means." Now, or in the near future, people may be able to prevent cancer or reduce their risk, not only by stopping smoking but also by reducing the fat in their diets, increasing their intake of dietary fiber, and participating in regimens of micronutrient and macronutrient supplementation (DeWys et al., 1986).

An overview of nutrition and nutritional epidemiology has been presented by Micozzi (1989), Newberne et al. (1989), and others in Moon and Micozzi (1989). Trock et al. (1990a,b) recently reviewed data regarding high fiber diets and colon cancer. They concluded that the data support a reduction in colon cancer risk of about 40% among people consuming diets with high vegetable and grain content. Prentice and Sheppard (1990, p. 213) projected that a lifetime low-fat diet could

---

**Current affiliation*: Duke Comprehensive Cancer Center, Durham, North Carolina.
Supported in part by NIH Grant No. 7201-06 awarded to Fox Chase Cancer Center.

be projected to reduce cancer incidence rates by 41% and cancer mortality rates by 29% among U.S. women aged 55–69 based on anticipated reductions in cancer rates of breast, colon, rectum, ovary and endometrium. Howe et al. (1990) projected that 16% of breast cancers in premenopausal women and 24% in postmenopausal women could be prevented through dietary modification. Previous chapters in this volume also discuss these issues. In this chapter, we discuss several specific methodologic issues related to participation in dietary macronutrient programs, including recruitment, enrollment, and compliance with recommended regimens.

Importance of Behavioral Factors

The data for planning cancer prevention trials have come from studies in epidemiology, carcinogenesis, and biology (Olsen and Love, 1986). Epidemiologic studies have shown that environmental factors are important in the etiology of most human cancers, dietary factors and tobacco being the most important in the United States. Behavioral factors are equally important in the implementation of trials to modify risk through macronutrient manipulation. People must be convinced that participating in risk-reduction trials is worth the effort. They also must be motivated to adhere to and remain on prevention trials for long periods of time, perhaps indefinitely. Where there are tangible benefits, such as losing weight as a consequence of participating in a low fat dietary trial (Glanz, 1985), participation may be more appealing than when no personal benefits are perceived other than the avoidance of a null event, i.e., not getting a cancer one might not have gotten anyway. There is always the threat that the large costs of inconvenience and side effects may overwhelm the perceived benefits of adherence (Turk, 1990). As Leventhal et al. (1989, p. 3) cautioned, behavioral factors can affect trial outcomes in a number of ways: "The goals of participants are a source of variance that can affect recruitment response to randomizations, adherence to various components of trial protocols and disease detection."

The theme that runs through all aspects of participation is *adherence*. The word adherence is preferred to compliance because it seems to suggest more self-motivated perseverance with a dietary and lifestyle (Turk et al., 1986) versus compliance with a therapeutic intervention. As Epstein and Cluss (1982) noted, the effectiveness of a treatment depends both on its efficacy and on adherence to the regimen. Adherence to recommended cancer control guidelines requires active participation of individuals in preventive practices that are intended to reduce their risk of mortality from cancer. In the case of macronutrients, this may mean either adding (e.g., fiber), subtracting (e.g., alcohol or dietary fat), or substituting (low fat for high fat foods) nutrients. As we will discuss later in this chapter, it is easier to ask people to add than subtract. The degree to which a person's behavior is in accordance with recommended practices is defined as *adherence*

(Hays and Dimatteo, 1987; Lerman et al., 1990a). Earlier chapters summarized the efficacy issues. This chapter will focus on adherence and related issues.

RECRUITMENT

One of the most pressing tasks in macronutrient research is recruitment of appropriate subjects into the trials. As Agras and Bradford (1982) noted, the study of the recruitment process, the complexities and difficulties of which have often been underestimated by investigators, is being established as an area of enquiry in its own right. In macronutrient trials, subjects are generally not ill (Stevens et al., 1989). They may be persons at high risk for cancer, for example, because of family history. They might also be members of the population at large, although they could be cancer patients trying to prevent a cancer recurrence or second primary cancer.

The appropriate participants for chemoprevention trials will vary depending on the phase of the trial. Phase I participants might include cancer patients. High risk persons, such as those with precancerous lesions, are especially appropriate for phase II trials where the goals are to define such factors as appropriate study population and compliance rates and measurement. Phase III trials conduct the comparison in subjects that volunteer from a preselected group. In phase IV trials, the participants must be from defined populations, and phase V trials are aimed at widespread dissemination. Here, participants would be those from the general community (Moon, 1990). Recruitment is predicted upon the existence of a pool of potential participants (Agras and Bradford, 1982). Recruitment is of major importance to the methodologic rigor of the trial; failure to recruit a sufficient number of participants could jeopardize power (Hunninghake et al., 1987). Because prevention trials often require large numbers of subjects for adequate statistical power (Greenwald et al., 1986; Zelen, 1988), recruitment is a critical step in the conduct of trials. Moreover, it is vital that subjects be enthusiastic about and committed to participating in the trial since dropouts can adversely affect the conduct of prevention trials and the ability to reach conclusions about impact (Hansen et al., 1985). Hunninghake et al. (1987) stressed the importance of recruitment administration. A good data management system and clear delineation of responsibilities are essential.

As Gritz et al. (1989) noted, a number of factors influence recruitment. These include participants' sociodemographic characteristics, biomedical variables, population size, and location. In smoking cessation research, community blood pressure and similar kinds of programs, men tend to be underrepresented, as do blacks and other minority groups. Usually, married white persons with higher educational status are easier to recruit (Agras and Bradford, 1982). Participants who enter a trial because they want to avoid a recurrence of cancer or because they are at high familial risk may be quite different and much more motivated than the population at large. Patients may be willing to accept risks in order to prevent recurrence of disease that others would not. Volunteers tend to differ from nonvolunteers: The former often have higher education levels, higher occupational status, and are likely to be disproportionately female (Gritz et al., 1989). Mettlin (1989) offered people participation in a hypothetical dietary trial: Those most interested were likely to be regular vitamin users, to believe that cancer risk could be modified by diet, and to feel more vulnerable to cancer. It is of interest that three fourths of those interviewed were receptive to participating in the trial.

Recruitment may be especially difficult when one is trying to recruit healthy members of the public and screen them for a potentially premalignant disorder (Arnold et al., 1989) or ask them to participate in a prolonged prevention trial. The evidence from a polyp trial is that even among people with serious conditions, such as colon neoplasms, agreement to participate may still be limited (Stevens et al., 1989). Stevens et al. (1989) concluded that the ideal participants for prevention trials have the following characteristics:

In good health and able to comply physically with the demands of the trial
Socially connected, that is, live with a spouse or family and unlikely to leave the area
Knowledgeable about the trial
Motivated at least in part by altruism
Willing to forgo the intervention if so assigned and willing to take the placebo

The recruitment phase of participation in primary prevention trials is fraught with problems and therefore offers great challenges. Investigators must temper their optimism with realism when planning their recruitment schedules since the evidence suggests that recruitment usually takes longer than expected. A major review of clinical trials conducted by Hunninghake et al. (1987) showed that recruitment rarely occurred in the expected duration and frequently was a cause for trial termination. Most studies not only recruit more slowly than anticipated, but also require additional sources over and above those initially planned. This is partly because researchers often overestimate the potential study populations. Estimates of the approximate number of annual patients with the prerequisite medical condition are not good predictors of actual recruitment. Moreover, because prevention trials are demanding in terms of patient time, perhaps without immediate perceived benefits, patient refusal rates may be higher than those to which researchers and clinicians may be accustomed. Leventhal et al. (1989) have argued that the repeated failure of investigators to gauge the time needed for recruitment is a clear indicator of failure to consider the behavioral dynamics of trials.

The evidence also suggests the importance of attention to human factors. Participants' perceptions of the disease, treatment, and trial are all important (Leventhal et al., 1989). Participants need to feel valued by the study steam; attention to building rapport and providing support is especially important when participation of 5–10 years is required, as in the case in some dietary modification trials. This may be particularly important since a significant proportion of subjects in at least one chemoprevention trial participated for altrustic reasons (Arnold et al., 1989). Finally, there is evidence that recruitment deteriorates over time (e.g., Agras and Bradford, 1982; Arnold et al., 1989), so it is necessary to maintain a constant vigilance and to plan ways to maintain the commitment of participants over time. These factors will be discussed further with regard to adherence.

Strategies for Recruitment

A variety of strategies have been used for recruitment in prevention trials, in general, and in chemoprevention and dietary change programs, particularly. As Gritz et al. (1989) cautioned, investigators should use multiple recruitment modalities, aiming for sources with high efficiency. Efficiency is defined as the proportion of initial contacts who arrive at the first protocol visit (Agras and Bradford, 1982). Sources differ in both their volume and efficiency. Promising recruitment methods include such diverse strategies as advertisements and articles in the mass media; solicitation through patient databases and identification of at-risk persons through tumor registries (Table 1).

Mass Media

Researchers conducting dietary and smoking cessation trials have had good experience with use of the mass media for recruitment (Lando, 1990). Both articles and targeted advertisements may be effective. Appearances on television by the principal investigator or a participant can raise the visibility of a study. Arnold et al. (1989) estimated that newspapers accounted for 50% of early contacts, but 65% of all participants eventually randomized to a heavy smokers trial of a chemopreventive agent. Overall, newspapers, television, and radio accounted for 93% of randomizations with a mean efficiency of about 10%; other sources had a mean efficiency of 3%. Lando (1990) also did well using radio and television announcements for recruitment to smoking cessation trials: 15% of the recruits came through television announcements and 11% through radio. For a smoking cessation trial aimed at older smokers (aged 50–64), we recruited 2800 eligible smokers through a brief announcement in *Modern Maturity*, the magazine of the American Association of Retired Persons (AARP). In fact, we received over 8000 inquiries as a result of that notice. Over 250 smokers were accrued to the trial when one of the PIs appeared on a local news show. Advertisements also may be a good source: 11% of the women enrolled in a cervical cancer chemoprevention trial first heard about it through a print ad (Loescher, 1990). So the mass media can be an important and effective source of recruitment. However, many of the inquiries may come from persons who are not appropriate for the trial,

Table 1 Recruitment Sources

Mass media
Television
Radio
Newspapers and newsletters
Paid advertisement or PSAs
Geographic areas
States, cities, neighborhoods, or other geograhic areas
Community groups
Women's clubs
Churches or synagogues
Self-help groups
Direct mail
Worksites
Health professional referral
Health and health-related organizations
HMOs, health insurance subscribers
Tumor registries
Professional groups

so considerable selection may be required. Staff must be available not only to communicate with representatives of the media but also to respond to inquiries and to provide referrals for people who need other assistance, but are not eligible for participation.

Geographic Areas

Some studies have attempted to recruit residents with a certain characteristic within a defined geographic area. For example, some of the breast screening trials in Europe have used such methods (Tabar, 1989). This approach was also used in the Hypertension Detection and Follow-up Program (Ford, 1987). The COMMIT and ASSIST smoking prevention and cessation trials sponsored by the NCI are geographically focused as well.

Community Group Recruitment

Another source of recruitment are special groups in the community where at-risk or eligible people are likely to be found. Such groups might include women's groups as a source of recruitment for dietary fat-reduction trials. We have recruited older adults to cancer detection trials (Keintz, 1988) and to an older smoker trial through presentations at churches, senior centers, and AARP meetings. Community presentations can have the beneficial impact of raising the visibility of the program; however, they are extremely labor-intensive. Self-help groups, e.g., weight loss, smoking cessation, persons with diseases (such as colitis) also are potentially powerful sources of recruitment.

Direct Mail

Eligible subjects can also be recruited through direct mail solicitations, if appropriate lists can be used to identify people. Direct mail is most effective when the potential subjects can be identified with some efficiency. McLarty (1990) recruited 50% of the asbestos workers in his trial through direct mailings to asbestos workers. Recruitment to the Physicians Health Study was conducted by mail among 22,071 male physicians (Hennekens, 1984). In this case, the AMA provided a list of all AMA male physicians, thus facilitating a methodologically sound approach to recruitment. Schmid et al. (1989) evaluated mass mailing recruitment strategies for smoking and weight correspondence programs as part of the Minnesota Heart Health Program. Overall, announcements were sent to over 6000 persons. In general, the more money spent per household, the higher the recruitment. Also, it was more economical when residents first had to return an interest card. Crude recruitment rates for communities ranged from 1.8 to 4.6% of the households contacted. Ho et al. (1987) had good success in recruiting participants for a fiber trial by conducting follow-up telephone interviews with subjects who had returned questionnaires in a mailed survey.

Worksites

Worksites have been used as the basis for recruiting employees into a variety of prevention studies, including those aimed at dietary change and smoking cesssation (Glanz, 1988). Unions are a source of workers exposed to carcinogenic substances. McLarty (1990) recruited participants for a β-carotene, retinol, and lung cancer chemoprevention study, in part, by presentations at union meetings. He attributed 20% of his recruitment to this method. Worksites have the advantage of providing a defined population, offering the possibility of continuity and also creating a climate in which there is social support for participation. Worksite recruitment requires managerial and supervisory level support and the designation of a liason at the worksite to coordinate with the study team. The support of occupational physicians and nurses should be sought. Goodman et al. (1985) noted that such professionals were essential in boosting recruitment to the CARET (β-carotene and retinol efficacy trial).

Health Professional Referral

Most trials depend to some extent on referral of potentially eligible patients through health professionals. Arnold et al. (1989) sent promotional materials regarding the Concerned Smoking Study to local physician offices, and announcements were made at rounds. In spite of these efforts, this source of recruitment did not prove effective, and the investigators turned instead to mass media and community advertising. Seventy-three percent of the women enrolled in a cervical dysplasia trial first heard about it from their physicians (Loescher et al., 1990). HMOs and other large organizations might be more efficient sources than individual providers. Reliance on physicians' hospital records or clinical laboratories alone has generally been unsuccessful (Hunninghake et al., 1987).

Health and Health-Related Organizations

Health insurance companies and health maintenance organizations can be excellent sources of recruitment to prevention trials. A large study of self-help smoking cessation methods was conducted among members of Group Health Cooperative (GHC) in Seattle, Washington. We have used HMO PA/NJ, an IPA-model HMO, to recuit women aged 50–74 into a secondary cancer prevention study and are now canvassing these women regarding their interest in a tomoxifen trial (Rimer et al., 1989; Lerman, 1990a). Goodman et al. (1985) recruited potential subjects to the CARET trial through an announcement in *View*, the magazine of GHC. Final randomization from this source was about 3%. Clearly, this is not a very efficient means of recruitment, but it is inexpensive. Romney et al. (1985) recruited subjects to a cervical cancer chemoprevention trial through physicians' offices and family planning clinics. Clark (1985) recruited hospital patients for a selenium trial. Loescher et al. (1990) used an HMO pathology department as a recruitment source.

Professional Groups

Studies of macronutrient effects can also be conducted within professional groups. The Physicians Health Trial (Hennekens, 1984) found physicians to be a highly compliant group in a micronutrient trial. Investigators using nurses as study subjects have had similarly positive experiences (Willett, 1989, 1990; Stampfer et al., 1989).

Tumor Registry Recruitment

Newcombe et al. (1990) demonstrated that a statewide tumor registry can be used to identify potential subjects for a trial. They used the Wisconsin Cancer Reporting System to identify 3585 women who met the study criteria with regard to age, stage, and previous therapy. When cases were identified, physicians were notified and permission was obtained to contact their patients. Ultimately, 140 (58%) women enrolled in the placebo-controlled, double-blind tamoxifen toxicity trial. Patients to a polyposis trial were recruited through a cancer center's registry (Miller et al., 1986–87).

ENROLLMENT

Once patients have been recruited to a prevention trial, enrollment is the next goal. Enrollment includes, first of all, assessing the patient's eligibility in relation to the goals of the trial and criteria specified in the protocol. The evidence (e.g., Arnold et al., 1989) suggests that, generally, only a small proportion of persons who respond to mass media or other forms of recruitment will be eligible according to the trial's criteria. For example, in the Women's Health Trial, eligible women were those who derived 38% or more of their calories from fat and had one or more risk factors for breast cancer (Nixon, 1988). Many people who expressed interest in the Concerned Smoker Trial were really looking for a smoking cessation program (Arnold et al., 1989) and were therefore not appropriate. In a pilot tamoxifen study conducted in England, only about 12% of the women who were recruited subsequently enrolled in the trial. Reasons for failure to enroll included a variety of sociodemographic and health-related factors (Powles et al., 1989). Stevens et al. (1989) estimated that only half of the patients eligible for their skin cancer prevention and polyp trials actually enrolled.

Informed Concent

Attention should be paid to the ethical issues involved in cancer prevention trials and to the risk/benefit ratio for participants (Weed, 1983). An important step in the enrollment process is the solicitation of the participants' informed consent. DHHS regulations require that participants in trials funded by the government give their informed consent to participate. This means they must be given information about the purpose of the trial, the risks and benefits, what is expected of the participant, the alternatives, and the right to ask questions. True informed consent requires a dialogue between the potential participant and the investigator. The participant must comprehend what he or she is expected to do, as well as the other elements that define informed consent. Research among cancer patients shows that only a small proportion of the information in the protocol is transmitted to the patient, and most of that is either not comprehended or is forgotten quickly (Rimer et al., 1984).

In the case of informed consent to macronutrient trials, it is especially important that participants understand the personal benefits, if any, the risks, number of visits they are expected to make, any study-related costs, and the length of time they are expected to participate. Because study attrition can have a devastating effect on trial outcomes (Hansen et al., 1985; Weiss, 1987), the last point is especially important. There are no data regarding participants' comprehension of information provided during the consent phase of macronutrient trials.

There is little information about refusal rates for chemoprevention trials, generally, or macronutrient trials, specifically. However, the available data suggest that many of these eligible for participation in prevention trials do not consent to do so. For example, about 47% of the eligible patients for a tamoxifen trial subsequently enrolled; 23% refused consent (Powles et al., 1989). Ho et al. (1987) asked people in a retirement community about their interest in a fiber trial. The main reasons for lack of interest were: lack of belief in the scientific evidence, behavioral inconvenience, old age, and health barriers. Miller et al. (1986–87) surveyed 61 participants and 28 nonparticipants in a chemoprevention trial for familial polyposis patients. Participants were younger, closer in time to diagnosis, more likely to be Catholic, and living further away. They were also more likely than nonparticipants to be happy with their marriage and to score at either extreme on the happiness scale used.

Dermatis et al. (1988) is the only reported study to have examined the issue of consent to chemoprevention regimens. A consent study was conducted after women had made a decision to participate in a double-blind chemoprevention study; 118 women entered the consent study. Most were married, white, and upper middle to upper SES. They were also proactive with regard to their health. The consenters did not differ from the refusers on demographic characteristics, objective risk status, components of the Health Belief Model, or psychosocial indices. However, the two groups differed in terms of what factors influenced their decision making. Refusers were concerned about the study demands and safety of the agent. Consenters focused more on potential benefits of participation, including altruism. Thus, the refusers emphasized the negative aspects of participation, whereas the consenters were more influenced by the positive aspects.

The literature on risk (e.g. Weinstein, 1979; Kahneman and Tversky, 1984; Slovic, 1987) suggests that some people may be unduly influenced by negative risk information. Studies by Meyerowitz and Chaiken (1987) and Lerman (1990b) with breast cancer patients and women who have received abnormal mammograms are testing the effect that positive or negative framing has on women's decisions and adherence. Data from Meyerowitz and Chaiken (1987) suggest that people are most influenced by a desire to avoid negative outcomes. Thus, the way information about macronutrient trials is presented to potential participants may influence strongly whether or not they decide to participate. Further research is needed to examine these issues specifically within the context of primary prevention trials.

It is important that means be found to both recruit and enroll lower SES persons in primary prevention trials to study the impact of macronutrients. If only those with higher education and incomes participate, the data will have limited generalizability. To attract lower SES participants may require a focus on community-level recruitment using credible sources (e.g., church leaders), study materials, including consent forms that are comprehensible to persons with low literacy, and perhaps, reimbursement for transportation, time lost from work, and other costs associated with participating in trials.

Finally, consent applies not only to potential participants, but sometimes to their physicians as well. Newcombe et al. (1990) reported that 61.5% of the physicians they contacted regarding eligible patients for a tamoxifen trial never responded; 2.1% of the 35% who responded were unwilling to give permission for the study team to contact their patients.

Run-In Periods

Run-in periods have been used as a way to identify persons who will be adherent participants in prevention trials. While run-in periods may reduce the number of subjects in a trial, those that remain will be likely to comply (Stampfer et al., 1989). Most noncompliers evidence this early during a trial, certainly within the first 3–4 months (although very long-term trials may experience nonadherence further into the trial). In the Physicians' Health Trial (Hennekens, 1984), about one third of the physicians who were enrolled initially dropped out prior to randomization, thus producing a stable population of proven compliers. In polyp prevention trials, from 3 to 7% of subjects did not proceed beyond a placebo run-in period (Stevens et al., 1989). Of 506 patients invited to a clinic for possible enrollment in the Concerned Smoker Study, 122 did not complete the study run-in requirements, provision of sputum samples (Arnold et al., 1989). Berenson et al. (1989) used a run-in period to assess compliance in a chemoprevention trial for patients with familial polyposis with placebo only used during the run-in period. It is not clear how many subjects were dropped during the run-in period due to poor compliance.

COMPLIANCE/ADHERENCE

One of the most challenging aspects of participation in primary prevention trials aimed at behavior change is adherence. Motivating people to make long-term, perhaps lifelong, changes in their diets, intake of alcohol, stopping smoking, all require a major commitment by participants. Adherence should be viewed as a complex, dynamic phenomenon that can change over time (Meichenbaum and Turk, 1987). Typically, health professionals overestimate their patients' compliance, no matter what the regimen. As Turk et al. (1986) summarized, adherence rates are generally low: 20–50% of patients do not appear for scheduled appointments; 20–80% make medication errors; 25–60% of patients drop out of lifestyle change programs. Compliance with smoking cessation and dietary change programs is especially low, with over 75% of participants in both groups relapsing within 6 months. There are dropout rates of 20–80% lifestyle change programs designed to treat obesity, smoking, and stress management (Meichenbaum and Turk, 1987). Overall, patient nonadherence may range from 20 to 80% (Stewart and Cluff, 1972). Nonadherence seems to occur regardless of patient gender, age, or other SES characteristics (Svarstad, 1986). In this section, we will discuss factors that affect adherence, strategies for enhancing adherence, and methodologic issues related to adherence. A comprehensive review of compliance is beyond the scope of this chapter (see Meichenbaum and Turk, 1987; Becker and Rosenstock, 1984).

As Meichenbaum and Turk (1987, p. 12) concluded, "The sheer magnitude of the problem suggests that adherence cannot be expected to occur on its own or because we wish it, and it is too important to leave to chance. Instead of bemoaning the fact that nonadherence is prevalent, we must plan measures to reduce its frequency." A note of caution is in order. As Turk et al. (1986) observed, compliance tends to be treated as a generic concept when, in fact, compliance must be viewed in the specific context of the behavioral regimen. For example, a program of fat reduction to 15% of daily calories requires that the participant understand how to calculate her desirable daily intake and substitute lower fat for higher fat dietary selections. The regimen thus requires both substitution behaviors and detection behaviors. Adherence to a fiber regimen might require remembering to take the fiber supplements provided by the investigators or *increasing* the intake of whole grain breads, fruits, and cruciferous vegetables. *Adding* these foods requires different skills and carries different barriers and facilitators from adherence to a very low fat diet, which requires *decreasing* overall fat intake and *substituting* low fat for high fat food choices. In the case of macronutrient trials, adherence also means agreeing not to self-medicate with the experimental treatment (Stampfer et al., 1989). In the case of readily available macronutrients, this is a serious concern (Stevens et al., 1989).

Theoretical Models of Adherence

A number of theoretical models have been developed to describe adherence. Most of these were developed in the course of studying screening or chronic disease behavior. There has been little theoretical work with regard to compliance with macronutrient programs for reducing cancer risk. However, we believe that the Health Belief Model should be investigated as a useful explanatory model for people's behaviors in this area. The HBM was developed originally during the 1950s by investigators working within the U.S. Public Health Service to explain what influenced people to seek screening for tuberculosis (Rosenstock, 1990). Over the ensuing years, the HBM has been applied to both preventive health and chronic disease behaviors and appears to be a robust, useful framework for describing health behavior. Here, we discuss the HBM and several other theoretical models that can be used singly or in combination to enhance compliance with macronutrient change regimens.

According to the HBM, people will take action when (1) they perceive a threat to be serious, (2) they feel that they are personally at risk or susceptible, (3) they believe one can have the disease in the absence of symptoms, (4) they have overcome the barriers to action, (5) they feel that they can perform the behavior, and (6) they have received a cue to action (Rosenstock, 1990). Thus, a woman in her 40s might adopt an extremely low fat diet if she believes she could be diagnosed with breast cancer, and breast cancer would be serious. She must have overcome the psychological, access, and skill barriers related to such dietary change and been exposed to a cue to action. The cue could be an article in the newspaper, an educational program or a strong recommendation from her personal physician. The HBM can be used both to design educational intervention and to select appropriate items for evaluating the impact of a primary prevention program.

Other theoretical approaches can be used to supplement the HBM. Social Learning Theory (Bandura, 1982; Perry et al., 1990; Rimer, 1990) posits that behavior is determined through a triadic, dynamic, and reciprocal model in which behavior, personal factors, and environmental influences all interact. According to SLT, participants must believe that a given behavior will lead to a given outcome and they must feel *efficacious*—capable of performing the behavior in question (Meichenbaum and Turk, 1987). Particularly important are the individual's abilities to symbolize the meanings of behavior, to foresee outcomes, to learn by observing others, to regulate behavior and to reflect and learn from experience (Perry et al., 1990). Behavior can be changed through observational learning and modeling, vicarious learning, and reinforcement (Strecher et al., 1986). Excellent reviews of Social Learning Theory can be found in Bandura (1982), Strecher et al. (1986), and Perry et al. (1990).

Another promising, relatively new theoretical approach is Prochaska and DiClemente's (1985) Transtheoretical Stages of Change Model. Their model is particularly useful in segmenting target audiences and matching the appropriate behavior change strategy to the person's stage of change. The model describes a cycle of change: People may be precontemplators (e.g., they have not even thought about adopting a low fat diet, perhaps they are not even aware of the role of fat), contemplators (they are thinking about a low fat diet; they may need both information and motivation), determinators (they are ready to take action to change their diets; they may need skill development, they may need help shopping), action (they have begun a low fat diet), and maintenance (they are now embarked on a new lifestyle but could slip or relapse anytime thus reentering the process at an earlier stage).

Gritz et al. (1989) have posited a six-factor model of adherence which includes: (1) effective communication of information (knowledge of the treatment and what is expected); (2) rapport with health professionals; (3) client's beliefs and attitudes (including some of the HBM variables described earlier); (4) participant's social climate and norms (family, friends, social class, and ethnicity are the major source of cultural beliefs and norms); (5) behavioral intentions (shaped by communication of information, rapport, beliefs, and attitudes); and (6) supports for and barriers to adherence.

When planning macronutrient programs, investigators should start with a theoretical model that is used to inform both program intervention and evaluation. In the absence of a theoretical model, the investigator may fail to recognize potential participants' barriers to participation and to plan accordingly. Likewise, the set of variables selected for measurement may be incomplete.

Reported Compliance in Chemoprevention and Macronutrient Trials

The literature on compliance is extensive, although there is still little experience with cancer macronutrient trials. However, research in the areas of chemoprevention and dietary intervention offers guidance regarding compliance issues that can be generalized to macronutrient trials.

The run-in periods used in most reported chemoprevention trials serve to eliminate at least short-term noncompliers from chemoprevention trials. For example, Romney et al. (1985) excluded from their cervical cancer chemoprevention trial patients thought to be unreliable or potentially noncompliant. Similarly, noncompliant physicians were dropped from the Physicians Health Trial during the run-in period (Steering Committee, 1989). So, while most reports indicate high levels of compliance, the participants have been generally highly motivated, white, middle to upper-middle–class persons (e.g., Dermatis et al., 1988). This means that ultimately the external validity of such data is limited.

Dermatis et al. (1988) found mean levels of adherence to supplements (ω-3 fatty acids or placebo) to be above 80% and continued to be high even at 12 months, although adherence had declined so that one third of participants were below the 80% level according to capsule counts. Arnold et al. (1989) reported compliance rates in excess of 85% while return of follow-up sputum samples was over 95%. In the intervention group, 91.6% of the serum samples were positive for etretinate compared to 2.8% in the placebo group (Browman et al., 1989). The authors noted that noncompliers had been eliminated during the run-in period. Dropout rates for different dosage levels ranged from 0 to 25%. Compliance in the Physicians Health Trial was also very high, partly because nonadherers were dropped during the run-in period. According to self-reports, compliance in both groups was nearly 86% (Steering Committee, 1989). Dropout rates with a retinol acetate gel to reduce the risk of cervical cancer ranged from 0 to 25%. About one half of the participants missed zero out of 21 days of usage, 22.5% missed 1 day, 12.5% missed 2 days, and 12.5% missed 3 or more days (Romney et al., 1985; Berenson et al., 1989).

Surveys indicate that current dietary practices of Americans fall far below recommended standards. Many studies have been conducted to alter eating behaviors (Stunkard, 1980; Brownell, 1982, 1984). In the MRFIT study (Caggiula et al., 1981; Gorder et al., 1986), educational strategies included group education, counseling, family involvement, monitoring, and reinforcement. The nutrition intervention resulted in average cholesterol reductions of 7.5%; notably, these changes were sustained for 6 years (Glanz, 1988). According to a national survey, average fat consumption in the United States is approximately 40% of total daily calories; average fiber consumption is only about 11 g/day (*Med. World News*, 1984). Similarly, a recent analysis of national survey data indicates that only a small proportion of Americans regularly consume cruciferous vegetables (21%) and high fiber breads and cereals (16%). Moreover, a substantial percentage of persons surveyed ate pork and lunch meats (43%) (Patterson and Block, 1988). While these statistics are quite discouraging, data from a recent low fat dietary trial for women with mammographic dysplasia suggest that adherence to dietary restrictions may be attainable in a high-risk population (Boyd et al., 1988). Dietary fat and fiber trials are now underway at a number of locations (Bright-See and Levy, 1985; Boyd et al., 1988).

Berenson et al. (1989) assessed compliance with dietary fiber and vitamin supplements in a randomized trial. Subject-reported compliance was validated using biologic markers, calendars, and returned fiber boxes. For the first 2 years, while vitamin compliance was above 85% overall, fiber compliance varied but generally tended to decrease sharply by month 9. Two thirds of the variance in fiber compliance was accounted for by four variables: an overall fiber product rating, interaction between having someone to prepare meals and eat breakfast, a psychosocial measure of internal control of health, and a measure of negative affect. At the end of 4 years, the control group showed a greater decline in compliance for both vitamins and fiber than did the high fiber group. Mean compliance for fiber decreased from 84.8 to 43.5% in the control group, from 79.1 to 38.9% in the vitamin group, and from 66.8 to 62% in the high fiber group (DeCosse et al., 1989). The data from this trial serve to reinforce what is generally known—that it is easier to motivate people to take pills than to make more complex behavioral changes, such as decreasing dietary fat or increasing fiber intake.

The preliminary evidence from fat-reduction trials aimed at reducing breast cancer risk is that high adherence rates can be achieved (Prentice and Sheppard, 1989; Boyd et al., 1990). Boyd et al. (1990) recruited 595 women with extensive mammographic dysplasia to a randomized study of dietary advice alone or the experimental group in which women were taught to reduce dietary fat intake to a target of 15% of calories. The experimental group performed extremely well: 4–12 months after randomization, about 60% of the experimental group had an intake of dietary fat that was within 5% of the target of 15% of calories, and about 80% were within 10% of target. High levels of adherence were documented through 24 months. It is noteworthy that the participants selected were at high risk for cancer and thus may have had increased levels of motivation to comply compared to the general population. Chlebowski et al. (1990) reported on a cooperative group trial in women with breast cancer and eligible for adjuvant treatment assigned randomly to a control (information about nutritional adequacy) or intervention group (also information on dietary fat reduction). Adherence was high: At 3, 6, and 12 months postentry, women in the intervention group showed significant differences compared to the control in percent of calories derived from fat; they also reduced daily fat intake 56% at 3 months. Serum cholesterol and weight also were reduced significantly.

In 1990, the National Cancer Institute (NCI) began a pilot study of a low fat intervention program among healthy women aged 45–69. The goal was for women in the intervention group to reduce fat from about 39% of calories to 20% of calories. Women in the intervention group (dietary and behavioral education and counseling) reduced their fat intake by about 60%. Most of this change occurred within the first 3 months of the program and has been largely maintained for 3 years. A follow-up study with an additional 1761 women showed similar results (Prentice and Sheppard, 1989). These data suggest that educational and behavioral methods can be used to help women dramatically reduce their fat intake to reduce breast cancer risk.

Strategies for Improving Compliance

People fail to adhere to recommended health professional advice, whether preventive or medical care–oriented, for a variety of reasons. For example, in one breast cancer chemoprevention trial, women cited memory problems (e.g. forgetting when to take the capsules and how many to take) as a reason for noncompliance. Patients may deviate from recommendations because they want to avoid side effects or they believe the advice no longer applies. They may lack essential knowledge or skills needed for compliance. Barriers, such as food costs, access, or the skill, time, and effort needed for preparation may act as barriers to compliance to macronutrient regimens (Glanz, 1985). Dietary change may be especially difficult to implement for older adults, especially those living alone and/or on fixed incomes (Benedict et al., 1989). Taste is important in dietary trials (Ho et al., 1987). Stevens et al. (1989) found that noncompliance often occurred when high risk patients continued to manifest endpoints or if they developed illnesses which they attributed (often incorrectly) to the study medication.

Adherence is a complex process. Nonadherence likewise is complex and may result from characteristics of the participant, the regimen, the participant's environment, the participant–professional relationship or an interaction among these elements. Behavioral change can be facilitated by instituting changes at the point of cognitive structures (changing beliefs and meaning systems), cognitive processes (changing automatic thoughts, images and coping skills), behavioral acts, and/or environmental characteristics and consequences (Turk et al., 1986). There is evidence from a number of cardiovascular disease studies that adherence rates above 90% can be achieved when considerable attention is paid to enhancing adherence through tangible and intangible support, creating a positive atmosphere and involving family members (Bell et al., 1985).

Before planning a macronutrient or other prevention trial, the investigators should examine carefully all the elements of adherence associated with the requirements of the trial and plan accordingly. Participants almost always need information to comply, but they often need skills as well (Morisky, 1986). Considering the specific protocol can help investigators to tailor their adherence-enhancing strategies accordingly to both the regimen and to the needs of the participants. In general, compliance rates tend to be lower with more complex regimens and with no longer ones (Higbee et al. 1982; Becker and Rosenstock, 1984), so an early concern should be with regimen simplication. For example, a chemopreventive approach using a single fiber supplement is simpler and requires less behavior change than asking people to increase fiber from a variety of dietary sources (Ho et al., 1987). While the latter may be an appropriate long-term goal, it may be difficult to achieve in the short term. Also, as noted earlier, it is harder to ask people to give up things they like (e.g., cigarettes) than to substitute (e.g., replace butter with sunflower oil, replace no-bran cereal with all-bran). It must be noted that to date no systematic studies of nutrition education to reduce cancer risk have been completed (Glanz, 1985). Therefore, we must rely on promising leads from cardiovascular and other risk reduction studies. In this section, we provide a number of different strategies that could be used to enhance compliance with macronutrient trials (Table 2).

Strategies for Improving the Participant–Researcher Relationship to Motivate Adherence

A substantial literature attests to the importance of the patient–physician relationship in facilitating adherence (see Hays and Dimatteo, 1987). In prevention trials, we may be talking not about patients but about participants who are often healthy individuals who choose to participate in prevention trials for any number of reasons. Their ongoing relationship might be with a physician, health educator, nurse, epidemiologist, or some other person on the study team, but the relationship is just as important as for patients. Berenson et al. (1989) highlighted the importance of trust, rapport, and integrity between the participant and study team in a polyposis trial. Loescher et al. (1990) concluded that many of their participants remained in the cancerprevention study because they liked the study team. Romney et al. (1985, p. 115) suggested that later recruits into their retinoid trial had better compliance despite a higher dosage of gel, because the participants had greater rapport with their study team and "were often willing to complete their participation in spite of the difficulties and discomforts encountered." Gritz et al. (1989) stressed that the quality of the practitioner–client relationship is a primary ingredient in therapeutic change. Both verbal and nonverbal communication of caring and warmth can improve rapport. Any attempt to increase long-term adherence requires a collaborative framework with responsibility shared by participants and investigators (Turk et al., 1986). Active collaboration can be facilitated by

Table 2 Strategies for Improving Adherence

Improve the quality of the participant–investigator relationship	*Behavioral strategies for enhancing adherence*
Establish trust and rapport	Goal setting
Show caring and warmth	Contracting
Develop collaborative relationship	Stimulus control
	Self-monitoring
	Relapse prevention
Strategies for memory enhancement	*Strategies for enhancing social support*
Simplify regimen	Family member involvement—show *how* to help
Telephone reminders, tip sheets, medication timers	Participant meetings
Once-a-day dose pack	
Mailed reminders	
Strategies for improving knowledge and skills	*Access strategies for enhancing adherence*
Present most important information first or last	Provide transportation
Categorize information	Flexible hours
Provide written information for reinforcement	Reduce waiting time
Assess participant's comprehension and correct misinformation	*Strategies for enhancing problem-solving skills*
Ask participants to practive new skills	Ask participants to model behaviors
Demonstrate the desired behavior	Counsel regarding barriers
Strategies for enhancing motivation	
Performance feedback	
Regular contact through personal interaction	
Small gifts or other incentives	
Appeal to altruism	
Telephone calls, birthday cards, newsletters	

encouraging and answering patient questions, being friendly rather than businesslike, and avoiding medical jargon (Meichenbaum and Turk, 1987).

Strategies for Improving Knowledge and Skills of Participants

As Morisky (1986) concluded, knowledge and skills are necessary but not sufficient for adherence. Some nonadherence may occur simply because participants do not understand what they are expected to do (Hays and Dimatteo, 1987). Providing information to help participants comprehend the regimen is an important first step. One-to-one counseling by a nutrionist may be essential when asking people to make dietary changes (Chlebowski et al., 1990). Written directions should supplement oral discussions, and key points should be repeated. Written instructions (Morris and Halperin, 1979; Morisky, 1986) can have a more sustained impact on both knowledge and behavior. Attention to several techniques can help to improve comprehension. Ley (1986) has shown that simplifying technical information and organizing it so that the most important information is first or last in both written and oral communications is helpful. People understand best information that is provided in specific categories (Ley, 1986), so it might be useful to say, "First, we'll talk about how you'll increase the fiber in your daily diet. Then, we'll talk about the vitamin supplements I have asked you to take." Participants should be given clear directions about what they are expected to do. It may be helpful for participants to be asked to restate the regimen in their own words. Then misunderstanding can be addressed. The use of self-help materials has been shown to achieve modest positive changes in smoking and dietary behaviors (Davis et al., 1984; Altman and King, 1986; Ley, 1986; Orleans, 1988). In large-scale programs, print and broadcast media cn be used (Altman and King, 1986).

Knowledge about colon cancer was the best predictor of subjects' willingness and ability to increase dietary fiber in a survey conducted by Ho et al. (1987). In a randomized study, participants who received fiber supplements and a comprehensive compliance enhancement intervention showed a doubling in compliance over those who received fiber alone (Ho et al., 1987). Nutrition information is probably best understood when presented in terms of foods rather than nutrients. Emphasis on brand-specific choices may be helpful in stimulating adherence to low fat and high fiber diets (Glanz, 1988). Women in a low fat trial could be accompanied on a food shopping trip and shown what items to select. In addition, demonstration of how to prepare appealing low fat or high fiber foods may not only impart skills. Such strategies may also help to maintain the morale of participants in macronutrient trials.

Behavioral Strategies for Increasing Adherence

Experience with a number of behavior change strategies from weight loss to smoking cessation suggests a number of specific behaivoral techniques for enhancing adherence. Specifics include asking the patient to set specific goals, signing contracts, keeping food records, and relapse prevention (Turk et al., 1986, 1988; Gritz et al., 1989). Turk et al. (1986) recommended contingency contracting as an especially effective means of producing initial adherence. Then the emphasis might be shifted to more intrinsic motivations. As yet, there have been no reports of systematic efforts aimed at behavioral modification of dietary patterns related to cancer risk, although work is currently in progress at several institutions to reduce the risk of breast cancer by reducing dietary fat (Bright-See and Levy, 1985; Boyd et al., 1988). However, behavioral strategies have been applied widely to weight reduction with some promising results (Brownell, 1984). The most popular approaches in this regard include self-monitoring of food intake, behavioral contracting (e.g., generating a written weight loss agreement with a family member or physician), incentives (e.g., gift or monetary reward), and modeling (Glanz, 1985). Other behavioral techniques used to promote smoking cessation oculd be considered for application to dietary cancer risks, as well as to adherence to early detection regimens. However, as Fisher et al. (1982) cautioned, detailed understanding of the peculiarities of the disease or risk factors must ultimately influence the nature of psychological approaches that are applied.

Strategies for Memory Enhancement

Refrigerator tip sheets, medication timers, special calendars, other visual cues, and mailed or telephone reminders can help to improve compliance by reminding and cuing patients. There is evidence from other trials that a one-time-a-day dosing greatly enhances long-term compliance Black et al., 1987; Cramer et al., 1989). If a calendar pack is used for distributing the medication, there is a much higher likelihood of compliance. The calendar pack has the additional value of providing a method to monitor treatment compliance at follow-up visits.

Strategies for Enhancing Problem-Solving Skills

One strategy for motivating long-term adherence is to engage in active problem solving with participants to help them overcome obstacles to adherence. Asking participants to model the recommended behavior is a first step. For example, a woman may decide she cannot adhere to a low fat diet because the regimen is boring. A demonstration and sampling of appetizing, easy-to-make low fat foods could help to reaffirm her commitment to adherence. We have used telephone counselors to make brief calls to people eligible for screening to help them identify their personal barriers and develop a plan to overcome them: 38% of the women have then adhered to the recommended behavior.

Access Strategies for Enhancing Participation and Adherence

One strategy for motiving long-term adherence is to engage in active problem solving with participants to help them overcome obstacles to adherence. Asking participants to model the recommended behavior is a first step. For example, a woman may decide she cannot adher to a low fat diet because the regimen is boring. A demonstration and sampling of appetizing, easy-to-make low fat foods could help to reaffirm her commitment to adherence. We have used telephone counselors to make brief calls to people eligible for screening to help them identify their personal barriers and develop a plan to overcome them: 38% of the women have then adhered to the recommended behavior.

Access Strategies for Enhancing Participation and Adherence

Some persons, especially poorer and older people, may fail to adhere because they lack transportation to the medical center or the hours are incompatible with their schedules. Providing transportation, lodging expenses, and flexible hours may help to decrease barriers to participation (Bell et al., 1985). Loescher et al. (1990) asked what changes would make it easier for women to participate in a cancerprevention trial: 27% responded "more flexible scheduling" and 8% said "provide transportation." For some populations, these tangible supports may be needed.

Strategies for Enhancing Social Support

There is evidence that people find it easier to change behaviors and to adhere to regimens when others around them are supportive (Colletti and Brownell, 1982; Morisky, 1986). Acceptance of dietary change requires family support (Glanz, 1985). Berenson et al. (1989) found high fiber compliance when a family member prepared breakfast. However, the data are not entirely consistent and suggest that health professionals may need to show family members *how* they can be most helpful. For smoking cessation programs, we have developed tip sheets to tell people how they can be helpful to the person engaged in behavior change. Likewise, occasional meetings where participants can help one another may also be useful. Such groups can help to reinforce new dietary norms (Carmody, 1987).

Strategies for Preventing Relapse

Most behavioral change programs experience high rates of relapse among participants. Often, as in the case of smoking cessation and dietary change, this occurs soon after initial change attempts. Relapse Prevention Theory (Marlatt and Gordon, 1985) address this important problem. Relapse Prevention Theory (RPT) is a generic term that refers to a wide range of strategies designed to prevent relapse. RPT focuses on changing patterns through the use of self-management and self-control techniques. It is especially important that people engaged in dietary change not regard a slip as a reason to forgo the regimen. In view of the length of participation time required for macronutrient trials, participants must be armed with strategies to avoid relapse. The best approach is to teach participants a combination of cognitive and self-management techniques. Particularly important is the recognition that an occasional lapse does not mean one has to give up. Marlatt and Gordon (1985) summarize RPT and provide detailed advice about specific techniques that can be used.

Strategies for Improving Participants' Long-Term Motivation

As we discussed earlier in this chapter, participants in prevention trials must be motivated for long periods of time. Thus, special thought must be given to participant's motivations. Feedback on performance (You've taken the fiber supplement every day for 6 months. That's great!) can be helpful (Marty et al., 1983). Birthday or holiday cards, participant newsletters (perhaps with special regimen and older health tips), and letters also may be useful. Positive reinforcement from the study team is essential. Eligibility for small gifts, lotteries, or other incentives can help to increase motivation for compliance; a rose was especially appreciated (Stevens et al., 1989). It is important that all participants be contacted regularly. Toll-free telephone numbers, provision of stamped, self-addressed cards and mailed reminders can aid in maintaining participants' cooperation over the 5 or more years often required in prevention trials at every contact, asking participants how they are doing, and overcoming any specific barriers. Brief counselor contact improves adherence and outcomes in self-help programs (Hoyt and Janis, 1975; Glascow et al., 1981; Prue et al., 1983; Davis et al., 1984). In one study, three to four brief counselor calls 6–8 months after receiving a self-help guide boosted quit rates 50% (Orleans, 1986). Winchester et al. (1983) found that the use of mailed reminders and telephone counseling resulted in an 85% appointment-keeping rate following FOBT testing in the community. These techniques can be used to sustain motivation in long-term trials. However, active involvement of participants in the process is at the very core of motivation (Russell, 1984).

Finally, as Gritz et al. (1989) suggested, motivation also can be enhanced by appealing to the value placed on health or on other values, such as attractiveness and weight loss, in a low fat dietary cancer prevention trial. Stevens et al. (1989) emphasized the importance of stressing contributions to medical knowledge over personal benefit.

Measurement of Adherence

Meichenbaum and Turk (1987) have identified 11 different methods to measure compliance. These include:

Interviews (careful attention must be paid to developing reliable and valid instruments)
Self-report
Self-monitoring
Pill counts of unused tablets
Tallies of refills of medications
Clinical ratings
Biochemical indicators
Marked-sign techniques (inactive or false markers embedded in treatment package)
Record of broken appointments
Clinical improvement or stability in medical conditions or symptoms
Collateral reports by others who are in a position to observe the participants behavior (Hays and Dimatteo, 1987; Gritz et al., 1989)

The best strategy is to use multiple measures of adherence over multiple points in time in order to overcome deficits in any one method. Macronutrient trials might include a combination of participants' dietary records, clinical measures, such as cholesterol, appointment keeping, and self-report. Objective reports using pharmacologic markers or a variety of other validation measures are considered the gold standard for documenting adherence (Baron, 1984). However, there are a number of limitations on the use or interpretation of serum or urine drug/nutrient levels: pharmacokinetic differences between drugs and between patients, environmental exposure or contamination, expense or cumbersome nature of the measure, promotion of an adversarial relationship between provider and patient, and time delay between patient visit and test results leading to poor feedback.

Biochemical or other markers that reliably reflect specific dietary changes may be especially useful in monitoring nutritional compliance (Taylor et al., 1989). Drug markers can provide feedback to both patient and investigator (Russell, 1984). For example, investigators might monitor plasma cholesterol levels. The use of serum plasma concentrations of an agent can be used to supplement other reports (Plezia et al., 1989). Stool samples might be used in fiber studies (Taylor et al., 1989). These methods and others have been discussed in considerable detail in Moon and Micozzi (1989). Collateral reports are another source of data. They consist of verifying observations from health professionals, family, friends, or coworkers and include attendance at scheduled meetings, completion of questionnaires, pill counts, dietary assessments, and behavioral verification.

Accurate assessment of macronutrient or micronutrient intake requires careful selection of methods. In addition to biochemical validation, where possible, Hunter and Willett (1989) have recommended the food-frequency method. Block and Hartman (1989) have discussed the advantages and disadvantages of different dietary assessment methods, including 24-hour recalls, diet records, and frequency questionnaires. Since biochemical markers are, at best, imperfect measures of eating behaviors, multipe measures are essential (Carmody et al., 1987).

Investigators conducting macronutrient trials must consider the possibility that the control group may well have access to the treatment and change their behavior during the course of the trial. Thus, careful dietary assessments are especially important. As Leventhal et al. (1989) cautioned, the fact that control group participants may be more health-oriented than randomly selected members of the general population may be a problem in clinical trials. Power estimates must reflect this possibility to ensure adequate sample size for testing study hypotheses.

Effects of Adherence on Sample Size and Interpretation of Results

Determination of sample size is a critical issue in cancer prevention studies, because the reduction in risk, due to any factor, is likely to be small, perhaps in the order of 20–30% (Peto, 1982). Randomized trials are by far the most powerful tool to identify these small to moderate effects. However, the trial must be sufficient sample size to minimize the probability that observed differences are due to chance. A randomized trial of sufficient sample size will ensure adequate statistical power to detect such effects if they truly exist and will also help to ensure that both known and unknown confounders will be evenly distributed among the treatment groups.

In designing chemoprevention trials, investigators often spend much time and effort on increasing the total number of participants enrolled. However, the effective sample size of a trial and, thus, the power of the study is proportional not simply to the number of participants enrolled, but specifically to two critical factors: (a) the total number of endpoints experienced by the study population and (b) the square of the difference in compliance between the treatment group (Buring and Hennekens, 1989). Nearly every prospectively randomized chemoprevention trial has required longer follow-up time than initially intended in order to accumulate sufficient endpoints to achieve statistical significance. One method for guaranteeing sufficient events is to select a high risk population such as familial polyposis subjects for the study.

Another major consideration in designing and implementing prevention trials is the need to assure near complete adherence in the study populations; deviations from complete adherence have serious implications for sample size. Buring and Hennekens (1984) developed power curves to calculate various reductions in risk of cardiovascular mortality in the Physician Health Trial among aspirin takers and aspirin avoiders. They showed that strategies to increase compliance maximize the power of the clinical trial to detect small to moderate differences for any given sample size. In any macronutrient trial, all subjects randomized must be analyzed to test the hypothesis under consideration. To limit the analysis to a subsample of compliant subjects would introduce post hoc observations that could be considered exploratory at best. Similarly, if the study was accomplished only in a highly compliant subject population, one could learn about the efficacy of the intervention, but the design would limit the generalizability.

CONCLUSION

The efficacy and full impact of macronutrient manipulation will not be known unless appropriate participants can be recruited, enrolled in trials, and motivated to participate for long periods of time. Ultimately, the health benefit can be determined only by the efficacy of the regimen (Green et al., 1980). However, macronutrient trials, like other cancer prevention and early detection programs, require the active collaboration of the participant in the treatment program. A variety of educational and behavioral strategies can be used to improve informed adherence at each step in the process. The true potential of cancerprevention will not be realized without the full commitment of those whom we recruit to participate in prevention trials.

REFERENCES

Agras, W. S., and Bradford, R. H. Recruitment: An introduction. *Circulation 66*(Suppl IV): 2-5 (1982).

Altman, D. G., and King, A. C. Approaches to compliance in primary prevention. *J. Compliance Health Care 1*(1): 55-73 (1986).

Arnold, A., Johnstone, B., Stoskopf, B., et al. Recruitment for efficacy study in chemoprevention—The concerned smoker study. *Prev. Med. 18*: 700-710 (1989).

Bandura, A. Self-efficacy mechanism in human agency. *American Psychologist 37*: 121-147 (1982).

Baron, J. A. *Compliance Issues/Biological Markers in Chemoprevention Clinical Trials: Problems and Solutions* (M. A. Sestilli, ed.), NIH Publication No. 85-2715.

Becker, M. H., and Rosenstock, I. M. Compliance with medical advice. In *Health Care and Human Behavior* (A. Steptoe and A. Mathews, eds.), Academic Press, New York, 1984.

Bell, R. L., Curb, J. D., Friedman, L. M., McIntyre, K. M., et al. Enhancement of visit adherence in the national beta-blocker heart attack trial. *Controlled Clinical Trials 6*: 89-101 (1985).

Benedict, J., Atwood, J. R., Ho, E. E., Sheehan, E. T. An exploratory investigation of elders'views on diet, nutrition and cancer prevention. *J. Nutr. for the Elderly* (December, 1989).

Berenson, M. Groshen, S., Miller, and H., DeCosse, J. Subject-reported compliance in a chemoprevention trial for familial adenomatous polyposis. *J. Behavioral Med. 12*(3): 233-247 (1989).

Berger, E. S., Hendee, W. R. The expression of health risk information. *Arch. Intern. Med. 149*: 1507-1508 (1989).

Black, D. M., Brand, R. J., Greenlick, M., Hughes, G., Smith, J. Compliance to treatment for hypertension in elderly patients: THe SHEP pilot study. *J. Gerontol. 42*: 552-557 (1987).

Block, G., Hartman, A. M. Dietary assessment methods. In *Nutrition and Cancer Prevention—Investigating the Role of Micronutrients*, Marcel Dekker, Inc., New York, 1989, pp. 159-180.

Boyd, N. F., Cousins, M., Beaton, M., Fishell, E., et al. Clinical trial of low-fat, high-carbohydrate diet in subjects with mammographic dysplasia: Report on early outcomes. *JNCI 80*: 1244-1248 (1988).

Boyd, N. F., Cousins, M., Lockwood, G., Tritchler, D. The feasibility of testing experimentally the dietary fat-breast cancer hypothesis. In *Recent Progress in Research on Nutrition and Cancer* (C. J. Mettlin and K. Aoki, eds.), Wiley-Liss, Inc., New York, 1990, pp. 231-241.

Bright-See, E., Levy, S. Dietary intervention in cancer prevention trials and clinical practice: Some methodological issues. In *Cancer, Nutrition, and Eating Behavior: A*

Biobehavioral Perspective (T. Burish, S. Levy, and B. Beyerwitz, eds.) Erlbaum, Hillsdale, NJ, 1985.

Browman, G. P., Arnold, A., Booker, L., Johnstone, B., Skingley, P., Levine, M. N. Etretinate blood levels in monitoring of compliance and contamination in a chemoprevention trial. *JNCI 81*: 795–798 (1989).

Brownell, K. D. Obesity: Understanding and treating a serious, prevalent, and refractory disorder. *J. Consult. Clin. Psychol. 50*: 820–840 (1982).

Brownell, K. D. The psychology and physiology of obesity: Implications for screening and treatment. *J. Am. Diet. Assoc. 84*: 406–414 (1984).

Buring, J. E., Hennekens, C. H. *Sample Size and Compliance in Randomized Trials in Chemoprevention Clinical Trials: Problems and Solutions* (M. A. Sestill, ed.). NIH Publication No. 85-275, 1984.

Buring, J. E., Hennekens, C. H. Methodologic issues in the design of primary prevention trials. In *Advances in Cancer Control: Innovations and Research* (P. Anderson, P. Engstrom, L. Mortenson, eds.), 1989.

Caggiula, A. W., Christakis, G., Farrand, M., et al. The multiple risk factor intervention trial (MRFIT). VI. Intervention on blood lipids. *Prev. Med. 10*: 443–475 (1981).

Carmody, T. P. Promoting adherence to heart-healthy diets: A review of the literature. *The Journal of Compliance in Health Care 2*(2): 105–124 (1987).

Chlebowski, R. T., Blackburn, G. L., Buzzard, I. M., et al. Current sttus: Evaluation of dietary fat reduction as secondary breast cancer prevention. In *Applications of Social Sciences to Clinical Medicine and Health Policy* (L. H. Aiken, D. Mechanic, eds.), Rutgers University Press, New Brunswick, NJ, 1990, pp. 201-209.

Colletti, G., Brownell, L. D. The physical and emotional benefits of social support: Application to obesity, smoking, and alcoholism. In *Progress in Behavior Modification* (M. Hersen, R. Eisler, and P. H. Miller, eds.), Academic Press, New York, 1982, pp. 109-178.

Cramer, J. A., Mattson, R. H., Prevey, M. L., Scheyer, R. D., Ouellette, V. L. How often is medication taken as prescribed? A novel assessment technique. *JAMA 261*: 3273-3277 (1989).

Davis, A. L., Faust, R., Ordenlich, M. Self-help smoking cessation and maintenance programs: A comparative study with 12-month follow-up by the American Lung Association. *Am. J. Public Health 74*: 1212–1217 (1984).

DeCosse, J. J., Miller, H. H., Lesser, M. L. Effect of wheat fiber and vitamins C and E on rectal polyps in patients with familial adenomatous polyposis. *JNCI 81*(17): 1290–1297 (1989).

Dermatis, H., Rowland, J., Miransky, J., Kerner, J., Osborne, M., Holland, J. Consent and complilance in chemoprevention trials. In *Proceedings: The First International Breast Cancer Chemoprevention Workshop*, New York, November 20, 1987. Marcel Dekker, New York, 1988, pp. 633–635.

DeWys, W. D., Malone, W. F., Butrum, R. R., Sestili, M. A. Clinical trials in cancer prevention. *Cancer 58*: 1954–1962 (1986).

Doll, R., Peto, R. *The Causes of Ancer.* Oxford University Press, New York, 1981.

Epstein, L. H., Cluss, P. A. A behavioral medicine perspective on adherence to long-term medical regimens. *J. Consult. Clin. Psychol. 50*: 950–971 (1982).

Fisher, E. B., Jr., Delamater, A., Berelson, A., Kirkley, B. Psychological factors in diabetes and its treatment. *J. Consult. Clin. Psychol.* *50*: 993–1003.

Ford, C. E., Langford, H. G., Palmer, M. J. Recruitment in the hypertension detection and follow-up program. *Controlled Clinical Trials* (Supplement) *8*: 54–67 (1987).

Glanz, K. Nutrition education for risk factor reduction and patient education: A review. *Prev. Med.* *14*: 721–752 (1985).

Glanz, K. Patient and public education for cholesterol reduction: A review of strategies and issues. *Patient Education and Counseling* *12*: 235–257 (1988).

Glascow, R., Schafer, L., O'Neill, H. L. Self-help books and amount of therapist contact in smoking cessation programs. *J. Consult. Clin. Psychol.* *49*: 449–455 (1981).

Goodman, G. E., Omenn, G. S., Feigl, P., et al. Chemoprevention of lung cancer with retinoids/beta-carotene. Second International Conference on the Modulation and Mediation of Cancer by Vitamins and Micronutrients, Tucson, AZ (Abstract), 1985.

Gorder, D. D., Dolecek, T. A., Coleman, G. G., et al. Dietary intake in the multiple risk factor intervention trial (MRFIT) *J. Am. Diet. Assoc.* *86*(6): 744–751 (1986).

Greenwald, P., Sondik, E. J., Young, J. L. Emerging roles for cancer registries in cancer control. *Yale J. Biol. Med.* *59*: 561–566 (1986).

Gritz, E. R., Dimatteo, M. R., Hays, R. D. Methodological issues in adherence to cancer control regimens. *Prev. Med.* *18*: 711–720 (1989).

Hansen, W. B., Collins, L. M., Malotte, C. K., et al. Attrition in prevention research. *J. Behav. Med.* *8*(3): 261–275 (1985).

Hays, R., Dimatteo, M. R. Key issues and suggestions for patient compliance assessment. *J. Compliance Health Care* *2*: 37–53 (1987).

Hennekens, C. H., Stampfer, M. J., Willett, W. Micronutrient and cancer chemoprevention. *Cancer Detect. Prevent.* *7*: 147–158 (1984).

Higbee, M., Dukes, G., Bosso, J. Patient recall of physician's prescription instructions. *Hospital Formulary* *17*: 553–556 (1982).

Ho, E. E., Atwood, J. R., Meyskens, Jr., F. L. Methodological development of dietary fiber intervention to lower colon cancer risk. *Advances in Cancer Control: The War on Cancer—15 Years of Progress*, Alan R. Liss, 1987, pp. 263–281.

Howe, G. R., Hirohata, T., Hislop, T. G., et al. Dietary factors and risk of breast cancer: Combined analysis of 12 case-control studies. *JNCI* *82*(7): 561–569 (1990).

Hoyt, M. F., Janis, I. L. Increasing adherence to a stressful decision via a motivational balance sheet procedure: a field experiment. *J. Pers. Soc. Psychol.* *31*: 833–839 (1975).

Hunninghake, D. B., Darby, C. A., Probstfield, J. L. Recruitment experience in clinical trials: Literature summary and annotated bibliography. *Controlled Clinical Trials* *8*(Supplement): 6–30 (1987).

Keintz, M. K., Rimer, B., Fleisher, L., Engstrom, P. Educating older adults about their increased cancer risk. *The Gerontologist* *28*(4): 487–490 (1988).

Lando, H. (1990). Comparative evaluation of American Cancer Society and American Lung Association smoking cessation clinics. *Am. J. Public Health* *80*(5): 554–559 (1990).

Lerman, C., Rimer, B., Engstrom, P. F. Reducing avoidable cancer motality through prevention and early detection regimens. *Cancer Res.* *49*: 4955–4962 (1989).

Lerman, C., Rimer, B., Trock, B., Balshem, A., Engstrom, P. F. Factors associated with repeat adherence to breast cancer screening. *Prev. Med.* (May, 1990a).

Lerman, C., Rimer, B., Trock, B., Jepson, C., Boyce, A., Engstrom, P. Implications of abnormal screening mammograms. Presented at the annual meeting of the American Society of Preventive Oncology, Bethesda, MD, March 19-21, 1990b.

Leventhal, H., Nerenz, D. R., Leventhal, E. A., Love, R. R., Bendena, L. M. The behavioral dynamics of clinical trials. Presented at Tamoxifen Conference, Madison, WI, November, 1989.

Ley, P. Cognitive variables and noncompliance. *J. Compliance Health Care 1*: 171–188 (1986).

Loescher, L. J., Graham, V. E., Meyskens, F. L., Jr., Surwit, E. A. Development of a contingency recruitment plan for a phase III chemoprevention trial of cervical dysplasia. In *Applications of Social Sciences to Clinical Medicine and Health Policy* (L. H. Aiken, D. Mechanic, eds.), Rutgers University Press, New Brunswick, NJ, 1990, pp. 151-163.

Marlatt, G. A., Gordon, J. R. *Relapse Prevention.* Guilford Press, New York, 1985.

Marty, P. J., McDermott, R. J., Christiansen, K. Evaluation of two pedagogical techniques for enhancing knowledge, attitudes and frequency of practice related to breast self-examination. *Health Educ.* 25–28 (Nov.-Dec. 1983).

McLarty, J. Recruitment strategies for asbestos workers in a beta-carotene, retinol and lung cancer chemoprevention study. Presented at The 14th Annual Meeting of the American Society of Preventive Oncology, Bethesda, MD, March 19-21, 1990.

Med. World News. 125–126 (March 24, 1980).

Meichenbaum, D., Turk, D. C. (eds.) *Facilitating Treatment Adherence—A Practitioner's Guidebook.* Plenum Press, New York, 1987.

Mettlin, C. J. The effects of subject selection factors in cancer prevention trials. In *Nutrition and Cancer Prevention—Investigating the Role of Micronutrients* (T. E. Moon and M. S. Micozzi, eds.), Marcel Dekker, New York, 1989, pp. 483–490.

Meyerowitz, B. E., Chaiken, S. The effect of message framing on breast self-examination attitudes, intentions and behavior. *J. Personality and Social Psychology 52*(3): 500–510 (1987).

Micozzi, M. S. Foods, micronutrients and reduction of human cancer. In *Nutrition and Cancer Prevention-Investigating the Role of Micronutrients* (Moon, T. E. and Micozzi, M. S., eds.), Marcel Dekker, Inc., New York, 1989, pp. 213-241.

Miller, H. H., Bauman, L. J., DeCosse, J. J. Psychosocial adjustment of familial polyposis patients and participation in a chemoprevention trial. *Int. J. Psychiatry in Medicine 16*(3): 211-230 (1986-87).

Moon, T. E. Approach to selection of agents for cancer prevention trials. In *Nutrition and Cancer Prevention—Investigating the Role of Micronutrients* (T. E. Moon and M. S. Micozzi, eds.), Marcel Dekker, Inc., New York, 1989, pp. 423–439.

Moon, T. E., Micozzi, M. S. (Eds.). *Nutrition and Cancer Prevention—Investigating the Role of Micronutrients*, Marcel Dekker, Inc., New York, 1989.

Morisky, D. E. Nonadherence to medical recommendations for hypertensive patients: Problems and potential solutions. *J. Compliance Health Care 1*: 5–20 (1986).

Morris, L., Halperin, J. Effects of written drug information on patient knowledge and compliance: A literature review. *Am. J. Public Health 69*: 47–52 (1979).

Newberne, P. M., Schrager, T. F., Conner, M. W. Experimental evidence on the nutritional prevention of cancer. In *Nutrition and Cancer Prevention-Investigating the Role of Micronutrients* (T. E. Moon and M. S. Micozzi, eds.), Marcel Dekker, Inc., New York, 1989, pp. 33-82.

Newcombe, P. A., Love, R. R., Phillips, J. L., Buckmaster, B. J. Using a population-based cancer registry for recruitment in a pilot cancer control study. *Prev. Med.* 1-5 (1990).

Nixon, D. W. The relevance of risk of breast cancer to chemoprevention trials. In *Proceedings: The First International Breast Cancer Chemoprevention Workshop*, New York, November 20, 1987. Marcel Dekker, Inc., New York, 1988, pp. 587–588.

Olsen, S. J., Love, R. R. A new direction in preventive oncology: Chemoprevention. *Seminars in Oncology Nursing* 2(3): 211–221 (1986).

Orleans, C. T. Smoking cessation in primary care setting. *N. Engl. J. Med. 85*: 116–126 (1988).

Patterson, B. H., Block, G. Food choices and the cancer guidelines. *Am. J. Public Health 78*: 282–286 (1988).

Perry, C. L., Baranowski, T., Parcel, G. S. How individuals, environments and health behavior interact: Social learning theory. In *Health Behavior and Health Education: Theory, Research, and Practice*. (K. Glanz, F. M. Lewis, B. K. Rimer, eds.), Jossey-Bass, Inc., San Francisco, CA, 1990, pp. 161-186.

Peto, R. Statistical aspects of cancer trials. In *Treatment of Cancer* (K. E. Halman, ed.), Chapman and Hall, London, 1982, pp. 867–870.

Piantadosi, S., Byar, D. P. Design of prevention trials. In *Nutrition and Cancer Prevention—Investigating the Role of Micronutrients* (T. E. Moon and M. S. Micozzi, eds.), Marcel Dekker, Inc., New York, 1989, pp. 441–472.

Plezia, P. M., Alberts, D. S., Peng, Y. M., et al. The role of serum and tissue pharmacology studies in the design and interpretation of chemoprevention trials. *Prev. Med. 18*: 680–687 (1989).

Powles, T. J., Davey, J., McKinna, A. Chemoprevention of breast cancer. *Acta Oncologica 28*: 865–867 (1989a).

Powles, T. J., Hardy, J. R., Ashley, S. E., et al. Chemoprevention of breast cancer. *Breast Cancer Research and Treatment 14*: 23–31 (1989b).

Prentice, R. L., Sheppard, L. Feasibility and importance of clinical trials of a low fat diet to reduce cancer risk. In *Recent Progress in Research on Nutrition and Cancer* (C. J. Mettlin and K. Aoki, eds.), Wiley-Liss, New York, 1990, pp. 205–215.

Prochaska, J. O., DiClemente, C. C. Common processes of self-change in smoking, weight control and psychological distress. In *Coping and Substance Use* (S. Shiffman and T. Wills, eds.), Academic Press, Orlando, FL, 1985, pp. 345–364.

Prue, D. M., Davis, C. J., Martin, J. E., Moss, R. A. An investigation of a minimal contact brand fading program for smoking treatment. *Addict. Behav. 8*: 307–310 (1983).

Rimer, B. K., Jones, W. L., Keintz, M. K., Catalano, R. B., Engstrom, P. F. Informed consent: A crucial step in cancer patient education. *Halth Education Quarterly 10* (Special Supplement): 30–42 (1984).

Rimer, B., Keintz, M. K., Kessler, H. B., Engstrom, P. F., Rosan, J. Why women resist

mammograms: Understanding patient-related barriers to acceptance of screening mammography. *Radiology 172*: 243–246 (1989).
Rimer, B. K. Perspectives on interpersonal theories in health education and health behavior. In *Health Behavior and Health Education: Theory, Research and Practice* (K. Glanz, F. M. Lewis, and B. K. Rimer, eds.), Jossey-Bass, Inc., San Francisco, CA, 1990.
Romney, S. L., Dwyer, A., Slagle, S., Duttagupta, C., et al. Chemoprevention of cervix cancer: Phase I-II: A feasibility study involving the topical vaginal administration of retinyl acetate gel. *Gynecol. Oncol. 20*: 109–119 (1985).
Rosenstock, I. M. The Health Belief Model: Explaining health behavior through expectancies. In *Health Behavior and Health Education: Theory, Research and Practice* (K. Glanz, F. M. Lewis, and B. K. Rimer, eds.), Jossey-Bass, Inc., San Francisco, CA, 1990, pp. 39–62.
Russell, M. L. Behavioral aspects of the use of medical markers in clinical trials. *Controlled Clinical Trials 5*: 526–534 (1984).
Schmid, T. L., Jeffrey, R. W., Hellerstedt, W. L. Direct mail recruitment to home-based smoking and weight control programs: A comparison of strategies. *Prev. Med. 18*: 503–517 (1989).
Slovic, P. Informing and educating the public about risk. *Risk Analysis 6*(4): 403–415 (1987).
Stampfer, M. J., Willett, W. C., Hennekens, C. H. Choice of populations for cancer prevention trials. In *Nutrition and Cancer Prevention—Investigating the Role of Micronutrients* (T. E. Moon and M. S. Micozzi, eds.), Marcel Dekker, Inc., New York, 1989, pp. 473–482.
Steering Committee of the Physicians' Health Study Research Group. Final report on the aspirin component of the ongoing physicians' health study. *N. Engl. J. Med.*: 321 (1989).
Stevens, M., Greenberg, E. R., Baron, J. A. Practical aspects of cancer prevention trials. In *Nutrition and Cancer Prevention—Investigating the Role of Micronutrients* (T. E. Moon and M. S. Micozzi, eds.), Marcel Dekker, Inc., New York, 1989, pp. 513–532.
Stewart, R. B., Cluff, L. E. A review of medication errors and compliance in ambulant patients. *Clin. Pharmacol. Ther. 13*: 463–468 (1972).
Strecher, V. J., DeVellis, B. M., Becker, M. H., Rosenstock, I. M. The role of self-efficacy in achieving health behavior change. *Health Education Quarterly 13*: 73–92 (1986).
Stunkard, A. J. (ed.) *Obesity*. Saunders, Philadelphia, 1980.
Svarstad, B. L. Patient-practitioner relationships and compliance with prescribed medical regimens. In *Applications of Social Sciences to Clinical Medicine and Health Policy* (L. H. Aiken and D. Mechanic, eds.), Rutgers University Press, New Brunswick, NJ, 1986, pp. 438–459.
Taylor, P. R., Schatzkin, A., Patterson, B. H., et al. Clinical metabolic studies in cancer research. *Prev. Med. 18*: 194–202 (1989).
Trock, B. J., Lanza, E., Greenwald, P. High fiber diet and colon cancer: A critical review. In *Recent Progress in Research on Nutrition and Cancer* (C. J. Mettlin and K. Aoki, eds.), Wiley-Liss, New York, 1990a, pp. 145–157.
Trock, B., Lanza, E., Greenwald, P. Dietary fiber, vegetables and colon cancer: Critical

review and Meta-analyses of the epidemiologic evidence. *JNCI 82*(8): 650–661 (1990b).

Turk, D. C. Nonadherence to chemoprevention regimens: A ton of prevention. In *Applications of Social Sciences to Clinical Medicine and Health Policy* (L. H. Aiken and D. Mechanic, eds.), Rutgers University Press, New Brunswick, NJ, 1990, pp. 139–149.

Turk, D. C., Salovey, P., Litt, M. D. Adherence: A cognitive-behavioral perspective. In *Compliance, The Dilemma of the Chronically Ill* (K. E. Gerber, and A. M. Nehemkis, eds.), Springer, New York, 1986, pp. 44–72.

Weed, D. L. Ethics and chemoprevention research. *Seminars in Oncology X*(3): 355–359 (1983).

Weinstein, N. D. Seeking reassuring or threatening information about environmental cancer. *J. Behav. Med. 2*: 125–139 (1979).

Weiss, D. J. Dropout in patient compliance studies: A suggested analytic procedure. *The Journal of Compliance in Health Care 2*(1): 73–83 (1987).

Willett, W. C. Epidemiologic studies of diet and cancer. In *Recent Progress in Research on Nutrition and Cancer* (C. J. Mettlin and K. Aoki, eds.), Wiley-Liss, New York, 1990, pp. 159–168.

Wynder, E. L., Morabia, A., Rose, D. P., Cohen, L. A. Clinical trials of dietary interventions to enhance cancer survival. In *Recent Progress in Research on Nutrition and Cancer* (C. J. Mettlin and K. Aoki, eds.), Wiley-Liss, New York, 1990, pp. 217–229.

Zelen, M. Are primary cancer prevention trials feasible? *JNCI 80*: 1442–1444 (1988).

Index

Abdomen, 191
Aberration, dietary, 58
Absinthe, 250
Activity diaries, 141
Adaptation
  human, 56–58, 60, 74, 174
  obesity, 60–61
  thermogenesis, 139
Adenomatous polyps, 408
Adherence, 438–439, 447–450, 455, 458
Adipose tissue, 57, 183, 190, 193, 322 (*see also* Fat, body)
Affluence, 231
Africa
  breast cancer, 61, 246, 263-265
  carcinogenesis, 249
  diet, 41–42
  dose-response, 266
  energy, 68, 127–128
  fiber, 70,293, 348
  intake, 56, 58, 246
  interactions, 183
  liver cancer, 260
  maize, 250
  tobacco, 246, 250, 447
Albumin, serum, 283
Alcohol, 260
  Africa, 260
  breast cancer, 246, 263-265, 377
  California, 263-264
  carcinogenesis, 249, 251-252, 264
  China, 250
  colorectal cancer, 246, 251, 258-260
  Finland, 265
  France, 250, 256
  Italy, 256
  Japan, 262
  micronutrients, 251
  occupation, 254
  oral cancer, 246, 251, 253-257
  pancreas cancer, 261-262

[Alcohol]
prostate cancer, 265
stomach cancer, 257
tobacco, 246, 250, 447
validity, 247
vitamin A, 251
Alfalfa, 43
Amino acids, 57, 184
Ammonia, 302
Animal models, 14, 17, 34
Anthropometry
cancer, 321
definition, 159
dimensions, 161–162
limitations, 173–174
measurement side, 168
participation, 169
reliability, 165,169
value, 167,174
Antioxidants, 289, 347
Arachidonic acid, 41
Asia (*see* China, Japan)
Australia, 410

Barley, 296
Beef, 233
Beer, 258 (*see also* Alcohol)
Behavior, 438, 449 (*see also* Trials, intervention)
Betel nut, 347
Bias, measurement, 160–165, 169
Bile
acids, 68, 301, 348
fatty acids, 14
Bioavailability, 182, 322
Biochemical
epidemiology,160–169
markers, 182, 408, 458
Bladder, 265
Body fat (*see* Adipose tissue *and* Fat, body)
Body mass index, 137, 143, 165, 170–171, 214, 288, 321–322, 330
Body size, 137, 207, 332, 335 (*see also* Stature (height) *and* Weight, body)
Body weight (*see* Weight, body)
Breast cancer, 22, 23, 47, 212, 221, 232
alcohol, 246, 263–265, 377
analytical studies, 212–213, 232, 359–361
in Asian-Americans, 160–161, 169, 232, 323
body size, 322–330
calories, 128
carcinogenesis, 16–17, 221, 330
detection, 60, 310, 378, 389, 442–443
fat, 17–19, 47–49, 358–359
fiber, 303–304, 309
intervention, 372, 377
macronutrients,47–48
in migrants, 162
mortality, 377–378
nurses health study, 24–25, 63, 112, 360–361
trends, 164, 377, 389
trials, clinical, 377
types, 4, 322
weight, 164, 321
Breast tissue, 9, 12–16, 24, 59–67, 128, 191, 212, 221, 232, 263, 303, 322, 355
Breath markers, 183, 196–197
Brewery workers, 262
Buccal mucosa, 189, 347
Buttocks, and breasts, 191

Cadmium, 425
Calcium, 21, 286, 413–414, 407
California
alcohol study, 262–264
Japanese migrants, in, 162–163, 257
Seventh-Day Adventists, 233–235, 238, 240, 257–259, 263, 312, 413, 424

Calories, 39, 46, 126, 206
adjustment, 95, 101, 137
assessment, 283, 288
carbohydrates, 185–186
carcinogenesis, 46–47, 125
definitions, 136
intake, 137, 206–206
macronutrient collinearity, 219
restriction, 46, 349
total, 161, 206
Calorimetry, 140
Calvados (apple brandy), 250, 256
Carcinogenesis
alcohol, 249, 251–252, 264
calories, 46–47
dietary restriction, 22
genotoxicity, 14–17
iron, 289
mechanisms, 4–8
micronutrients, 344
phases,36–38
Carotenoids, 345, 424 (*see also* Vitamin A)
Case-control studies, 160–161, 168, 212–215, 232
Cellulose, 45, 196, 294
Cereals, 56, 296
Cervix, 265
Chemoprevention, vs. chemosuppression, 377
China (and People's Republic of), 215, 236
alcohol consumption (pai-kan), 250
breast cancer, 47
colon cancer, 237–238
ovarian cancer, 215, 240
Shanghai study, 47, 63
Taiwan, 284
Cholesterol, 57, 67, 263–363, 367, 372, 382, 459
Cigarettes (*see* Smoking)
Citrus, 44
Coconut oil, 39, 49
Cod liver oil, 188 (*see also* Fish oil)
Colo-rectal cancer
alcohol, 246, 251, 258–260
analytical studies, 213–215, 232, 360–361
body composition, 322–335
calories, 127
in Hawaii, 232, 332
in Hong Kong, 211, 348
fat, 409–410
fiber,41–42, 236, 301–303, 306–308, 411–412
protein,45–46
survival, 407
trials, clinical, 407
types, 4, 35
Community group
recruitment, 442
Copper, 286
Corn
bran, 44, 45
oil, 20, 38, 39, 49
Cultigens, 160

Dairy products, 14, 233
Dcutcrium, 142 143
Diet
adaptation, 56
assessment methods, 87, 89, 247, 296–297, 416
description, 89
errors, 90, 93, 102 ff
limitations, 160–161, 343
validity, 89, 93, 135, 219, 247
change, 366–367
constituents, 57
deficiencies, 70
etiology, 35
exposure, 58
factors, 258
fat, 35,47–48, 193, 231, 359
fiber, 293–294, 305
history, 91, 135, 136
reliability, 136
validity, 135

[Diet]
human, 55
individual, 88–89
intervention, 355
"original", 75
patterns, 193
prehistoric, 56, 245
purified, 43
recommendation, 231–241
records, 90–91, 367
restriction, 22–23
retrospective, 93
selected, 87
total, 87–88
U.S., 41, 298, 348
usual, 88
Western, 12
whole, 87
Direct mail, 443
DMBA, 17

Endometrial
cancer, 331–332, 369–370, 379, 385–386
tissue, 9, 17, 23, 59, 312, 331, 356
Energy
adjustments, 94–102, 349
balance, 216, 209, 220
by calorimetry,140
cancer, 205, 330, 337–338
estimates, 139–140
fecal energy loss,349
imbalance, 58
importance, 209
intake, 102, 125, 129–130, 136, 205, 210, 214, 216, 369
loss, 349
measurement, 129
mechanisms, 59–60
output, 59, 140
restriction, 207
total, 210
Enrollment, 445 (*see also* Trials, intervention)
Epidemiology, 8, 46, 55, 182, 232, 252, 284, 304, 321, 359, 428
Erythrocyte membrane, 187–188
Esophagus, 16, 67, 70, 255
Estrogens, 18, 23, 59, 68, 322, 331, 379
Exercise, 23, 144 (*see also*, Physical activity)

Famine, 22
Fat, body, 125, 170, 174, 191, 322 (*see also* Adipose tissue)
Fat, dietary
and cancer, 231
breast cancer 17–19, 47–49, 358–359
colon cancer, 19–21, 35
pancreas cancer, 21
prostate cancer, 428
residual, 98
saturated, 38, 48,56, 344
type, 38–39, 48–49, 361–362
Fatty acids, 18, 41, 49, 57, 67, 187, 190, 192–193, 286, 302, 344, 349
Fermentation, 56–58, 197, 250–251, 302–303, 349
Ferritin, serum, 284
Fiber
analysis, 296–298
breast cancer, 303–304, 309–311
calcium, 21–22
calories, 126, 194
citrus, 44
colon cancer, 301–303, 306–308, 410–411
compliance, 451
consumption, 298–300
definitions, 70, 294
diet, 41–45
intervention studies, 314–315, 366
as macronutrient, 70
and micronutrients, 347–349
stool samples, 459

Finland
  alcohol consumption, 265
  anthropometry,168
  diet, 12–13
  fiber, 106, 411
  food frequency, 103
  liver cancer, 260
Fish oil, 39, 49, 186
  cod liver, 188
  intake, 185–186
  omega-3 fatty acids, 39
  omega-6 fatty acids, 20, 21
Food frequency (*see also* Diet assessment)
4-day food records, 367 (*see also* Diet assessment)
France, 233, 237, 246, 256
Fruit, 25, 296, 311, 313, 513
  food, vs. nutrients, 455
  patterns, 92–93, 103, 367–368
  portion size, 91–92
  records, 91, 455
  validity, 93, 114,360–361

Genetic
  composition, 220
  toxicity, 14
Geography, 442
Globulin, 285, 322, 326, 331
Grains, 41, 56, 296, 312
Growth
  adapation, 74–75, 174
  and calories, 138, 142
  cellular, 57, 166, 221, 346, 380, 428
  changes, 171–172
  control, 166
  curves, 163
  energy balance, 59
  human, 57, 161, 166–167, 283
  migrants, 12, 161
  sensitivity, 167
Guar gum, 45, 294

Hawaii
  body composition, 321
  breast cancer, 330
  diet, 232, 234, 438
  Japanese, 165, 214, 238, 257, 321, 332
Head and neck, 253, 255
Health belief model, 446, 448–450
Height, standing (*see* Stature)
Hemicellulose, 294
Hemoglobin, 288
Hepatitis B, 260–261
Hippocrates, 205, 293
History, 3, 91, 139,162, 205, 245, 344 (of diet and cancer studies)
Hong Kong, 211, 348 (*see also* China)
Hormones, 18, 57, 68, 312, 322, 326, 331, 365
Hormone replacement therapy, 378–379
Hydrogen, breath, 196–197

Immunity, 221, 288, 346
Induction, tumor, 36
Informed consent, 445
Initiation, 4, 38
Insulin, 57, 186–187
Interferon, 189
Intermediate
  endpoints, 314
  markers, 408
Intervention trials, 355, 428 (*see also* Trials, intervention)
Iron, 284, 289, 346
Israel, 233, 321, 344
Italy
  alcohol consumption, 256
  colon cancer, 414
  diet, 12
  ovarian cancer, 240

Japan
  alcohol, 262

[Japan]
breast cancer, 211
colon cancer, 238
diet, 9, 14, 348
liver cancer,261
migrants, 162, 165, 214, 257, 335
ovarian cancer, 211
prostate cancer, 424
westernization, 12–13
Japanese-Americans (*see* California *and* Hawaii)

Kidney, 239

Lamb, 235
Lard, 38
Larynx, 254 (*see also* Oral cancer)
Lean body mass, 164, 170
assessment, 288
calories, 138
prostate cancer 321, 423
Leg length, 163
Legumes, 296
Lifestyle, 33
Lignin, 196, 294, 296
Limitations,
dietary assessment, 160–161
of quantifying intake, 181
Lineoleic acid, 41, 48, 183, 191
albumin, 289
conjugated, 289
definition, 183
erythocytes, 187
macronutrients, 344
margarine, 188, 193
Linkage, statistical, 106
Lipoproteins, 183, 188, 344–345, 383
Liver
albumin, 286
cancer, 262
cod, 188
disease, 252
metabolism, 183
tamoxifen, 384
Lung, 71, 329, 265, 346

Macronutrients, 23–24, 189 (*see also* Cholesterol, Diet, Energy, Fat, Fiber, Food, Protein)
Margarine, 193
Marseilles, 237
Mass media,439
Memory, exact, 92
Metabolism
adipose tissue, 322
albumin, 286
amino acid, 185
carbohydrates, 183
effects, 343
lipids, 183
liver, 183
of nutrients, 181
protein, 183
rate, 138
resting, 140
Metabolizable formula diet, 143
Metals, 286
Methane, breath, 196–197
Migrant studies, 9–10,161, 361–365
diet, 161, 182
growth factors, 12, 161, 321

Micronutrients, 39 (*see also* Vitamins A, C, D, E)
alcohol, 251
fats, 344–345
fiber, 304
interactions, 343
macronutrients, 183, 343
prostate cancer, 425
supplements, 410–411, 451
Mormons (*see* Utah)
Mucilage, 294
Mucosa
buccal,189–190, 347
rectal, 314
Multiple sites, 221
Myeloma, multiple, 288

Natural selection, 58
Neoteny, 59

Neoplasia, 4
Nickle, 286
NMU, 17
Nutrient
  density, 95
  imbalance, 59

Oats, 296
Obesity (*see* Adipose tissue, Fat, body, Weight)
Occupation
  alcohol consumption, 254, 262
  physical activity, 144
Oils, 48, 193
  corn, 20, 38, 49
  fish, 39, 49, 186
  olive, 39, 48
  safflower, 20, 39
  vegetable, 41
Omega-3 fatty acids
  breast cancer, 49
  fish oil, 39
  microsomal uptake, 41
Omega-3 polyunsaturated fats, 39, 41, 49
Omega-6 polyunsaturated fats, 20, 21
Oral cancer
  alcohol,246, 251, 253–257
  carcinogenesis, 16
Ornithine decarboxylase, 410
Osmosis, 286
Ovarian cancer, 215, 240
  carcinogenesis, 17
  dietary fat, 239–240
  fiber, 311
  intervention, 370
  tamoxifen, 386

Pancreas cancer, 99, 23, 50, 215, 240, 313
  alcohol, 261–262
  anthropometry and, 164
  calories, 215
  carcinogenesis, 16–17
  dietary fat, 21, 63, 239–240
  macronutrients, 50–51
  vegetables, 71
Pasta, 312
Pectin, 43, 196, 294
Physical activity, 23, 59, 141, 144
Plants, 73, 294
Polymers, 294
  nonpolysaccharide, 294
Polysaccharide,
  noncelulose, 196
ω-3 Polyunsaturated fats, 39, 41, 49
ω-6 Polyunsaturated fats, 20, 21
Progression, 5
Promotion, 4–5, 36, 39
Prostate cancer
  alcohol, 265
  anthropometry and, 164, 335
  dietary fat, 239
  etiology, 423
  fiber, 312
  in Hawaii, 232
  Japanese, 24, 424
Prostate tissue,, 9, 12, 23, 232, 265, 288, 312, 335, 423
Protein, 9, 39, 45, 49, 50, 61, 161, 206
  breast cancer, 49–50
  diet, 45–46, 283
  foods, 289
  independent effect, 45–46
  nutritional status, 283, 288
Public health education, 25, 267, 315

Quetelet index, 326 (see also Body mass index)

Recommended dietary allowances
  assessment, 58
  energy, 126
  fat, 184
  fiber, 315
Recruitment, 368, 392, 438–439, 442, 444

Rectum, 35, 63, 751, 356
Referral, health professional, 443
Retinoids, 345
Retinol (*see* Vitamin A)
Retrospective diet, 93 (*see also* Diet)
Rice, 45
Run-in, 447

Safflower oil, 20, 39
Sample size, 113, 136, 168, 459–460
Saturated fat, 38, 48 56, 344
Seaweed
  carrageenan, 44
  fiber, 296
Secular trend, 164, 362
Seventh-Day Adventists (*see* California)
Singapore, 237, 256
Smoking
  cigarette, 183, 220
  control, 358
  interactions, 183
  weight, 164, 220
Social learning theory, 449
Soybean, 45
Stature (height),
  cancer, 162–164
  breast cancer, 322
  protein intake, 283
  reliability, 169–170, 322
  variations, 166
Stomach cancer
  alcohol, 257
  calories, 215
  carcinogenesis, 16
  fiber, 313
  micronutrients, 346
Stomach tissue, 67, 71, 346

Tamoxifen, 380–389, 447
Therapeutic drugs, 286
Thermic effects, 138, 139, 142
Threshold
  diet and cancer, 161
  stature and cancer, 163
Thrifty gene hypothesis, 60
Thymidine, 410
Time
  activity, 141
  intake duration, 218
Tobacco, 253, 254, 255
  and alcohol, 246, 250, 447
Toronto, 240
Trials, intervention, clinical
  breast cancer, 377, 389
  colon cancer, 407
  compliance, 396–397, 450
  cost, 373, 392, 397
    and benefit, 397
  design, 368–369
  eligibility, 395–396
  endpoint, 396
  feasibility, 366, 390, 432
  fiber, 314–315, 366
  participation, 437
  population, 389–390
  power, 368–369, 439
  prostate cancer, 428
Triglycerides, 49, 193
"True" relative risk, 108–109
Tumor Registry, 444
24-hour recall, diet, 89–90, 135 (*see also* Diet assessment)

Undressing
  in frigid, 168
  participation in, 172
  willingness for, 169
Utah, 236, 256, 263

Validity
  alcohol, 247
  dietary intake, 219
  history, 93
Variety, food, 56
Vegetables, 25, 71, 296, 311, 313, 346
Vegetarians (*see* Seventh-Day Adventists)

Vitamin A (retinol), 345
  alcohol, 251
  ambiguity,, 8–9
  assessment, 92, 106
  breast cancer, 309
  fiber correlation, 94
  macronutrients, 395–397
  mechanisms, 7
  portion size, 91–92
  prostate cancer, 424–425
Vitamin C, 425
Vitamin D, 414–415
Vitamin E, 347

Weight, body, 164, 331
  albumin, 288
  calories, 127
  cancer, 164, 216
    breast, 322
    prostate, 335
  loss, 367, 438
  reliability, 169–170, 322
  replacement, 143
  stabilization, 143
  variations, 166
Wheat, 43–45, 196
Women's Health Trial, 355–356, 366–367, 391, 445, 452
Worksite, 443

Yanomamo (Indians), 287

Zinc, 286

About the Editors

MARC S. MICOZZI is Director of the National Museum of Health and Medicine, Associate Director of the Armed Forces Institute of Pathology in Washington, D.C., and Clinical Professor of Pathology at the Uniformed Services University of the Health Sciences in Bethesda, Maryland. An author or editor of five books, including *Nutrition and Cancer Prevention: Investigating the Role of Micronutrients* (Marcel Dekker, Inc.), and author of over 135 articles, book chapters, and abstracts, he has served as Chairman of the National Cancer Institute Source Evaluation Group for Preclinical Toxicology of Chemopreventive Agents. He is a member or Fellow of the American Public Health Association, American Society for Preventive Oncology, Society for Applied Anthropology, and College of American Pathologists. Dr. Micozzi received the B.A. degree (1974) in chemistry and zoology from Pomona College, Claremont, California, and M.D. degree (1979) and Ph.D. degree (1986) in epidemiology and anthropology from thc University of Pennsylvania, Philadelphia. He is board-qualified in pathology.

THOMAS E. MOON is Director of the Arizona Disease Prevention Center and Professor of Epidemiology at the University of Arizona Health Sciences Center, Tucson. He serves on the Prevention, Diagnosis, and Therapy review committee of the American Cancer Society. An associate editor of the journal *Cancer Epidemology, Biomarkers and Prevention*, Dr. Moon is the coeditor of *Nutrition and Cancer Prevention: Investigating the Role of Micronutrients* (Marcel Dekker, Inc.) and author of over 135 articles. The principal investigator on two retinoid skin cancer prevention trials and two diet and cancer analytic epidemology studies, and a consultant for diet and prevention trials of cervical, colon, and breast cancer, he is President of the American Society of Preventive Oncology and a member of the American College of Epidemilogy, Society for Epidemiologic Research, International Epidemilogy Institute, International Biometrics Society, and American Association for Cancer Research. Dr. Moon received the B.S. degree (1965) in mathematics from Northern Illinois University, DeKalb, M.S. degree (1967) in statistics from the University of Chicago, Illinois, and Ph.D. degree (1973) in biostatistics/epidemiology from the University of California, Berkeley.